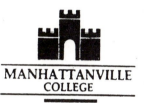

Second Edition

Neuroanatomy
Text and Atlas

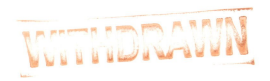

Second Edition

Neuroanatomy
Text and Atlas

John H. Martin, PhD
Center for Neurobiology & Behavior
Department of Psychiatry
College of Physicians & Surgeons
of Columbia University
New York

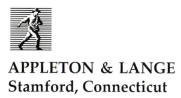

APPLETON & LANGE
Stamford, Connecticut

Copyright © 1996 by Appleton & Lange
A Simon & Schuster Company
Copyright © 1989 by Appleton & Lange

96 97 98 99 00 / 10 9 8 7 6 5 4 3 2 1

Prentice Hall International (UK) Limited, *London*
Prentice Hall of Australia Pty. Limited, *Sydney*
Prentice Hall Canada, Inc., *Toronto*
Prentice Hall Hispanoamericana, S.A., *Mexico*
Prentice Hall of India Private Limited, *New Delhi*
Prentice Hall of Japan, Inc., *Tokyo*
Simon & Schuster Asia Pte. Ltd., *Singapore*
Editora Prentice Hall do Brasil Ltda., *Rio de Janeiro*
Prentice Hall, *Upper Saddle River, New Jersey*

Library of Congress Cataloging-in-Publication Data

Martin, John H. (John Harry). 1951–
    Neuroanatomy: text and atlas / John H. Martin.—2nd ed.
        p.   cm.
    Companion v. to: Principles of neural science / edited by Eric R.
Kandel, James H. Schwartz, Thomas M. Jessell. 3rd ed. c1991.
    ISBN 0-8385-6694-4 (case : alk. paper)
    1. Neuroanatomy.   2. Neuroanatomy—Atlases.   I. Principles of
neural science.   II. Title.
    [DNLM: 1. Central Nervous System—anatomy & histology.   2. Central
Nervous System—anatomy & histology—atlases.   WL 300 M381n 1996]
    QM451.M27 1996
    611'.8—dc20
    DNLM/DLC
    for Library of Congress   95-50401

Photographs copyright © 1988 Howard J. Radzyner (unless otherwise credited)

Managing Editor: John J. Dolan
Development Editor: Gregory   Huth
Art Coordinator: Gregory   Huth
Designer: Susan Schmidler
Cover Designer: Janice Barsevich Bielawa

ISBN 0-8385-6694-4
90000

PRINTED IN THE UNITED STATES OF AMERICA

To my mother and father

Box Features

Contents

I The Central Nervous System

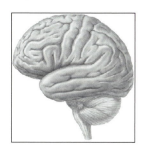

Sensory Systems

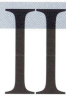

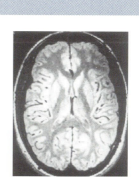

Motor Systems

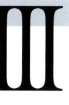

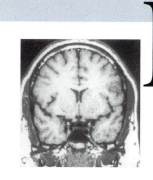

The Brain Stem

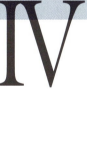

12   General Organization of the Cranial Nerve Nuclei and the Trigeminal System   353

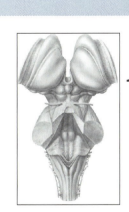

13 The Somatic and Visceral Motor Functions of the Cranial Nerves   383

Integrative Systems

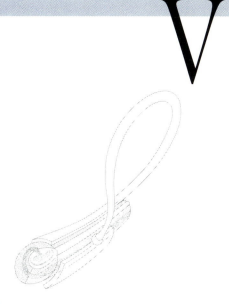

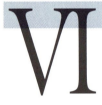

VI

Atlas

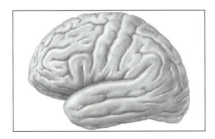 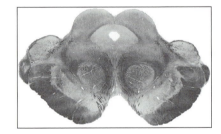

Preface

Neuroanatomy has always played a crucial role in the health science curriculum, particularly as a means of preparing students for understanding the anatomical basis of clinical neurology. The advent of high-resolution brain imaging techniques—magnetic resonance imaging and positron emission tomography—has underscored the importance of studying human neuroanatomy. These techniques provide detailed information about the structure, chemistry, and function of the living brain.

The particular brain regions where drugs may be acting to produce their neurological and psychiatric effects can now be mapped. Thus, these brain imaging techniques provide the neuroscientist and clinician with powerful tools to elucidate and localize function in the human brain, to study the biological substrates of disordered thought and behavior, and to identify traumatized brain regions with unprecedented clarity. Nevertheless, to interpret the information obtained requires a high level of neuroanatomical competence.

Neuroanatomy is helping to provide key insights into disease by providing a bridge between molecular and clinical neural science. We now know the distribution of many different gene products, such as neurotransmitter receptor subtypes, in the normal human brain. By knowing how this distribution changes in the brains of patients with neurological and psychiatric disease, neuroanatomy is helping us to better understand how pathological changes in brain structure alter brain function.

An important goal of *Neuroanatomy: Text and Atlas* is to prepare the reader for interpreting this new wealth of images by developing an understanding of the *anatomical localization of brain function*. To provide a workable focus, this book is restricted to a treatment of the central nervous system. It takes a traditional approach to gaining neuroanatomical competence: because the basic imaging picture is a two-dimensional slice through the brain, the locations of structures are examined on two-dimensional *myelin-stained sections through the human central nervous system*.

Newly featured in the second edition of *Neuroanatomy: Text and Atlas* are drawings of selected key brain structures that are based on computer reconstructions of thinly sliced gross material. The structures chosen for illustration have particularly complex shapes and are the most difficult for students to learn. Neuroanatomical information is better consolidated when the three-dimensional shape of brain structures is correlated with their locations on two-dimensional sections.

Neuroanatomy: Text and Atlas is written as a companion to *Principles of Neural Science,* edited by Eric R. Kandel, James H. Schwartz, and Thomas Jessell (Appleton & Lange). In fact, the sequence of chapters on functional neural systems in *Neuroanatomy: Text and Atlas* parallels those in *Principles of Neural Science. Neuroanatomy: Text and Atlas* is aimed at medical, dental, physical therapy, and other allied health science students. Designed as a self-study guide and resource for information on the structure and function of the human central nervous system, this book could serve as both text and atlas for an introductory laboratory course in human neuroanatomy. Here at the College of Physicians and Surgeons, we use this book in conjunction with a parallel series of weekly laboratory exercises.

Acknowledgments

I take this opportunity to recognize the help I received in the preparation of the second edition of *Neuroanatomy: Text and Atlas*. I am grateful to the following friends and colleagues who have read portions of the manuscript or have provided radiological or histological materials: David Amaral, Jim Ashe, Richard Axel, Brian Boycott, Bill Byne, Mike Crutcher, Christine Curcio, Richard Defendini, John Dowling, Gary Duncan, Susan Folstein, Peter Fox, Apostolos Georgopoulos, Suzanne Haber, David Hubel, Sharon Juliano, Joe LeDoux, Marge Livingstone, Randy Marshall, Bill Merigan, D. Kent Morest, InKi Mun, Jesús Pujol, Pat Goldman-Rakic, Neal Rutledge, David Ruggiero, John Scott, David Smith, Roger Tootell, Bob Vassar, Bob Waters, Torsten Wiesel, and Semir Zeki. I also would like to thank Alice Ko for help with the three-dimensional reconstructions that provided the basis for various illustrations in this edition.

I would like to extend a special note of thanks to Gay Holstein, Craig Bailey, Sam Schacher, and Larry Borden and other members of the neuroanatomy teaching faculty at the College of Physicians and Surgeons for many helpful discussions. To John Rapoport, thanks for his expert advice. I am indebted to Gregory R. Huth first for reading, editing, and improving the clarity of the text and then for overseeing much of the production of the book. For the illustrations in this text, I credit Michael Leonard. Finally, I thank Carol S. Martin for editorial assistance and untiring support during the preparation of this book and to Caitlin E. Martin, Rachel A. Martin, and Emma V. Martin for help with many of the illustrations.

Guide to Using This Book

Neuroanatomy: Text and Atlas takes a combined regional and functional approach to teaching neuroanatomy: knowledge of the spatial interrelations and connections between brain regions is developed in relation to the functions of the brain's various components. Divided into six sections, this book first introduces the major concepts of central nervous system organization. The next four sections consist of chapters that consider neural systems subserving particular sensory, motor, and integrative functions. The last section comprises an atlas of surface anatomy of the brain and histological sections stained for the presence of the fatty myelin sheath that surrounds axons.

Overview of Chapters

The general structural organization of the mature and developing central nervous system is surveyed in Chapters One and Two. This material provides the background for the third chapter, in which the functional organization of the central nervous system is introduced. Here, we consider how different neural circuits, spanning the entire central nervous system, serve particular functions. The circuits for touch perception and voluntary movement control are used as examples.

Central nervous system vasculature and cerebrospinal fluid are the topics of Chapter Four. By considering vasculature early in the book, the reader can better understand why particular functions can become profoundly disturbed when brain regions are deprived of nourishment. These four chapters are intended to provide a synthesis of the *basic concepts* of the structure of the central nervous system and its functional architecture. A fundamental neuroanatomical vocabulary is also established in these chapters.

The remaining 11 chapters examine the major functional neural systems: sensory, motor, and integrative. In these chapters, we reexamine the views of the surface and internal structures of the central nervous system presented in the introductory chapters, but from the perspective of the different functional neural systems. As these latter chapters on functional brain architecture unfold, the reader gradually builds a neuroanatomical knowledge of the regional and functional organization of the spinal cord and brain.

These chapters on neural systems have a different organization from that of the introductory chapters: each is divided into two parts, functional and regional neuroanatomy. The initial part, on *functional neuroanatomy*, considers how particular brain regions work together to produce their intended functions. This part of the chapter presents an "overall view" of *function in relation to structure* before considering the detailed anatomical organization of the neural system. Together with descriptions of the functions of the various components, diagrams illustrate each system's anatomical organization, including key connections that help to show how the particular system accomplishes its tasks. Neural circuits that run through various divisions of the brain are depicted in a standardized format: representations of myelin-stained sections through selected levels of the spinal cord and brain stem are presented with the neural circuit superimposed.

Regional neuroanatomy is emphasized in the latter part of the chapter. Here, structures are depicted on myelin-stained histological sections through the brain. These sections reveal the locations of major pathways and neuronal integrative regions. Typically, we examine a sequence of myelin-stained sections that are ordered according the flow of information processing in the system. For example, for hearing we begin with the ear, where sounds are received and initially processed, and end with the cerebral cortex, where research suggests that our perceptions are formulated. In keeping with the overall theme of the book, the relation between the structure and the function of discrete brain regions is emphasized.

To illustrate the close relationship between neuroanatomy and radiology, magnetic resonance imaging (MRI) scans, positron emission tomography (PET) scans, and angiograms are included in many of the chapters. These scans are intended to facilitate the transition from learning the actual structure of the brain, as revealed by histological sections, to the "virtual structure," as depicted on the various imaging modalities. This is important in learning to "read" the scans, an important clinical skill.

Atlas of the Central Nervous System

This book's atlas, in two parts, offers a complete reference of anatomical structure. The first part presents key views of the surface anatomy of the central nervous sytem. This collection of drawings is based on actual specimens, but emphasizes features shared by each specimen. Thus, no single brain has precisely the form illustrated in this appendix. The second part of the atlas presents a complete set of photographs of myelin-stained sections through the central nervous system in three anatomical planes.

With few exceptions, the same surface views and histological sections used in the chapters are also present in the atlas. In this way, the reader does not have to cope with anatomical variability and is thus better able to develop a thorough understanding of a limited, and sufficiently complete, set of materials. Moreover, brain views and histological sections shown in the chapters have identified only the key structures and those important for the topics discussed. In the atlas, all illustrations are comprehensively labeled. The atlas also serves as a useful guide during a neuroanatomy laboratory.

Didactic Boxes

Selected topics that complement material covered in the chapters are presented in boxes. Neuroradiological and functional circuitry are two topics that are emphasized. In many of the boxes, a new perspective on neuroanatomy is presented, one that has emerged only recently from research. The neuroscience community is enthusiastic that many of these new perspetives may help explain changes in brain function that occur following brain trauma.

Study Aids

This book offers three features that can be used as aids in learning neuroanatomy initially as well as in reviewing for examinations, including professional competency exams. These features are:

- Summaries at the end of each chapter, which present very concise descriptions of key structures in relation to their functions.
- Listing of key terms, which can serve as a self-test allowing the reader to think about what a particular structure does, its location in the central nervous system, from where it receives its inputs, and to where it projects.
- The atlas of key brain views and myelin-stained histological sections, which juxtapose unlabeled and labeled views. The unlabeled image can also be used for self-testing, such as for structure identification.

These study aids are designed to help the reader assimilate the extraordinary amount of detail required to develop a thorough knowledge of human neuroanatomy.

Second Edition

Neuroanatomy
Text and Atlas

1

Introduction to the Central Nervous System

T*HE HUMAN NERVOUS SYSTEM CARRIES OUT* an enormous number of functions, and it does so by means of many subdivisions. Indeed, the complexity of the brain has traditionally made the study of neuroanatomy a notoriously demanding task. This task can be greatly simplified, however, by approaching the study of the nervous system from the dual perspectives of its functional and regional anatomy. **Functional neuroanatomy** examines those parts of the nervous system that work together to accomplish a particular task, for example, in visual perception. An understanding of the neural architecture underlying behavior is readily achieved by considering functional neuroanatomy. In contrast, the study of **regional neuroanatomy** examines the spatial relations between brain structures in a portion of the nervous system. By knowing the local, neighborhood, relationships of brain structures together with the functions that they subserve, a unique solution can be achieved for the clinical problem of determining the location of damage to the nervous system of a neurologically impaired patient.

In this chapter, we introduce the anatomical organization of the nervous system and the means to study it. We establish a working knowledge of the structure of the nervous system and develop the vocabulary needed to study its functional and regional anatomy. Later in the chapter, we consider techniques for examining the microscopic anatomy of the nervous system. Box 1–1 introduces two modern approaches for imaging the living human brain. This background prepares us to explore in detail the functional and regional organization of the nervous system in the chapters that follow.

Neurons and Glia Are the Two Principal Cellular Constituents of the Nervous System

The nerve cell, or **neuron**, is the functional cellular unit of the nervous system: neurons process and store information. Neuroscientists strive to understand the myriad functions of the nervous system in terms of the morphology, physiology, and biochemistry of neurons and their interconnections. The other major cellular constituent of the nervous sys-

1

tem is the neuroglial cell, or **glia**. Glia do not participate directly in signaling information. Rather, they provide structural and metabolic support for neurons both during development and in the mature brain.

All Neurons Have a Common Morphological Plan

Although neurons come in different shapes and sizes, each has four morphologically specialized regions that serve a particular function (Figure 1–1A): dendrites, cell body, axon, and axon terminals. **Dendrites** receive information from other neurons. The **cell body** contains the nucleus and cellular organelles critical for the neuron's vitality. The cell body also receives information from other neurons and serves important integrative functions as well. The **axon** conducts information, which is encoded in the form of action potentials, to the **axon terminal**.

Despite a wide range of shapes and sizes, we can distinguish three classes of neuron based on the configuration of their dendrites and axons: unipolar, bipolar, and multipolar. Examples of the three neuron types are shown in Figure 1–1B. These neurons were drawn by the distinguished Spanish neuroanatomist Santiago Ramón y Cajal at the beginning of the twentieth century.

Unipolar neurons (Figure 1–1B1) are the simplest in shape. They have no dendrites; the cell body of unipolar neurons receives and integrates incoming information. A single axon, which originates from the cell body, gives rise to multiple processes at the terminal. In the human nervous system, unipolar neurons control exocrine gland secretions and smooth muscle contractility.

Bipolar neurons (Figure 1–1B2) have two processes that arise from opposite poles of the cell body. Despite the name, the flow of information (i.e., action potential conduction) in bipolar neurons is from one of the processes, which functions like a dendrite, across the cell body to the other process, which functions like an axon. A morphological subtype of bipolar neuron is a pseudounipolar neuron (see Figure 5–3). During development, the two processes of the embryonic bipolar neuron fuse into a single process in the pseudounipolar neuron, which bifurcates a short distance from the cell body. Sensory neurons, such as those that transmit information about odors or touch to the brain, are bipolar and pseudounipolar neurons.

Multipolar neurons (Figure 1–1B3) feature a complex array of dendrites on the cell body and a single axon. Most of the neurons in the brain and spinal cord are multipolar. Multipolar neurons that have long axons, with axon terminals located in distant sites, are termed **projection neurons**. Projection neurons mediate communication between brain regions, and much of the study of human neuroanatomy focuses on the origins, paths, and terminations of these neurons. The long axon of a projection neuron is particularly susceptible to damage. For example, mechanical trauma of a particular part of the nervous system can destroy the axons of these neurons and produce paralysis. The neuron in Figure 1–1B3 is a projection neuron. The terminals of this neuron are not shown because they are located so far from the cell body that Cajal could not represent them in the same illustration. Indeed, for this type of neuron the axon may be up to 1 meter long, about 50,000 times the width of the cell body! Other multipolar neurons have short axons; these neurons are commonly called **interneurons**. The axon terminals of interneurons remain in the same brain region in which the cell body is located. Interneurons help to process and integrate neuronal information within a local brain region.

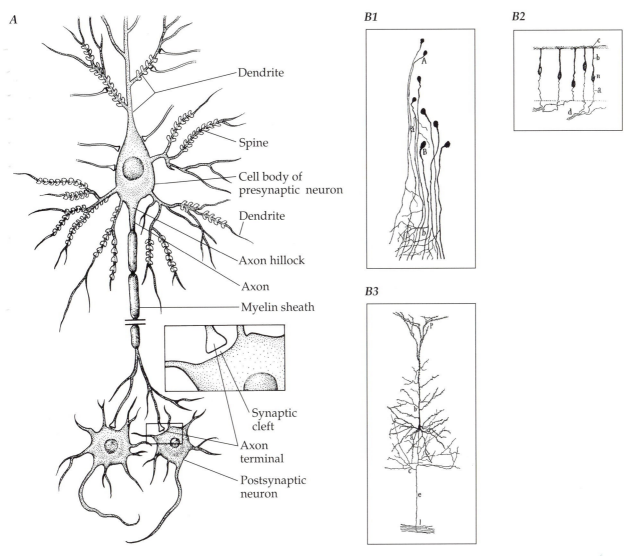

A

Dendrite

Spine

Cell body of
presynaptic neuron

Dendrite

Axon hillock

Axon

Myelin sheath

Synaptic
cleft

Axon
terminal

Postsynaptic
neuron

B1

B2

B3

Figure 1–1. Neurons are the functional cellular unit of the nervous system. *A.* A schematic nerve cell is shown, illustrating the dendrites, cell body, and axon. Dendritic spines are located on dendrites. These are sites of excitatory synapses. Inhibitory synapses are located on the shaft of the dendrites, the cell body, and axon hillock. The axon can be seen to emerge from the cell body. The presynaptic terminals of the neuron are shown synapsing on the cell bodies of the postsynaptic neurons. The inset shows the spatial relations of three components of the synapse, the axon terminal, the synaptic cleft, and the cell body of the postsynaptic neuron. *B.* Selected examples of three neuron classes: (B1) unipolar, (B2) bipolar, and (B3) multipolar. (*A,* Adapted from Kandel, E. R., Schwartz, J. H., and Jessell, T. J. (eds.) 1991. Principles of Neural Science, 2nd ed. New York: Elsevier. *B,* Reproduced from Cajal, S. Ramón y. 1909, 1911. Histologie du système nerveux de l'homme et des vertébres. 2 vols. Paris: Maloine.)

Neurons Communicate With Each Other at Specialized Sites

Information flow along a neuron is polarized. The dendrites and cell body receive and integrate incoming information, which is transmitted along the axon to the terminals. Communication of information from one neuron to another also is polarized and occurs at sites of contact called **synapses**. We call the neuron that sends information the **presynaptic neu-**

ron and the one that receives the information the **postsynaptic neuron**. The information carried by the presynaptic neuron is transduced at the synapse into a chemical signal that is received by the dendrites and cell body of the postsynaptic neuron. Postsynaptic neurons do, however, communicate with presynaptic neurons. This retrograde communication serves important regulatory functions, including maintaining and modulating the strength of synaptic connections.

The synapse consists of three distinct elements: (1) the **presynaptic terminal**, the axon terminal of the presynaptic neuron; (2) the **synaptic cleft**, the narrow intercellular space between the neurons; and (3) the **receptive membrane** of the postsynaptic neuron, typically located either on the dendrites or on the cell body. The axon terminals of certain neurons, instead of contacting postsynaptic neurons, contact muscle cells (e.g., striated limb muscle cells) or exocrine gland cells (e.g., cells of the salivary gland). Synapses are also present at other sites on neurons besides dendrites and the cell body. One such site is the portion of the axon closest to the cell body, the **axon hillock** or **initial segment**. Another site is the presynaptic terminal.

To send a message to its postsynaptic target neurons, a presynaptic neuron releases a **neurotransmitter** into the synaptic cleft. Neurotransmitters are small molecular weight compounds; among these are acetylcholine and monoaminergic compounds such as norepinephrine and serotonin. Amino acids (e.g., glutamate, glycine, and γ-aminobutyric acid, or GABA) and larger molecules, such as peptides (e.g., enkephalin and substance P) also function as neurotransmitters.

When the presynaptic neuron releases the neurotransmitter into the synaptic cleft, two important actions occur. First, the molecules diffuse across the cleft and bind to receptors on the postsynaptic membrane. Second, the neurotransmitter changes the permeability of the membrane to certain ions. The resulting change in ion permeability either excites or inhibits the postsynaptic neuron, depending on the particular ion and its intracellular and extracellular concentrations. For example, excitation (i.e., depolarization) can be produced by a neurotransmitter that increases the flow of sodium ions into a neuron, and inhibition (i.e., hyperpolarization), by a neurotransmitter that increases the flow of chloride ions into a neuron. Glutamate and acetylcholine typically excite neurons, whereas GABA and glycine typically inhibit neurons. Some neurotransmitters, like serotonin, have more complex actions, exciting some neurons and inhibiting others.

Although chemical synaptic transmission is the most common way of sending messages from one neuron to another, purely electrical communication can occur between neurons. At such **electrical synapses**, there is direct cytoplasmic continuity between the presynaptic and postsynaptic neurons.

Glial Cells Provide Structural and Metabolic Support for Neurons

Glial cells comprise the other major cellular constituent of the nervous system and outnumber neurons by 10 to 1. The structural and metabolic support that glial cells provide for neurons must be a formidable task given the 10:1 ratio! There are two major classes of glia: microglia and macroglia. **Microglia** subserve a phagocytic or scavenger role, responding to nervous system infection or damage. **Macroglia**, of which there are four separate types—oligodendrocytes, Schwann cells, astrocytes, and ependymal cells—subserve a variety of support and nutritive functions. **Oligodendrocytes** and **Schwann cells** form the **myelin sheath** (Figure 1–1A) around axons. The myelin sheath, which serves to increase the velocity of action potential conduction, is whitish in appearance because it is rich in a fatty substance called **myelin**. **Astrocytes** subserve important structural and metabolic functions. For example, in the developing nervous system astrocytes act as scaffolds for growing axons. **Ependymal cells** line fluid-filled cavities in the central nervous system (see below).

The Nervous System Consists of Separate Peripheral and Central Components

Neurons and glial cells of the nervous system are organized into two anatomically separate but functionally interdependent parts: the **peripheral** and the **central nervous systems** (Figure 1–2A). The peripheral nervous system is subdivided into **somatic** and **autonomic** divisions that are actually controlled by the central nervous system. The somatic division contains the sensory neurons that innervate the skin, muscles, and joints; these neurons detect all stimuli. This division also contains the axons that innervate skeletal muscle. These axons transmit control signals to muscle to regulate the force of contraction. The autonomic division contains the neurons that innervate the glands and the smooth muscle of the viscera and blood vessels (see Chapter 14). This division, with its separate **sympathetic**, **parasympathetic**, and **enteric** subdivisions, regulates body functions based, in part, on information about the internal state of the organism. The autonomic nervous system was once thought not to be under conscious control. We now know that many autonomic functions can indeed be controlled, but with greater difficulty than controlling skeletal muscles.

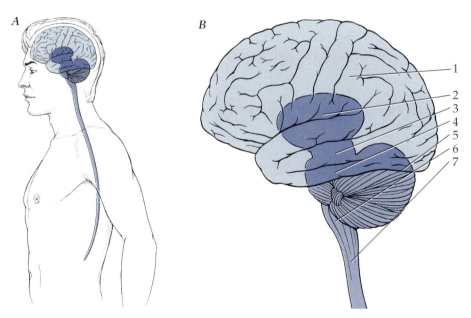

Figure 1–2. **A.** Location of the central nervous system in the body. **B.** There are seven major divisions of the central nervous system: (1) cerebral hemispheres, (2) diencephalon, (3) midbrain, (4) pons, (5) cerebellum, (6) medulla, and (7) spinal cord. The midbrain, pons, and medulla comprise the brain stem.

The central nervous system consists of the **spinal cord** and **brain** (Figure 1–2A), and the brain is further subdivided into the medulla, pons, cerebellum, midbrain, diencephalon, and cerebral hemispheres (Figure 1–2B). Within each of the seven central nervous system divisions resides a component of the **ventricular system**, a labyrinth of fluid-filled cavities that serve various supportive functions.

Neuronal cell bodies and axons are not distributed randomly within the nervous system. In the peripheral nervous system, cell bodies collect in peripheral **ganglia** and axons are contained in **peripheral nerves**. The central nervous system also shows a clear distinction between regions containing predominantly neuronal cell bodies and dendrites and regions that contain axons. Neuronal cell bodies and dendrites in the central nervous system are located in **cortical** areas, which are large flattened sheets of cells (or laminae) usually located on the surface of the central nervous system and in **nuclei**, which are clusters of neurons typically located beneath the surface. Nuclei come in various sizes and shapes, commonly spherical and oval and sometimes in small flattened sheets. Regions of the central nervous system that contain axons have an unwieldy number of names, the most common of which is **tract**. In fresh tissue, nuclei and cortical areas appear gray and tracts appear white, hence the familiar terms **gray matter** and **white matter**. The whitish appearance of tracts is caused by the presence of the myelin sheath surrounding the axons (Figure 1–1A). In the peripheral nervous system **Schwann cells** form the myelin sheath, whereas in the central nervous system, the myelin sheath is formed by **oligodendrocytes**.

The Spinal Cord Displays the Simplest Organization of All Seven Major Divisions

The spinal cord (Figure 1–3) participates directly in body movement control, in regulating visceral functions, and in processing sensory information from the limbs, trunk, and many internal organs. It also provides a conduit for the longitudinal flow of information to and from the brain. The spinal cord is the only part of the central nervous system that has a clear external **segmental** organization (Figure 1–3, inset), reminiscent of its embryonic and phylogenetic origins (see Chapter 2). The significance of this organization is that every spinal cord segment (Figure 1–3) has basically the same structure.

Each spinal cord segment is dominated by the presence of a pair of nerve roots (and associated rootlets) called the **dorsal** and **ventral** roots. (The terms dorsal and ventral describe the spatial relations of structures; these and other anatomical terms are explained later in this chapter.) Dorsal roots contain only **sensory axons** and thus transmit sensory information into the spinal cord. By contrast, ventral roots contain **motor axons** and therefore transmit the motor commands to muscle. Dorsal and ventral roots exemplify the separation of function in the nervous system, a principle that we will reexamine in subsequent chapters. These sensory and motor axons, which are part of the peripheral nervous system, become intermingled in the **spinal nerves** (Figure 1–3) en route to their peripheral targets.

The Brain Stem and Cerebellum Regulate Body Functions and Movements

The next three divisions—medulla, pons, and midbrain—comprise the **brain stem** (Figure 1–4). The brain stem has three general functions. First, it receives sensory information from cranial structures and controls

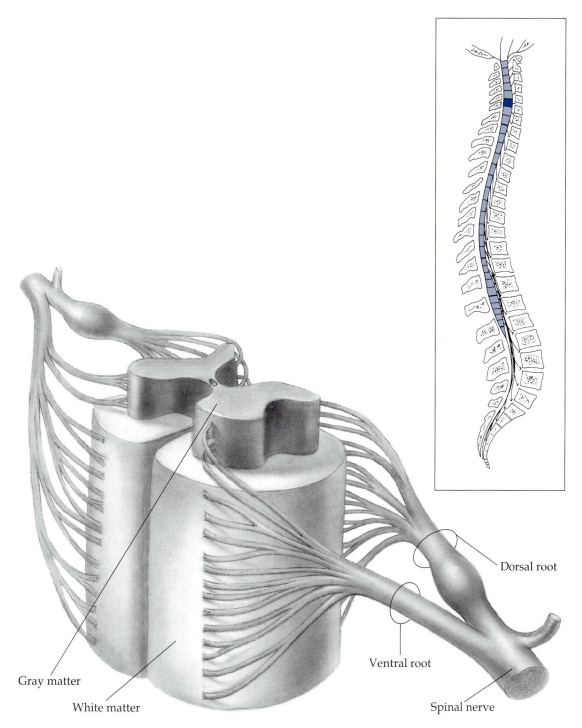

Gray matter

White matter

Dorsal root

Ventral root

Spinal nerve

Figure 1–3. Surface topography and internal structure of the spinal cord. The inset shows the segmental arrangement of the spinal cord (light blue) and vertebral column and the location of a single spinal segment (dark blue).

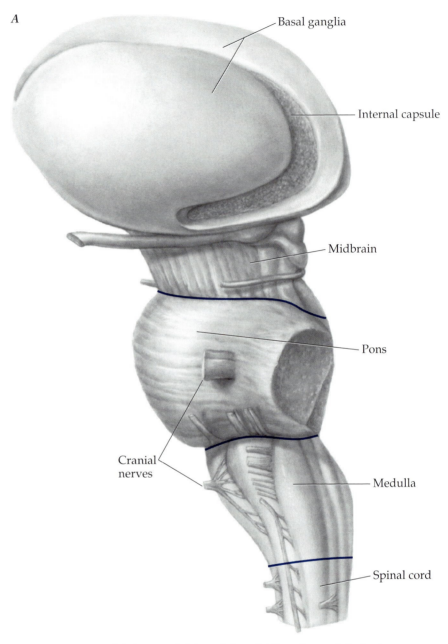

Figure 1–4. Lateral *(A)*, ventral *(B)*, and dorsal *(C)* surfaces of the brain stem. The thalamus and basal ganglia are also shown.

the muscles of the head. This function is similar to that of the spinal cord. **Cranial nerves**, the nerve roots that enter and exit the brain stem (Figure 1–4), are the parts of the peripheral nervous system that provide the sensory and motor innervation of the head. The cranial nerves are therefore analogous to the spinal nerves. Second, the brain stem contains neural circuits that transmit information from the spinal cord up to other brain regions, and down, from the brain to the spinal cord. Finally, through the integrated actions of the medulla, pons, and midbrain, the brain stem regulates arousal. This function is mediated by the central portion, or core, of the brain stem, termed the **reticular formation**.

In addition to these three general functions, the various divisions of the brain stem subserve specific sensory and motor functions. The

B

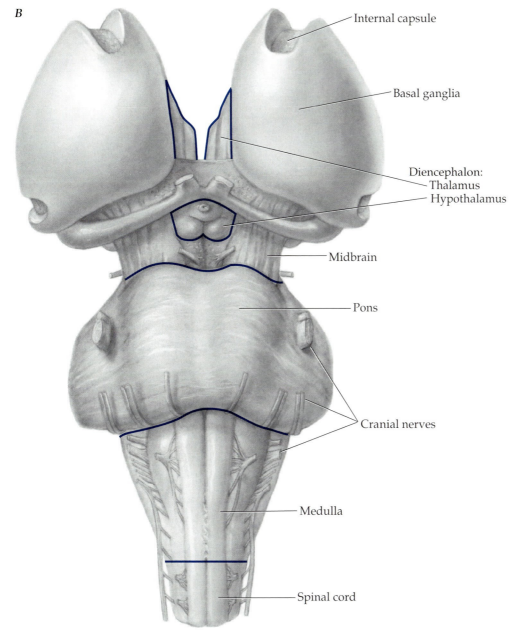

Internal capsule

Basal ganglia

Diencephalon:
Thalamus
Hypothalamus

Midbrain

Pons

Cranial nerves

Medulla

Spinal cord

Figure 1–4. (continued)

medulla and the **pons** participate in essential blood pressure and respiratory regulatory mechanisms. Indeed, damage to these parts of the brain is almost always life threatening. The **midbrain** plays a key role in the control of eye movement.

The **cerebellum** (Figure 1–5) regulates movements of our eyes and limbs and helps us to maintain posture and balance. When this important movement control structure becomes damaged, for example when a portion of its blood supply is interrupted, limb movements become erratic and poorly coordinated. The cerebellum and pons are sometimes considered to be parts of the same division of the mature brain because they develop from the same embryonic brain division (see Chapter 2) and many of their motor control functions are closely related.

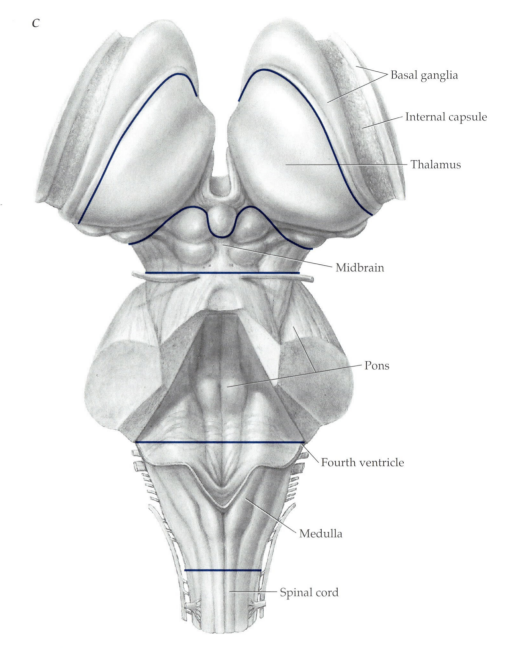

C

Basal ganglia

Internal capsule

Thalamus

Midbrain

Pons

Fourth ventricle

Medulla

Spinal cord

Figure 1–4. (continued)

The Diencephalon Consists of the Thalamus and Hypothalamus

The **diencephalon** and the **cerebral hemispheres** are the most highly developed portions of the human central nervous system. The diencephalon consists of two major components. One, the **thalamus** (Figures 1–4C, 1–5, 1–6, and 1–7B), is a key structure for transmitting information to the cerebral hemispheres. Neurons in separate thalamic nuclei transmit information to different cortical areas. In most brains, a small portion of the thalamus in each half adheres at the midline, the **thalamic adhesion** (or massa intermedia). The other component, the **hypothalamus** (Figures 1–7B and 1–8A), integrates the functions of the autonomic nervous system and controls endocrine hormone release from the pituitary gland. Techni-

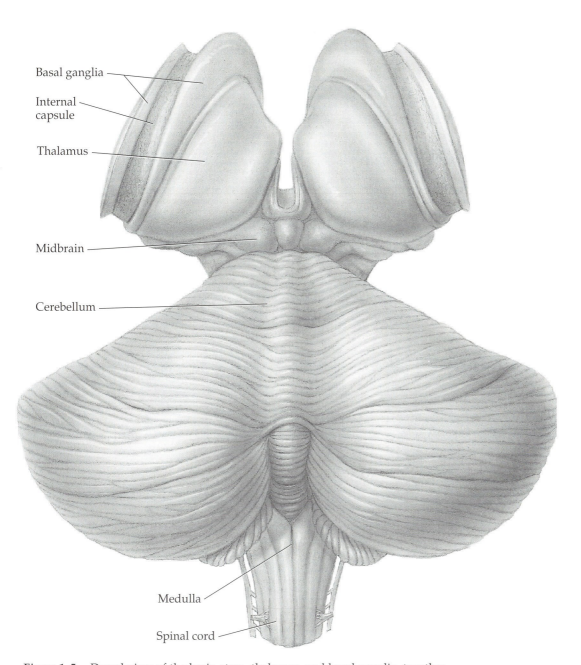

Basal ganglia

Internal capsule

Thalamus

Midbrain

Cerebellum

Medulla

Spinal cord

Figure 1–5. Dorsal view of the brain stem, thalamus, and basal ganglia, together with the cerebellum.

cally, the diencephalon is part of the brain stem. It is discussed together with the cerebral hemispheres because of the important role diencephalic structures play in the functions of the cerebral hemispheres.

The Cerebral Hemispheres Have the Most Complex Three-dimensional Configuration of All Central Nervous System Divisions

The **cerebral hemispheres** have four major components: cerebral cortex, hippocampal formation, amygdala, and basal ganglia. Together, these structures mediate the most sophisticated of human behaviors. The **cere-**

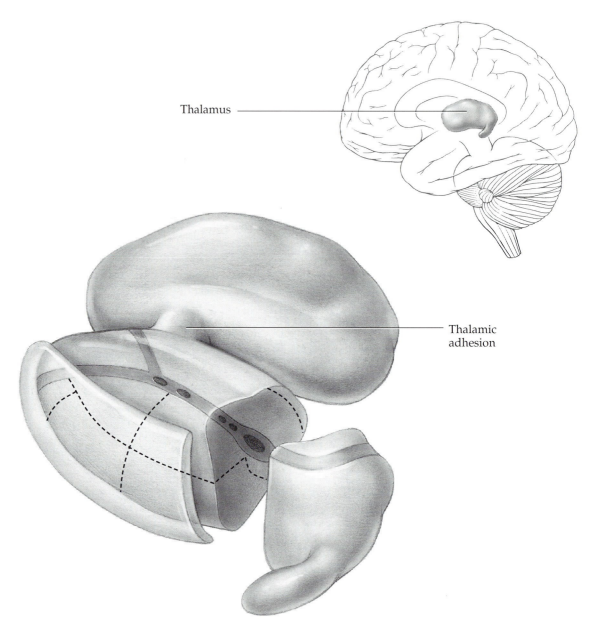

Thalamus

Thalamic
adhesion

Figure 1–6. The three-dimensional structure of the thalamus. The inset is a view
of the lateral surface of the cerebral hemisphere and brain stem, illustrating the
location of the thalamus.

bral cortex, which is located on the surface of the brain (Figures 1–7 and
1–8), is highly convoluted. Convolutions are an evolutionary adaptation to
fit a greater surface area within the confined space of the cranial cavity. In
fact, only one quarter to one third of the cerebral cortex is exposed on the
surface. The elevated convolutions, called **gyri**, are separated by grooves
called fissures or sulci. **Fissures** are deep grooves that are consistently present from one brain to the next. For example, the cerebral hemispheres are
separated into two halves by the **sagittal** (or interhemispheric) **fissure**
(Figure 1–8). **Sulci** are not as deep as fissures, and their precise form and
location are not reliably consistent.

The Cerebral Cortex is Divided Into Four Lobes

The four **lobes** (Figure 1–7, inset) of the cerebral cortex are named after the cranial bones that overlie them: frontal, parietal, occipital, and temporal. The functions of the different lobes are remarkably distinct as are the functions of individual gyri within each lobe. The **frontal** and **parietal** lobes, important for motor control and for bodily senses such as touch or pain, are separated by the **central sulcus**. The **temporal** lobe, important for various sensory functions including hearing, is separated from the frontal and parietal lobes by the **lateral sulcus** (or **Sylvian fissure**) (Figure 1–7A). The **occipital** lobe, essential for sight, is separated from the parietal and temporal lobes by an imaginary line connecting the **preoccipital notch**, on the lateral surface (Figure 1–7A), and the tip of the **parieto–occipital sulcus**, on the medial brain surface (Figure 1–7B). The major sulci and fissures are surprisingly deep. In fact, we will see in Chapter 3 that the cortex within the lateral sulcus is so extensive that it rivals that of an entire lobe.

The **frontal lobe** is essential for motor behavior, not only for regulating the simple mechanical actions of movement, such as strength, but also for deciding which movements are performed to achieve a particular goal. These functions are accomplished by the **motor cortex**, which is located on the **precentral gyrus**, and the premotor areas, which are located adjacent to the motor cortex. On the lateral surface, most of the remaining portions of the frontal lobe are important in cognitive functions and emotions. These portions, which collectively are termed the **prefrontal association cortex**, consist of the superior, middle, and inferior frontal gyri. The cingulate gyrus (Figure 1–7B), a prominent gyrus on the medial surface, is important for emotional functions. The **corpus callosum** can also be seen on the view of the medial brain surface. To integrate the functions of the two halves of the cerebral cortex, axons of this structure course through each of its four principal parts (Figure 1–7B): rostrum, genu, body, and splenium. The olfactory sensory organ, the **olfactory bulb**, is located on the inferior surface of the frontal lobe (Figure 1–8A). Portions of the **orbital gyri** and the **basal forebrain**, both of which are on the ventral surface of the frontal lobe, are important in processing olfactory information.

The **parietal lobe** not only plays a unique role in our perceptions of touch, pain, and limb position but also integrates our sensory experiences from skin, muscles, and joints, enabling us to perceive the size and shape of grasped objects. These functions are carried out primarily by the **somatic sensory cortex**, which is located in the **postcentral gyrus**. The remaining portion of the parietal lobe on the lateral brain surface consists of the superior and the inferior parietal lobules, which are separated by the intraparietal sulcus. The **superior parietal lobule** is essential for a complete self-image and mediates behavioral interaction with the world around us. A lesion in this portion of the parietal lobe can produce bizarre neurological signs that include neglecting a portion of the body on the side opposite the lesion. For example, a patient may not shave half of his face or dress half of her body. The **inferior parietal lobule** is involved in integrating diverse sensory information for speech and perception.

The **occipital lobe** is the most singular in function; it subserves visual perception. The **visual cortex** is located in the walls and depths of the **calcarine fissure** (Figure 1–7B) on the medial brain surface. While the visual cortex is important in the initial stages of visual processing, the surrounding cortex plays a role in elaborating the sensory message that enables us to see the form and color of objects. On the medial brain surface, hidden from view by the brain stem and cerebellum, is a portion of

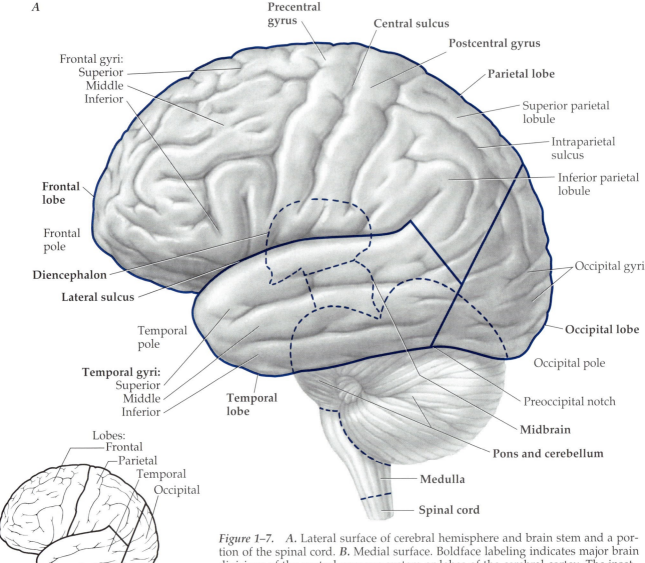

Figure 1–7. **A.** Lateral surface of cerebral hemisphere and brain stem and a portion of the spinal cord. **B.** Medial surface. Boldface labeling indicates major brain divisions of the central nervous system or lobes of the cerebral cortex. The inset shows the four lobes of the cerebral cortex.

the occipital lobe important for recognizing faces. Patients with a lesion of this area can confuse faces with inanimate objects. The **parieto–occipital sulcus** (Figure 1–7B) separates the occipital and parietal lobes.

The **temporal lobe** mediates a variety of sensory functions as well as participating in memory and emotions. The **auditory cortex**, located on the **superior temporal gyrus**, works with surrounding areas within the lateral sulcus and on the middle temporal gyrus to help us perceive and localize sounds (Figure 1–7A). An important cortical center for recognizing speech, termed Wernicke's area, is located in the superior temporal gyrus. This region is interconnected with the frontal speech area, termed Broca's area, which is important for articulating speech. The **inferior temporal gyrus** (Figures 1–7A and 1–8A) serves the perception of visual form and

B

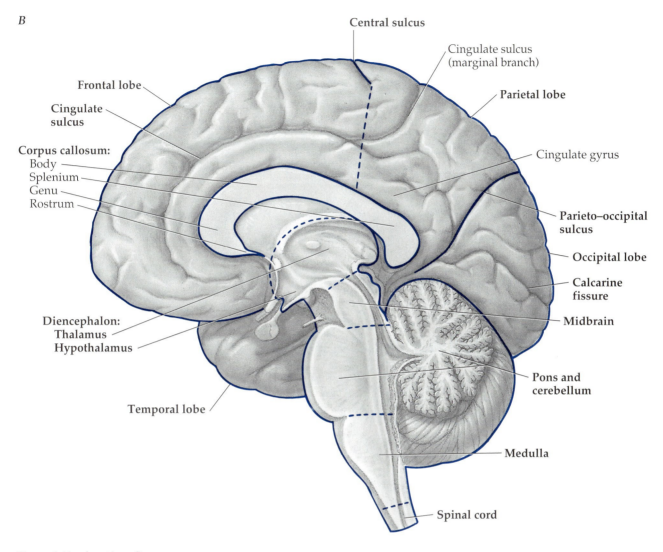

Figure 1–7. (continued)

color. Emotions are mediated by the cortex located at the temporal pole (Figure 1–8A), together with adjacent portions of the medial temporal lobe and inferior and medial frontal lobe.

The Other Components of the Cerebral Hemispheres Are Located Beneath the Cortex

The second and third major components of the cerebral hemisphere are located beneath the cortical surface: the **hippocampal formation** and the **amygdala** (Figure 1–9A). The hippocampal formation is important in learning and memory, whereas the amygdala not only participates in emotions but also helps to coordinate our body's response to stressful and threatening situations, such as preparing to fight. These two structures are part of the **limbic system**, which includes other parts of the cerebral hemi-

A

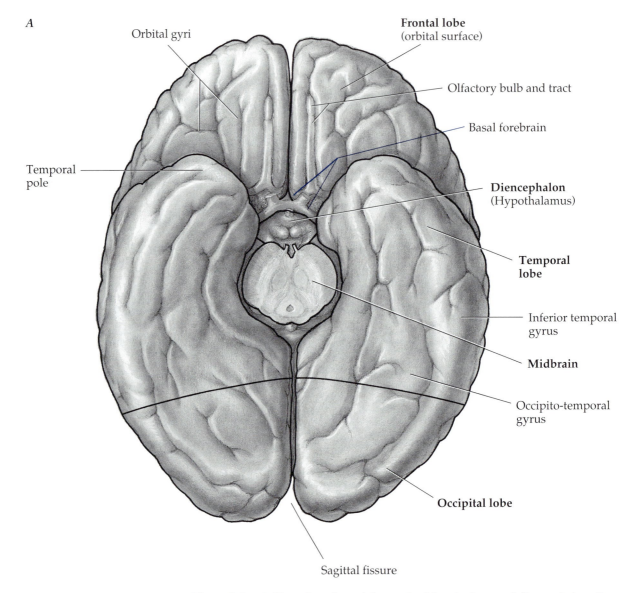

Orbital gyri

Frontal lobe
(orbital surface)

Olfactory bulb and tract

Basal forebrain

Temporal
pole

Diencephalon
(Hypothalamus)

**Temporal
lobe**

Inferior temporal
gyrus

Midbrain

Occipito-temporal
gyrus

Occipital lobe

Sagittal fissure

Figure 1–8. *A.* Ventral surface of the cerebral hemisphere and diencephalon; the
midbrain is cut in cross section. *B.* Dorsal surface of cerebral hemisphere.

spheres, diencephalon, and midbrain (see Chapter 15). Because the limbic
system plays a key role in mood, it is not surprising that psychiatric disorders are often associated with limbic system dysfunction.

The fourth major component of the cerebral hemisphere is the **basal
ganglia**, deeply located collections of neurons. One portion of the basal
ganglia, called the **striatum**, is illustrated in Figure 1–9B along with portions of the ventricular system (see below). The basal ganglia participate in
many higher brain functions in concert with the cerebral cortex. For example, the role of the basal ganglia in the control of movement is clearly
revealed when they become damaged, as in Parkinson's disease. Tremor
and a slowing of movement are some of the overt signs of this disease. The
basal ganglia also participate in emotion and cognition.

B

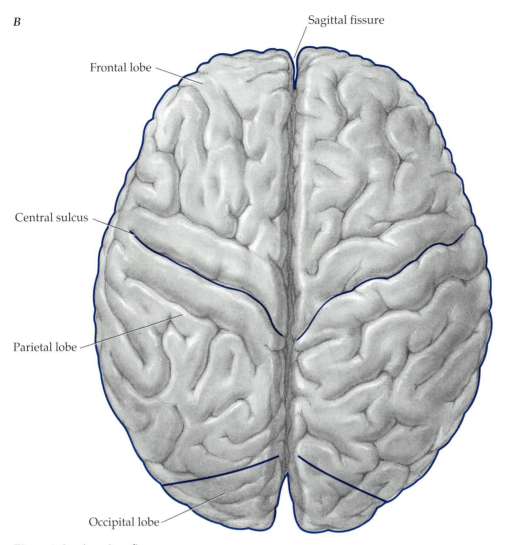

Sagittal fissure

Frontal lobe

Central sulcus

Parietal lobe

Occipital lobe

Figure 1–8.   (continued)

Cavities Within the Central Nervous System Contain Cerebrospinal Fluid

The central nervous system is basically tubular in organization. Within it are cavities, collectively termed the **ventricular system** (Figure 1–10), that contain **cerebrospinal fluid**. Cerebrospinal fluid is a watery fluid that cushions the central nervous system from physical shocks and is a medium for chemical communication. An intraventricular structure, the **choroid plexus**, secretes most of the cerebrospinal fluid. We will consider cerebrospinal fluid production in Chapter 4.

Within the ventricular system, cerebrospinal fluid accumulates in the ventricles. The two **lateral ventricles** are located within each half of the cerebral hemisphere. Between the two halves of the diencephalon is the **third ventricle**, forming a midline cavity. The **fourth ventricle** is located between the brain stem and cerebellum: the medulla and pons form the

A

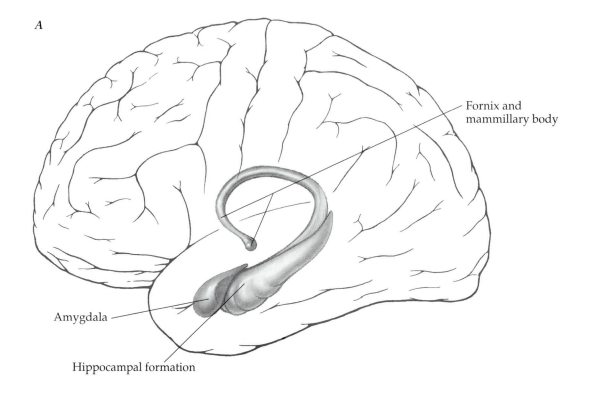

Fornix and
mammillary body

Amygdala

Hippocampal formation

B

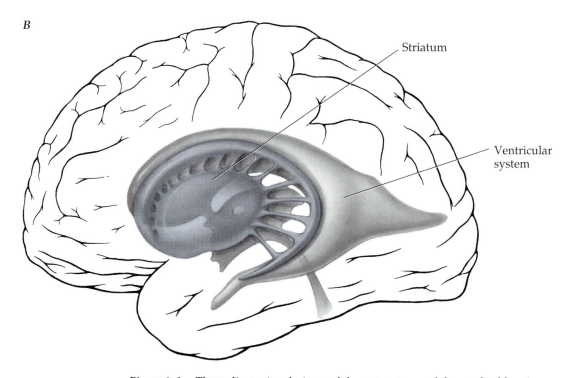

Striatum

Ventricular
system

Figure 1–9. Three-dimensional views of deep structures of the cerebral hemi-sphere. *A.* The hippocampal formation and amygdala. The fornix and mammil-lary body are structures that are anatomically and functionally related to the hip-pocampal formation. *B.* Striatum, a component of the basal ganglia. The ventricular system is also illustrated. Note the similarity in overall shapes of the striatum and the lateral ventricle.

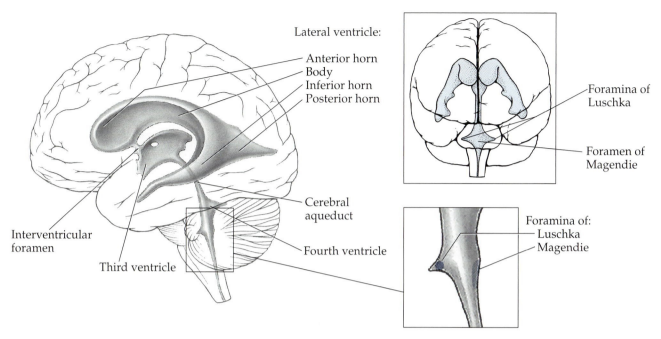

Lateral ventricle:
- Anterior horn
- Body
- Inferior horn
- Posterior horn

Interventricular foramen

Third ventricle

Cerebral aqueduct

Fourth ventricle

Foramina of Luschka

Foramen of Magendie

Foramina of:
- Luschka
- Magendie

Figure 1–10. Ventricular system. The lateral ventricles, third ventricle, cerebral aqueduct, and fourth ventricle are seen from the lateral brain surface. The lateral ventricle is divided into four main components: anterior (or frontal) horn, body, inferior (or temporal) horn, and the posterior (or occipital) horn. The interventricular foramen (of Monro) connects each lateral ventricle with the third ventricle. The cerebral aqueduct connects the third and fourth ventricles. The insets show the approximate locations of the formina of Luschka and Magendie in the fourth ventricle viewed from the ventral surface (top inset) and lateral surface (bottom inset).

floor of the fourth ventricle and the cerebellum, the roof. The third and fourth ventricles are relatively simple in configuration; however, the lateral ventricles are further subdivided into a **body** and three compartments termed **horns** (Figure 1–10). The ventricles are interconnected by narrow conduits: the **interventricular foramina** (of Monro) connect each of the lateral ventricles with the third ventricle, and the **cerebral aqueduct** (of Sylvius), in the midbrain, connects the third and fourth ventricles. The ventricular system extends into the spinal cord as the **central canal**.

Cerebrospinal fluid not only bathes the interior of the brain via the ventricular system, but flows over the surface of the entire central nervous system. Cerebrospinal fluid exits the ventricular system through three small apertures in the roof of the fourth ventricle: the two laterally placed **foramina of Luschka** and the **foramen of Magendie**, which is located at the midline (Figure 1–10, inset).

The Central Nervous System Is Covered by Three Meningeal Layers

The **meninges** consist of the dura mater, the arachnoid mater, and the pia mater (Figure 1–11). The **dura mater** is the thickest and outermost of these membranes and serves a protective function. (Dura mater means "hard mother" in Latin.) It is composed of fibroblastlike cells which secrete abundant collagen to produce a tough protective membrane. Ancient surgeons knew that patients could survive even severe skull fractures if the dura was not penetrated by bone fragments.

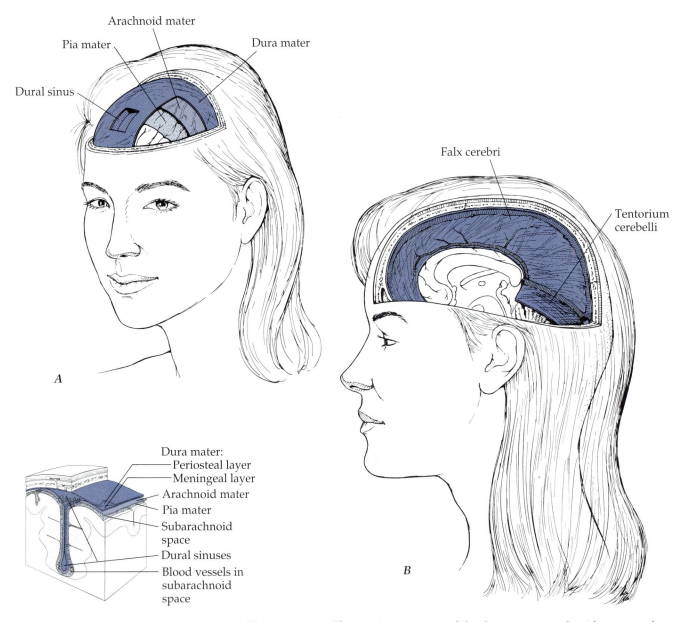

Figure 1–11. **A.** The meninges consist of the dura mater, arachnoid mater, and the pia mater. **B.** The two major dural flaps are the falx cerebri, which incompletely separates the two cerebral hemispheres, and the tentorium cerebelli, which separates the cerebellum from the cerebral hemisphere. The inset shows the dural layers. (*A*, Adapted from Snell, R. S. 1987. Clinical Neuroanatomy for Medical Students. Boston: Little-Brown.)

The portion of the dura overlying the cerebral hemispheres and brain stem contains two separate layers: an outer **periosteal layer** and an inner **meningeal layer** (Figure 1–11). The periosteal layer is attached to the inner surface of the skull. Two important partitions arise from the meningeal layer and separate different components of the cerebral hemispheres and brain stem (Figure 1–11B): (1) the **falx cerebri** separates the two cerebral hemispheres; (2) the **tentorium cerebelli** separates the cerebellum from the cerebral hemispheres. The dura mater that covers the spinal cord is continuous with both the meningeal layer of the cranial dura and the epineurium of peripheral nerves.

The **arachnoid mater** adjoins but is not tightly bound to the dura mater, thus allowing a potential space to exist between them. This potential space, called the **subdural space**, is important clinically. Because the dura mater contains blood vessels, breakage of one of its vessels can lead to subdural bleeding and to the formation of a blood clot (a **subdural hematoma**). In this condition, the blood clot pushes the arachnoid away from the dura mater, fills the subdural space, and compresses underlying neural tissue.

The innermost meningeal layer, the **pia mater**, is very delicate and adheres to the surface of the brain and spinal cord. (Pia mater means "tender mother" in Latin.) The space between the arachnoid mater and pia mater is the **subarachnoid space**. Filaments of arachnoid mater pass through the subarachnoid space and connect to the pia mater, giving this space the appearance of a spider's web. (Hence the name **arachnoid**, which derives from the Greek word *arachne*, meaning spider.) After leaving the fourth ventricle, cerebrospinal fluid circulates over the surface of the brain and spinal cord within the subarachnoid space. In Chapter 4, we will see the path through which cerebrospinal fluid is returned to the venous circulation.

The meninges also serve an important circulatory function. The veins and arteries that overlie the surface of the central nervous system are located in the subarachnoid space. Moreover, within the dura are large, low-pressure blood vessels, which are part of the return path for cerebral venous blood. These vessels are termed the **dural sinuses** (Figure 1–11, inset; see also Chapter 4).

An Introduction to Neuroanatomical Terms

The complex three-dimensional organization of the brain requires a precise method for describing both the absolute position of structures and their position relative to other structures. The terminology of neuroanatomy is specialized to meet this need. Although using more intuitive descriptions of the positions of structures may at first make neuroanatomy easier to understand, the lack of precision quickly results in confusion. The terms describing spatial relations and the major axes of the nervous system are briefly described next. This nomenclature may seem arbitrary at first, but in Chapter 2, we will see that it follows logically from the developmental plan of the central nervous system.

Two Major Axes Describe the Organization of the Central Nervous System

The central nervous system is organized along the **rostral–caudal** and the **dorsal–ventral** axes of the body (Figure 1–12). These axes are most easily understood in animals with a central nervous system that is more simple than that of humans, for example, the rat (Figure 1–12A). Here, the rostral–caudal axis runs approximately in a straight line from the nose to the tail. This axis is also the **longitudinal axis** of the nervous system and is often termed the **neuraxis** because the central nervous system has a predominant longitudinal organization. In Chapter 3, we will examine major neural systems that have a longitudinal organization. The dorsal–ventral

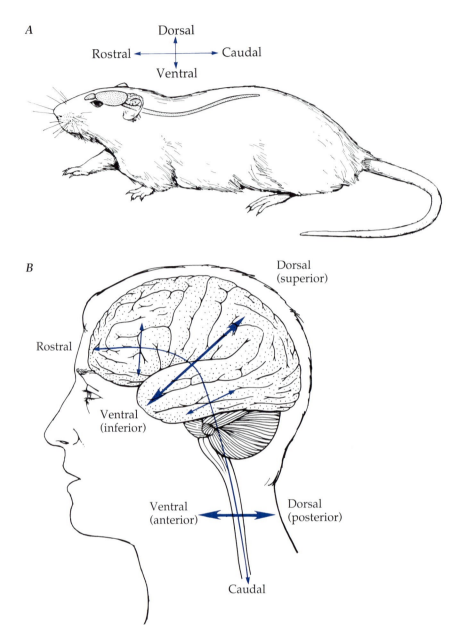

Figure 1–12. The axes of central nervous system are illustrated for the rat *(A)*, an animal whose central nervous system is organized in a linear fashion, and the human *(B)*, whose central nervous system has a prominent flexure at the midbrain. (Adapted from Kandel, E. R., and Schwartz, J. H. (eds.) 1985. Principles of Neural Science. New York: Elsevier.)

axis, which is perpendicular to the rostral–caudal axis, runs from the back to the abdomen. The terms **posterior** and **anterior** are synonymous with dorsal and ventral, respectively.

The longitudinal axis of the human nervous system is not straight as it is in the rat (Figure 1–12B). During development, the brain—and therefore its longitudinal axis—undergoes a prominent bend, or **flexure**, at the midbrain. Instead of describing structures located rostral to this flexure as dorsal or ventral, we typically use the terms **superior** and **inferior**.

*There Are Three Major Planes of Section
Through the Central Nervous System*

We also name the planes in which anatomical sections, or slices, are made through the brain and spinal cord (Figure 1–13). We define three principal planes relative to the longitudinal axis of the nervous system: hori-

A   *B*   *C*

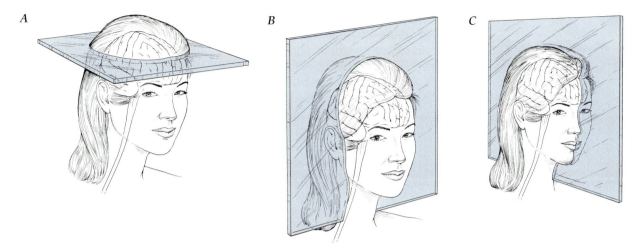

Figure 1–13. The three main anatomical planes: *(A)* horizontal, *(B)* coronal, and *(C)* sagittal.

zontal, transverse, and sagittal. **Horizontal** sections are cut parallel to the longitudinal axis, from one side to the other. **Transverse** sections are cut perpendicular to the longitudinal axis, between the dorsal and ventral surfaces. Transverse sections through the cerebral hemisphere are roughly parallel to the coronal suture and, as a consequence, are also termed **coronal** sections. **Sagittal** sections are cut parallel both to the longitudinal axis of the central nervous system and to the midline, between the dorsal and ventral surfaces. A **midsagittal** section divides the central nervous system into two symmetrical halves, whereas a **parasagittal** section is cut off the midline.

Techniques for Studying the Regional Anatomy and Interconnections of the Central Nervous System

Historically, the earliest methods for studying normal regional neuroanatomy involved selective staining of different portions of the neuron: either the cell body or the axon. The **Nissl** method uses a dye that binds to acid groups, in particular to ribonucleic acids of the ribosomes located within the cell body. The **Weigert** method, for example, is an axonal staining method that uses a dye that binds to the myelin sheath. Tissues prepared with either a **cell stain** or a **myelin stain** have a different appearance (Figure 1–14). This is because nuclei and tracts are found in separate parts of tissue in the central nervous system. Stains that use silver, for example the **Golgi** method (see Figure 10–13), may show not only the cell body of the neuron but its dendrites and axon as well. Silver is thought to bind to filamentous proteins within the cytoplasm. Unlike the Nissl and Weigert methods, which stain either the cell body or axon of all neurons exposed to the dye, silver stains an entire neuron (or glial cell) but, curiously, only a small number of cells in an area.

The various staining methods are used to reveal different features of the cellular organization of the nervous system. For example, myelin stains are used to reveal the general topography of brain regions, and cell stains are used to characterize the cellular architecture of nuclei and cortical areas. Silver stains are used to study the detailed morphology of neurons.

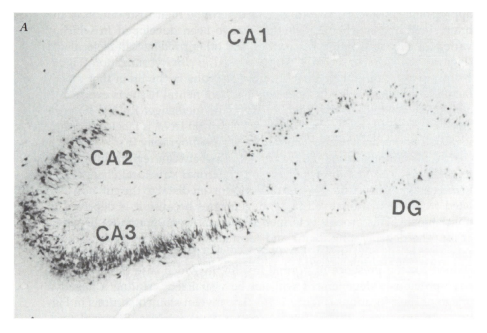

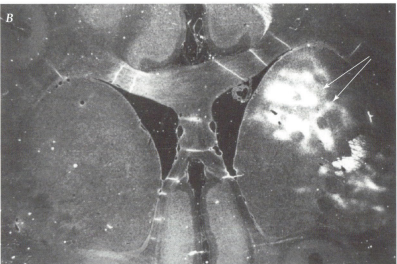

Figure 1–17. Retrograde and anterograde labeling in the central nervous system. *A.* Retrogradely labeled neurons in the hippocampal formation after injection of tracer in the paraventricular nucleus of the thalamus. The tracer used was pseudorabies virus, which is taken up by axon terminals and retrogradely transported to neuronal cell bodies the CA regions of the hippocampal formation. The tracer is then transported transneuronally to presynaptic neurons in the DG region of the hippocampal formation. *B.* Autoradiograph showing axon terminal labeling in the striatum, a portion of the basal ganglia. Radioactive tracer, consisting of a mixture of ³H proline and ³H leucine, was injected into the prefrontal cortex of a rhesus monkey. (*A,* Courtesy of Dr. David Ruggiero; *B,* Courtesy of Dr. Patricia Goldman-Rakic; Goldman-Rakic, P.S. 1978. Science 202:768–770.)

transported to other parts. Some materials are taken up by axon terminals and transported **retrogradely** to the cell body. Other compounds are taken up by neuronal cell bodies and transported **anterogradely** to the axon terminals. Many compounds are transported in both retrograde and anterograde directions. Chemicals commonly used to trace axonal connections between brain regions include horseradish peroxidase, the plant lectin wheat germ agglutinin, amino acids, certain fluorescent dyes, and neurotoxins.

Retrograde transport of the tracer molecules is used to examine the distribution of neurons projecting their axons to a particular region (Figure 1–17A). In contrast, anterograde transport is used to examine where neurons in a particular region project their axons (Figure 1–17B). Depending on the material used, tracer molecules are visualized by special histochemical reactions, fluorescence microscopy, or autoradiography. Certain compounds used for tracing brain connections are transported across the synapse (i.e., through transneuronal transport) and thereby offer the opportunity to probe the anatomical organization of neural pathways. For example, the tracer used in the experiment shown in Figure 1–17A is a virus that is taken up by neuronal terminals in the thalamus and transported back to the cell bodies located in the regions marked CA of the hippocampal formation. The tracer is then transported transneuronally to presynaptic neurons located in the region DG of the hippocampal formation. (The various portions of the hippocampal formation are discussed in detail in Chapter 15.) Moreover, the transneuronal transport of some of these compounds is believed to be dependent on the activity of neurons in the pathway. Activity-dependent transport reveals the anatomy of particular sets of functional connections.

Two radiological techniques now permit remarkably precise examination of regional and functional anatomy of the living human brain. The first technique, **magnetic resonance imaging** (MRI), probes the regional anatomy of the brain, principally by measuring the water content of tissues. This technique can also provide an image of brain function by measuring changes in the oxygenated state of hemoglobin. The second technique, **positron emission tomography** (PET), provides an image of brain function by computing the distribution of radiolabeled compounds involved in neuronal metabolism or cerebral blood flow. In Box 1–1, we explore, in a general way, components of the human central nervous system that participate in **visual perception**.

Box 1–1. Structure and Function Can Be Imaged in the Living Brain

The components of the central nervous system that are important for visual perception are schematically illustrated in Figure 1–18A. (The visual system is discussed in detail in Chapter 6.) Briefly, the visual pathway begins in the **retina**, where sensory receptors that convert visual energy to neuronal events are located. Here, receptor neurons synapse on interneurons, which in turn synapse on projection neurons. The axon terminals of the projection neurons terminate in the **thalamus**. The thalamus functions as a gateway for information flow to the cerebral cortex.

From the thalamus, the next processing stage in the visual pathway is the **primary visual cortex**. Each sensory modality has a **primary** cortical area, so termed because it receives sensory information directly from the thalamus. A cascade of intracortical projections that are important for perception is initiated from the primary sensory cortex. These projections terminate in the **secondary sensory cortex**, where another set of connections lead to the **tertiary sensory cortex**. Each sensory modality has numerous

Figure 1–18. Structures that are important for visual perception are illustrated in this figure. *A.* Drawing of the medial surface of the cerebral hemisphere schematically illustrating the visual pathway from the retina to the cerebral cortex. *B.* Magnetic resonance imaging (MRI) scan of the midsagittal human central nervous system. *C.* Positron emission tomographic (PET) scan of the human brain. This is a ^{15}O-labeled water PET scan of a midsagittal slice. The scan was obtained while the subject viewed a visual stimulus (presented to the central, or macular, region of the retina). The distribution of ^{15}O-labeled water approximates that of cerebral blood flow, which correlates with neuronal activity. This image reflects the calculated difference between cerebral blood flow at rest and cerebral blood flow during visual stimulation. (*B,* Courtesy of Dr. Neal Rutledge, University of Texas at Austin; *C,* Courtesy of Dr. Peter Fox, University of Texas at San Antonio; adapted from Fox et al. 1987. J. Neurosci. 7:913–922.

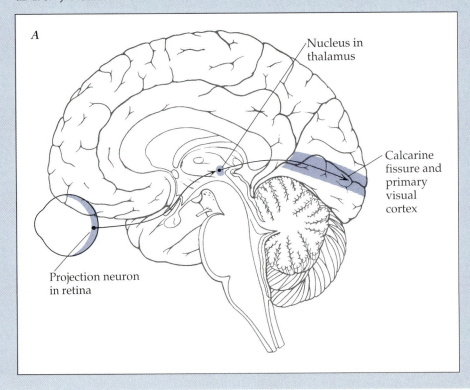

A

Nucleus in thalamus

Calcarine fissure and primary visual cortex

Projection neuron in retina

Box 1–1. (continued)

Thalamus   Calcarine
fissure

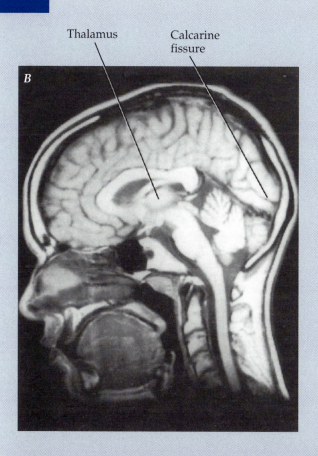

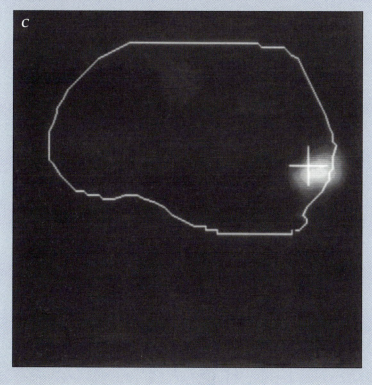

higher-order areas. In the human brain, the primary visual cortex is located in the occipital lobe, in the banks and depth of the **calcarine fissure** (Figure 1–18A). The higher-order visual areas are also located in the occipital lobe, adjacent to the primary visual cortex.

Regional anatomy of parts of the brain important for vision can be viewed on the MRI scan of the midsagittal plane of the central nervous system (Figure 1–18B). The key structures of the path for visual perception, including the thalamus and the cortex adjacent to the calcarine fissure, are clearly revealed. The PET scan in Figure 1–18C presents a functional image of the primary visual cortex. This PET scan reflects the increase in cerebral blood flow (probed by measuring the distribution of ^{15}O-labeled water) that accompanies neuronal activation. The bright region corresponds to the part of the primary visual cortex that is active when a visual stimulus is presented to a particular portion of the retina.

Summary

Cellular Organization of the Nervous System

The cellular constituents of the nervous system are **neurons** (Figure 1–1) and **glia**. Neurons have four specialized regions: (1) the **dendrites**, which receive information, (2) the **cell body**, which receives and integrates information, (3) the **axon**, which transmits information to (4) the **axon terminals**. There are three neuron classes: **unipolar**, **bipolar**, and **multipolar**. Intercellular communication occurs at **synapses**. The glia include the four types of **macroglia** (**oligodendrocytes** and **Schwann cells**, which form the myelin sheath in the central and peripheral nervous systems, respectively; **astrocytes**, which serve as structural and metabolic support for neurons; and **ependymal cells**, which line the ventricular system) and **microglia**, which are phagocytic.

Regional Anatomy of the Nervous System

The nervous system contains two separate divisions, the **peripheral nervous system** and the **central nervous system** (Figure 1–2). Each system may be further subdivided. The **autonomic** division of the peripheral nervous system controls the glands and smooth muscle of the viscera and blood vessels, whereas the **somatic** division provides the sensory innervation of body tissues and the motor innervation of skeletal muscle. There are seven separate components of the central nervous system (Figures 1–2 through 1–9): (1) **spinal cord**, (2) **medulla**, (3) **pons**, (4) **cerebellum**, (5) **midbrain**, (6) **diencephalon**, which contains the **hypothalamus** and **thalamus**, and (7) **cerebral hemispheres**, which contain the **basal ganglia**, **amygdala**, **hippocampal formation**, and **cerebral cortex**. The external surface of the cerebral cortex is characterized by **gyri** (convolutions), **sulci** (grooves), and **fissures** (particularly deep and consistent grooves). The cerebral cortex consists of four lobes: **frontal**, **parietal**, **temporal**, and **occipital**.

Ventricular System

Cavities comprising the **ventricular system** are filled with **cerebrospinal fluid** and are located within the central nervous system (Figure 1–10). Two **lateral ventricles** are located in each of the cerebral hemispheres, the **third ventricle** is located in the diencephalon, and the **fourth ventricle** is between the brain stem (pons and medulla) and the cerebellum. The **central canal** is the component of the ventricular system in the spinal cord. The **interventricular foramina** connect the two lateral ventricles with the third ventricle. The **cerebral aqueduct** is in the midbrain and connects the third and fourth ventricles. Cerebrospinal fluid exits from the ventricular system to the subarachnoid space via three aper-tures in the roof of the fourth ventricle, the two lateral foramina of **Luschka** and the foramen of **Magendie**, located at the midline (Figure 1–10, inset).

Meninges

The central nervous system is covered by three meningeal layers (Figure 1–11), from outermost to innermost: **dura mater**, **arachnoid mater**, and **pia mater**. Arachnoid mater and pia mater are separated by the **subarachnoid space**, which also contains cerebrospinal fluid. Two prominent flaps in the dura separate brain structures: **falx cerebri** and the **tentorium** cerebelli (Figure 1–11). Also located within the dura are the **dural sinuses**, low-pressure blood vessels (Figure 1–11).

Axes and Planes of Section

The central nervous system is oriented along two major axes (Figure 1–12): the **rostral–caudal axis**, which is also termed the **longitudinal axis**, and the **dorsal–ventral axis**, which is perpendicular to the longitudinal axis. Sections through the central nervous system are cut in relation to the rostral–caudal axis (Figure 1–13). **Horizontal** sections are cut parallel to the rostral–caudal axis, from one side to the other. **Transverse** or **coronal** sections are cut perpendicular to the rostral–caudal axis, between the dorsal and ventral surfaces. **Sagittal** sections are cut parallel to the longitudinal axis and the midline, also between the dorsal and ventral surfaces.

Techniques for Visualizing Components of the Central Nervous System

Cell staining methods (e.g., Nissl) reveal the location of neuronal cell bodies (Figure 1–14A); **myelin staining methods** (e.g., Weigert)

KEY STRUCTURES AND TERMS

neuron
   dendrites
   cell body
   axon
   axon terminal
synapse
   presynaptic terminal
   synaptic cleft
   receptive membrane
ganglion
nucleus
cortex
glia
   microglia
   macroglia
      oligodendrocytes
      Schwann cells
      astrocytes
      ependymal cells
myelin sheath
peripheral nervous system
   somatic
   autonomic
      sympathetic
      parasympathetic
      enteric
central nervous system
   spinal cord
   medulla
   pons
   cerebellum

midbrain
diencephalon
   thalamus
   hypothalamus
cerebral hemispheres
   cerebral cortex
   hippocampal formation
   amygdala
   basal ganglia
corpus callosum
limbic system
olfactory bulb
gray matter
white matter
gyri
fissures
sulci
ventricular system
   lateral ventricles
      body
      anterior horn
      posterior horn
      inferior horn
   third ventricle
   fourth ventricle
   interventricular foramina
   cerebral aqueduct
   central canal
   foramina of Luschka
   foramen of Magendie
cerebrospinal fluid

choroid plexus
meninges
   dura mater
   arachnoid mater
   pia mater
falx cerebri
tentorium cerebelli
subarachnoid space
dural sinuses
magnetic resonance imaging (MRI)
positron emission tomography (PET)

Cortical Lobes and Key Gyri and Sulci
frontal lobe
   precentral gyrus
   central sulcus
   orbital gyri
parietal lobe
   postcentral gyrus
   superior parietal lobule
   inferior parietal lobule
temporal lobe
   lateral sulcus
   superior temporal gyrus
   inferior temporal gyrus
occipital lobe
   parietal–occipital sulcus
   calcarine fissure
cingulate sulcus and gyrus

reveal the locations of tracts and are excellent for distinguishing white matter from gray matter (Figure 1–14B); and **silver staining methods** (e.g., Golgi) reveal the detailed morphology of neurons. Other staining methods reveal the locations of **specific neuronal chemicals** and **biochemical processes** (Figure 1–15). Anatomical connections are demonstrated by **degeneration** techniques (Figure 1–16) as well as by **axonal transport** (anterograde and retrograde; Figure 1–17). **Magnetic resonance imaging** (MRI) reveals brain structure (Figure 1–18B) or function, whereas only brain function is probed with **positron emission tomography** (PET) (Figure 1–18C). ■

Selected Readings

Duvernoy, H. M. 1988. The Human Hippocampus. Munich: J. F. Bergmann Verlag.

Jones, E. G., and Cowan, W. M. 1983. Nervous tissue. In Weiss, L. (ed.), Histology: Cell and Tissue Biology, 5th ed. New York: Elsevier Biomedical, pp. 283–370.

Kandel, E. R., Schwartz, J. H., and Jessell, T. M. (eds.) 1991. Principles of Neural Science, 3rd ed. New York: Elsevier.

Moonen, C. T. W., van Zihl, P. C. M., Frank, J. A., et al. 1990. Functional magnetic resonance imaging in medicine and physiology. Science 250:53–61.

Oldendorf, W. H. 1980. The Quest for an Image of Brain. New York: Raven Press.

Sawchenko, P. E., and Gerfen, C. R. 1985. Plant lectins and bacterial toxins as tools for tracing neuronal connections. Trends in Neurosci. 8:378–384.

Sigal, R., Doyon, D., Halimi, P., and Atlan, H. 1988. Magnetic Resonance Imaging. Berlin: Springer-Verlag.

Zeki, S. 1993. A Vision of the Brain. Oxford: Blackwell Scientific Publications.

References

Cajal, S. Ramón y. 1909, 1911. Histologie du système nerveux de l'homme et des vertèbres. 2 vols. Paris: Maloine.

Carpenter, M. B., and Sutin, J. 1983. Human Neuroanatomy. Baltimore: Williams & Wilkins.

Fox, P. T., Miezin, F. M., Allman, J. M., et al. 1987. Retinotopic organization of human visual cortex mapped with positron emission tomography. J. Neurosci. 7:913–922.

Goldman, P.S. 1978. Neuronal plasticity in primate telencephalon: anomalous projections induced by prenatal removal of frontal lobe. Science 202:768–770.

Nieuwenhuys, R., Voogd, J., and Van Huijzen, C. 1988. The Human Central Nervous System: A Synopsis and Atlas, 3rd ed. Berlin: Springer-Verlag.

Vassar, R. Chao, S.K., Sticheran, R., Nuñex, J.M., Vosshall, L.B., and Axel, R. 1994. Topographic organization of sensory projections to the olfactory bulb. Cell 79:981–991.

2

Development of the Central Nervous System

THE KEY TO UNDERSTANDING THE COMPLEX ANATOMY of the mature brain is to understand how it develops. Principles that govern the regional anatomy of the brain are more easily appreciated in its simpler, embryonic form. Knowing how the central nervous system develops also is essential for understanding how congenital abnormalities and intrauterine events, such as birth trauma or fetal drug exposure, affect brain function. In fact, early defects in the formation of the central nervous system are the most common cause of perinatal mortality, and babies who survive often have multiple handicaps. In this chapter, we examine those aspects of central nervous system development that provide insight into the complex three-dimensional structure of the mature brain. First we consider how the nervous system forms from the ectoderm of the embryo. Then we examine how key components of each major division of the central nervous system and the ventricular system develop from their earliest stages through maturity.

The Neurons and Glial Cells Derive from Cells of the Neural Plate

Similar to all vertebrates, the human embryo has three principal cell layers: **ectoderm**, the outer layer; **mesoderm**, the middle layer; and **endoderm**, the inner layer. The cellular constituents of the central nervous system, neurons and glial cells, are formed from a specialized region of the ectoderm called the **neural plate**. **Neural induction**, the process by which the neural plate becomes committed to the formation of the nervous system, depends on signals from the underlying mesoderm that originate from the **notochord** (Figure 2–1).

The neural plate lies along the **dorsal** midline of the embryo (Figure 2–1). Proliferation of cells is greater along the margin of the neural plate than along the midline, resulting in the formation of the **neural groove**. This midline indentation deepens gradually and closes (see below) to form a hollow structure, the **neural tube** (Figure 2–1). Lining the neural tube is the **neuroepithelium**, which consists of the epithelial cells that

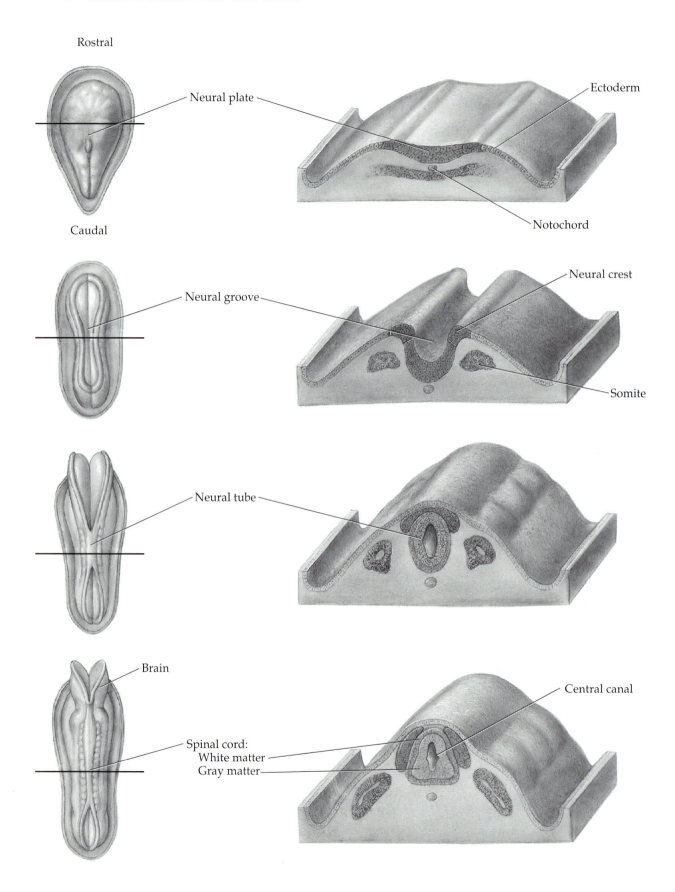

Rostral

Neural plate

Ectoderm

Caudal

Notochord

Neural groove

Neural crest

Somite

Neural tube

Brain

Central canal

Spinal cord:
White matter
Gray matter

◁ *Figure 2–1.* The neural tube forms from the dorsal surface of the embryo. The left side of the figure presents dorsal views of the developing embryo during the third and fourth weeks after conception. The right side illustrates transverse sections through the developing nervous system. The levels at which the sections are taken are indicated by the bold lines on the left. The notochord is first present at about the fourth gestational week. Prior to this, it exists as the notochordal plate, which is less well organized than the notochord. (Adapted from Cowan, W. M. 1979. The development of the brain. Sci. Am. 241:112–133.)

generate virtually all the neurons of the **central nervous system**. After neural tube formation, important developments occur that establish the normal structure of the nervous system. The caudal portion of the neural tube forms the spinal cord whereas the rostral portion becomes the brain. Glial cells (macroglia) of the central nervous system also develop from the neuroepithelium, and the cavity within the neural tube forms the **ventricular system**.

Closure of the neural plate to form the neural tube occurs first at the location where the neck will form, then proceeds both caudally and rostrally. The location at which the rostral end of the neural tube closes is termed the **lamina terminalis**, a landmark that will form the rostral wall of the ventricular system (see Figure 2–15D). There are important clinical implications to neural tube closure. For example, when the caudal portion of the neural plate fails to close, the functions subserved by the caudal spinal cord are severely disrupted. This results in varying degrees of lower limb paralysis and defective bladder control. This developmental abnormality is one of a wide range of neural tube defects, collectively termed **spina bifida**, that are often associated with herniation of the meninges and neural tissue to the body surface. When the rostral neural plate fails to close, **anencephaly** may occur, resulting in gross disturbance of the overall structure of the brain.

Whereas the central nervous system develops from the epithelial cells lining the neural tube, many of the key components of the peripheral nervous system develop from a population of cells called the **neural crest** (Figure 2–1). This collection of cells emerges from the dorsal region of the neural tube to migrate peripherally and give rise to all of the neurons whose cell bodies lie outside of the central nervous system. These neurons include the sensory neurons that innervate body tissues and peripheral components of the autonomic nervous system. The neural crest also gives rise to nonneural cells, including the chromaffin cells of the adrenal medulla and the Schwann cells, which form the myelin sheath of peripheral nerves. The two inner meningeal layers, the arachnoid and pia mater, also derive from the neural crest. However, the outermost (and toughest) meningeal layer, the dura mater, derives from the mesoderm.

The developing central nervous system is laminated, as are many regions of the mature central nervous system. Progressing outward from the cavity within the neural tube, there are three principal layers (Figure 2–2). The neuroepithelium is located in the ventricular or **ependymal layer**. Immature nerve cells arise from the division of neuroependymal cells and migrate to the intermediate or **mantle layer**. Specialized glial cells are located in the mantle layer. These cells form a scaffolding along which much of this migration takes place. The **marginal layer** contains the axonal processes of developing neurons. In the mature brain, the ependymal layer remains one-cell thick, is ciliated, and lines the ventricular system. The mantle layer becomes the gray matter and the marginal layer, the white matter.

Figure 2–2. Schematic diagram of a transverse section through the developing spinal cord illustrating the three cell layers of neural tube—the marginal, mantle, and ependymal layers—and the roof and floor plates.

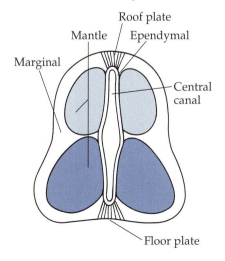

The Neural Tube Forms Five Brain Vesicles and the Spinal Cord

In early stages of development, the rostral portion of the neural tube forms three primary vesicles (Figure 2–3A): (1) the **prosencephalon** or **forebrain**, (2) the **mesencephalon** or **midbrain**, and (3) the **rhombencephalon** or **hindbrain**. From the prosencephalon two secondary vesicles emerge later in development, the **telencephalon** (or cerebral hemisphere) and the **diencephalon** (or thalamus and hypothalamus). Whereas the mesencephalon remains undivided throughout further brain development, the rhombencephalon gives rise to the **metencephalon** (or pons) and the **myelencephalon** (or medulla). The five brain vesicles and primitive spinal cord, already identifiable by the sixth week of fetal life, give rise to the seven major divisions of the central nervous system (see Figure 1–2B).

Figure 2–3. Schematic illustration of the three- and five-vesicle stages of the neural tube. The top portion of the figure shows dorsal views of the neural tube drawn without flexures. The bottom portion of the figure presents lateral views. **A.** Three-vesicle stage. **B.** Five-vesicle stage. The inset illustrates the location of the interventricular foramen on one side in the five-vesicle stage. (Adapted from Kandel, E. R., Schwartz, J. H., and Jessell, T. M. (eds.) 1991. Principles of Neural Science, 3rd ed. New York: Elsevier.)

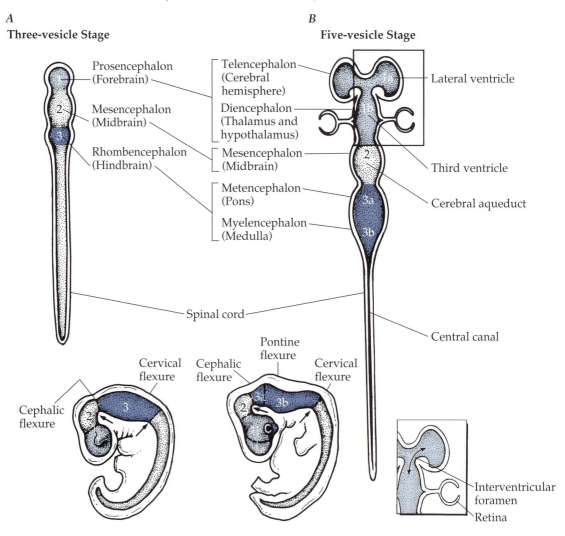

A
Three-vesicle Stage

Prosencephalon (Forebrain)

Mesencephalon (Midbrain)

Rhombencephalon (Hindbrain)

Spinal cord

Cephalic flexure

Cervical flexure

B
Five-vesicle Stage

Telencephalon (Cerebral hemisphere)

Diencephalon (Thalamus and hypothalamus)

Mesencephalon (Midbrain)

Metencephalon (Pons)

Myelencephalon (Medulla)

Lateral ventricle

Third ventricle

Cerebral aqueduct

Central canal

Cephalic flexure

Pontine flexure

Cervical flexure

Interventricular foramen

Retina

The Longitudinal Axis of the Developing Brain Bends at the Midbrain–Diencephalic Juncture

The complex configuration of the mature brain is determined, in part, by how the developing brain bends, or **flexes**. Flexures occur because proliferation of cells in the brain stem and cerebral hemispheres is enormous, and the space that the developing brain occupies in the cranium is constrained. At the three-vesicle stage there are two prominent flexures: the **cervical flexure**, at the junction of the spinal cord and the caudal hindbrain (or future medulla), and the **cephalic flexure**, at the level of the midbrain (Figure 2–3). At the five-vesicle stage a third flexure becomes prominent, the **pontine flexure**. By birth, both the cervical and pontine flexures have straightened out. The cephalic flexure, however, remains prominent and causes the longitudinal axis of the forebrain to deviate from that of the midbrain, hindbrain, and spinal cord.

The Ventricular System Develops From the Cavities in the Neural Tube

The large cavities within the cerebral vesicles develop into the ventricular system of the brain, and the caudal cavity becomes the central canal of the spinal cord (Figures 2–2 and 2–3). The ventricular system contains **cerebrospinal fluid**, which is produced mainly by the **choroid plexus**. Here we examine how the ventricular system develops. Later we will consider the part of the ventricular system with the most complex three-dimensional structure, the lateral ventricle.

As the five brain vesicles develop, the forebrain cavity divides into the two **lateral ventricles** (i.e., the first and second ventricles) and the **third ventricle** (Figure 2–3). The lateral ventricles, which develop as out-pouchings from the rostral portion of the third ventricle, are each interconnected with the third ventricle by an **interventricular foramen** (of Monro; Figure 2–3, inset). The lamina terminalis, located immediately rostral to the two interventricular foramina (see Figure 2–15D), forms the rostral wall of the third ventricle.

The **fourth ventricle**, the most caudal ventricle, develops from the cavity within the hindbrain. It is connected to the third ventricle by the **cerebral aqueduct** (of Sylvius). The cerebral aqueduct is more dilated in the embryonic brain than in the mature brain. Throughout development, proliferation of cells in the dorsal region of the midbrain, termed the **tectum**, compresses the cerebral aqueduct and constricts its diameter (for example, compare Figures 2–10A1 and A3). The midbrain tectum of the mature brain, as we will see in Chapter 3, contains separate collections of neurons that are important in processing auditory information and controlling rapid eye movements. Similar to the cerebral aqueduct, the central canal of the caudal medulla and spinal cord becomes much smaller during development (see Figure 2–6). In the mature nervous system, the central canal is thought to be partially occluded.

Recall that cerebrospinal fluid normally exits from the ventricular system into the subarachnoid space through the foramina of Luschka and Magendie in the fourth ventricle (see Figure 1–10). (The central canal does not have such an aperture for the outflow of cerebrospinal fluid.) Pathological processes can close the interventricular foramina or the cerebral aqueduct, effectively damming the flow of cerebrospinal fluid, which continues to be produced by the choroid plexus, out of the foramina of Luschka and Magendie. This can happen because the interventricular foramina and the cerebral aqueduct are narrow, they are more vulnerable than other parts of the ventricular system to the constricting effects of tumors, inflammation, or swelling from trauma. If occlusion occurs before the bones of the skull are fused (i.e., in embryonic life or in infancy) the increasing ventricular size will cause head size to increase, a condition called **hydrocephalus**. If occlusion of the interventricular foramina or the cerebral aqueduct occurs after the bones of the skull are fused, ventricular size cannot increase without increasing intracranial pressure. This is a life-threatening condition.

The Choroid Plexus Forms When Blood Vessels Penetrate the Brain Surface at Selected Dorsal Sites

As the neural tube thickens, the nutritional requirements of the central nervous system are supplied by the vasculature rather than by diffusion. At this time the blood vessels, which overlie the pia (Figure 2–4A), penetrate the brain surface, carrying the pia into the brain. In most locations this pial sheath over the vasculature disappears close to the surface (see Figure 4–15). At the roofs of the developing ventricles neural and glial cells do not proliferate. Here, the pia remains apposed to the penetrating blood vessels (Figure 2–4). At these sites, the **choroid plexus** develops. The cellular constituents of embryonic, as well as mature, choroid plexus are, from inside to outside (i.e., the ventricular surface): a central core of **blood vessels**, **pia**, and **ependymal cells**. (These ependymal cells, which are specialized to secrete cerebrospinal fluid, are called choroidal epithelium.) Choroid plexus is present only in the ventricles. In the mature brain the choroid plexus remains in the roof of the third and fourth ventricles. In the lateral ventricles, the choroid plexus is located in both the ventricular roof and floor.

The Spinal Cord and Hindbrain Have a Segmented Structure

Repeated modules or **segments** characterize the developing spinal cord and brain stem. Whereas segmentation in the spinal cord also is present in maturity, in the brain stem segmentation is apparent only during early development. Spinal segmentation is dependent on mesodermal tissue, which breaks up into 38 to 40 pairs of repeating units, called **somites**. The muscles, bones, and other structures of the neck, limbs, and trunk develop from these somites, which are organized from rostral to caudal. There are 8 cervical, 12 thoracic, 5 lumbar, 5 sacral, and 8 to 10 coccygeal somites. For each of these somites there is a corresponding spinal cord **segment**. Each segment provides the sensory and motor innervation of the skin and muscle of the body part derived from its associated somite. Neural connections between the developing somite and spinal cord are made by the axons of primary sensory neurons and motor neurons (i.e., peripheral nervous system). Traveling together in spinal nerves (Figure 2–5A), the sensory and motor axons enter and leave the spinal cord via the dorsal and ventral roots, respectively. The mature spinal cord is shown in Figure 2–5B; its segmentation is apparent as the series of dorsal and ventral roots emerging from its surface. The cervical segments innervate the skin and muscles of the back of the head, neck, and arms. The thoracic segments innervate the trunk, and the lumbar and sacral segments innervate the legs and perineal region. (Most of the coccygeal segments disappear later in development in the mature spinal cord.)

Throughout the first 3 months of development, the spinal cord grows at about the same rate as the vertebral column. During this period, the

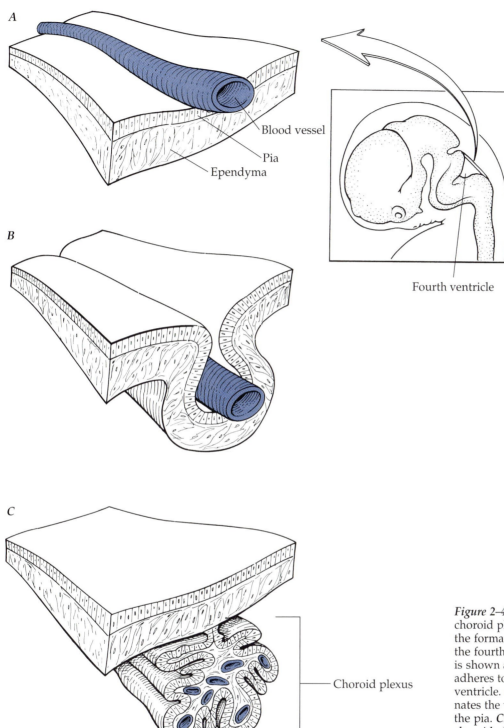

Figure 2–4. Development of the choroid plexus. This figure illustrates the formation of the choroid plexus in the fourth ventricle. *A.* A blood vessel is shown apposing the pia, which adheres to the ependyma lining the ventricle. *B.* The blood vessel invaginates the ventricle, carrying with it the pia. *C.* Later in development, the choroid plexus proliferates within the ventricle.

spinal cord occupies the entire **vertebral canal**, the space within the vertebral column. The dorsal and ventral roots associated with each segment pass directly through the intervertebral foramina (Figure 2–5B) to reach their target structures. Later, the growth of the vertebral column exceeds that of the spinal cord. In the adult, the most caudal spinal cord segment is located at the level of the **first lumbar vertebra**. There are two important

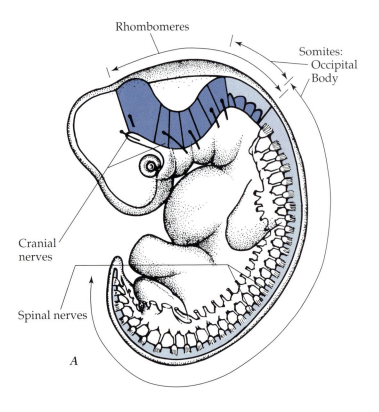

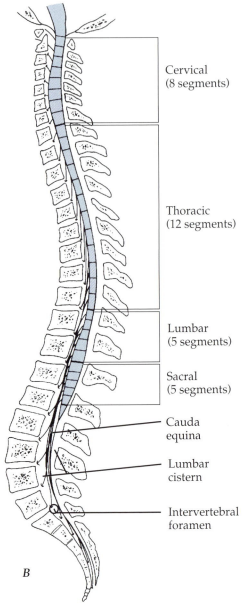

Figure 2–5. The hindbrain and spinal cord are segmented structures. In the caudal brain stem, the segments are called rhombomeres and, in the spinal cord, somites. There are four occipital somites that form structures of the head. These are shown in the caudal medulla. *A.* The position of the developing nervous system in the embryo is illustrated as well as the segmental organization of rhombomeres and somites. The cranial nerves that contain the axons of brain stem motor neurons are also shown. From rostral to caudal, the following cranial nerves are illustrated: IV, V, VI, VII, IX, X, and XII. The two mesencephalic segments and the segment between the metencephalon and mesencephalon are not shown. *B.* Lateral view of the mature spinal cord in the vertebral canal. Note that the spinal nerves exit from the vertebral canal through the intervertebral foramina. (*A,* Adapted from Lumsden, A. 1990. The cellular basis of segmentation in the developing hindbrain. Trends Neurosci. 13:329–335.)

anatomical consequences of the differential growth of the spinal cord and vertebral column. First, a space, the **lumbar cistern**, forms within the caudal portion of the spinal canal that is part of the subarachnoid space (Figure 2–5B; see Figure 4–18). Cerebrospinal fluid can be withdrawn from the lumbar cistern without risk of damaging the spinal cord by inserting a needle through the space between the third and fourth (or the fourth and fifth) vertebrae. This procedure is known as a **spinal** or **lumbar tap**. Second, the dorsal and ventral roots subserving sensation and movement of the legs must travel a long distance before exiting the vertebral canal (Figure 2–5B). These roots resemble a horse's tail, hence the name **cauda equina**.

The eight segments of the hindbrain, termed **rhombomeres**, provide sensory and motor innervation for most of the head through the peripheral projections of the cranial nerves. However, there is a more complex relationship between hindbrain segmentation and peripheral innervation patterns. In contrast to the spinal cord, where each segment contains a pair of dorsal and ventral roots, each rhombomere is not associated with a single pair of sensory and motor cranial nerve roots. We will take up the question of the segmental organization of the pons and medulla when we consider the organization of the cranial nerves in Chapter 12. There is a segment between the metencephalon and mesencephalon (termed the isthmus) as well as two segments in the mesencephalon. The relationship between these segments in the rostral brain stem and the third and fourth cranial nerves is, however, not understood.

Segmentation may be a mechanism for establishing a basic plan of organization for the various parts of the spinal cord and hindbrain. In maturity, this segmental plan remains in the spinal cord. In the brain stem, however, segmentation is obscured by later elaboration of neural interconnections. It is not yet understood whether the forebrain also uses a similar developmental strategy.

The Spinal Cord and Brain Stem Develop From the Caudal and Intermediate Portions of the Neural Tube

The spinal cord receives sensory information from the limbs and trunk and provides the motor innervation of the muscles of these structures via the **spinal nerves**. The sensory and motor innervation of the head is provided by the **cranial nerves**, which enter and exit from the brain stem. An important principle governs the organization of spinal cord and the brain stem gray matter: nuclei that directly mediate sensory and motor functions form longitudinally oriented columns of cells. Keeping this in mind, we will first discuss the development of the spinal cord and then turn to the development of the brain stem.

Dorsal and Ventral Regions of the Spinal Cord Mediate Somatic Sensation and Motor Control of the Limbs and Trunk

During development, there are two zones of proliferating neuroblasts which are separated by the **sulcus limitans**: the alar plate and the basal plate. The **alar plate** (Figure 2–6A) is located in the dorsal portion of the wall of the neural tube and mediates sensory functions. Developing neurons from the alar plate form the interneurons and projection neurons of the **dorsal horn** of the mature spinal cord (Figure 2–6B). Dorsal horn neurons mediate somatic and visceral sensations, such as pressure and pain. These neurons receive sensory information from the primary sensory neurons, whose axons enter the spinal cord through the **dorsal roots** (Figure 2–6A; see Figure 1–3). The **basal plate** (Figure 2–6A) is located in the ventral portion of the neural tube wall and mediates motor function. Most of the basal plate neurons give rise to the interneurons and motor neurons of the **ventral horn** of the mature spinal cord (Figure 2–6B). The motor neurons project their axons to the periphery via the **ventral roots** (Figure 2–6A).

The sensory and motor innervation of somatic and visceral structures is mediated by separate primary sensory neurons and motor neurons. The axons of sensory neurons innervating somatic and visceral structures are intermingled in peripheral nerves but terminate in separate regions of the spinal gray matter and white matter. Axons of the somatic and visceral motor neurons are similarly intermingled in peripheral nerves, but their cell bodies are located in different portions of the spinal

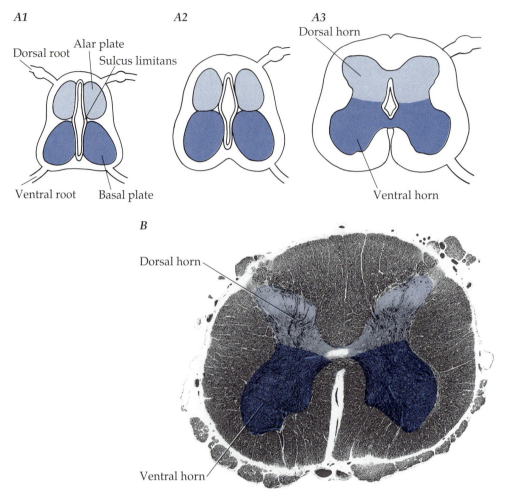

Figure 2–6. **A.** Schematic drawing of transverse sections of the spinal cord at three stages of development. **B.** Myelin-stained section through spinal cord of mature nervous system.

cord gray matter. A nomenclature (labeling system) describes the organization of peripheral nerves and the sensory and motor nuclei of the central nervous system. For peripheral nerves, this is based on two criteria: (1) the direction information travels along the axons, and (2) the peripheral targets innervated.

Information in peripheral nerves can travel toward or away from the central nervous system. The term **afferent** means that the axons carry information **toward the central nervous system**; this is different from the functional term **sensory**, which implies that the information is consciously perceived. The term **efferent**, which indicates that axons transmit information **away from the central nervous system**, is different from the functional term **motor**, which indicates the functional connection of a nerve with a peripheral effector organ, such as a muscle or a gland. Because information carried by some axons to the central nervous system is not perceived, sensory and afferent are not equivalent terms. We generally use the term afferent, not sensory, to describe information in peripheral nerves. On the other hand, because all axons projecting to the periphery transmit motor control signals, the terms motor and efferent are equivalent and we use the term motor, not efferent. The second criteria for describing peripheral nerves is whether the axons innervate somatic or visceral structures. The terms afferent and efferent are also used to describe the direction of information flow within the central nervous system.

There are four categories of spinal nerves (Table 2–1): (1) **somatic afferent**, (2) **visceral afferent**, (3) **somatic motor**, and (4) **visceral motor**. Somatic afferent nerves innervate skin, muscles, and joints, whereas visceral afferent nerves innervate blood vessels and body organs. The two motor nerve classes also innervate distinct structures. The somatic motor nerves innervate skeletal muscle; whereas the visceral motor nerves innervate neurons of the autonomic nervous system located in the periphery, which, in turn, innervate blood vessels and glands. There is a corresponding nomenclature for regions of the spinal cord based on whether neuronal cell bodies receive input *from* somatic or visceral structures (i.e., afferent or sensory) or transmit motor control signals *to* these structures (i.e., efferent or motor). For example, somatic motor nuclei are located in the ventral horn.

The Somatic and Visceral Cell Columns in the Brain Stem Are Further Differentiated Than Those in the Spinal Cord

The developmental plan of the brain stem is similar to that of the spinal cord. Gray matter of the brain stem consists of separate alar and basal plates that extend from the medulla to the midbrain. These plates form columns of neurons (see Figures 2–7 through 2–10) that, in the mature nervous system, subserve sensory and motor functions. In the brain stem, dorsal and ventral roots are replaced by cranial nerves and the dorsal and ventral horns are replaced by the cranial nerve sensory and motor nuclei. Cranial nerve sensory nuclei contain neurons that receive afferent information from cranial structures; cranial nerve motor nuclei contain motor neurons. The cranial nerve nuclei are connected with peripheral structures, such as sensory receptors or striated muscle, by the cranial nerves.

Despite these similarities, there are four important differences between the developmental plans of the spinal cord and the brain stem. First, rather than being oriented in the dorsal–ventral axis, as in the spinal cord, the alar and basal plate cell columns of the caudal brain stem are aligned roughly from the lateral brain stem margin to the midline. This is because, in the caudal medulla, it is as if the central canal "opens up" at its

Table 2–1. Functional classes of spinal nerves.

Classification	Function	Structure innervated
Afferent Fibers		
General somatic	Tactile, proprioception, pain/temperature	Skin, mucous membranes, skeletal muscles
General visceral	Mechanical, pain/temperature	Viscera, cardiovascular, respiratory, genitourinary tract
Motor Fibers		
General somatic	Skeletal muscle control (somites)	Limb and axial musculature
General visceral	Autonomic control	Sweat glands, gut

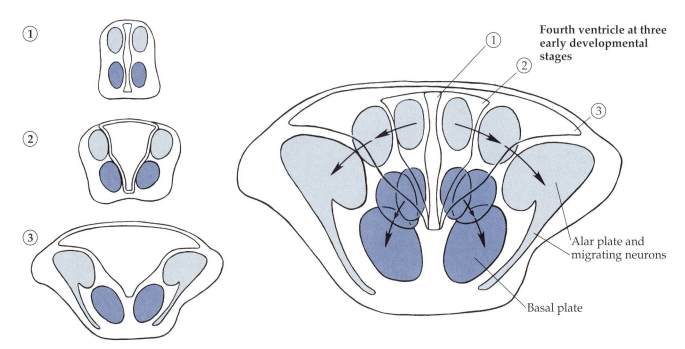

Figure 2–7. At the junction of the spinal cord and medulla, it is as if the central canal opens along its dorsal margin. This has the effect of transforming the dorsoventral nuclear organization of the spinal cord into the lateromedial organization of nuclei in the caudal brain stem (medulla and pons).

dorsal surface to form the fourth ventricle (Figure 2–7). Second, in brain stem development, immature neurons migrate from the alar and basal plates on the ventricular floor to reach more dorsal or ventral destinations (see next section). Extensive neuroblast migration also characterizes the developmental plan of the cerebellum and forebrain. Third, the visceral and somatic cell columns of the alar and basal plates of the brain stem are further differentiated, and the nuclei mediating these functions are completely distinct (see Figure 2–8A3).

Fourth, as a consequence of specialized sensory and motor structures of the head, there is further differentiation of cranial nerve nuclei and a resultant increase in the number of categories of cranial nerves. The special sensory (afferent) structures include the olfactory epithelium, the retina, the cochlea, the labyrinth, and the taste buds. The special motor structures are the muscles of **branchiomeric** (gill arch) origin (Table 2–2). These unique cranial structures are innervated by axons of the **special afferent** and **special motor** categories.

There are seven functional categories of axons in cranial nerves (Figure 2–8; Table 2–2) and there are separate cranial nerve nuclei where axons in these nerves either terminate (e.g., afferent or sensory nuclei) or take origin (e.g., efferent or motor nuclei). The cell column that contains the cranial nerve nuclei that innervate skeletal muscles derived from body somites is located most medially. This column is called the **general somatic motor** column. The next two cell columns are the **special visceral motor** column, which contains the motor neurons that innervate the branchiomeric skeletal muscle, and the **general visceral motor** column, which contains autonomic preganglionic neurons. The sulcus limitans separates the motor columns from the afferent or sensory columns, which are located more laterally. The afferent column closest to the sulcus limitans

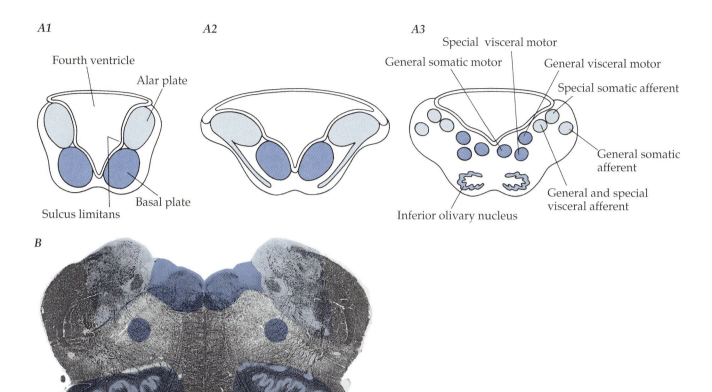

Figure 2–8. The alar and basal plates are subdivided in the medulla. **A.** Schematic drawing of transverse sections of the medulla at three stages of development. **B.** Myelin-stained section through medulla of mature nervous system.

Table 2–2. Functional classes of cranial nerves.[1]

Classification	Function	Structure innervated	Cranial nerve
Afferent Fibers			
General somatic	Tactile, pain/temperature proprioception	Skin, mucous membranes, skeletal muscles of head and neck	V, VII, IX, X
General visceral	Mechanical, pain/temperature proprioception	Oral cavity, pharynx, larynx	V, VII, IX, X
Special somatic	Audition, balance	Cochlea, labyrinth	VIII
Special visceral	Taste, olfaction	Taste buds, olfactory epithelium	I, VII, IX, X
Motor Fibers			
General somatic	Skeletal muscle control (somites)	Extraocular and tongue muscles	III, IV, VI, XII
General visceral	Autonomic control	Tear glands, sweat glands, gut	III, VII, IX, X
Special visceral	Skeletal muscle (branchiomeric)	Facial expression, jaw, pharynx, larynx	V, VII, IX, X, XI

[1]The optic nerve (II) is not considered in this table because it does not contain the axons of primary sensory neurons but rather those of third-order neurons in the visual pathway. The visual system is, however, considered to be part of the special somatic afferent class.

contains neurons that process **general** (i.e., mechanoreception and chemoreception) and **special visceral afferent information** (taste). While taste and some visceral mechanoreception is perceived, much of visceral chemoreception is not. The two most lateral afferent cell columns mediate sensation from structures of somatic origin. Tactile stimulation of the face is mediated by the **general somatic afferent** column; audition and balance are mediated by the **special somatic afferent** column. In the adult, the sulcus limitans remains as a landmark on the floor of the fourth ventricle (see Figure AI–7).

The Complex Morphology of the Brain Stem Is Determined by the Migratory Patterns of Developing Neurons

Cranial nerve nuclei have relatively simple roles in processing afferent information or transmitting motor control signals. However, most brain stem nuclei have more complex integrative functions. Whereas brain stem integrative nuclei also derive from alar and basal neuroblasts on the ventricular floor, the immature neurons that give rise to these structures **migrate** from the ventricular floor to their destinations in more dorsal or ventral regions (see Figures 2–8 through 2–10).

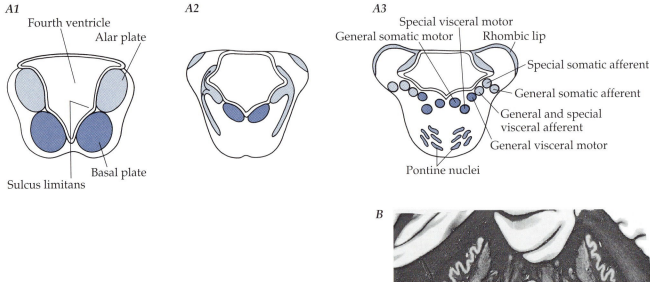

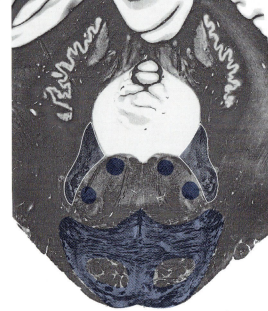

Figure 2–9. Immature neurons migrate from the alar plate and form the pontine nuclei. *A.* Schematic drawing of transverse sections of the pons at three stages of development. *B.* Myelin-stained section through pons of mature nervous system.

Neuroblasts migrate along paths established by glial cells (i.e., astrocytes). Some of the more prominent nuclei that develop from migrating neuroblasts include the inferior olivary nucleus in the medulla (Figure 2–8A3) and the pontine nuclei (Figure 2–9A3). Both of these nuclei integrate sensory information and motor control signals from diverse brain areas and transmit this information to the cerebellum. The inferior olivary and pontine nuclei, together with the cerebellum, are thought to form important circuits for the learning of motor skills (see Chapter 10). In the midbrain, the red nucleus and substantia nigra (Figure 2–10A3) also develop from immature neurons that migrate from more dorsal portions. These two midbrain structures are part of the motor system.

Now that we have considered general principles determining how the brain stem develops, we can compare schematic sections through the developing medulla, pons, and midbrain with myelin-stained sections through the same divisions of the mature brain stem (Parts B in Figures 2–8 through 2–10). Knowledge of how the brain stem alar and basal plates are organized provides an essential framework for understanding the mature brain stem. During development, the visceral and somatic cell columns maintain constant relative positions with respect to the midline and the floor of the fourth ventricle. Because cranial nerve nuclei that serve similar functions are aligned in the same rostral–caudal columns, knowledge of the locations of these columns will aid in understanding their function. The longitudinal organization of the various cell columns forming the cranial nerve nuclei in the mature brain stem is shown in Figure 2–11. Table 2–3 lists the locations and general functions of the cranial nerves.

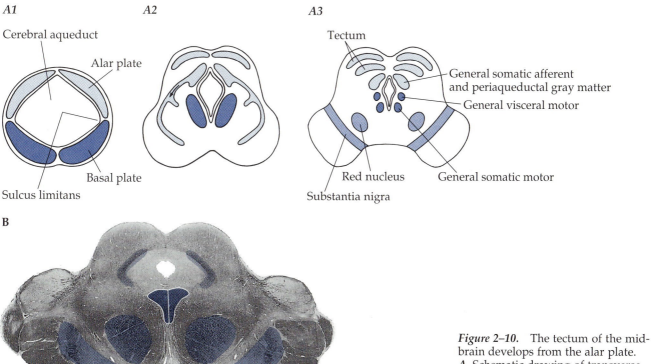

Figure 2–10. The tectum of the midbrain develops from the alar plate. *A.* Schematic drawing of transverse sections of the midbrain at three stages of development. *B.* Myelin-stained section through midbrain of mature nervous system.

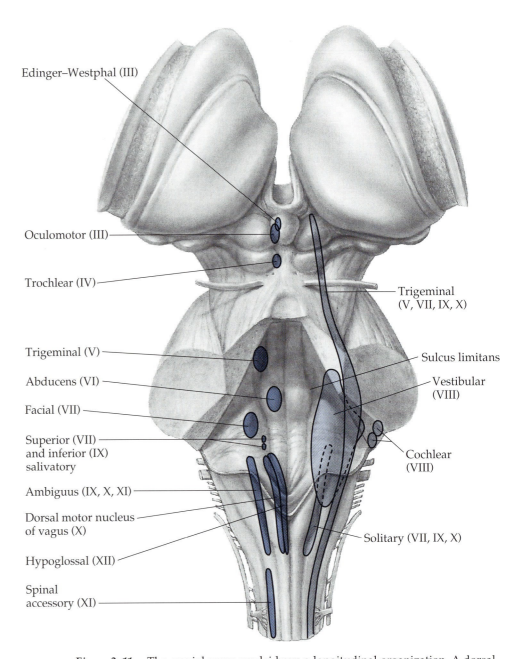

Edinger–Westphal (III)

Oculomotor (III)

Trochlear (IV)

Trigeminal (V)

Abducens (VI)

Facial (VII)

Superior (VII)
and inferior (IX)
salivatory

Ambiguus (IX, X, XI)

Dorsal motor nucleus
of vagus (X)

Hypoglossal (XII)

Spinal
accessory (XI)

Trigeminal
(V, VII, IX, X)

Sulcus limitans

Vestibular
(VIII)

Cochlear
(VIII)

Solitary (VII, IX, X)

Figure 2–11. The cranial nerve nuclei have a longitudinal organization. A dorsal view of the brain stem of the mature central nervous system is illustrated, with the locations of the various cranial nerve nuclei indicated.

The Cerebellum Develops From the Rhombic Lips

The cerebellum plays a key role in controlling movement. Without the cerebellum, even simple and routine movements would be uncoordinated. Indeed, patients with damage to the cerebellum reach inaccurately and display a characteristically unsteady gait. The cerebellum develops from neuroblasts located in a specialized region of the alar plate of the dorsolateral metencephalon (pons) termed the **rhombic lips** (Figure 2–9). Initially the rhombic lips are widely separated from each other, but eventually they fuse at the midline. This midline region forms the **vermis** (Figure 2–12C), the portion of the mature cerebellum that is concerned with

Table 2–3. Cranial nerves and their functions.

Cranial nerve		Central nervous system division	Sensory or motor	Major function
I	Olfactory	Cerebral hemispheres	Sensory	Olfaction (smell)
II	Optic	Thalamus	Sensory	Vision
III	Oculomotor	Midbrain	Motor	Eye muscle control
IV	Trochlear	Midbrain	Motor	Eye muscle control
V	Trigeminal	Pons	Sensory and motor	Touch and pain; facial muscle control
VI	Abducens	Pons	Motor	Eye muscle control
VII	Facial	Pons	Sensory and motor	Facial muscle control; taste
VIII	Vestibulocochlear	Pons/medulla	Sensory	Balance and hearing
IX	Glossopharyngeal	Medulla	Sensory and motor	Visceral sensation; taste; visceral motor
X	Vagus	Medulla	Sensory and motor	Visceral sensation; visceral motor
XI	Spinal accessory	Medulla/spinal cord	Motor	Neck muscle control
XII	Hypoglossal	Medulla	Motor	Tongue muscle control

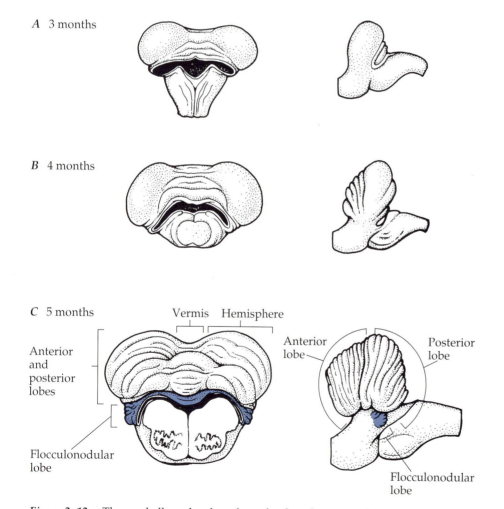

A 3 months

B 4 months

C 5 months

Vermis   Hemisphere

Anterior and posterior lobes

Flocculonodular lobe

Anterior lobe

Posterior lobe

Flocculonodular lobe

Figure 2–12. The cerebellum develops from the dorsal portion of the metencephalon, a region termed the rhombic lip. Caudal views (*left*) and lateral views (*right*) are shown at three stages of development. (Adapted from Keibel, F., and Mall, F. P. [eds.]. 1910–1912. Manual of Human Embryology. 2 vols. Philadelphia: Lippincott.)

balance and posture. The paired lateral regions form the **cerebellar hemispheres**, which participate in the control of limb movements, such as reaching. Later in development, fissures form on the cerebellar surface. The most prominent of these fissures are oriented from medial to lateral and divide the cerebellum into three lobes: anterior, posterior, and flocculonodular (named for its two components, the flocculus and nodulus). The organization of the cerebellum will be considered in Chapter 10.

The Rostral Portion of the Neural Tube Gives Rise to the Diencephalon and Cerebral Hemispheres

More than any other brain region, the structure of the cerebral hemispheres is markedly transformed during development (Figure 2–13). Whereas the brain stem and spinal cord retain their longitudinal organization in the mature brain, the cerebral hemispheres have a more complex three-dimensional shape. This is largely the result of the enormous proliferation of cells of the cerebral cortex. The development of the diencephalon is discussed with that of the cerebral hemispheres because they are functionally related and are typically presented together in slices through the mature central nervous system.

The Lateral Margin of the Diencephalon Fuses With the Telencephalon

Early in development, at the five-vesicle stage, the diencephalon and third ventricle lie medial to the cerebral hemispheres and lateral ventricles (Figures 2–3B and 2–14A). At this early stage, three components of the diencephalon are apparent: the **epithalamus**, which forms the pineal gland, important in diurnal rhythms; the **thalamus**, a collection of nuclei that communicate directly with the cerebral cortex; and the **hypothalamus**, a major brain structure for regulating visceral functions and their emotional counterparts (Figure 2–14A). (The retina also develops from the diencephalon [Figure 2–3, inset]. Despite its peripheral location, the retina is actually a portion of the central nervous system.)

In Figure 2–14, we also see the spatial relationships between the developing telencephalon and diencephalon. Two components of the basal ganglia, the **caudate nucleus** and the **putamen**, are of telencephalic origin. They develop from neuroblasts collected in the **corpus striatum**, in the floor of the lateral ventricle. The third major component of the basal ganglia, the **globus pallidus**, is of diencephalic origin. Immature neurons of the developing globus pallidus migrate from the ventricular surface, near the interventricular foramina, to a more lateral location. The **amygdala** also develops from the corpus striatum. Although the amygdala is adjacent to the caudate nucleus and putamen, both during development (Figure 2–14) and in maturity (see Figure 2–17A), these structures mediate distinct functions. The caudate nucleus and putamen participate in cognition and motor function, whereas the amygdala is important in visceral function and emotions.

The development of the **cerebral cortex** (see below) results first in the apposition and subsequent fusion of parts of the telencephalic and diencephalic surfaces (Figure 2–14B2). This fusion results in two important consequences. First, despite separation early in development (Figure 2–14A2) the caudate nucleus and the thalamus later become adjacent, an arrangement that continues into brain maturity. Second, after fusion there is a proliferation of ascending projections from the thalamus to the cortex and descending projections from the cortex to subcortical structures,

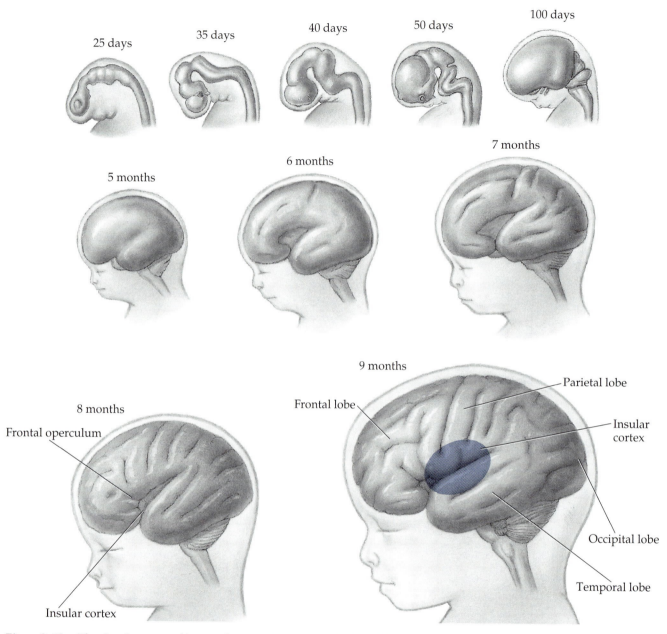

25 days 35 days 40 days 50 days 100 days

5 months 6 months 7 months

8 months

Frontal operculum

Insular cortex

9 months

Frontal lobe

Parietal lobe

Insular cortex

Occipital lobe

Temporal lobe

Figure 2–13. The development of human brain is shown from the lateral surface in relation to the face and the general shape of the cranium. (Adapted from Cowan, W. M. 1979. The development of the brain. Sci. Am. 241:112–133.)

including the thalamus, brain stem, and spinal cord. These axons connecting the cortex with other parts of the central nervous system form the **internal capsule** (Figure 2–14B2; see also Figure 3–12). The caudate nucleus and the putamen, which both develop from the corpus striatum, are incompletely separated by axons of the internal capsule. In the mature brain, the caudate nucleus and the putamen often are collectively called the **striatum**.

As development of the ascending and descending connections of the cerebral cortex proceeds, so too does that of the **corpus callosum**, the large fiber path that interconnects the cerebral cortex of the two hemi-

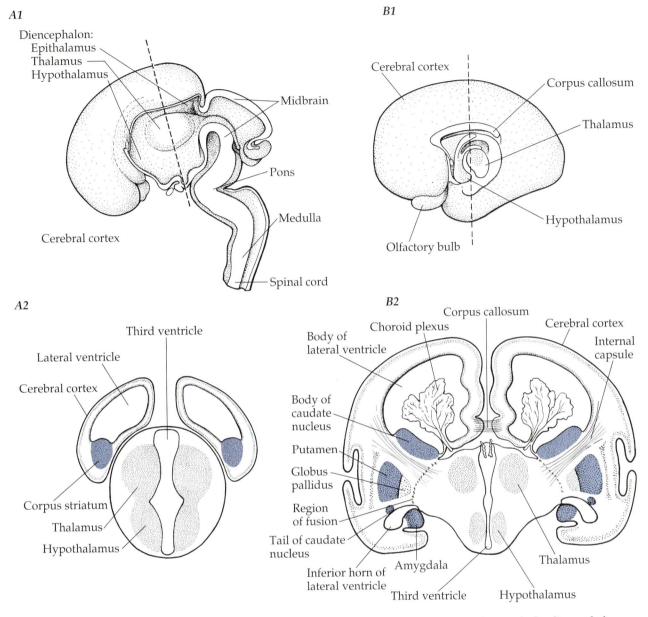

A1

Diencephalon:
Epithalamus
Thalamus
Hypothalamus

Midbrain

Pons

Medulla

Cerebral cortex

Spinal cord

B1

Cerebral cortex

Corpus callosum

Thalamus

Hypothalamus

Olfactory bulb

A2

Third ventricle

Lateral ventricle

Cerebral cortex

Corpus striatum

Thalamus

Hypothalamus

B2

Corpus callosum

Choroid plexus

Body of
lateral ventricle

Cerebral cortex

Internal
capsule

Body of
caudate
nucleus

Putamen

Globus
pallidus

Region
of fusion

Tail of caudate
nucleus

Inferior horn of
lateral ventricle

Amygdala

Third ventricle

Thalamus

Hypothalamus

Figure 2–14. Portions of the cerebral hemispheres fuse with the diencephalon. The top portions of this figure illustrate medial views of brain during an early *(A)* and a later *(B)* stage of development. The bottom portion of the figure shows schematic transverse sections through the brain in the planes indicated on top *(dashed lines)*. (Adapted from Patten, B. M. 1968. Human Embryology. New York: McGraw-Hill [Blackston Division].)

spheres (Figure 2–14, right). Collections of axons that interconnect the two halves of the central nervous system are termed **commissures**; the corpus callosum is the largest such commissure. Remarkably, when this structure is surgically transected to ameliorate the most severe symptoms of epilepsy, the two halves of the cerebral hemisphere function independently. The right hand may reach for an item only to be intercepted by the left hand!

The Cerebral Cortex Encircles the Diencephalon

During development, the **cerebral cortex** acquires a laminated structure and its surface area greatly increases. Initially, the cerebral cortex consists of a thin sheet of immature neurons and axonal processes that overlie the lateral ventricles. Neuroblasts migrate from this sheet along a glial scaffold. The earliest neuroblasts to migrate give rise to the deeper layers of the cerebral cortex; those that migrate later form the superficial layers.

As the cerebral cortex develops, it encircles the diencephalon and takes on a **C-shape**. First, there is an increase in the surface area of the parietal lobe, followed by an increase in the frontal lobe. Next, the cortex expands posteriorly and inferiorly, forming the occipital and temporal lobes (Figure 2–13). Because the cranial cavity does not increase in size in proportion with the increase in cortical surface area, this expansion is accompanied by tremendous infolding. As we saw in Chapter 1, about one third of the cerebral cortex is exposed, with the remainder located within sulci.

The Lateral Ventricle and the Caudate Nucleus
Are Subcortical C-shaped Structures

As the surface area of the cerebral cortex increases, it forces many of the underlying subcortical structures to assume a C-shape (Figure 2–15). Here we will consider two such structures, the lateral ventricle and the caudate nucleus, a component of the basal ganglia (Figure 2–15, left). We will examine the development and structure of the other major C-shaped structures, the hippocampal formation and fornix, in Chapter 15 when we consider its functional anatomy.

At 2 months of intrauterine life, the lateral ventricle is located lateral to the interventricular foramen and is roughly spherical in shape. The transformation of the lateral ventricle into the characteristic C-shape of the mature brain begins at about 3 months. As the cortex develops, the lateral ventricle expands anteriorly to form the **anterior** (or frontal) **horn**, caudally to form the **body** and **posterior** (or occipital) **horn**, and inferiorly to form the **inferior** (or temporal) **horn**. The region of confluence of the body, posterior horn, and inferior horn is the **atrium**. All of the parts of the lateral ventricle are present by the fifth month of development (Figure 2–15C; see also Figure 1–10).

The anterior horn and body of the two lateral ventricles remain close to the midline. The medial walls of each lateral ventricle are formed by a separate **septum pellucidum**, (Figure 2–15E, right). The choroid plexus located in the lateral ventricle also has a C-shape (Figure 2–16): it runs along the **floor of the body of the lateral ventricle** and then along the **roof of the inferior horn**. Its configuration is thus similar to that of the lateral ventricle. The choroid plexus in each lateral ventricle is continuous with that in the third ventricle, running through the interventricular foramina.

The developing C-shape of the caudate nucleus closely parallels that of the lateral ventricle. At 2 months, the caudate nucleus lies along the ventricular floor. It, too, expands rostrally to form the **head**, caudally to form the **body**, and inferiorly to form the **tail** of the nucleus. The caudate nucleus lies in the floor of the anterior horn and body but in the roof of the inferior horn. The configuration of the caudate nucleus in the mature brain is also shown in Figure 2–15E.

The lateral ventricle and caudate nucleus are important landmarks throughout most of the mature cerebral hemispheres. The key to under-

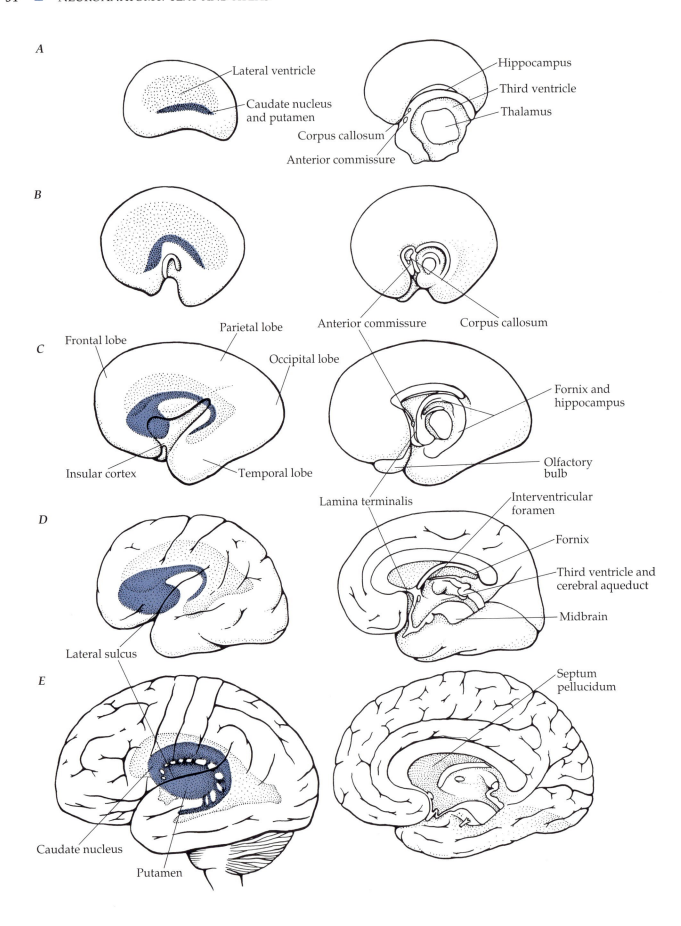

A

Lateral ventricle

Caudate nucleus
and putamen

Hippocampus

Third ventricle

Thalamus

Corpus callosum

Anterior commissure

B

Anterior commissure

Corpus callosum

C

Frontal lobe

Parietal lobe

Occipital lobe

Fornix and
hippocampus

Insular cortex

Temporal lobe

Olfactory
bulb

Lamina terminalis

Interventricular
foramen

Fornix

D

Third ventricle and
cerebral aqueduct

Midbrain

Lateral sulcus

E

Septum
pellucidum

Caudate nucleus

Putamen

◁ *Figure 2–15.* Various components of the telencephalon acquire a C-shape during development. Lateral views of the cerebral hemisphere, with the lateral ventricle lightly stippled and the striatum tinted blue are shown on the left; medial views are shown on the right. Five stages of development are illustrated: 2, 3, 5, 7, and 9 months. (Adapted from Keibel, F., and Mall, F. P. (eds.). 1910–1912. Manual of Human Embryology. 2 vols. Philadelphia: Lippincott.)

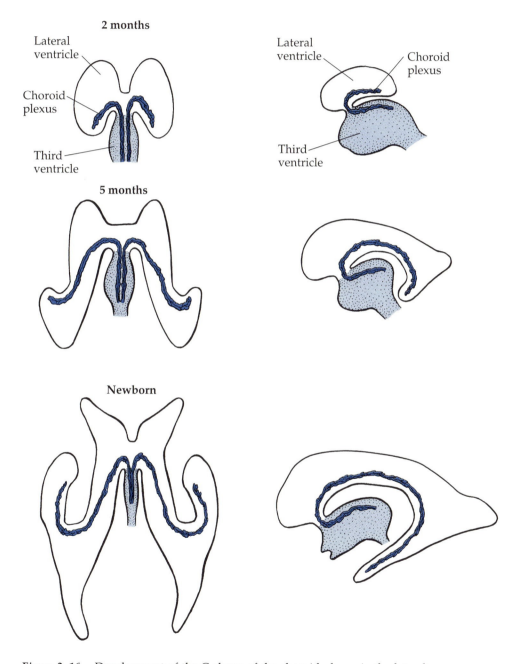

Figure 2–16. Development of the C-shape of the choroid plexus in the lateral ventricle. Three stages of development are shown: 2 months (*top*); 5 months (*middle*); and newborn (*bottom*). The left column illustrates a dorsal view of the lateral ventricles and third ventricle; the right column, the lateral view.

standing their locations in two-dimensional slices is knowing that they are located **dorsally** and **ventrally**. Myelin-stained transverse sections through the mature brain are shown in Figure 2–17. The body of the lateral ventricle is revealed in the dorsal portion of each section, in the frontal lobe; ventrally, the inferior horn of the lateral ventricle is seen in the temporal lobe. The caudate nucleus is also present in two locations: dorsally, in the lateral wall of the body of the lateral ventricle, and ventrally, in the roof of the inferior horn. The partial separation of the caudate nucleus and putamen by the fibers of the internal capsule is reflected in the thin cell bridges that link these two structures (Figure 2–17). The constituent parts of the caudate nucleus will be reexamined in Chapter 11.

Figure 2–17. Coronal sections (myelin-stained) through the cerebral hemisphere of the mature brain illustrate that portions of the lateral ventricle and caudate nucleus are located dorsally and ventrally. The inset shows the shape of the lateral ventricle and the planes of section. The caudate nucleus follows the C-shaped course of the lateral ventricle. *A.* Rostral section through the anterior horn of the lateral ventricle and the head of the caudate nucleus. *B.* Caudal section through the body of the lateral ventricle and caudate nucleus (dorsomedially), the inferior horn of the lateral ventricle, and the tail of the caudate nucleus (ventrolaterally).

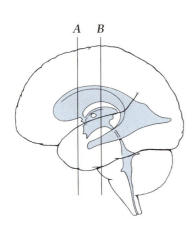

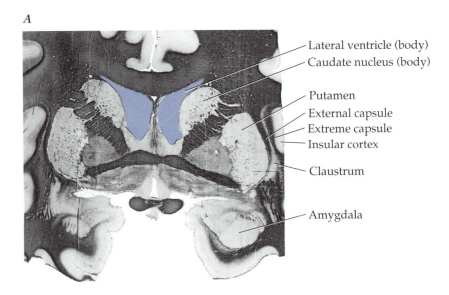

A

Lateral ventricle (body)
Caudate nucleus (body)

Putamen
External capsule
Extreme capsule
Insular cortex

Claustrum

Amygdala

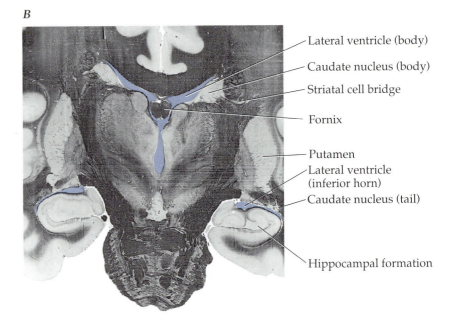

B

Lateral ventricle (body)

Caudate nucleus (body)

Striatal cell bridge

Fornix

Putamen
Lateral ventricle (inferior horn)
Caudate nucleus (tail)

Hippocampal formation

The Insular Cortex Is Hidden Beneath the Operculum
of the Frontal, Parietal, and Temporal Lobes

Before most of the gyri and sulci are present on the cortical surface, a lateral region becomes buried by the developing frontal, parietal, and temporal lobes (Figures 2–13 and 2–15). This region, the **insular cortex** (see Figure 2–13, 9 months), is located deep within the lateral sulcus (Sylvian fissure), one of the earliest grooves to form on the lateral surface. In the mature brain, the insular cortex is revealed only when the banks of the lateral sulcus are partially separated or when the brain is sectioned. The portions of the frontal, parietal, and temporal cortices that cover the insular cortex are termed the **opercula**. The frontal operculum of the dominant hemisphere (typically the left hemisphere in right-handed individuals) is important in motor mechanisms for speech. The parietal and temporal opercular regions and the insular cortex are important in sensory function. Beneath the insular cortex is the **claustrum** (Figure 2–17A), which is a thick sheet of neurons thought to derive from migrating neuroblasts in the overlying cortex. The claustrum is separated from the cortex by the **extreme capsule** and from the putamen by the **external capsule** (Figure 2-17A). Although we know many of the anatomical connections of the claustrum, we understand little of its function.

Early Development of the Central Nervous System

Nerve cells and glial cells are derived from a specialized portion of the ectoderm termed the **neural plate** (Figure 2–1). The edges of the neural plate fold, ultimately appose, and form the **neural tube** (Figure 2–1). The cerebral hemispheres and the brain stem develop from the rostral and intermediate portions of the neural tube, and the spinal cord develops from the caudal portions. The **neuroepithelium** (Figure 2–2) lines the neural tube and forms the cellular constituents of the central nervous system. Immature neurons arise from the neuroepithelium. The neural tube has two additional layers: the **mantle layer**, which becomes the gray matter of the central nervous system, and the **marginal layer**, which becomes the white matter (Figure 2–2). The cavity within the neural tube forms the ventricular system.

Summary

Development of Major Central Nervous System Divisions

Three brain vesicles first form from the rostral neural tube (Figure 2–3): (1) **prosencephalon (forebrain)**, (2) **mesencephalon (midbrain)**, and (3) **rhombencephalon (hindbrain)**. The prosencephalon divides into the **telencephalon (cerebral cortex, hippocampal formation, basal ganglia, and amygdala)** and **diencephalon (thalamus and hypothalamus)**, and the rhombencephalon divides into the **metencephalon (pons and cerebellum)** and **myelencephalon (medulla)**. The **spinal cord**, like the mesencephalon, remains undivided throughout development. A persistent bend called the **cephalic flexure** occurs at the juncture of the mesencephalon and diencephalon (Figure 2–3). The **choroid plexus** is formed by the apposition of brain vasculature, overlying the ventricles, with the **pia** and subsequent invagination of blood vessels of the pia and **ependyma** into the ventricle (Figure 2–4).

Spinal Cord and Brain Stem Development

The spinal cord is segmented, both during development and in maturity. There are **8 cervical**, **12 thoracic**, **5 lumbar**, and **5 sacral** segments. The hindbrain is segmented only during development. The eight hindbrain segments, termed **rhombomeres**, provide the sensory and motor innervation of most of the cranium. Immature neurons in the developing brain stem and spinal cord organize into rostrocaudally oriented columns of cells (Figures 2–6 through 2–10). There are two such columns in the spinal cord: the **alar plate** forms the **dorsal horn**, and the **basal plate** forms the **ventral horn** (Figure 2–6). In the brain stem, the alar and basal plates become oriented mediolaterally (Figure 2–7) as if the central canal opens up to form the fourth ventricle. The alar and basal plates are divided into separate **somatic** and **visceral** columns, from which the cranial nerve nuclei derive (Figures 2–8 through 2–11). Other sensory and motor nuclei of the brain stem derive from immature neurons that migrate from the alar and basal plates. The cerebellum forms from a particular portion of the alar plate, the **rhombic lip** (Figures 2–9 and 2–12).

Development of the Diencephalon and Cerebral Hemispheres

The diencephalon (Figure 2–14) remains roughly **spherical** in shape throughout development. Structures of the cerebral hemispheres take on a **C-shape** (Figures 2–13 through 2–15), including the cerebral cortex and the **caudate nucleus**. The **lateral ventricle**, which is located within the cerebral hemisphere, and **choroid plexus** have a C-shape as well (Figure 2–16). C-shaped structures appear twice on transverse sections through the cerebral hemisphere (Figure 2–16): dorsal and ventral. ■

KEY STRUCTURES AND TERMS

ectoderm
mesoderm
endoderm
neural plate
neural induction
neural groove
neural tube
neuroepithelium
lamina terminalis
neural crest
ependymal layer
mantle layer
marginal layer
primary vesicles
   prosencephalon (forebrain)
   mesencephalon (midbrain)
   rhombencephalon (hindbrain)
      rhombic lips
cephalic flexure
somites
spinal segment
rhombomeres

cauda equina
spinal nerves and nuclei
sulcus limitans
alar plate
dorsal horn
dorsal roots
basal plate
ventral horn
ventral roots
cranial nerves and nuclei
   general somatic motor
   special visceral motor
   general visceral motor
   general visceral afferent
   special visceral afferent
   general somatic afferent
   special somatic afferent
septum pellucidum

**Secondary vesicles
and brain divisions**
telencephalon

cerebral cortex
   insular cortex
   operculum
   hippocampal formation and fornix
   amygdala
   caudate nucleus and putamen
   claustrum
   lateral ventricle
diencephalon
   thalamus
   hypothalamus
   third ventricle
mesencephalon
   cerebral aqueduct
metencephalon
   pons
   medulla
   cerebellum
   fourth ventricle
myelencephalon
   central canal

Selected Readings

Bonner-Fraser, M. 1993. Crest density. Current Biology 3:201–203.
Copp, A. J. 1993. Neural tube defects. Trends Neurosci. 16:381–383.
Cowan, W. M. 1979. The development of the brain. Sci. Am. 241:112–133.
Jacobson, M. 1978. Developmental Neurobiology, 2nd ed. New York: Plenum Press.
Jones, E. G., and Cowan, W. M. 1983. Nervous tissue. In Weiss, L. (ed.), Histology: Cell and Tissue Biology, 5th ed. New York: Elsevier Biomedical, pp. 283–370.
Langman, J. 1981. Medical Embryology. Baltimore: Williams & Wilkins.
Lumsden, A. 1990. The cellular basis of segmentation in developing hindbrain. Trends Neurosci. 13:329–335.
O'Rahilly, R., Müller, F. 1994. The Embryonic Human Brain. New York: Wiley-Liss.
Puelles, L., Rubenstein, L. R. 1993. Expression patterns of homeobox and other putative regulatory genes in the embryonic mouse forebrain suggest a neuromeric organization. Trends Neurosci. 16:472–479.

References

Heimer, L. 1983. The Human Brain and Spinal Cord. New York: Springer-Verlag.
Keibel, F., and Mall, F. P. (eds.) 1910–1912. Manual of Human Embryology. 2 vols. Philadelphia: Lippincott.
Keynes, R. J., and Stern, C. D. 1990. Mechanisms of vertebrate segmentation. Development 103:423–429.
Lumsden, A., and Keynes, R. 1989. Segmental patterns of neuronal development in the chick hindbrain. Nature 337:424–428.
O'Rahilly, R., Müller, F. 1990. Ventricular system and choroid plexuses of the human brain during the embryonic period proper. Am. J. Anat. 189:285–302.
Pansky, B. 1982. Review of Medical Embryology. New York: Macmillan.
Patten, B. M. 1968. Human Embryology. New York: McGraw-Hill (Blackston Division).
Shuangoshoti, S., Netsky, M.G. 1966. Histogenesis of choroid plexus in man. Am. J. Anat. 188:283–315.
Tuchmann-Duplessis, H., Auroux, M., and Haegel, P. 1974. Illustrated Human Embryology. Vol III. Nervous System and Endocrine Glands. New York: Springer-Verlag.

3

Internal Organization of the Central Nervous System

I N CHAPTER 2, WE SAW THAT THE COMPLEX three-dimensional organization of the central nervous system is explained by its developmental plan. In the cerebral hemispheres, the enormous proliferation of cells forces many structures into a C-shape. By contrast, the brain stem and spinal cord remain relatively undifferentiated. In fact, the brain stem and spinal cord in the mature brain closely resemble their embryonic counterparts.

In this chapter, we begin to focus on internal organization of the central nervous system from the dual functional and regional perspectives. We examine functional neural systems that have a component at **each level of the neuraxis** together with anatomical structures that characterize the various divisions of the central nervous system. Two such neural systems are the dorsal column–medial lemniscal system, the principal pathway for perceiving touch, and the corticospinal tract, the principal pathway for voluntary movement control. These two pathways are good examples of the complex interrelations between structure and function. Although the regional anatomy of the brain is extraordinarily complex and difficult to learn, we can simplify the task somewhat by looking at only a limited number of new structures at each level. We also reexamine the ventricular system because these fluid-filled cavities are present at all levels of the central nervous system. Knowledge of the overall anatomy of the ventricular system helps us understand the anatomy of individual brain divisions by providing a framework for remembering the locations of other structures.

We first survey the longitudinal organization of the neural systems and ventricular system, from the spinal cord to the cerebral hemispheres, and then examine the key levels of the neuraxis using sections through the central nervous system. Our goal is to obtain an overall view of the organization of the central nervous system as we identify components of these three systems in each brain division. In the course of examining the various regions of the central nervous system, we correlate the three-dimensional configuration of brain structures with their appearance in myelin-stained sections, which are two-dimensional slices.

In addition to containing circuits that mediate particular functions, such as touch or voluntary movement, the central nervous system also contains neural circuits that subserve the generalized function of **regulating neuronal**

excitability. Our level of attention during waking hours or how easily we are aroused from sleep are examples of aspects of behavior that involve more integrated neural functions. Consider how the quiescent state of a mother's brain can be mobilized by the sound of her infant's cry during the night. The neural systems mediating such generalized functions involve the integrated actions of different parts of the brain stem, collectively called the **reticular formation**, as well as populations of neurons that use particular neurotransmitters and have extraordinarily diffuse axonal projection patterns. These neurotransmitter-specific regulatory systems are particularly important in human behavioral dysfunction. In this chapter, we also survey the key brain regions that are involved in these functions.

Longitudinally Oriented Systems Have a Component at Each Level of the Neuraxis

The dorsal column–medial lemniscal system and the corticospinal tract each have a longitudinal organization, spanning virtually the entire neuraxis. The dorsal column–medial lemniscal system is termed an **ascending pathway** because it brings information from sensory receptors in the periphery to lower levels of the central nervous system, such as the brain stem, and then to higher levels, such as the thalamus and cerebral cortex. In contrast, the corticospinal tract, a **descending pathway**, carries information from the cerebral cortex to a lower level of the central nervous system, the spinal cord.

The dorsal column–medial lemniscal system (Figure 3–1A) consists of a three-neuron circuit that links the periphery with the cerebral cortex. In doing so it traverses the spinal cord, brain stem, diencephalon, and cerebral hemispheres. Its name derives from two of its components: the axonal pathway in the spinal cord, called the **dorsal column**, and the pathway in the brain stem, the **medial lemniscus**. The first neurons in the circuit are the **dorsal root ganglion cells**, the class of neurons that innervate the peripheral sensory receptors. Dorsal root ganglion cells link the periphery, where stimuli are received, with the spinal cord and brain stem, where stimulus information is first processed. This component of the system is a fast transmission line that is visible on the dorsal surface of the spinal cord as the dorsal column.

The first synapse is made in a **relay nucleus** in the medulla. A relay nucleus processes incoming signals and transmits this information to the next component of the circuit. The signal emerging from the relay nucleus is different from the incoming signal, reflecting the particular feature of sensory processing performed by the nucleus. For example, the somatic sensory relay nucleus in the medulla is the **dorsal column nucleus**, and it plays a role in enhancing the spatial resolving capacity of the somatic sensory system. The cell bodies of the second neurons in the pathway are located in the dorsal column nucleus. The axons of these second-order neurons cross the midline, or **decussate**. Because of this decussation, sensory information from the right side of the body is processed by the left side of the brain. Most sensory (and motor) pathways decussate at some point along their course. Surprisingly, we do not know why neural systems decussate!

After crossing the midline, the axons ascend in the brain stem pathway, the **medial lemniscus**, to synapse in a relay nucleus in the **thalamus**. From here, third-order neurons send their axons through the white matter underlying the cortex, in the **internal capsule**. These axons synapse on

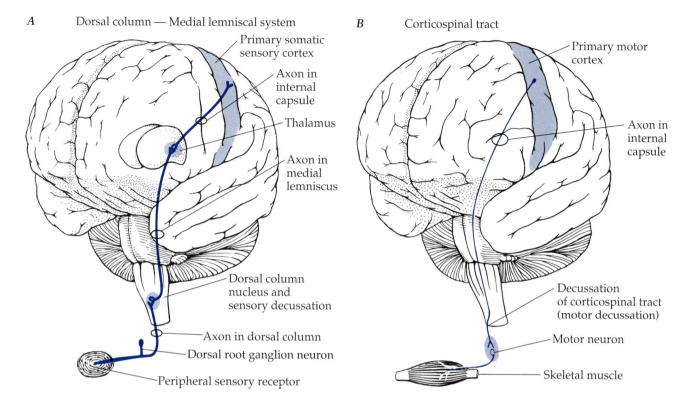

A Dorsal column — Medial lemniscal system

- Primary somatic sensory cortex
- Axon in internal capsule
- Thalamus
- Axon in medial lemniscus
- Dorsal column nucleus and sensory decussation
- Axon in dorsal column
- Dorsal root ganglion neuron
- Peripheral sensory receptor

B Corticospinal tract

- Primary motor cortex
- Axon in internal capsule
- Decussation of corticospinal tract (motor decussation)
- Motor neuron
- Skeletal muscle

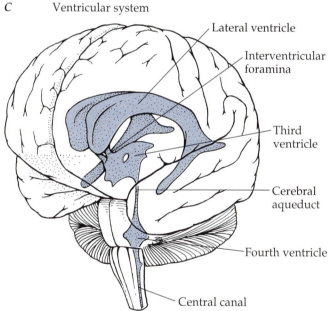

C Ventricular system

- Lateral ventricle
- Interventricular foramina
- Third ventricle
- Cerebral aqueduct
- Fourth ventricle
- Central canal

Figure 3–1. The dorsal column–medial lemniscal system *(A)*, the corticospinal tract *(B)*, and the ventricular system *(C)* are longitudinally organized.

neurons in the **primary somatic sensory cortex**, which is located in the postcentral gyrus of the parietal lobe (Figure 3–1A). Each sensory system has a primary cortical area and several higher-order areas. The primary area receives input directly from the thalamus, whereas the higher-order areas receive input predominantly from the primary and other cortical areas. When the primary somatic sensory cortex is damaged, patients have impaired touch and limb position sense, two sensory modalities mediated by the dorsal column–medial lemniscal system. Before antibiotics, it was common to see patients with damage to the dorsal column–medial lemniscal system resulting from advanced syphilitic infection, a condition termed tabes dorsalis.

The corticospinal tract descends from the cerebral cortex to terminate on motor neurons in the spinal cord. In contrast to the dorsal column–medial lemniscal system, in which fast transmission lines are interrupted by relay nuclei in the brain stem and thalamus, the corticospinal tract consists of single neurons that link the cortex with the spinal cord. The cell bodies of many corticospinal tract neurons are located in the primary motor cortex on the precentral gyrus of the frontal lobe just rostral to the primary somatic sensory cortex on the postcentral gyrus (Figure 3–1B). The axons of these neurons leave the motor cortex and travel in the **internal capsule**.

The corticospinal tract emerges from the cerebral hemisphere to course on the ventral surface of the midbrain. The axons disappear below the ventral surface of the pons and reappear on the ventral surface of the medulla as the **pyramid**. In the caudal medulla, most corticospinal axons decussate (pyramidal, or motor, decussation). Once in the spinal cord, descending cortical axons run along the lateral margin in the white matter before terminating on motor neurons in the gray matter. These motor neurons innervate skeletal muscle; hence, the motor cortex directly influences movements of our limbs and trunk. For example, patients with corticospinal tract damage, commonly caused by interruption of the blood supply to the internal capsule, demonstrate muscle weakness and impaired fine motor skill.

The brain ventricles and the central canal of the spinal cord contain cerebrospinal fluid (Figure 3–1C). The **lateral ventricles** and **third ventricle** are located within the cerebral hemisphere and diencephalon, respectively. They are connected by the interventricular foramina. The cerebral aqueduct, located in the midbrain, connects the **third** and the **fourth ventricles**. The fourth ventricle is located in the pons and medulla. The **central canal** is the most caudal portion of the ventricular system, extending directly from the fourth ventricle into the spinal cord.

The rest of this chapter focuses on the internal structure of the central nervous system. We learn the functions and locations of nuclei and tracts of the brain and spinal cord by examining drawings and photographs of sections through key levels of the central nervous system. Many of these sections are stained for the presence of myelin (see Figure 1–14). We also examine magnetic resonance imaging (MRI) scans of the living brain. Because the central nervous system is so complex, we limit our discussion in this chapter to (1) structures directly associated with the dorsal column–medial lemniscal system, the corticospinal tract, and the ventricular system, and (2) surface and internal landmarks that characterize the level of a particular slice.

Locating particular structures on myelin-stained sections or radiological images is often difficult, because neighboring structures are stained or imaged similarly. This problem calls attention to how we identify structures in normal myelin-stained sections. Many structures are distinguished clearly from their neighbors because of morphological changes at boundaries; for example, a nucleus–which stains lightly–is clearly identifiable when it is surrounded by axons–which stain darkly. Note the myelin-stained section in Figure 3–3, where we can distinguish the lightly stained dorsal horns, which contain mostly neuronal cell bodies, from the darkly stained dorsal columns, which contain myelinated axons. Unfortunately, functionally different structures that have similar staining properties are often intermingled. Thus, we can localize the corticospinal tract only to a general region in the white matter, because it is surrounded by other myelinated axons. In humans, the location of such a structure is determined by comparing normal and lesioned material (see Chapter 1, Figure 1–16). In laboratory animals, axon tracing methods are used to localize structures.

The Spinal Cord Has a Central Cellular Region Surrounded by a Region That Contains Myelinated Axons

The gray matter of the spinal cord (Figure 3–2A) contains two functionally distinct regions, the **dorsal** and **ventral horns**, each containing columns of neurons oriented rostrocaudally. Recall from Chapter 2 that the dorsal horn develops from the alar plate and the ventral horn develops from the basal plate. The white matter of the spinal cord, which surrounds the gray matter, contains three rostrocaudally oriented columns—the **dorsal**, **lateral**, and **ventral** columns—in which axons ascend or descend.

Figure 3–2. Three-dimensional schematic view of a spinal cord segment showing key spinal cord structures and the branching pattern of dorsal root ganglion cells in the spinal cord *(A)* and the circuit for the knee-jerk reflex *(B)*. The afferent fiber in part B carries information from muscle and the efferent fiber transmits signals to contract muscle.

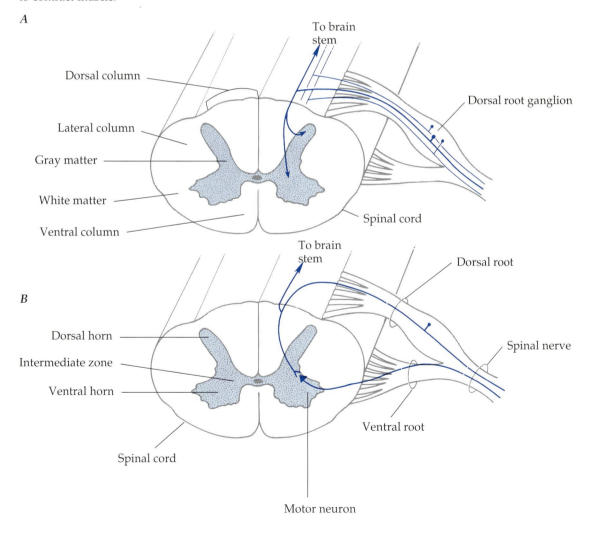

A

To brain stem

Dorsal column

Dorsal root ganglion

Lateral column

Gray matter

White matter

Ventral column

Spinal cord

B

To brain stem

Dorsal root

Dorsal horn

Intermediate zone

Ventral horn

Spinal nerve

Spinal cord

Ventral root

Motor neuron

Dorsal horn neurons subserve the bodily senses: pain, touch, temperature sense, and limb position sense. These sensory neurons receive sensory information from the periphery from the somatic sensory receptor neurons, dorsal root ganglion cells. The axons of the ganglion cells enter the spinal cord through the **dorsal root**. The dorsal root ganglion neurons also branch into the **dorsal column**. These axon branches transmit sensory information to the brain stem (Figure 3–2) and are part of the **dorsal column–medial lemniscal system**.

Neurons of the ventral horn subserve limb and trunk movement. Motor neurons located here have axons that exit from the spinal cord through the **ventral root**. Motor neurons receive direct connections from the **corticospinal tract**, whose axons course in the **lateral column** of the white matter. The ventral column contains the axons of both ascending sensory and descending motor pathways and will be considered in later chapters.

Although the dorsal and ventral horns have different functions, interconnections between them integrate our sensory experiences with movement. For example, monosynaptic connections occur between a certain type of dorsal root ganglion cell that innervates stretch receptors, called primary muscle spindle receptors, and motor neurons (Figure 3–2B). In certain segments of the lumbar spinal cord, this contact mediates the **knee-jerk reflex**. A tap to the patella tendon stretches the quadriceps muscle, thereby stretching primary spindle receptors in the muscle. The central branches of dorsal root ganglion cells that innervate these receptors synapse on quadriceps motor neurons. Because this synapse is excitatory, the quadriceps motor neurons are discharged and the muscle contracts.

Integration of the sensory and motor functions of the spinal cord is also accomplished by neurons located in the **intermediate zone** (Figure 3–2B), between the dorsal and ventral horns. These neurons transmit sensory information from dorsal horn neurons to motor neurons, in the ventral horn. Many spinal reflexes have numerous neurons interposed between the sensory and motor neurons, and many of these neurons are located in the intermediate zone. Interneurons in the intermediate zone of the cervical spinal cord enable you to reflexively withdraw your hand away from a hot stove after touching it. In the thoracic and lumbar segments of the spinal

Figure 3–3. Myelin-stained transverse section through the cervical spinal cord. The three parts of the spinal gray matter, the dorsal horn, intermediate zone, and ventral horn, are distinguished.

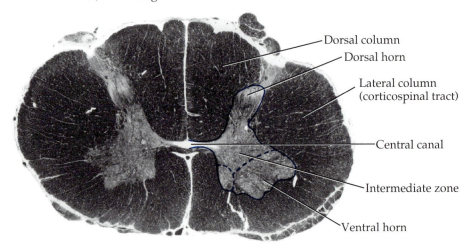

Dorsal column

Dorsal horn

Lateral column
(corticospinal tract)

Central canal

Intermediate zone

Ventral horn

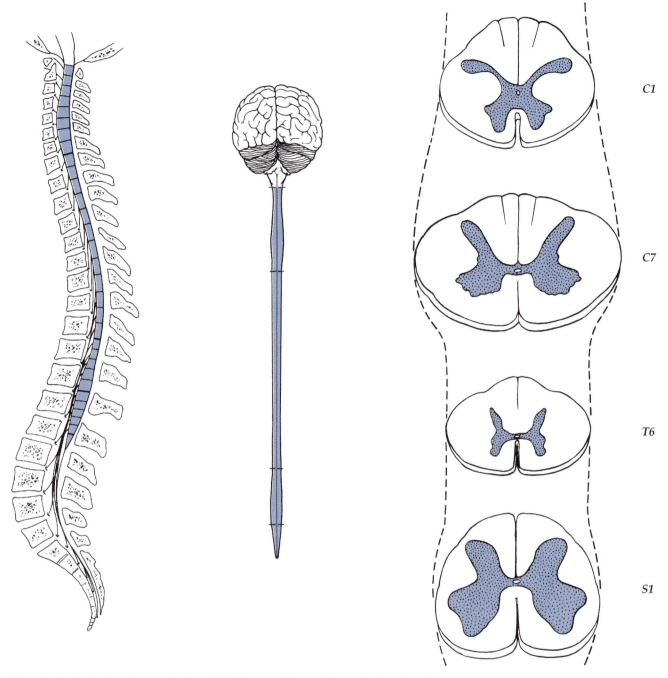

Figure 3–4. Spinal cord organization. (*Left*) A lateral view of the spinal cord and the vertebral column. (*Middle*) A dorsal view of the central nervous system. (*Right*) Drawings of myelin-stained sections through the spinal cord. The levels of sections are indicated by the horizontal lines on the dorsal view of the central nervous system. The dashed line indicates schematically the width of the spinal cord, emphasizing the expansion of segments in the caudal cervical cord (cervical enlargement) and the lumbosacral cord (lumbosacral enlargement).

cord, the intermediate zone also mediates visceral motor function, because autonomic preganglionic neurons are located there (see Chapter 14).

The slice through the spinal cord shown in Figure 3–3 is stained for myelinated axons. Unfortunately, in myelin-stained material the white matter of the central nervous system stains black and the gray matter stains light! (The terms "white matter" and "gray matter" derive from

A

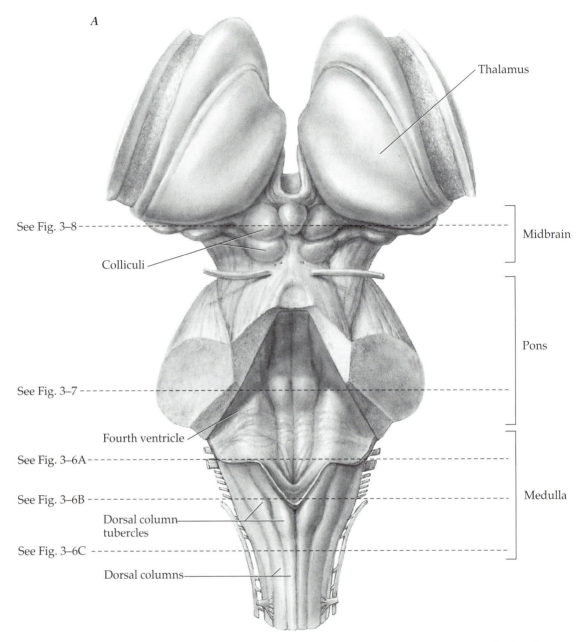

Thalamus

See Fig. 3–8

Colliculi

Midbrain

Pons

See Fig. 3–7

Fourth ventricle

See Fig. 3–6A

See Fig. 3–6B

Dorsal column
tubercles

See Fig. 3–6C

Medulla

Dorsal columns

Figure 3–5. Dorsal *(A)* and ventral *(B)* surfaces of the brain stem. Dashed lines indicate the approximate levels through which sections in Figures 3–6 through 3–8 were obtained.

their appearance in fresh tissue.) Between the intermediate zones on the two sides of the spinal cord is the **central canal**, a component of the ventricular system. (It is believed that in the adult the central canal is not an open channel for its entire rostral–caudal extent.)

There are two characteristic changes in morphology at different levels of the spinal cord. First, the amount of white matter increases from caudal (Figure 3–4, S1) to rostral (Figure 3–4, C1) to accommodate a greater number of both ascending and descending axons. Second, the gray matter is enlarged between the fifth cervical and first thoracic segments (**cervical enlargement**; Figure 3–4, C7), as well as between the first lumbar and second

B

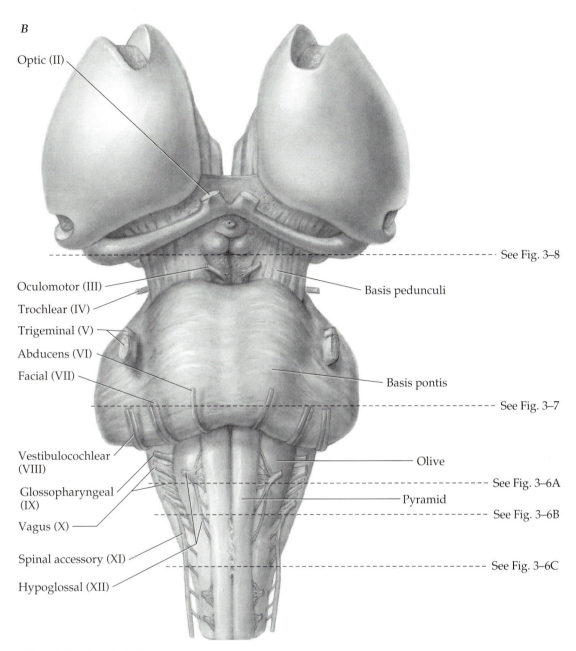

Optic (II)

Oculomotor (III)

Trochlear (IV)

Trigeminal (V)

Abducens (VI)

Facial (VII)

Vestibulocochlear (VIII)

Glossopharyngeal (IX)

Vagus (X)

Spinal accessory (XI)

Hypoglossal (XII)

See Fig. 3–8

Basis pedunculi

Basis pontis

See Fig. 3–7

Olive

See Fig. 3–6A

Pyramid

See Fig. 3–6B

See Fig. 3–6C

Figure 3–5. *(continued)*

sacral segments (**lumbosacral enlargement**; Figure 3–4, S1). These enlargements accommodate the increased numbers of neurons in these levels that
are needed to provide the sensory and motor innervation of the limbs.

Surface Features of the Brain Stem
Mark Key Internal Structures

The rostral spinal cord merges with the brain stem, as can be seen in
Figure 3–5, which illustrates the dorsal and ventral surfaces of these structures. The cerebellum has been removed in this figure, revealing the fourth

ventricle on the dorsal brain stem surface. While the spinal cord surface is basically the same at different levels, the surface of the brain stem has many nerve roots and distinctive landmarks, imaginatively named for their appearance by early anatomists. Thin sections through the brain stem reveal many of these surface features. Knowledge of the surface features of the brain stem therefore can help in recognizing the level of a particular section.

On the dorsal brain stem surface (Figure 3–5A), we can identify four important landmarks: dorsal columns, dorsal column tubercles, the fourth ventricle, and the colliculi. Where the spinal cord meets the brain stem, the **dorsal columns** merge with swellings, **dorsal column tubercles**, that signify underlying nuclei. Two dorsal column nuclei on each side of the medulla process sensory information from different body parts (see Chapter 5). The first neurons in the dorsal column–medial lemniscal system, the primary sensory neurons, synapse on neurons in the dorsal column nuclei that form these tubercles.

With the cerebellum removed, the floor of the **fourth ventricle** can be identified by its rhomboid shape. The key tubercles and sulci on the floor of the fourth ventricle will be examined in Chapter 12. The **colliculi** are four bumps located on the dorsal surface of the midbrain. The rostral pair of bumps, termed the superior colliculi, are important in controlling eye movements and the caudal pair, the inferior colliculi, process sounds.

We also identify four important landmarks on the ventral surface (Figure 3–5B) and, remarkably, all are key components of the motor system: pyramids, olives, basis pontis, and basis pedunculi. In the medulla, the axons of the corticospinal tract are located in the **pyramids**. The **olives** are located lateral to the pyramids. Neurons in the olives together with those in the **basis pontis**, the large basal surface of the pons, are major sources of afferent information to the cerebellum. Using this information, the cerebellum controls the accuracy of movement. Finally, the **basis pedunculi** are on the ventral surface of the midbrain. Many of the axons that are immediately beneath the ventral midbrain surface in the basis pedunculi are part of the corticospinal tract. These axons course through the basis pontis and emerge on the medullary surface in the pyramid.

Another characteristic of the brain stem is the presence of the cranial nerves (Figure 3–5). Knowledge of their locations helps us develop a general understanding of brain stem anatomy. There are 12 pairs of **cranial nerves**, which, like the spinal nerves, mediate sensory and motor function, but of cranial structures (see Table 2–3). The cranial nerves and their major functions will be considered in detail in Chapters 12 and 13.

In the next part of the chapter, we approach brain stem anatomy by examining transverse sections through five key levels: (1) the spinal cord–medullary junction, (2) the caudal medulla, (3) the middle medulla, (4) the caudal pons, and (5) the rostral midbrain. To better understand structure at these levels, we correlate the surface features observed earlier with internal anatomy.

The Caudal Medulla and Spinal Cord Have a Similar Organization

The first of three key sections through the medulla that we will examine is shown in Figure 3–6C. This section is at the transition between the spinal cord and medulla. The corticospinal tract is located in the ventral portion of the section, and it decussates at this level. The **pyramidal (or motor) decussation** is visible on the ventral brain stem surface (Figure 3–5B). As a result of this decussation, one side of the brain controls mus-

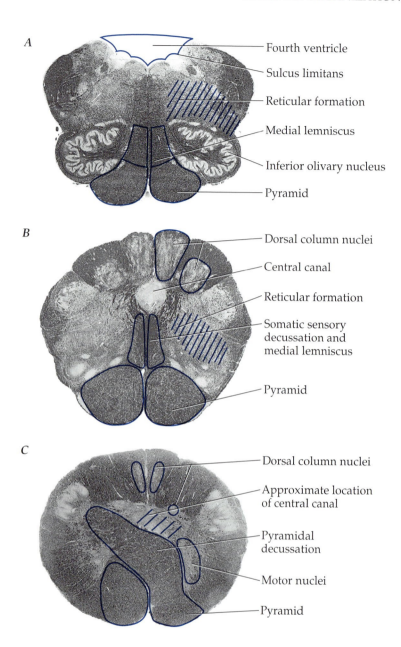

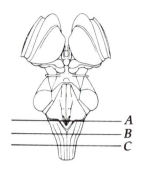

A
- Fourth ventricle
- Sulcus limitans
- Reticular formation
- Medial lemniscus
- Inferior olivary nucleus
- Pyramid

B
- Dorsal column nuclei
- Central canal
- Reticular formation
- Somatic sensory decussation and medial lemniscus
- Pyramid

C
- Dorsal column nuclei
- Approximate location of central canal
- Pyramidal decussation
- Motor nuclei
- Pyramid

Figure 3–6. Myelin-stained sections through three levels of the medulla. From rostral to caudal: inferior olivary nucleus *(A)*, dorsal column nuclei *(B)*, and pyramidal decussation *(C)*. Levels of sections are indicated in the inset and in Figure 3–5. Key medullary structures are highlighted.

cles of the opposite side of the body. Because this section is stained for myelin, the corticospinal axons appear dark, just as the lateral column of the spinal cord does.

Many of the nuclei of the brain stem are analogous to the three regions of spinal cord gray matter–the dorsal horn, the ventral horn, and the intermediate zone. *First*, the brain stem sensory nuclei (Figure 3–6C), which receive sensory input directly from the receptor neurons innervating cranial structures, have general functions similar to neurons of the dorsal horn. The **dorsal column nuclei**, a pair of nuclei on each side of the dorsal medulla, are small in this section compared with more rostral levels (e.g., Figure 3–6B). Their position within and at the base of the dorsal columns helps us understand their afferent connections: the dorsal column nuclei receive their major input from the axons of somatic sensory receptors in the dorsal columns.

Second, the cranial nerve motor nuclei (Figure 3–6C), which contain motor neurons innervating cranial muscles, are analogous to the spinal

motor nuclei in the ventral horn. *Third*, the **reticular formation** (Figure 3–6C), like the spinal intermediate zone, plays a role in sensory–motor integration. The reticular formation also regulates arousal by affecting the excitability of neurons throughout the central nervous system. Receiving input from all of the sensory modalities, neurons of the reticular formation can affect neuronal excitability directly through diffuse projections, or indirectly by contacting neurons with diffuse projections. A particularly important path by which the reticular formation affects the excitability of cerebral cortical neurons is through connections with certain thalamic nuclei (see below). At the level of the spinal cord–medulla junction, the central canal is located at the midline within the reticular formation (Figure 3–6C).

Dorsal Column Nuclei Relay Somatic Sensory Information to the Thalamus

The dorsal column nuclei are located in transverse sections through most of the medulla because they are elongated in the rostrocaudal direction. The largest portion of the dorsal column nuclei lies rostral to the junction of the spinal cord and the medulla (Figure 3–6B); here, the nuclei bulge to form the dorsal surface landmarks, the dorsal column tubercles. The second order neurons of the dorsal column–medial lemniscal system originate in these nuclei. Their axons decussate and ascend to the thalamus in the **medial lemniscus** (Figure 3–6B). Because of this decussation, sensory information from one side of the body is processed by the other side of the brain. The corticospinal tract is located ventral to the medial lemniscus, in the medullary **pyramid** (Figure 3–5B) and the central canal is located more dorsally, on the midline (Figure 3–6B).

The Inferior Olivary Nucleus Sends Axons to the Cerebellum

The **olive**, a bulge located on the ventral medullary surface lateral to the medullary pyramid (Figure 3–5B), marks the position of the **inferior olivary nucleus** (Figure 3–6A). As we saw in Chapter 2, this nucleus develops from neurons of the alar plate that migrate from the ventricular surface to the ventral medulla. In the mature brain, neurons in the inferior olivary nucleus project to the cerebellum, where they form one of the strongest excitatory synapses in the entire central nervous system (see Chapter 10). A single action potential in an olivary neuron evokes a burst of activity in its postsynaptic target neurons in the cerebellum. The medial lemniscus and pyramid are both medial to the inferior olivary nuclei (Figure 3–6A).

At this level, the first clear view of the ventricular system of the brain finally becomes apparent. The central canal expands to form the **fourth ventricle**, whose floor is formed by the medulla. The ventricular roof consists of a thin tissue formed by the apposition of the pia and ependyma during development. Recall that during development the expansion of the central canal to form the fourth ventricle transforms the dorsal–ventral organization of the alar and basal plates into a lateral–medial organization (see Figure 2–7). Both during development and in maturity, the **sulcus limitans** separates cranial sensory and motor nuclei on the ventricular floor (Figure 3–6A).

The Pontine Nuclei Surround the Axons of the Corticospinal Tract in the Base of the Pons

The dorsal surface of the pons forms part of the floor of the fourth ventricle; the cerebellum forms the roof (Figure 3–7). The medial lemniscus, which is less distinct than in the medulla because neighboring myelinated fibers obscure its borders, is displaced dorsally by the **pontine**

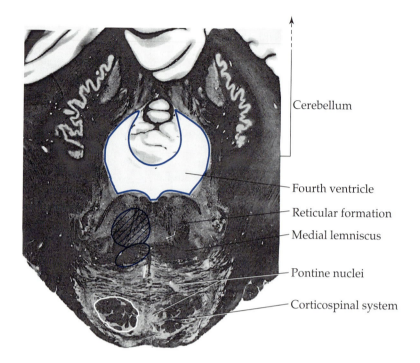

Cerebellum

Fourth ventricle

Reticular formation

Medial lemniscus

Pontine nuclei

Corticospinal system

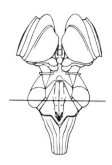

Figure 3–7. Myelin-stained section through pons. The level of section is indicated in the inset and in Figure 3–5. The reticular formation, medial lemniscus, and corticospinal system are outlined on the left side of the section.

nuclei. Like the inferior olivary nucleus, the pontine nuclei derive from immature neurons that migrate ventrally from the ventricular floor. Neurons in the pontine nuclei, which transmit information from the cerebral cortex to the cerebellum, participate in skilled movements. The pontine nuclei surround the corticospinal axons; both nuclei and axons are located within the base of the pons, or **basis pontis** (Figure 3–5).

The Dorsal Surface of the Midbrain Contains the Colliculi

The midbrain can be divided into three regions, moving from the dorsal to ventral (Figure 3–8): (1) the **tectum** (Latin for "roof"), (2) the **tegmentum** (Latin for "cover"), and (3) the **basis pedunculi**. The tegmentum and basis pedunculi comprise the **cerebral peduncle**. The colliculi are

Figure 3–8. Myelin-stained section through the rostral midbrain, at the level of the superior colliculus. The level of section is indicated in the inset and in Figure 3–5. The reticular formation, medial lemniscus, and corticospinal system are outlined on the left side.

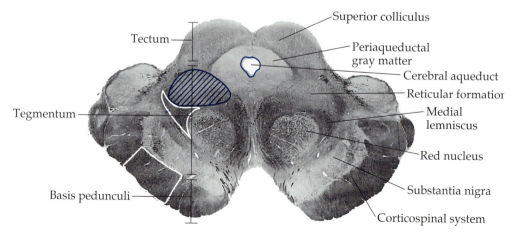

Tectum

Superior colliculus

Periaqueductal gray matter

Cerebral aqueduct

Reticular formation

Medial lemniscus

Red nucleus

Tegmentum

Substantia nigra

Basis pedunculi

Corticospinal system

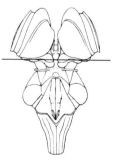

located in the tectum. The superior colliculi (Figure 3–8) play an important role in controlling eye movement and the inferior colliculi (located more caudally, see Figure 7–7) in hearing.

The tectum and tegmentum are separated by the **cerebral aqueduct**, which connects the third and fourth ventricles. This ventricular conduit is surrounded by a nuclear region, termed the **periaqueductal gray**, which contains neurons that are part of the circuit for endogenous pain suppression. For example, pain may be perceived as less severe during intense emotional experiences such as childbirth or military combat, and this neural system participates in this pain diminution. The medial lemniscus is located within the tegmentum.

The **corticospinal tract** is located in the basis pedunculi. This pathway is therefore seen on the ventral surfaces of both the midbrain (as the basis pedunculi) and the medulla (as the pyramid). A nucleus of major clinical significance, the **substantia nigra**, separates the corticospinal fibers and the medial lemniscus. The substantia nigra functions closely with the striatum (see Figure 1–9B) in control of movement. In patients with Parkinson's disease, neurons in the substantia nigra that use dopamine as a neurotransmitter are destroyed. Two major neurological signs of this disease are tremor and slowing of voluntary movements. The **red nucleus** is another midbrain nucleus that helps control movement.

The Thalamus Transmits Information From Subcortical Structures to the Cerebral Cortex

Most sensory information reaches the cortex indirectly by relay neurons in the **thalamus** (Figure 3–9). This is also the case for neural signals controlling movements, learning and memory, and emotions. Neurons in each half of the thalamus project to the cerebral cortex on the same (ipsilateral) side. Thalamic neurons are clustered into discrete nuclei. The organization of thalamic nuclei can be approached from an anatomical and a functional perspective. Based on their locations, six nuclear groups are distinguished in the thalamus (Figure 3–9). The four major groups are named according to their locations with respect to bands of myelinated axons, called the **internal medullary laminae**: (1) anterior nuclei, (2) medial nuclei, (3) lateral nuclei, and (4) intralaminar nuclei, which lie within the laminae. The two other nuclear groups are: (5) the midline nuclei, and (6) the reticular nucleus.

We divide the various thalamic nuclei into two major functional classes on the basis of the extent and functions of their cortical projections: (1) relay nuclei, and (2) diffuse-projecting nuclei. Table 3–1 lists the major thalamic nuclei. **Relay nuclei** are essential for all brain functions, and each relay nucleus serves a distinct role in perception, volition, or cognition. They transmit information from particular subcortical inputs to a **restricted portion of the cerebral cortex**.

The cortical projections of some of the major thalamic relay nuclei are shown in Figure 3–10. Relay nuclei that mediate sensation and movement are located in the lateral portion of the thalamus and project their axons to the sensory and motor cortical areas. For each sensory modality, there is a relay nucleus. The only exception is olfaction, where information from the periphery is transmitted directly to the cortex on the medial temporal lobe (see Chapter 8). We learned in Chapter 1 that each sensory modality has a primary area, which receives input directly from the thalamic relay nucleus for that modality. For example, the ventral posterior lateral nucleus is the relay nucleus for the dorsal column–medial lemniscal system. It transmits somatic sensory information from the medial lemniscus

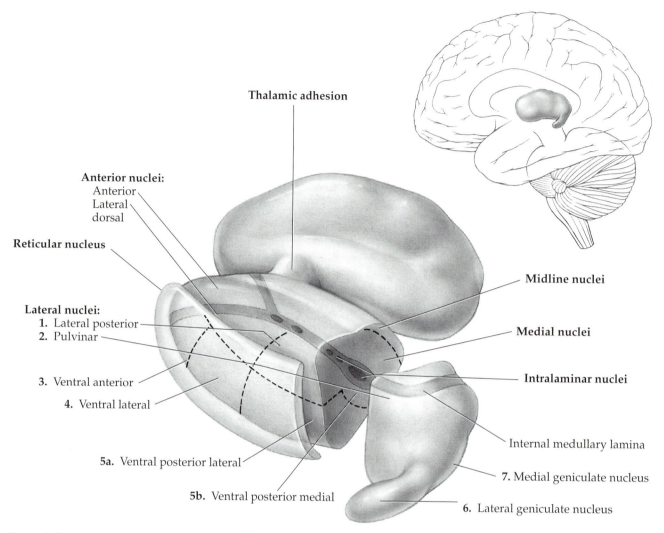

Figure 3–9. A three-dimensional view of the thalamus as well as its approximate location in cerebral hemispheres. The major nuclei are labeled. Nuclei of the lateral group of nuclei are numbered.

to the somatic sensory cortex for touch (Figure 3–10, dark gray). The different motor areas also receive input directly from motor relay nuclei. An important nucleus for controlling voluntary movement, the ventral lateral nucleus, transmits signals from the cerebellum to the motor cortex, which gives rise to the corticospinal tract (Figure 3–10, dark blue stipple).

Relay nuclei located in the anterior, medial, and lateral parts of the thalamus project to the **association cortex**, the cortical regions that lie outside the sensory and motor areas. There are three major regions of association cortex, which subserve distinct sets of functions: the parietal–temporal–occipital cortex, the prefrontal cortex, and the limbic cortex. The **parietal–temporal–occipital association cortex**, which is located at the juncture of these lobes (Figure 3–10, blue), receives information from the pulvinar nucleus as well as from different sensory areas. This area is crucial for perception. The **prefrontal association cortex** is important for cognitive functions and for organizing behavior, including the memories and motor plans that are necessary for interacting with our environment (Figure 3–10, light stipple). For example, patients with damage to the prefrontal cortex blindly repeat motor acts irrespective of their efficacy. The prefrontal association cortex receives a projection from the medial dorsal nucleus. The **limbic association cortex**

Table 3–1. Thalamic nuclei: major connections and functions.

Nucleus	Functional class	Major imputs	Major outputs	Functions
Anterior Group				
Anterior	Relay	Hypothalamus (mammillary body), hippocampal formation	Cingulate gyrus (limbic association cortex)	Learning, memory, and emotions
Lateral dorsal	Relay	Hippocampal formation; pretectum	Cingulate gyrus	?
Medial Group				
Medial dorsal	Relay	Basal ganglia, amygdala, olfactory system, hypothalamus	Prefontal association cortex	Emotions, cognition, learning, and memory
Lateral Group				
Ventral anterior	Relay	Basal ganglia	Supplementary motor cortex	Movement planning
Ventral lateral	Relay	Cerebellum	Premotor and primary motor cortex	Movement planning and control
Ventral posterior	Relay	Spinal cord, brain stem, medial lemniscus, trigeminal lemniscus	Primary somatic sensory cortex	Touch, limb position sense, pain, and temperature sense
Lateral geniculate	Relay	Retina	Primary visual cortex	Vision
Medial geniculate	Relay	Inferior colliculus	Primary auditory cortex	Hearing
Pulvinar	Relay	Superior colliculus; parietal, temporal, occipital lobes	Parietal, temporal, occiptal association cortex	Sensory integration, perception, language
Lateral posterior	Relay	Superior colliculus, pretectum, occipital lobe	Posterior parietal association cortex	Sensory integration
Intralaminar Nuclei				
Centromedian	Diffuse-projecting	Brain stem, basal ganglia, spinal cord	Cerebral cortex, basal ganglia	Regulation of cortical activity
Central lateral	Diffuse-projecting	Spinal cord, brain stem	Cerebral cortex, basal ganglia	Regulation of cortical activity
Parafascicular	Diffuse-projecting	Spinal cord, brain stem	Cerebral cortex, basal ganglia	Regulation of cortical activity
Midline Nuclei	Diffuse-projecting	Reticular formation, hypothalamus	Cerebral cortex, basal forebrain, allocortex	Regulation of fore-brain neuronal excitability
Reticular Nucleus		Thalamus, cortex	Thalamus	Regulation of thalamic neuronal activity

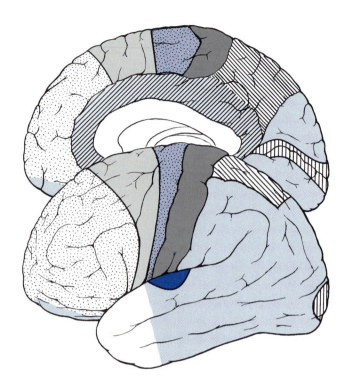

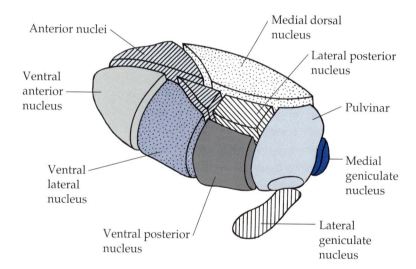

Figure 3–10. The relationship between the major thalamic nuclei and the cortical regions to which they project.

is essential for emotions as well as for learning and memory. It is located primarily on the medial brain surface (Figure 3–10, blue hatching), in the cingulate gyrus, and on the orbital surface of the frontal lobe. Patients with structural or functional abnormalities of the limbic cortex, such as temporal lobe epilepsy, often also have mood disorders, such as depression. Part of the limbic association cortex receives input from the anterior nucleus.

Diffuse-projecting nuclei are thought to function in arousal and in regulating the excitability of wide regions of the cerebral cortex. They receive input from many converging sources and in turn project widely to the cerebral cortex. The **intralaminar** and **midline thalamic nuclei** are the nuclei in this class (Table 3–1). The patterns of termination of neurons in diffuse-projecting nuclei are described as **regional** because they may cross

functional boundaries in the cortex. By contrast, the terminations of an individual relay nucleus are confined to a **single functional cortical area**. The thalamic **reticular nucleus** sends its axons to other thalamic nuclei. It coordinates the activity of neurons within the thalamus and may play a role, together with the intralaminar nuclei, in regulating arousal.

The Internal Capsule Contains Ascending and Descending Axons

Thalamic neurons project to the cerebral cortex via the **internal capsule**. The internal capsule is a two-way path, not only for transmission of information from the thalamus to the cerebral cortex, but also from the cerebral cortex to subcortical structures, including the basal ganglia, thalamus, brain stem, and spinal cord. Whereas the ascending thalamocortical fibers are located entirely in the internal capsule, the descending cortical fibers course within and through the internal capsule and appear to condense in the midbrain to form the basis pedunculi. The internal capsule looks like a curved fan (Figure 3–11). When the cerebral hemispheres are sliced horizontally (Figure 3–12), the internal capsule resembles an arrowhead with the tip pointing medially. The internal capsule separates the thalamus and caudate nucleus from the putamen and globus pallidus. Figure 3–12 also shows the nomenclature for the basal ganglia, a topic we will consider in Chapter 11.

Figure 3–11. Three-dimensional view of the internal capsule. The descending cortical axons collect into a discrete tract in the brain stem. Lines indicate planes of horizontal (e.g., Figure 3–12) and coronal (e.g., Figure 3–13) sections. (Adapted from Carpenter, M. B., and Sutin, J. 1983. Human Neuroanatomy. Baltimore: Williams & Wilkins.)

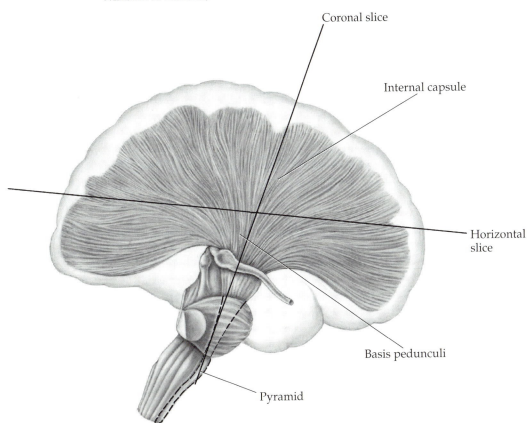

Coronal slice

Internal capsule

Horizontal slice

Basis pedunculi

Pyramid

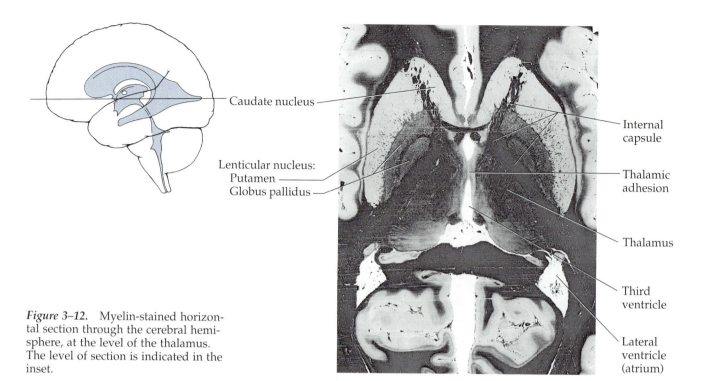

Caudate nucleus

Internal capsule

Thalamic adhesion

Lenticular nucleus:
Putamen
Globus pallidus

Thalamus

Third ventricle

Lateral ventricle (atrium)

Figure 3–12. Myelin-stained horizontal section through the cerebral hemisphere, at the level of the thalamus. The level of section is indicated in the inset.

The structures we have just identified in Figure 3–12 are also sectioned in the coronal slice shown in Figure 3–13. The axons of the thalamic neurons that receive input from the medial lemniscus pass through the internal capsule en route to the primary somatic sensory cortex. The corticospinal axons descend through the internal capsule. In fact, in this coronal slice (Figure 3–13) the entire course of the corticospinal tract in the cerebral hemispheres and brain stem can be traced: the internal capsule, the basis pedunculi, the pontine base, and the pyramid. In the human

Figure 3–13. Myelin-stained coronal section through the cerebral hemisphere, at the level of the thalamus. The inset shows the plane of section.

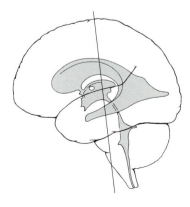

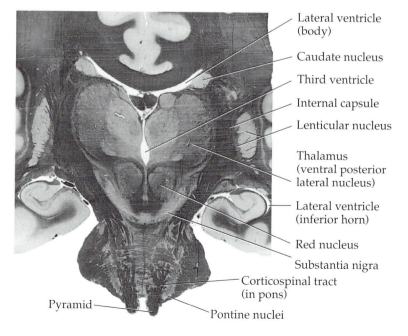

Lateral ventricle (body)

Caudate nucleus

Third ventricle

Internal capsule

Lenticular nucleus

Thalamus (ventral posterior lateral nucleus)

Lateral ventricle (inferior horn)

Red nucleus

Substantia nigra

Corticospinal tract (in pons)

Pyramid

Pontine nuclei

Box 3–1. *The Major Deep Structures Are Revealed on Magnetic Resonance Imaging (MRI) Scans*

Routine MRI of the nervous system reveals the proton constituents of neural tissues and fluids; most of the protons are contained in water. Protons in different tissue and fluid compartments, when placed in a strong **magnetic field**, have slightly different properties. MRI takes advantage of such differences to construct an image of brain structure or even function.

MRI relies on the simple property that protons can be made to emit signals that reflect the local tissue environment. Hence, protons in different tissues or fluids emit different signals. This is done by exciting protons with low levels of energy, which is carried by electromagnetic waves emitted from a coil placed over the tissue. Once excited, protons emit a signal that has three components, or parameters. These signals depend on tissue charactersitics. The first parameter is related to the **density of protons** (i.e., primarily water content) in the tissue. The second and third parameters are related to proton **relaxation times**; that is, the times it takes protons to return to the energy state they were in before excitation by electromagnetic waves. The two relaxation times are termed T1 and T2. **T1 relaxation time** (or spin–lattice relaxation time) is related to the overall tissue environment and T2 relaxation time (or spin–spin relaxation time), to interactions between

protons. The MRI signal, which is used to generate the image, reflects these three parameters. When an image is generated, it can be made to be dominated by one of these parameters. This differential dependence is accomplished by fine-tuning the electromagnetic waves that are used to excite the tissue. The choice of whether to have an image reflect proton density, T1 relaxation time, or T2 relaxation time depends on the purpose of the image. For example, in **T2-weighted images**, which are dominated by T2 relaxation time, watery constituents of the brain produce a stronger signal than fatty constituents (e.g., white matter). These images can be used to distinguish an edematous region of the white matter from a normal region.

Four constituents of the central nervous system are distinguished using MRI: cerebrospinal fluid, blood, white matter, and gray matter. The exact appearance of these central nervous system constituents depends on whether the image reflects proton density, T1 relaxation time, or T2 relaxation time. The images shown in Figure 3–14 reflect T2 relaxation times. The signals produced by protons in cerebrospinal fluid are strong and, on this image, cerebrospinal fluid is shaded white. Cerebrospinal fluid in the ventricles and overlying the brain surface, in the subarachnoid space, has the same bright appearance. On

the other hand, protons in blood in arteries and veins produce a weak signal and these tissue constituents appear black. The weak signal in blood derives from two factors: tissue motion (i.e., nonstatic blood flow) and the presence of hemoglobin, an iron-containing protein that attenuates the MRI signal because of its paramagnetic properties. The gray and white matter are also distinct because their protons emit signals of slightly different strengths. On these T2-weighted images, white matter appears darker than gray matter.

The imaging planes are shown in the inset. The plane of the horizontal MRI scan (Figure 3–14A) is close to that of the section shown in Figure 3–12, and for the coronal image (Figure 3–14B) is similar to the plane of section in Figure 13–13. The major deep structures, the thalamus, striatum, lenticular nucleus, and internal capsule can all be seen on these images. In fact, on this type of image the subcortical white matter does not appear homogeneous. Portions, including the internal capsule and the visual pathway, are darker. The weak signal produced by these parts of the white matter is due to the presence of iron (probably as ferritin), which attenuates the MRI signal (Figure 3–14A). Neurons and axons in the red nucleus (Figure 3–14B) also contain iron and this nucleus appears dark.

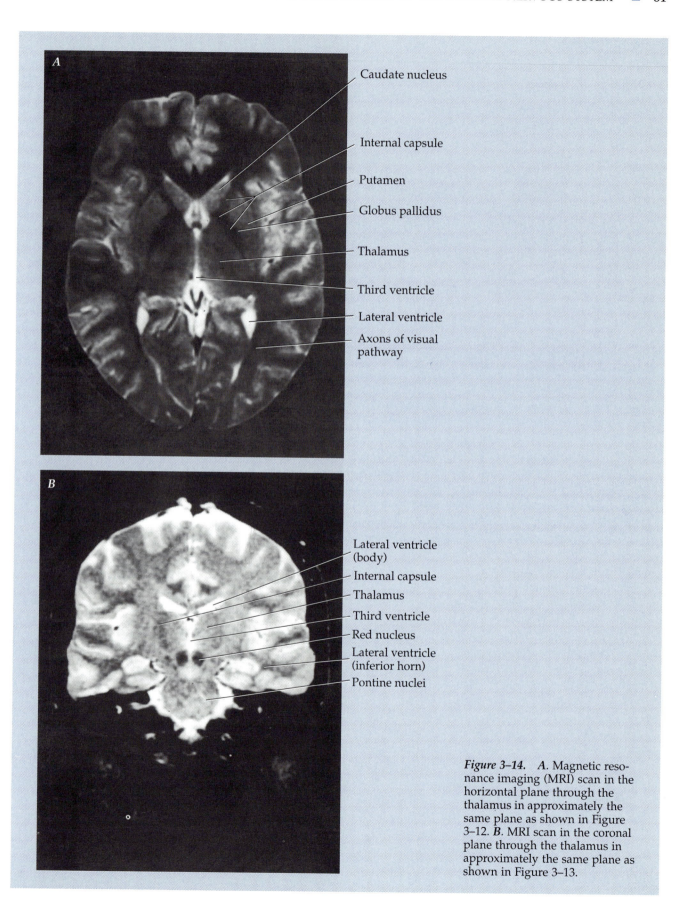

Caudate nucleus

Internal capsule

Putamen

Globus pallidus

Thalamus

Third ventricle

Lateral ventricle

Axons of visual
pathway

Lateral ventricle
(body)

Internal capsule

Thalamus

Third ventricle

Red nucleus

Lateral ventricle
(inferior horn)

Pontine nuclei

Figure 3–14. **A.** Magnetic resonance imaging (MRI) scan in the horizontal plane through the thalamus in approximately the same plane as shown in Figure 3–12. **B.** MRI scan in the coronal plane through the thalamus in approximately the same plane as shown in Figure 3–13.

brain, the locations of these structures are revealed on magnetic resonance imaging (MRI) scans (Box 3–1; see Figure 3–14).

Cerebral Cortex Neurons Are Organized Into Layers

The dorsal column–medial lemniscal system projects to the cerebral cortex, which is also the origin of the corticospinal tract. Its neurons are organized into discrete layers (Figure 3–15). Lamination is a feature of all cortical regions, although different cortical regions characteristically contain different numbers of layers. Most of the cerebral cortex contains at least six cell layers; this cortex is termed **isocortex**. Because isocortex dominates the cerebral cortex of phylogenetically higher vertebrates, such as mammals, it is also called **neocortex** (Figure 3–15A). Cortex with fewer than six layers is termed **allocortex** (Figure 3–15B). There are two major types of allocortex: **paleocortex** and **archicortex**, as well as various transitional forms with characteristics of both isocortex and allocortex. Although present in higher vertebrates, allocortex dominates the cortex of more primitive vertebrates, such as reptiles and amphibians. In higher vertebrates, paleocortex mediates the sense of smell as well as emotions, and archicortex, memories. In the human brain, approximately 95 percent of the cortex is neocortex and 5 percent, allocortex. The type of allocortex shown in Figure 3–15B is archicortex, which comprises the hippocampal formation. It contains only three cell layers. Here, we consider further the neocortex, because this is the type of cortex that comprises the major sensory, motor, and association areas. The paleocortical areas mediating olfaction are considered further in Chapter 8 and the archicortical areas mediating memory, in Chapter 15.

Each region of neocortex that subserves a different function has its own microscopic anatomy: the thickness of the six principal neocortical cell layers varies, as does the density of neurons in each layer. Areas that subserve sensation (e.g., primary visual cortex) have a thick layer 4 (Figure 3–16). This is the layer to which most thalamic neurons from the sensory

Figure 3–15. The neocortex *(A)* has six cell layers and the allocortex *(B)* has fewer than six layers. The drawing of a Nissl-stained section through the neocortex of the human brain is semischematic. The section through allocortex is of a portion of the hippocampal formation. This is archicortex and it has three cell layers. (*A*, Adapted from Brodmann, K. 1909. Vergleichende Lokalisationslehre der Grosshirnrinde in ihren Prinzipien dargestellt auf Grund des Zellenbaues. Leipzig: Barth.)

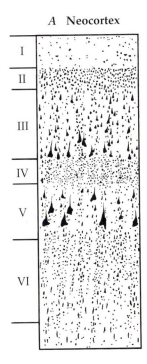

A **Neocortex**

I
II
III
IV
V
VI

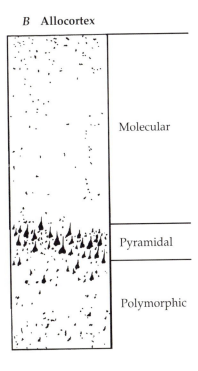

B **Allocortex**

Molecular

Pyramidal

Polymorphic

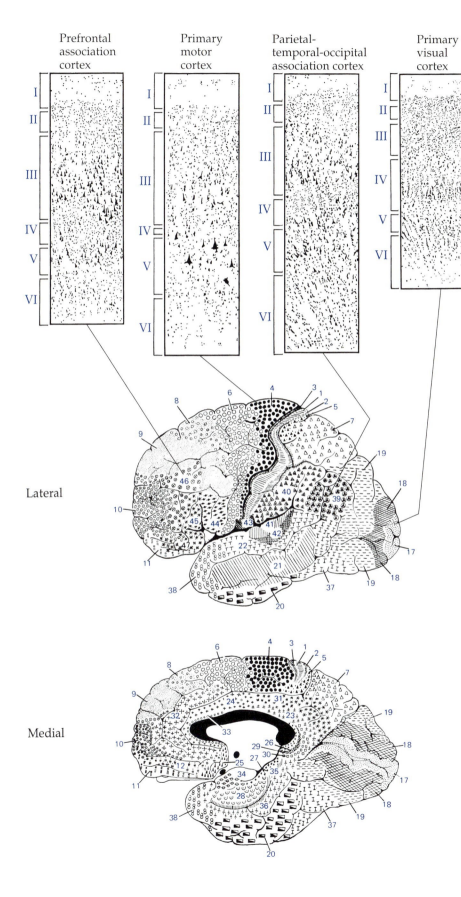

Prefrontal
association
cortex

Primary
motor
cortex

Parietal-
temporal-occipital
association cortex

Primary
visual
cortex

Lateral

Medial

Figure 3–16. Different regions of the cerebral cortex have a different cytoarchitecture. (*Top*) Nissl-stained sections through various portions of the cerebral cortex. (Adapted from Campbell, 1905.) (*Bottom*) Brodmann's cytoarchitectonic areas of the cerebral cortex. (Adapted from Brodmann, K. 1909. Vergleichende Lokalisationslehre der Grosshirnrinde in ihren Prinzipien dargestellt auf Grund des Zellenbaues. Leipzig: Barth, and Campbell, A. W. 1905. Histological Studies on the Localization of Cerebral Function. New York: Cambridge University Press.)

relay nuclei project. In contrast, the primary motor cortex has a thin layer 4 and a thick layer 5 (Figure 3–16). Layer 5 contains the neurons that project to the spinal cord, via the corticospinal tract. Association areas of the cerebral cortex, such as prefrontal and parietal–temporal–occipital association cortex, have a morphology that is intermediate between those of sensory cortex and motor cortex (Figure 3–16).

The Cytoarchitectonic Map of the Cerebral Cortex Is the Basis for a Map of Cortical Function

Based primarily on differences in the thickness of cortical layers and on the sizes and shapes of neurons, the German anatomist Korbinian Brodmann identified almost 50 divisions (now termed **Brodmann's areas**; Figure 3–16, bottom). These divisions are based only on the neuronal architecture, or **cytoarchitecture**, of the cortex, such as the size and shapes of neurons in the different laminae and their packing densities. It is remarkable that research on the functions of the cerebral cortex has shown that different functional areas of the cortex have a different cytoarchitecture. In humans, by noting the particular behavioral changes that follow discrete cortical lesions and using functional imaging approaches, such as positron emission tomography (PET; see Figure 1–18) and MRI, we have some insight into the functions of most of the cytoarchitectonic divisions identified by Brodmann (Table 3–2).

Neurons in the Brain Stem and Basal Forebrain Have Diffuse Projections and Regulate Central Nervous System Neuronal Excitability

Despite their vast numbers, most neurons in the mature brain have projections limited to a single central nervous system division or a restricted portion of the cerebral cortex. There are three major exceptions; the first two were considered earlier in this chapter, neurons of the reticular formation and those in diffuse-projecting thalamic nuclei. The third exception consists of groups of neurons in the basal forebrain and brain stem. Neurons in each group use a particular neurotransmitter. Because the projections of neurons in each of these groups can be so diffuse and the locations of the cell bodies somewhat dispersed, we characterize the systems on the basis of the neurotransmitter used.

There are four major neurotransmitter-specific projection systems, which use acetylcholine, dopamine, norepinephrine, and serotonin. Many of the neurons that use one of these neurotransmitters also contain other neuroactive compounds, such as neuropeptides, that are released at the synapse along with the particular neurotransmitter. We are beginning to unravel the postsynaptic actions of the various chemicals released by these systems. Some neuroactive compounds have prolonged actions on neurons and are therefore effective in regulating the long-term excitability of neurons, whereas others have more abbreviated effects for regulating short-term excitability. We are also beginning to discover that some of these compounds can affect metabolic and other functions of neurons by altering the expression of particular genes. Most portions of the central nervous system receives input from one or more of these systems.

Neurons in the Basal Nucleus of Meynert Contain Acetylcholine

The axons of acetylcholine-containing neurons at the base of the cerebral hemispheres project throughout the neocortex and the allocortex. Figure 3–17A shows the projection pattern of the system containing acetyl-

Table 3–2. Brodmann's areas.

Brodmann area	Functional area	Location	Function
1, 2, 3	Primary somatic sensory cortex	Postcentral gyrus	Touch
4	Primary motor cortex	Precentral gyrus	Voluntary movement control
5	Tertiary somatic sensory cortex; posterior parietal association area	Superior parietal lobule	Sterognosia
6	Supplementary motor cortex; supplementary eye field; premotor cortex; frontal eye fields	Precentral gyrus and rostral adjacent cortex	Limb and eye movement planning
7	Posterior parietal association area	Superior parietal lobule	Visuomotor; perception
8	Frontal eye fields	Superior, middle frontal gyri, medial frontal lobe	Saccadic eye movements
9, 10, 11, 12	Prefrontal association cortex; frontal eye fields	Superior, middle frontal gyri, medial frontal lobe	Thought, cognition, movement planning
17[1]	Primary visual cortex	Banks of calcarine fissure	Vision
18	Secondary visual cortex	Medial and lateral occipital gyri	Vision; depth
19	Tertiary visual cortex, middle temporal visual area	Medial and lateral occipital gyri	Vision, color, motion, depth
20	Visual inferotemporal area	Inferior temporal gyrus	Form vision
21	Visual inferotemporal area	Middle temporal gyrus	Form vision
22	Higher-order auditory cortex	Superior temporal gyrus	Hearing, speech
23, 24, 25, 26, 27	Limbic association cortex	Cingulate gyrus, subcallosal area, retrosplenial area, and parahippocampal gyrus	Emotions
28	Primary olfactory cortex; limbic association cortex	Parahippocampal gyrus	Smell, emotions
29, 30, 31, 32, 33	Limbic association cortex	Cingulate gyrus and retrosplenial area	Emotions
34, 35, 36	Primary olfactory cortex; limbic association cortex	Parahippocampal gyrus	Smell, emotions
37	Parietal–temporal–occipital association cortex; middle temporal visual area	Middle and inferior temporal gyri at junction temporal and occipital lobes	Perception, vision, reading, speech
38	Primary olfactory cortex; limbic association cortex	Temporal pole	Smell, emotions
39	Parietal–temporal–occipital association cortex	Inferior parietal lobule (angular gyrus)	Perception, vision, reading, speech
40	Parietal–temporal–occipital association cortex	Inferior parietal lobule (supramarginal gyrus)	Perception, vision, reading, speech
41	Primary auditory cortex	Heschl's gyri and superior temporal gyrus	Hearing
42	Secondary auditory cortex	Heschl's gyri and superior temporal gyrus	Hearing
43	Gustatory cortex (?)	Insular cortex, frontoparietal operculum	Taste
44	Broca's area; lateral premotor cortex	Inferior frontal gyrus (frontal operculum)	Speech, movement planning
45	Prefrontal association cortex	Inferior frontal gyrus (frontal operculum)	Thought, cognition, planning behavior
46	Prefrontal association cortex (dorsolateral prefrontal cortex)	Middle frontal gyrus	Thought, cognition, planning behavior, aspects of eye movement control
47	Prefrontal association cortex	Inferior frontal gyrus (frontal operculum)	Thought, cognition, planning behavior

[1]Areas 13, 14, 15, and 16 are part of the insular cortex.

A

Medial septal nucleus and nucleus of diagonal band

To neocortex

To hippocampus

Basal nucleus (of Meynert)

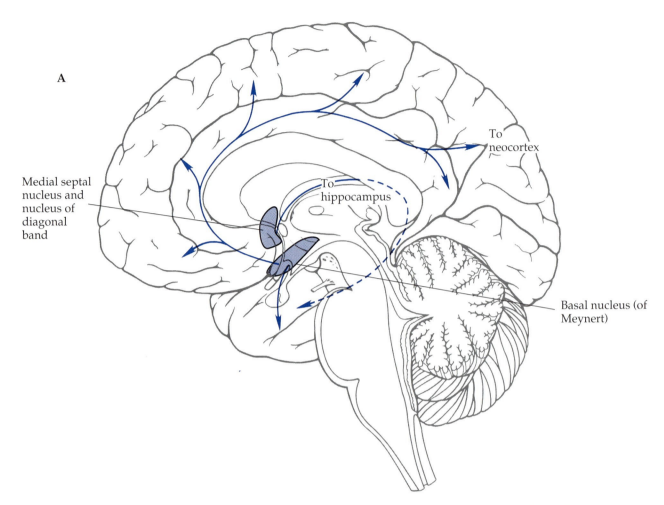

Figure 3–17. Groups of brain stem and forebrain neurons have diffuse projections throughout the central nervous system. *A*. Schematic illustration of the diffuse projection pattern of acetylcholine-containing neurons in the basal nucleus (of Meynert), septal nuclei, and nucleus of the diagonal band (of Broca). Many of the axons projecting to the hippocampal formation course in the fornix (*dashed line*). *B1*. Dopamine-containing neurons in the substantia nigra and ventral tegmental area. *B2*. Norepinephrine-containing neurons in the locus ceruleus. *B3*. Serotonin-containing neurons of the raphe nuclei.

choline. The **basal nucleus (of Meynert)** contains the cholinergic neurons that project to the neocortex (Figure 3–17A), both on the medial surface (e.g., the cingulate gyrus) and laterally (not shown in Figure 3–17A). The cholinergic projection to the allocortex, located medially in the temporal lobe, originates from neurons that are located medial to those in the basal nucleus (Figure 3–17A). These medial neurons are in the medial septal nucleus, near the septum pellucidum (Figure AII-23), and the nucleus of the diagonal band (of Broca). In **Alzheimer's disease**, a neurological disease in which individuals lose memories and cognitive functions, these cholinergic neurons degenerate.

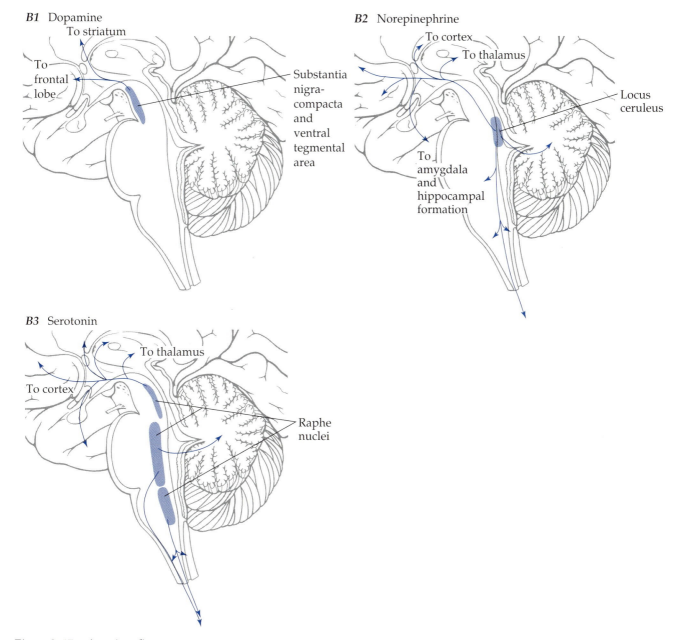

Figure 3–17. (continued)

The Substantia Nigra and Ventral Tegmental Area Contain Dopaminergic Neurons

More is known of the clinical consequences of damage to brain dopamine systems than of the other neurotransmitter-specific systems. The cells of origin of the dopaminergic system are located mostly in the midbrain (Figure 3–17B1), in the **substantia nigra** and **ventral tegmental area**; the major targets of these dopaminergic neurons are the striatum and portions of the frontal lobe. In **Parkinson's disease**, for example, there is a loss of the dopamine-containing neurons. Voluntary movements are dramatically slowed and patients develop a tremor (see Chapter 11). By replacing dopamine in these patients with a drug that acts like dopamine, movement control is improved.

The Locus Ceruleus Gives Rise to a Projection That Uses Norepinephrine

Although there are numerous brain stem nuclei with norepinephrine-containing neurons (Figure 3–17B2), the **locus ceruleus** has the most widespread projections. Based on the projection patterns and the physiological properties of locus ceruleus neurons, this noradrenergic projection is thought to play an important role in the response of the brain to stressful stimuli. The locus ceruleus, through its widespread noradrenergic projections to the cerebral cortex, has been implicated in depression and the anxiety disorder, panic attacks. Additional noradrenergic cell groups are located in the caudal pons and medulla (not shown in figure); these neurons are critically involved in maintaining the function of the sympathetic nervous system, especially in blood pressure regulation.

Neurons of the Raphe Nuclei Use Serotonin as Their Neurotransmitter

The **raphe nuclei** (Figure 3–17B3) consist of numerous distinct groups of brain stem neurons that are located close to the midline. They give rise to an ascending and descending projection. The ascending projection is targeted to the diencephalon and telencephalon and arises predominantly from the raphe nuclei that are located in the midbrain and rostral pons. Dysfunction of this ascending serotonergic projection has been implicated in certain mood disorders. The descending projection terminates in the medulla, cerebellum, and spinal cord and arises mainly from the raphe nuclei in the caudal pons and medulla. One function of the descending spinal serotonergic projections to the medulla and spinal cord is to control the transmission of information about pain from the periphery to the central nervous system.

Summary

Spinal Cord Organization

The spinal cord, the most caudal of the major central nervous system divisions, has a central region that contains predominantly cell bodies of neurons (gray matter), surrounded by a region that contains mostly myelinated axons (white matter) (Figures 3–2 and 3–3). Both of these regions can be further subdivided. The **dorsal horn** of the gray matter subserves somatic sensation and the **ventral horn**, skeletal motor function. The **intermediate zone** (Figure 3–2A) integrates sensory and motor functions and contains **autonomic preganglionic neurons**. The **dorsal column** of the white matter carries somatic sensory information to the brain, the **lateral** and **ventral columns** carry both sensory and motor information (Figure 3–2). The spinal cord is **segmented** (Figure 3–4) and the sizes and shapes of the gray and white matter are different for the various segments.

Brain Stem Organization

The caudal medulla (Figure 3–6C) is similar in its organization to the spinal cord. At a more rostral level (Figure 3–6B) the medulla contains nuclei on its dorsal surface that subserve tactile sensation—the **dorsal column nuclei**—and a pathway on its ventral surface that subserves voluntary movement—the corticospinal tract—which is located in the

pyramid. The **medial lemniscus** is located dorsal to the pyramid. At the level of the **inferior olivary nucleus** (Figure 3–6A), the fourth ventricle forms the dorsal surface of the medulla. The pons (Figure 3–7) contains nuclei in its ventral portion, the **pontine nuclei**, that transfer information from the cerebral cortex to the cerebellum. The midbrain (Figure 3–8) contains the **colliculi** on its dorsal surface and the motor pathway on its ventral surface, **basis pedunculi** (Figures 3–5B and 3–8). The **cranial nerves** (see Table 2–3; Figure 3–5) enter and exit from each division of the brain stem.

Organization of Diencephalon and Cerebral Hemispheres

The **diencephalon** and the **cerebral hemisphere** have a more complex organization than that of the brain stem or spinal cord. The **thalamus**, which relays information from subcortical structures to the cerebral cortex, contains two different functional classes of nuclei: **relay** and **diffuse-projecting**. Three of the four main **anatomical** divisions of the thalamus (Figure 3–9) serve relay functions (Table 3–2): (1) **anterior nuclei**, (2) **medial nuclei**, and (3) **lateral nuclei**. The fourth main anatomical division of the thalamus, **intralaminar nuclei**, contains diffuse-projecting nuclei. The anatomical divisions are based on the spatial location of nuclei with respect to the **internal medullary lamina**, bands of myelinated fibers in the thalamus. There is a **topographic relation** between the projections of the different thalamic nuclei and the cerebral cortex (Figure 3–10). Thalamocortical projections (as well as descending cortical projections) course through the **internal capsule** (Figures 3–11 and 3–12).

Two types of cortex are identified, based on the number of cell layers. **Neocortex** (or isocortex) has **six layers** (Figures 3–15A and 3–16), and the different layers have different thicknesses depending on the function of the particular cortical area. **Allocortex** (Figure 3–15B) has fewer than **six layers** and consists mainly of the **archicortex** of the **hippocampal formation** and the **paleocortex** of the **olfactory regions**. Based on cortical layering patterns as well as the sizes and shapes of cortical neurons, or **cytoarchitecture**, about 50 different areas of the cerebral cortex have been identified (Figure 3–16; Table 3–2). These are termed **Brodmann's areas**.

Diffuse-projecting Neurotransmitter-specific Systems

Four neurotransmitter-specific systems have diffuse projections throughout the central nervous system. **Cholinergic** neurons (1) in the **basal nucleus of Meynert**, on the ventral telencephalic surface, and in neurons on the ventromedial telencephalic surface project throughout the neocortex and allocortex (Figure 3–17A). Midbrain **dopaminergic** neurons (2), located mostly in the **substantia nigra** and **ventral tegmental area**, project to the basal ganglia and frontal lobes (Figure 3–17B1). The **locus ceruleus** (3) contains **norepinephrine** and projects throughout all central nervous system divisions (Figure 3–17B2). The **raphe nuclei** (4) contain **serotonin** and have ascending projections to the cerebral hemispheres and diencephalon and descending projections to the spinal cord (Figure 3–17B3). ■

KEY STRUCTURES AND TERMS

ascending pathway
   relay nucleus
   dorsal column–medial lemniscal
      system
descending pathway
   corticospinal tract
spinal cord
   dorsal root ganglion cells
   dorsal roots
   ventral root
   dorsal column
   lateral column
   ventral column
   dorsal horn
   intermediate zone
   ventral horn
   knee-jerk reflex
   cervical enlargement
   lumbosacral enlargement
brain stem tectum
brain stem tegmentum

brain stem base
medulla
   dorsal column nucleus
   dorsal column tubercles
   medial lemniscus
   pyramid
   pyramidal (motor) decussation
   inferior olivary nucleus (olive)
pons
   pontine nuclei
midbrain
   periaqueductal gray
   colliculi
   substantia nigra
   red nucleus
   basis pedunculi
   cerebral peduncle
thalamus
   internal medullary laminae
thalamic nuclei
   relay nuclei

ventral posterior
ventral lateral
ventral anterior
pulvinar
lateral posterior
anterior
medial dorsal
diffuse-projecting nuclei
   intralaminar nuclei
   reticular nucleus
Brodmann's areas
neurotransmitter-specific diffuse-
      projecting systems
   basal nucleus of Meynert
      (acetylcholine)
   raphe nuclei (serotonin)
   locus ceruleus (norepinephrine)
   substantia nigra (dopamine)
   ventral tegmental area (dopamine)

Selected Readings

Brodal, A. 1981. Neurological Anatomy. New York: Oxford University Press.

Jones, E. G. 1985. The Thalamus. New York: Plenum Press.

Kandel, E. R., Schwartz, J. H., and Jessell, T. M. (eds.) 1991. Principles of Neural Science, 3rd ed. New York: Elsevier.

Sigal, R., Doyon, D., Halimi, P., and Atlan, H. 1988. Magnetic Resonance Imaging. Berlin: Springer-Verlag.

References

Brodmann, K. 1909. Vergleichende Lokalisationslehre der Grosshirnrinde in ihren Prinzipien dargestellt auf Grund des Zellenbaues. Leipzig: Barth.

Campbell, A. W. 1905. Histological Studies on the Localisation of Cerebral Function. New York: Cambridge University Press.

Carpenter, M. B., and Sutin, J. 1983. Human Neuroanatomy. Baltimore: Williams & Wilkins.

Gorman, D. G., and Unützer, J. 1993. Brodmann's missing numbers. Neurology 43:226–227.

Hassler, R. 1982. Architectonic organization of the thalamic nuclei. In Shaltenbrand, G., and Warhen, W. W. (eds), Stereotaxy of the Human Brain. New York: G. Thieme Verlag, pp. 140–180.

Hirai, T., and Jones, E. G. 1989. A new parcellation of the human thalamus on the basis of histochemical staining. Brain Res. Rev. 14:1–34.

Jones, E. G. 1984. Organization of the thalamocortical complex and its relation to sensory processes. In Darian-Smith, I. (ed.), Handbook of Physiology, Section 1: The Nervous System, Vol. III. Sensory Processes. Bethesda, Md.: American Physiological Society, pp. 149–212.

Nieuwenhuys, R., Voogd, J., van Huijzen, C. 1988. The Human Central Nervous System: A Synopsis and Atlas, 3rd ed. Berlin: Springer-Verlag.

Pearson, J., Halliday, G., Sakamoto, N., Michel, J.-P. 1990. Catecholaminergic neurons. In Paxinos, G. (ed.), The Human Nervous System. San Diego: Academic Press, pp. 1023–1049.

Rexed, B. 1952. The cytoarchitectonic organization of the spinal cord in the cat. J. Comp. Neurol. 96:415–495.

Saper, C. 1990. Cholinergic system. In Paxinos, G. (ed.), The Human Nervous System. San Diego: Academic Press, pp. 1095–1113.

Saper, C. B. 1987. Diffuse cortical projection systems: Anatomical organization and role in cortical function. In Plum, F. (ed.), Handbook of Physiology. The Nervous System, Vol. V. Bethesda, Md.: American Physiological Society, pp. 169–210.

Törk, I., Hornung, J.-P. 1990. Raphe nuclei and the serotonergic system. In Paxinos, G. (ed.), The Human Nervous System. San Diego: Academic Press, pp. 1001–1022.

Zilles, K. 1990. Cortex. In Paxinos, G. (ed.), The Human Nervous System. San Diego: Academic Press, pp. 757–802.

4

Vasculature of the Central Nervous System and the Cerebrospinal Fluid

BRAIN VASCULATURE DISORDERS CONSTITUTE A MAJOR CLASS of nervous system disease. One reason for this is that the principal source of nourishment for the central nervous system is glucose, and neither glucose nor oxygen is stored in appreciable amounts. Thus, when the blood supply of the central nervous system is interrupted, even briefly, brain functions become severely disrupted.

Much of what we know about the arterial supply to the different parts of the central nervous system derives from three approaches. First, colored dye can be injected into a blood vessel in fixed, post mortem tissue, enabling us to see the areas supplied by the vessel. Second, in post mortem tissue or on radiological examination, one can infer which portion of the central nervous system is supplied by an artery by observing the extent of damage that occurs when the artery is occluded or ruptures. Third, **cerebral angiography** allows us to view the arterial and venous circulation radiologically, in the living brain. This important clinical tool permits localization of a vascular obstruction or other pathology.

In this chapter, we examine the blood supply of the central nervous system. Initially, we focus on arteries because of the importance of oxygenated blood to normal brain function. Next, we briefly consider venous drainage. Finally, we examine a related topic, the blood–brain barrier and the cerebrospinal fluid.

The Vertebral and Carotid Arteries Supply Blood to the Central Nervous System

The principal blood supply of the brain comes from two arterial systems that receive blood from different systemic arteries: the **anterior circulation**, fed by the **internal carotid arteries**, and the **posterior circulation**, which receives blood from the **vertebral arteries** (Figure 4–1, inset). The vertebral arteries join at the junction of the medulla and pons to form the **basilar artery**, which lies unpaired along the midline (Figure 4–1). The anterior circulation is also called the **carotid circulation**, and the posterior

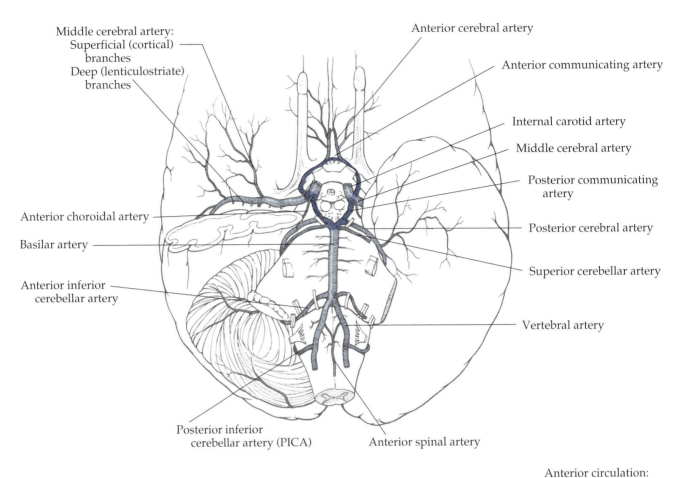

Middle cerebral artery:
Superficial (cortical) branches
Deep (lenticulostriate) branches

Anterior cerebral artery

Anterior communicating artery

Internal carotid artery

Middle cerebral artery

Posterior communicating artery

Anterior choroidal artery

Posterior cerebral artery

Basilar artery

Superior cerebellar artery

Anterior inferior cerebellar artery

Vertebral artery

Posterior inferior cerebellar artery (PICA)

Anterior spinal artery

Figure 4–1. Diagram of the ventral surface of the brain stem and cerebral hemispheres illustrating the key components of the anterior (carotid) circulation and the posterior (vertebral–basilar) circulation. The anterior portion of the temporal lobe of the right hemisphere is removed to illustrate the course of the middle cerebral artery through the lateral (Sylvian) fissure and the penetrating branches (lenticulostriate arteries). The circle of Willis (dark blue) is formed by the anterior communicating artery, the two posterior communicating arteries, and the three cerebral arteries. The inset (*right*) shows the extracranial and cranial courses of the vertebral, basilar, and carotid arteries.

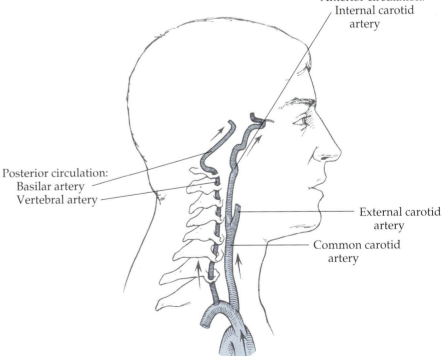

Anterior circulation:
Internal carotid artery

Posterior circulation:
Basilar artery
Vertebral artery

External carotid artery

Common carotid artery

circulation, the **vertebral–basilar circulation**. The anterior and posterior circulations are not independent, but are connected by networks of arteries on the cortical surface and on the ventral surface of the diencephalon and midbrain (see below).

Whereas the cerebral hemispheres receive blood from both the anterior and posterior circulations, the brain stem is supplied only from the posterior. The arterial supply of the spinal cord is provided by the systemic circulation and, to a lesser degree, by the vertebral arteries. Cerebral and spinal arteries drain into veins. Although spinal veins are part of the general systemic circulation, most cerebral veins drain first into the dural sinuses—a collection of large channels in the dura—before blood is returned to the major systemic veins.

The Spinal and Radicular Arteries Supply Blood to the Spinal Cord

The spinal cord receives blood from two sources. First are the **anterior** and **posterior spinal arteries** (Figure 4–1), branches of the vertebral arteries. Second are the **radicular arteries** (Figure 4–2), which are branches of segmental vessels, such as the cervical, intercostal, and lumbar. Neither anterior nor posterior spinal arteries typically form a single continuous

Figure 4–2. Schematic ventral (*left*) and dorsal (*right*) views of the spinal cord and brain stem are illustrated with the arterial circulation of the spinal cord. (Adapted from Carpenter, M. B., and Sutin, J. 1983. Human Neuroanatomy. Baltimore: Williams & Wilkins.)

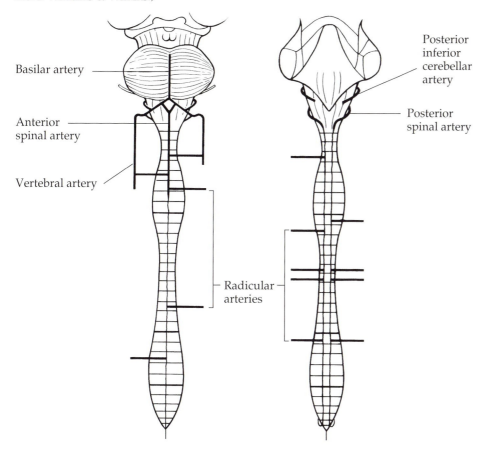

vessel along the entire length of the ventral or dorsal spinal cord. Rather, each forms a network of communicating channels that are oriented along the rostral–caudal axis of the spinal cord. The radicular arteries feed into this network along the entire length of the spinal cord.

Although both the spinal and radicular arteries supply blood to all spinal cord levels, different spinal cord segments are preferentially supplied by one or the other set of arteries. The cervical spinal cord, for example, is supplied primarily from the vertebral and radicular arteries (the ascending cervical artery). In contrast, the radicular arteries (the intercostal and lumbar arteries) nourish the thoracic, lumbar, and sacral segments. Particularly prominent is the **artery of Adamkiewicz**, the radicular artery that supplies the spinal cord segments that innervate the legs (lumbosacral enlargement).

When spinal cord segments are supplied by a single artery, they are particularly susceptible to injury after arterial occlusion. In contrast, segments that receive a redundant blood supply tend to fare better following such damage. Such redundant blood supply is termed **collateral circulation**. For example, individual rostral thoracic segments are supplied by fewer radicular arteries than more caudal segments. When a radicular artery that serves the rostral thoracic segments becomes occluded, serious damage is more likely to occur because there is no backup system for perfusion of oxygenated blood. Interrupting the blood supply to critical areas of the spinal cord can produce sensory and motor control impairments similar to those produced by traumatic mechanical injury, such as that resulting from an automobile accident. Collateral circulation also is key to understanding perfusion of the cerebral hemispheres (see below).

The Vertebral and Basilar Arteries Supply Blood to the Brain Stem

Each of the three major divisions of the brain stem and the cerebellum receives its arterial supply from the posterior circulation (Figure 4–3A). The medulla is nourished by the vertebral and spinal arteries, and the pons, by the basilar artery. In the medulla and pons, arterial branches perfuse regions of tissue that resemble wedge-shaped slices in transverse section (Figure 4–3B). The midbrain is supplied primarily by the posterior cerebral artery as well as the basilar artery. The cerebellum is supplied by branches of the vertebral and basilar arteries.

Even though the spinal arteries primarily supply the spinal cord, they also supply the caudal medulla. The spinal arteries lie close to the dorsal and ventral midline and nourish the most medial areas (Figure 4–3B3). The more lateral area is served by the vertebral arteries. At intermediate and rostral medullary levels, blood is supplied only by the vertebral arteries. Small branches exiting from the main artery supply the medial medulla, whereas the major laterally emerging branch from the vertebral artery, the **posterior inferior cerebellar artery** (PICA), nourishes the lateral region (Figure 4–3B2). The part of the medulla that is supplied by the posterior inferior cerebellar artery does not receive blood from any other artery. The absence of a collateral arterial supply makes this artery particularly important because occlusion almost always results is some damage to the dorsolateral medulla (Figure 4–3B2). When this occurs, patients commonly lose facial pain sensation on the side of the occlusion and sense of touch on the opposite side of the limbs and trunk. They may also become hoarse because of the loss of the motor neurons that innervate striated muscles of the larynx.

The vertebral arteries join to form the basilar artery at the pontomedullary junction. Three sets of branches of the **basilar artery** supply the pons: (1) paramedian, (2) short circumferential, and (3) long circumferential. The **paramedian branches** supply regions of the pons that are located close to the midline. The **short circumferential branches** supply lateral wedge-shaped regions, and the **long circumferential branches** supply the dorsolateral portions of the pons.

The dorsolateral portion of the caudal pons is supplied by a long circumferential branch of the basilar artery, termed the **anterior inferior cerebellar artery** (AICA). The region in the pons rostral to that supplied by the anterior inferior cerebellar artery is nourished by the **superior cerebellar artery**, another long circumferential branch of the basilar artery (Figure 4–3A).

Two sets of arteries nourish the midbrain: the basilar artery supplies the caudal midbrain and paired **posterior cerebral arteries**, the rostral midbrain. Proximal branches of each artery supply the base and tegmentum of the midbrain (see Figure 3–8). The tectum is primarily supplied by the posterior cerebral artery's more distal branches, as they course around the dorsolateral midbrain surface.

The cerebellum, like the three divisions of the brain stem, receives its blood supply from the posterior circulation. The **posterior inferior cerebellar artery** supplies the caudal portion of the cerebellum. More rostral portions of the cerebellum are supplied by the long circumferential branches of the basilar artery, the **anterior inferior cerebellar artery** and the **superior cerebellar artery** (Figures 4–1 and 4–3A).

The Anterior and Posterior Circulations Supply the Diencephalon and Cerebral Hemispheres

The three cerebral arteries supply the cerebral cortex, basal ganglia, and thalamus (Figures 4–4 through 4–7). Two of them, the **anterior cerebral** and **middle cerebral arteries**, are part of the anterior circulation; the third, the **posterior cerebral artery**, is part of the posterior circulation. In the embryo, the posterior cerebral artery derives from the anterior system, thereby receiving blood from the carotid arteries. But in maturity, much more blood comes from the basilar artery, making this artery functionally part of the posterior circulation.

These two arterial systems connect at two locations (see below; Figure 4–12): (1) at the terminal ends of the cerebral arteries on the convexity of the cerebral cortex (Figure 4–4A), and (2) on the ventral surface of the diencephalon and midbrain, where branches of the anterior and posterior circulations form a network of interconnected arteries, or an **anastomosis**, called the **circle of Willis** (Figure 4–1, dark blue). The connection of the two arterial systems becomes crucial in making up for reduced arterial perfusion when one system shuts down because of occlusion (see below).

In general, deep structures of the brain, for example, the basal ganglia and parts of the diencephalon, receive blood directly from branches of the internal carotid artery and the proximal portions of the cerebral arteries. In contrast, the gray matter of the cerebral cortex and the underlying white matter are supplied by branches of more distal portions of the cerebral arteries.

A

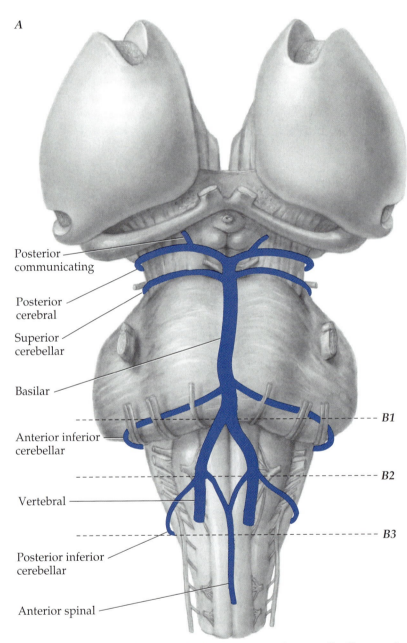

Posterior communicating

Posterior cerebral

Superior cerebellar

Basilar

- - - - - - - - - - - - - - - *B1*

Anterior inferior cerebellar

- - - - - - - - - - - - - - - *B2*

Vertebral

- - - - - - - - - - - - - - - *B3*

Posterior inferior cerebellar

Anterior spinal

Figure 4–3. ***A.*** Arterial circulation of the brain stem is schematically illustrated on a view of the ventral surface of the brain stem. ***B.*** Three transverse sections through the brain stem, illustrating wedge-shaped regions supplied by different arteries: (1) pons, (2) rostral medulla, (3) caudal medulla.

B1

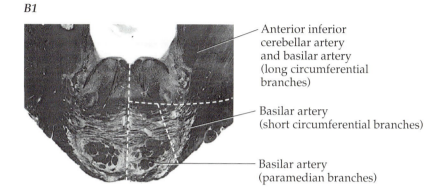

— Anterior inferior
cerebellar artery
and basilar artery
(long circumferential
branches)

— Basilar artery
(short circumferential branches)

— Basilar artery
(paramedian branches)

B2

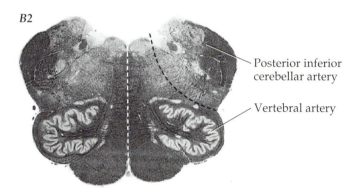

— Posterior inferior
cerebellar artery

— Vertebral artery

B3

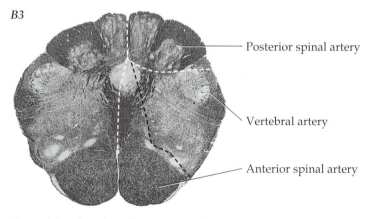

— Posterior spinal artery

— Vertebral artery

— Anterior spinal artery

Figure 4–3. (continued)

A

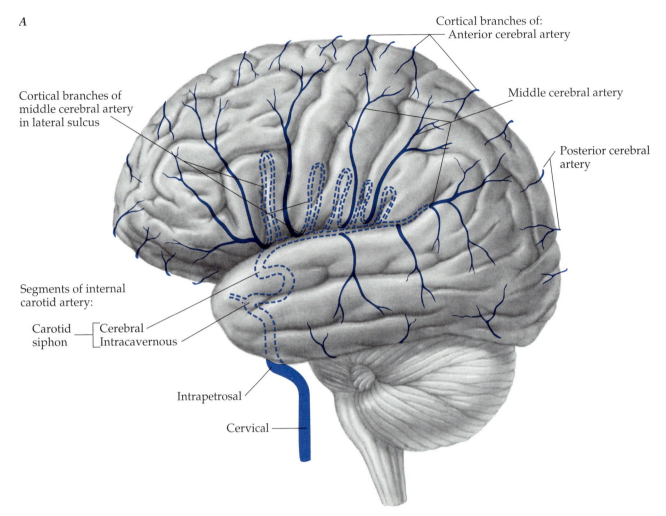

Cortical branches of:
Anterior cerebral artery

Middle cerebral artery

Posterior cerebral artery

Cortical branches of
middle cerebral artery
in lateral sulcus

Segments of internal
carotid artery:

Carotid
siphon — Cerebral
Intracavernous

Intrapetrosal

Cervical

Figure 4–4. The courses of the three cerebral arteries are illustrated in views of the lateral surface of the cerebral hemisphere *(A),* and the midsagittal surface *(B)*.

The Internal Carotid Artery Has Four Principal Portions

The **internal carotid artery** consists of four segments (Figure 4–4A). The **cervical segment** (1) extends from the bifurcation of the common carotid (into the external and internal carotid arteries; see Figure 4–1) to where it enters the carotid canal. The **intrapetrosal segment** (2) courses through the petrous portion of the temporal bone. The **intracavernous segment** (3) courses through the cavernous sinus, a venous structure overlying the sphenoid bone (see Figure 4-13B). The **cerebral segment** (4) extends to where the internal carotid artery bifurcates into the anterior and middle cerebral arteries. The intracavernous and cerebral portions form the **carotid siphon**.

We can observe cerebral vessels *in vivo* using **cerebral angiography**. First, radiopaque material is injected into either the anterior or the posterior arterial system. Then a series of skull x-ray films are taken in rapid repetition as the material circulates. Films obtained while the radiopaque material is within cerebral arteries are called angiograms. Films obtained later, after the radiopaque substance has reached the cerebral veins or the dural sinuses, are called venograms. The entire

B

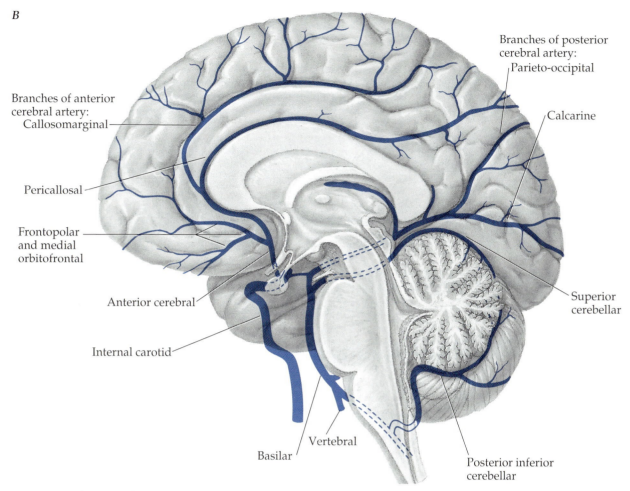

Branches of anterior
cerebral artery:
    Callosomarginal

Pericallosal

Frontopolar
and medial
orbitofrontal

Anterior cerebral

Internal carotid

Basilar

Vertebral

Branches of posterior
cerebral artery:
    Parieto-occipital

Calcarine

Superior
cerebellar

Posterior inferior
cerebellar

Figure 4–4. *(continued)*

course of the internal carotid artery is shown in cerebral angiograms in Figure 4–5. We can obtain images from different angles with respect to the cranium. Two views are common—from the side (lateral projection, Figure 4–5A) and from the front (frontal projection, Figure 4–5B). Box 4–1 shows how magnetic resonance imaging (MRI) can also be used to examine cerebral arteries.

Branches of the internal carotid artery supply cerebral and other cranial structures. The major branches of the **cerebral segment** of this artery (Figure 4–1), in caudal to rostral order, are: (1) the **ophthalmic artery**, which supplies the optic nerve and the inner portion of the retina, (2) the **posterior communicating artery**, which forms part of the circle of Willis and primarily nourishes diencephalic structures, and (3) the **anterior choroidal artery**, which supplies diencephalic and telencephalic structures. Intrapetrosal and intracavernous branches do not supply the central nervous system.

The Circle of Willis Is Formed by the Communicating and Cerebral Arteries

The internal carotid artery divides near the basal surface of the cerebral hemisphere to form the **anterior cerebral** and the **middle cerebral arteries** (Figures 4–1 and 4–4B). The **posterior cerebral artery** is part of the

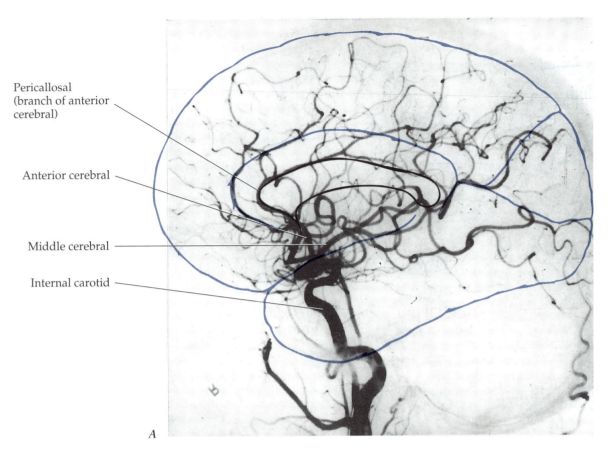

Pericallosal
(branch of anterior
cerebral)

Anterior cerebral

Middle cerebral

Internal carotid

A

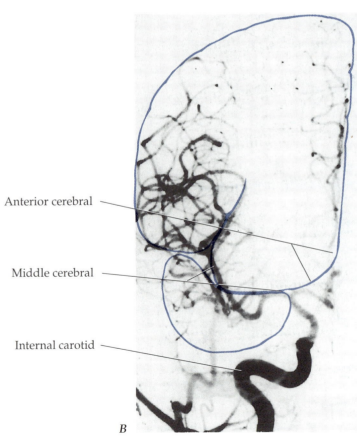

Anterior cerebral

Middle cerebral

Internal carotid

B

Figure 4–5. Cerebral angiograms of the anterior circulation are shown in a lateral projection (*A*) and a frontal projection (*B*). Overlaying each angiogram is a schematic drawing of the cerebral hemisphere, showing the approximate location of surface landmarks in relation to the arteries. (Angiograms courtesy of Dr. Neal Rutledge, University of Texas at Austin.)

Box 4–1. Magnetic Resonance Angiography

Cerebral angiography is an invasive procedure that involves intravascular injection of radio-opaque material. This material can produce neurological complications and therefore its use is not without risk. Recently, magnetic resonance imaging (MRI) has been applied to the study of brain vasculature because it can detect motion of water molecules. This application, termed **magnetic resonance angiography** (MRA), selectively images blood in motion (Figure 4–6). The entire cerebral circulation can be reconstructed from the locations of cerebral arteries or veins at multiple levels.

Figure 4–6A shows a dorsoventral reconstruction (i.e., as if looking up from the bottom). In this MRA the posterior communicating artery is present only on the left side. Part B shows an anteroposterior reconstruction (i.e., as if looking from front).

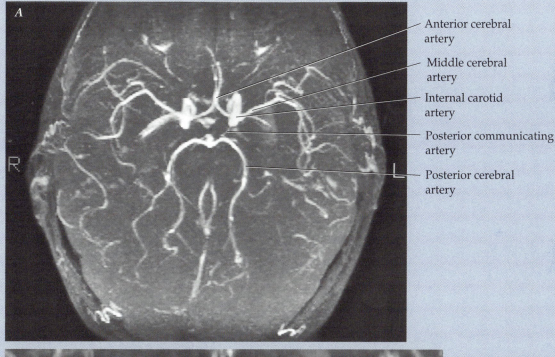

Anterior cerebral artery

Middle cerebral artery

Internal carotid artery

Posterior communicating artery

Posterior cerebral artery

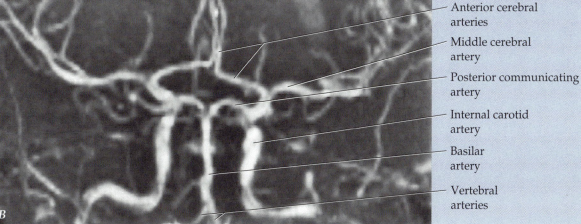

Anterior cerebral arteries

Middle cerebral artery

Posterior communicating artery

Internal carotid artery

Basilar artery

Vertebral arteries

Figure 4–6. Magnetic resonance angiogram.

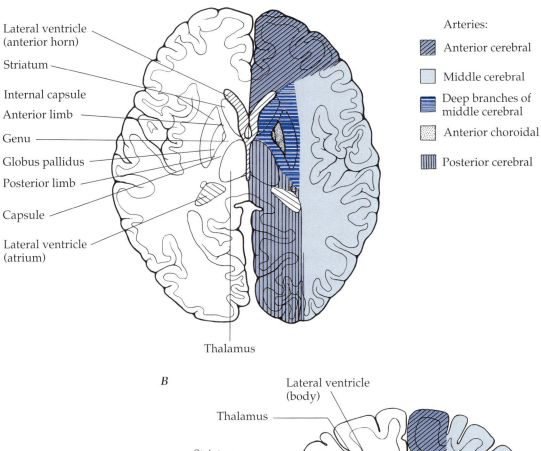

Figure 4–7. The arterial circulation of deep cerebral structures is illustrated in a schematic horizontal section (*A*) and a schematic coronal section (*B*). (Adapted from Fisher, C. M. 1975. Modern concepts of cerebrovascular disease. In Meyer, J. S. (ed.), The Anatomy and Pathology of the Cerebral Vasculature. New York: Spectrum Publications, pp. 1–41.)

vertebral–basilar system and originates at the bifurcation of the basilar artery at the midbrain (Figures 4–1 and 4–3A). These three cerebral arteries are interconnected by two communicating arteries. Together the proximal portions of the cerebral arteries and the communicating arteries form the **circle of Willis**. The **posterior communicating artery** (1) allows blood to flow between the middle and posterior cerebral arteries, and the **anterior communicating artery** (2) allows blood to flow between the anterior cerebral arteries on both sides of the cerebral hemispheres (Figure 4–1). The anterior communicating artery is the only artery of the circle of Willis that is unpaired. When either the posterior or anterior arterial circulation becomes occluded, collateral circulation may occur through the circle of Willis to rescue the region deprived of blood. Many individuals, however,

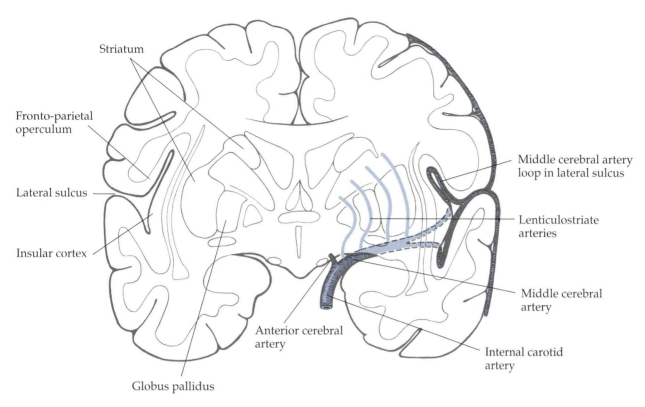

Striatum

Fronto-parietal
operculum

Lateral sulcus

Insular cortex

Middle cerebral artery
loop in lateral sulcus

Lenticulostriate
arteries

Middle cerebral
artery

Anterior cerebral
artery

Internal carotid
artery

Globus pallidus

Figure 4–8. The course of the middle cerebral artery through the lateral sulcus and along the insular and opercular surfaces of the cerebral cortex is shown in a schematic coronal section. (Adapted from DeArmond, S. J., Fusco, M. M., and Dewey, M. M. 1976. Structure of the Human Brain. New York: Oxford University Press.)

lack one of the components of the circle of Willis. In these individuals, a functional "circle" may not be achieved, resulting in incomplete cerebral perfusion by the surviving system.

Branches of the internal carotid artery and the proximal portions of the three cerebral arteries supply the diencephalon, basal ganglia, and internal capsule (Figures 4–7 and 4–8; Table 4–1). The **internal capsule**, which is the structure through which axons pass to and from the cerebral cortex (see Figure 3–11), contains three separate parts: the **anterior limb**, **genu**, and **posterior limb**. We will see in later chapters that axons with different functions course through the different components of the internal capsule. The different parts of the capsule also have a somewhat different arterial supply. The superior halves of the anterior and posterior limbs and the genu are supplied primarily by branches of the middle cerebral artery (Figure 4–7A). The inferior half of the internal capsule is supplied by the anterior cerebral (anterior limb) and choroidal arteries (posterior limb; Figure 4–7B). The inferior part of the genu is supplied by the anterior cerebral, middle cerebral artery, or posterior communicating artery. The **basal ganglia** also receive their arterial blood supply principally from the anterior choroidal artery and the middle cerebral artery (the lenticulostriate arteries) (Figures 4–7 and 4–8). The **thalamus** is nourished by branches of the posterior cerebral artery, posterior communicating artery, and the posterior choroidal artery. The **hypothalamus** is fed by branches of the anterior and posterior cerebral arteries and the posterior communicating artery.

Table 4–1. Blood supply of the central nervous system.

Brain division	Major artery
Spinal cord	Anterior, posterior spinal arteries, radicular arteries
Medulla	Vertebral
Pons	Basilar
Cerebellum	Vertebral, basilar
Midbrain	Basilar, posterior cerebral, anterior choroidal, posterior chorodial
Diencephalon	
Thalamus	Posterior communicating, posterior choroidal, posterior cerebral
Hypothalamus	Anterior cerebral, posterior communicating, posterior cerebral
Subthalamus	Anterior choroidal, posterior choroidal, posterior communicating, posterior cerebral
Basal ganglia	
Globus pallidus	Anterior choroidal
Striatum	Middle cerebral
Cerebral cortex	
Frontal lobe	Anterior cerebral
Parietal lobe	Anterior cerebral, middle cerebral
Occipital lobe	Posterior cerebral, middle cerebral
Temporal lobe	Middle cerebral, posterior cerebral, posterior choroidal
Internal capsule	
Anterior limb	Anterior cerebral, middle cerebral
Genu	Middle cerebral
Posterior limb	Middle cerebral, anterior choroidal
Retrolenticular	Anterior choroidal

Different Functional Areas of the Cerebral Cortex Are Supplied by Different Cerebral Arteries

The cerebral cortex is supplied by the distal branches of the anterior, middle, and posterior cerebral arteries (Figure 4–9). These branches are often termed "cortical" branches to differentiate from the deep branches supplying the diencephalon, basal ganglia, and internal capsule. The **anterior cerebral artery** is C-shaped, like many parts of the cerebral hemispheres. It originates where the internal carotid artery bifurcates, and courses within the sagittal fissure and around the rostral end (genu) of the corpus callosum (Figure 4–4B).

Knowledge of the approximate boundaries of the cortical regions that are supplied by the different cerebral arteries helps us understand the functional disturbances that follow vascular obstruction, or other pathology, of the cerebral vessels. As its gross distribution would suggest (Figure 4–4), the anterior artery supplies the dorsal and medial portions of the frontal and parietal lobes (Figure 4–9). The angiograms in Figure 4–5 illustrate the course of the anterior cerebral artery in the living brain. Its C-shape can be seen in the lateral view (A), and its position with respect to the midline is shown in the frontal view (B).

A

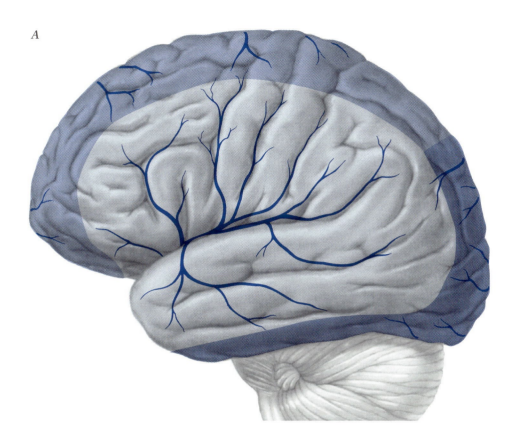

B

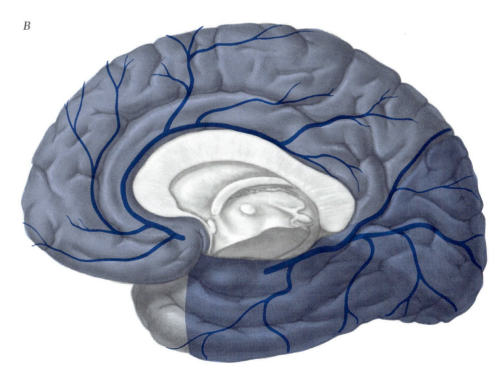

Figure 4–9. Cortical territories supplied by the anterior, middle, and posterior cerebral arteries are shown on lateral (*A*) and medial (*B*) views of the cerebral hemispheres. The distribution of the middle cerebral artery is indicated by light blue, the anterior cerebral artery by medium blue, and the posterior cerebral artery by dark blue.

The **middle cerebral artery** supplies blood to the lateral convexity of the cortex (Figure 4–9). The middle cerebral artery begins at the bifurcation of the internal carotid artery and takes an indirect course through the lateral sulcus (Figure 4–8), along the surface of the **insular cortex**, and over the inner opercular surface of the frontal, temporal, and parietal lobes. It finally emerges on the lateral convexity. This complex configuration of the middle cerebral artery can be seen in the angiograms in Figure 4–5. The rostrocaudal course of the middle cerebral artery, from the point at which it enters the lateral sulcus to the point at which it emerges and distributes over the lateral surface of the cerebral cortex, is revealed in Figure 4–5A. In Figure 4–5B, its course can be followed from medial to lateral. The middle cerebral artery forms loops at the dorsal junction of the insular cortex and the opercular surface of the frontal and parietal lobes (Figure 4–8). These loops serve as radiological landmarks that aid in estimating the position of the brain in relation to the skull.

The **posterior cerebral artery**, originating where the basilar artery bifurcates (Figures 4–1 and 4–3A), courses around the lateral margin of the midbrain. This artery supplies the occipital lobe and portions of the medial and inferior temporal lobe (Figure 4–9). A lateral view angiogram of the posterior circulation is shown in Figure 4–10. An angiogram of the posterior circulation is also shown in Figure 4–11. This view reveals the two vertebral arteries joining to form the basilar artery and the subsequent bifurcation of the basilar artery into the two posterior cerebral arteries.

Figure 4–10. Cerebral angiogram of the posterior circulation (lateral projection). The overlay drawing is a schematic illustration of the brain stem and cerebellum in relation to the distribution of the posterior circulation. (Angiogram courtesy of Dr. Neal Rutledge, University of Texas at Austin.)

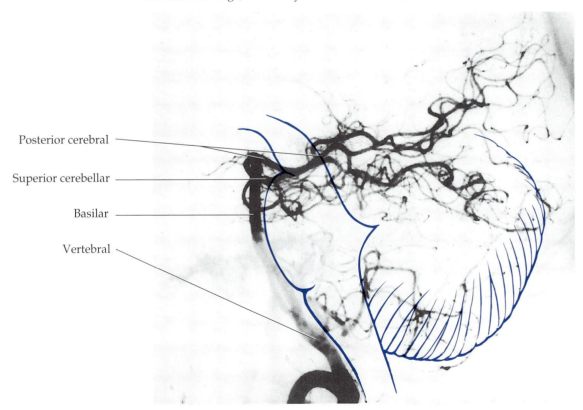

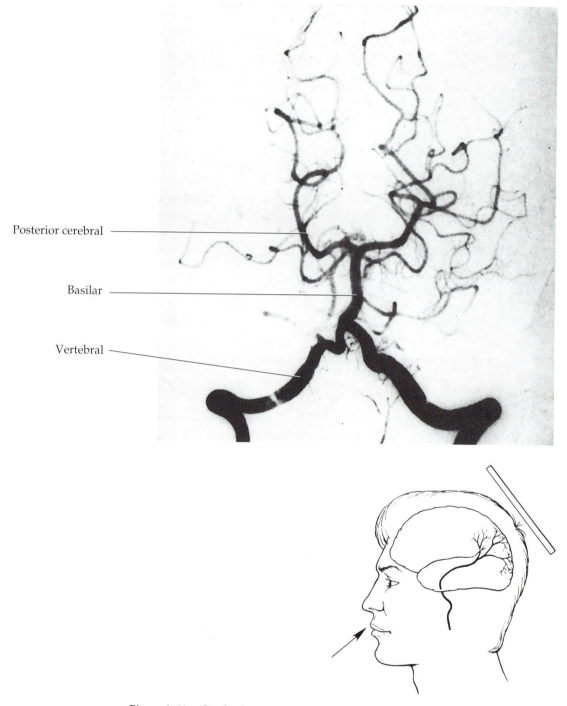

Posterior cerebral

Basilar

Vertebral

Figure 4–11. Cerebral angiogram of the posterior circulation, viewed anteriorly and inferiorly. The inset shows the head and selected cerebral vasculature on the left side (vertebral, basilar, and posterior cerebral arteries) in relation to the direction of transmitted x-rays and the imaging plane. (Angiogram courtesy of Dr. Neal Rutledge, University of Texas at Austin.)

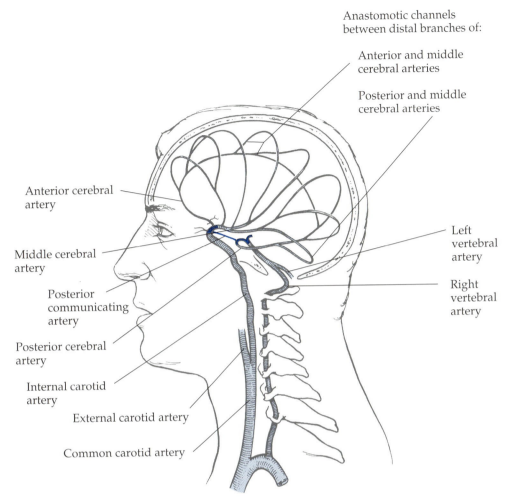

Anastomotic channels
between distal branches of:

Anterior and middle
cerebral arteries

Posterior and middle
cerebral arteries

Anterior cerebral
artery

Middle cerebral
artery

Posterior
communicating
artery

Posterior cerebral
artery

Internal carotid
artery

External carotid artery

Common carotid artery

Left
vertebral
artery

Right
vertebral
artery

Figure 4–12. Paths for collateral blood supply. Course of the major cerebral arteries over the lateral and medial cortical surfaces. Anastomotic channels between the middle and anterior cerebral arteries—one site for collateral circulation—are depicted. Part of the circle of Willis is shown (dark blue; see Figure 4–1). (Adapted from Fisher, C. M. 1975. Modern concepts of cerebrovascular disease. In Meyer, J. S. (ed.), The Anatomy and Pathology of the Cerebral Vasculature. New York: Spectrum Publications, pp. 1–41.)

On the lateral convexity of the cerebral hemisphere, the terminal ends of the various cerebral arteries anastomose (Figure 4–12). These interconnections or networks only occur between branches when they are located on the cortical surface, not when the artery has penetrated the brain. When a major artery becomes occluded, these anastomoses limit the extent of damage. For example, if a branch of the posterior cerebral artery becomes occluded, tissue with comprised blood supply in the occipital lobe may be rescued by collateral circulation from the middle cerebral artery that connects anastomotically with the blocked vessel.

This collateral circulation can rescue the gray matter of the cerebral cortex. In contrast, there is little collateral circulation between the regions perfused by the cerebral arteries in the white matter. Although collateral circulation provides the cerebral cortex with a margin of safety during arterial occlusion, the anastomotic network that provides such insurance also creates a vulnerability. When systemic blood pressure is reduced, the

region served by this anastomotic network is particularly susceptible to ischemia because such anastomoses occur at the terminal ends of the arteries, regions where perfusion pressure is lowest. The peripheral borders of the territory supplied by major vessels are termed **border zones** and an infarction occurring in these regions is termed a **border zone infarct**.

Cerebral Veins Drain Into the Dural Sinuses

Venous drainage of the cerebral hemispheres is provided both by superficial and deep cerebral veins (Figure 4–13). Superficial veins, arising from the cerebral cortex and underlying white matter, are variable in distribution. Among the more prominent and consistent are the superior anastomotic vein (of Trolard), lying across the parietal lobe, and the inferior anastomotic vein (of Labbé), on the surface of the temporal lobe. The **deep cerebral veins** drain the more interior portions of the white matter, including the basal ganglia and parts of the diencephalon. Many deep cerebral veins drain into the **great cerebral vein** (of Galen) (Figures 4–13 and 4–14).

Drainage of blood from the central nervous system into the major vessels emptying into the heart—the systemic circulation—is achieved through either a direct or indirect path. Spinal cord and caudal medullary veins drain directly, through a network of veins and plexes, into the systemic circulation. By contrast, the rest of the central nervous system drains by an indirect path: the veins first empty into the **dural sinuses** (Figures 4–14 and 4–15; see also Figure 1–12) before returning blood to the systemic circulation. The dural sinuses function as low-pressure channels for venous blood flow back to the systemic circulation. They are located between the periosteal and meningeal layers of the dura (Figure 4–15).

The superficial cerebral veins drain into the superior and inferior sagittal sinuses (Figures 4–13 and 4–14). The **superior sagittal sinus** runs along the midline of the cranial cavity at the superior margin of the falx cerebri. The **inferior sagittal sinus** courses along the inferior margin of the falx cerebri just above the corpus callosum. The inferior sagittal sinus, together with the **great cerebral vein (of Galen)**, return venous blood to the **straight** (sometimes called rectus) **sinus** (Figures 4–13 and 4–14). At the occipital pole, the superior sagittal sinus and the straight sinus join to form the two **transverse sinuses**. Finally, these sinuses drain into the **sigmoid sinuses**, which, in turn, return blood to the internal jugular veins. The cavernous sinus is also illustrated in Figure 4–14B.

Veins of the midbrain drain into the **great cerebral vein**, which empties into the **straight sinus**, whereas the pons and rostral medulla drain into the **superior petrosal sinus**. Cerebellar veins drain into both the **great cerebral vein** and **superior petrosal sinus** (Figure 4–14B).

The Blood–Brain Barrier Isolates the Chemical Environment of the Central Nervous System From That of the Rest of the Body

The intravascular compartment is isolated from the extracellular compartment of the brain and spinal cord. This feature, the **blood–brain barrier** (Figure 4–16A), was discovered when intravenous dye injection stained most tissues and organs but not the brain. This permeability barrier protects the brain from neuroactive compounds in the blood as well as rapid changes in the ionic constituents of the blood that can affect neuronal excitability.

The blood–brain barrier is thought to result from two characteristics of endothelial cells in the capillaries of the brain and spinal cord (Figure

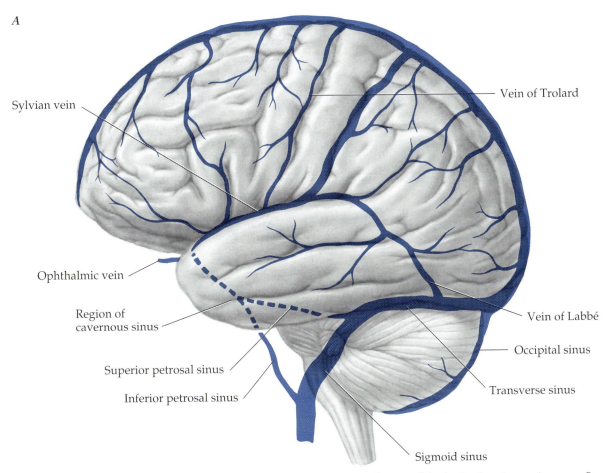

A

Sylvian vein

Vein of Trolard

Ophthalmic vein

Region of
cavernous sinus

Vein of Labbé

Occipital sinus

Superior petrosal sinus

Inferior petrosal sinus

Transverse sinus

Sigmoid sinus

Figure 4–13. Cerebral veins. *A.* Lateral view of the brain showing major superficial veins and the dural sinuses. *B.* Midsagittal view of brain showing dural sinuses and major deep cerebral veins.

4–16B). First, in peripheral capillaries endothelial cells have fenestrations (pores) that allow large molecules to flow into the extracellular space. Moreover, the intercellular spaces between adjacent endothelial cells are leaky. In contrast, in central nervous system capillaries adjacent endothelial cells are tightly joined, preventing movement of compounds into the extracellular compartment of the central nervous system. Second, there is little transcellular movement of compounds from the intravascular to extracellular compartments in the central nervous system because the endothelial cells lack the required transport mechanisms. Moreover, relatively nonselective transport may occur by pinocytosis in peripheral but not central nervous system capillaries.

A number of brain structures lack a blood–brain barrier. These structures are close to the midline and, because they are closely associated with the ventricular system, are collectively termed **circumventricular organs** (Figure 4–17). They include: (1) area postrema, (2) subcommisural organ, (3) subfornical organ, (4) vascular organ of the laminar terminalis, (5) median eminence, (6) neurohypophysis, (7) choroid plexus, and (8) pineal gland. At each of these structures, either neurosecretory products are secreted into the blood or local neurons detect blood-borne compounds as part of a mechanism for regulating the internal environment of the body.

B

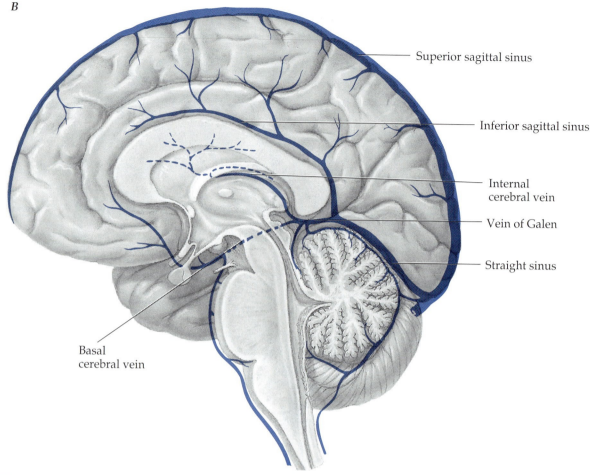

Superior sagittal sinus

Inferior sagittal sinus

Internal
cerebral vein

Vein of Galen

Straight sinus

Basal
cerebral vein

Figure 4–13. *(continued)*

Regions that lack a blood–brain barrier are isolated from the rest of the brain by specialized ependymal cells.

Cerebrospinal Fluid Serves Many Diverse Functions

Cerebrospinal fluid is a watery fluid that fills the ventricles and bathes the internal brain surface. It also fills the subarachnoid space and thus bathes the external brain surface. Together, the ventricles and subarachnoid space contain approximately 125 mL of cerebrospinal fluid (25 mL in the ventricles and 100 mL in the subarachnoid space).

Cerebrospinal fluid serves at least three essential functions. First, it provides physical support for the brain, which floats within the fluid. Second, it serves an excretory function and regulates the chemical environment of the central nervous system. (Because the brain has no lymphatic system, water-soluble metabolites, which have limited ability to cross the blood–brain barrier, diffuse from the brain into the cerebrospinal fluid.) Third, it acts as a channel for chemical communication within the central nervous system.

Neurochemicals released by neurons in the vicinity of the ventricles enter the cerebrospinal fluid and can be taken up at sites on the ventricu-

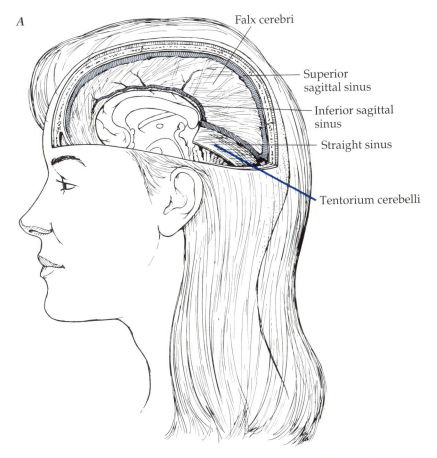

A

Falx cerebri

Superior
sagittal sinus

Inferior sagittal
sinus

Straight sinus

Tentorium cerebelli

Figure 4–14. Dural sinuses. *A.* Falx cerebri and superior sagittal sinus from a lateral perspective. *B.* View of the ventral surface of the anterior and middle cranial fossae, and the sinuses on the dorsal surface of the tentorium cerebelli and the ventral cranium.

lar floor and walls by specialized cells that line the ventricular cavities. Once in the cerebrospinal fluid, these compounds also have relatively free access to neural tissue adjacent to the ventricles. This is because, in contrast to the blood–brain barrier, most of the ventricular lining presents no barrier between the cerebrospinal fluid compartment and the extracellular compartment of the brain. In the following sections, we will survey the production and flow of cerebrospinal fluid and consider how it drains into the vascular system.

Most of the Cerebrospinal Fluid Is Produced by the Choroid Plexus

Cerebrospinal fluid is secreted mainly by the **choroid plexus**, which is located in the ventricles (Figure 4–18; see also Figure 2–16). A barrier imposed by the choroidal epithelium prevents the transport of materials from blood into the cerebrospinal fluid. This is the **blood–cerebrospinal fluid barrier** (see Figure 4–16A), analogous to the blood–brain barrier. The rest of the cerebrospinal fluid is secreted by brain capillaries. This extrachoroidal source of cerebrospinal fluid enters the ventricular system through ependymal cells, the ciliated cuboidal epithelial cells that line the ventricles. Total cerebrospinal fluid production by both sources is approx-

B

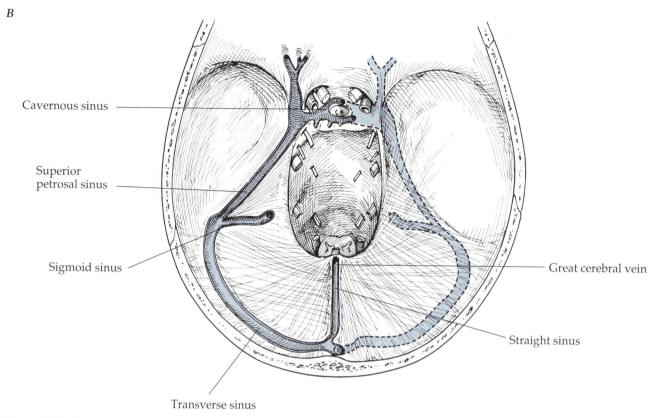

Cavernous sinus

Superior
petrosal sinus

Sigmoid sinus

Great cerebral vein

Straight sinus

Transverse sinus

Figure 4–14. (continued)

imately 500 mL per day. Although the principal function of the choroid
plexus is cerebrospinal fluid secretion, the plexus also serves a reabsorp-
tive function. Experiments have shown that a variety of compounds introduced into the ventricles are eliminated from the cerebrospinal fluid by
the choroid plexus.

Cerebrospinal Fluid Circulates Throughout
the Ventricles and Subarachnoid Space

Cerebrospinal fluid produced by the choroid plexus in the lateral
ventricles (Figure 4–18) flows through the interventricular foramina and
mixes with cerebrospinal fluid produced in the third ventricle. From here,
it flows through the cerebral aqueduct and into the fourth ventricle,
another major site for cerebrospinal fluid production because the choroid
plexus is also located there. Three apertures in the roof of the fourth ventricle drain cerebrospinal fluid from the ventricular system into the subarachnoid space (see Figure 1–10): the **foramen of Magendie**, located on
the midline, and the two **foramina of Luschka**, located at the lateral mar-
gins of the fourth ventricle.

The subarachnoid space is dilated in certain locations, termed **cis-**

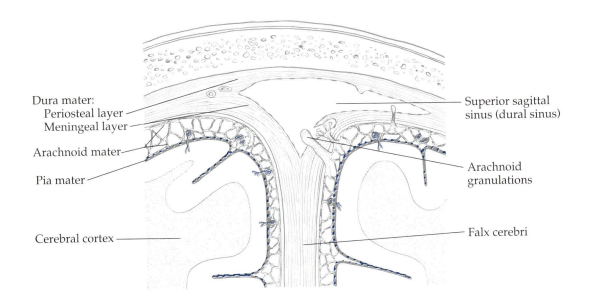

Dura mater:
Periosteal layer
Meningeal layer

Arachnoid mater

Pia mater

Cerebral cortex

Superior sagittal
sinus (dural sinus)

Arachnoid
granulations

Falx cerebri

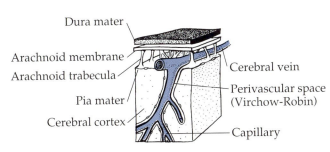

Dura mater

Arachnoid membrane
Arachnoid trabecula

Pia mater
Cerebral cortex

Cerebral vein

Perivascular space
(Virchow-Robin)

Capillary

Figure 4–15. A schematic cut through the superior sagittal sinus illustrating the arachnoid granulations, collections of arachnoid villi containing the unidirectional valves through which cerebrospinal fluid passes to the venous circulation. The inset shows the relationship between cerebral blood vessels and the meningeal layers. (Adapted from Davson, H., Keasley, W., and Segal, M. B. 1987. Physiology and Pathophysiology of the Cerebrospinal Fluid. Edinburgh: Churchill Livingstone. Insert from Kuffler, S. W., and Nicholls, J. G. 1976. From Neuron to Brain. Sunderland, Mass. Sinauer Associates Inc., Publishers.)

terns; cerebrospinal fluid pools here. Five prominent cisterns are located on the midline: (1) the **interpeduncular cistern**, between the basis pedunculi on the ventral midbrain surface; (2) the **quadrageminal cistern**, dorsal to the superior and inferior colliculi (the quadrageminal bodies is another name for the superior and inferior colliculi); (3) the **pontine cistern**, ventral to the pons; (4) the **cisterna magna**, dorsal to the medulla; and (5) the **lumbar cistern**, in the caudal vertebral canal (Figure 4–18). The subarachnoid space also contains the blood vessels of the central nervous system (Figure 4–15 inset). Blood vessels penetrate into the brain together with the pia creating a perivascular space between the vessel and pia. These spaces, termed the Virchow–Robin spaces, contain cerebrospinal fluid.

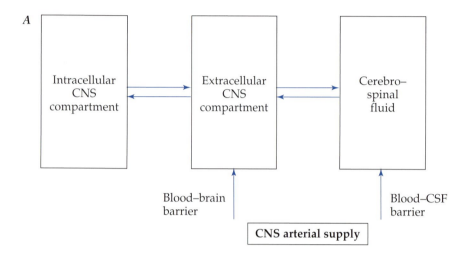

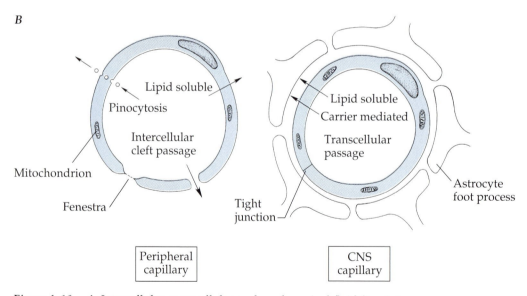

Figure 4–16. **A.** Intracellular, extracellular, and cerebrospinal fluid (i.e., intraventricular) compartments of the central nervous system. **B.** Schematic diagram of peripheral and central nervous system capillary. (**A,** Adapted from Rapoport, S. I. 1976. Blood–Brain Barrier in Physiology and Medicine. New York: Raven Press; **B,** Adapted from Oldendorf, W., et al. 1977. Ann. Neurology 1:409–417.)

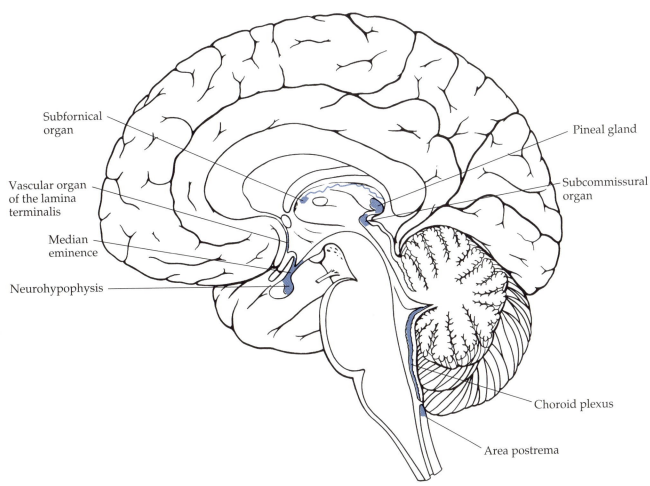

Subfornical organ

Pineal gland

Vascular organ of the lamina terminalis

Subcommissural organ

Median eminence

Neurohypophysis

Choroid plexus

Area postrema

Figure 4–17. Circumventricular organs are brain regions that do not have a blood–brain barrier. The locations of the eight circumventricular organs are shown on a view of the midsagittal brain.

The Dural Sinuses Provide the Return Path for Cerebrospinal Fluid

Cerebrospinal fluid passes from the subarachnoid space to the venous blood through small unidirectional valves, termed **arachnoid villi**. Arachnoid villi are microscopic evaginations of the arachnoid mater that protrude into the **dural sinuses** as well as directly into veins. The cerebrospinal fluid flows through a system of large vacuoles in the arachnoid cells of the villi, as well as through an extracellular path between cells of the villi. Numerous clusters of arachnoid villi are present over the dorsal (superior) convexity of the cerebral hemispheres in the superior sagittal sinus, where they form a macroscopic structure called the **arachnoid granulations** (Figures 4–15 and 4–18). The arachnoid villi are also present where the spinal nerves exit the spinal dural sac. These villi direct the flow of cerebrospinal fluid into the radicular veins.

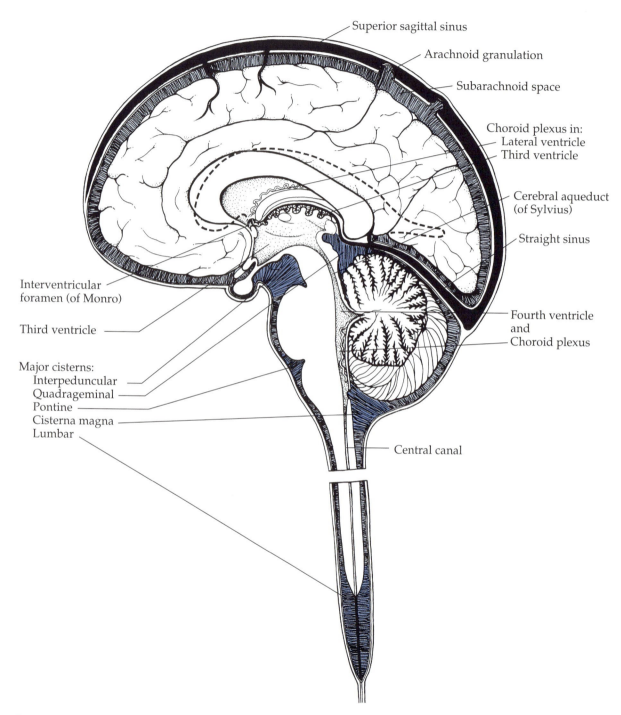

Figure 4–18. The flow of cerebrospinal fluid is shown on a view of the midsagittal surface of the central nervous system. (Adapted from Kuffler, S. W., and Nicholls, J. G. 1976. From Neuron to Brain. Sunderland, Mass.: Sinauer Associates Inc., Publishers.

Summary

Arterial Supply of the Spinal Cord and Brain Stem

The arterial supply of the spinal cord is provided by the **vertebral arteries** and the **radicular arteries** (Figures 4–1 and 4–2). The brain is supplied by the **internal carotid arteries (the anterior circulation)** and the **vertebral arteries**, which join at the pontomedullary junction to form the **basilar artery** (collectively termed the **posterior circulation**) (Figure 4–1). The brain stem and cerebellum are supplied only by the posterior system (Figure 4–3A; Table 4–1). The medulla receives blood directly from small branches of the **vertebral arteries** as well as from the **spinal arteries** and the **posterior inferior cerebellar artery** (PICA) (Figure 4–3A, 3B). The pons is supplied by **paramedian** and **short circumferential branches** of the **basilar artery**. Two major long circumferential branches are the **anterior inferior cerebellar artery** (AICA) and the **superior cerebellar artery** (Figure 4–3A). The midbrain receives its arterial supply primarily from the **posterior cerebral artery** as well as from the basilar artery (Figure 4–3A). The PICA supplies the caudal cerebellum, and both the AICA and the superior cerebellar artery supply the rostral cerebellum.

Arterial Supply of the Diencephalon and Cerebral Hemispheres

The diencephalon and cerebral hemispheres are supplied by both the **anterior** and the **posterior circulations** (Figure 4–9). The cerebral cortex receives its blood supply from the three cerebral arteries: the **anterior** and **middle cerebral arteries**, which are part of the anterior circulation, and the **posterior cerebral artery**, which is part of the posterior circulation (Figures 4–1 and 4–12). The diencephalon, basal ganglia, and internal capsule receive blood from branches of the **internal carotid artery**, the three **cerebral arteries**, and the **posterior communicating artery** (Figures 4–1, 4–4, 4–7, and 4–12; Table 4–1).

Collateral Circulation

The anterior and posterior systems are interconnected by two networks of arteries: (1) the **circle of Willis**, which is formed by the anterior, middle, and posterior **cerebral arteries**, the **posterior communicating arteries,** and the **anterior communicating artery** (Figure 4–1), and (2) terminal branches of the cerebral arteries, which anastomose on the superior convexity of the cerebral cortex (Figures 4–4 and 4–12).

Venous Drainage

The venous drainage of the spinal cord and caudal medulla is direct to the systemic circulation. By contrast, veins draining the cerebral hemispheres, diencephalon, midbrain, pons, cerebellum, and rostral medulla (Figure 4–13) drain into the **dural sinuses** (Figures 4–13, 4–14, and 4–15). The major dural sinuses are: **superior sagittal**, **inferior sagittal**, **straight**, **transverse**, **sigmoid**, **superior**, and **inferior petrosal**.

Blood–Brain Barrier

The internal environment of most of the central nervous system is protected from circulating neuroactive agents in blood by the **blood–brain barrier** (Figure 4–16A). The blood–brain barrier is formed by a number of specializations in the **capillary endothelium** of the central nervous system (Figure 4–16B). Brain regions without a blood–brain barrier, termed the **circumventricular organs** (Figure 4–17), include the: (1) **area postrema** in

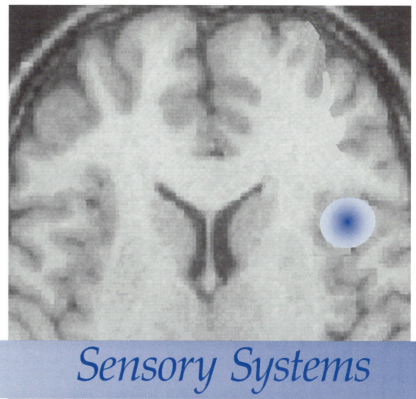

II

Sensory Systems

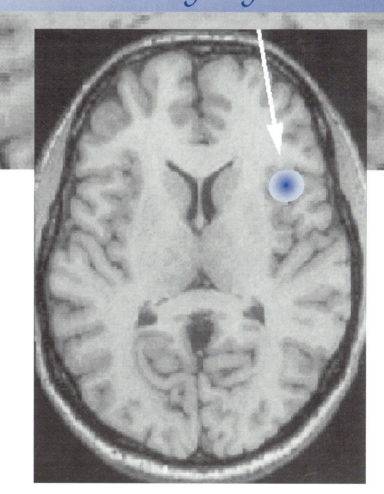

the medulla, (2) **subcommisural organ**, (3) **subfornical organ**, (4) **vascular organ of the lamina terminalis**, (5) **median eminence**, (6) **neurohypophysis**, (7) **choroid plexus**, and (8) **pineal gland**.

Production and Circulation of Cerebrospinal Fluid

Most of the cerebrospinal fluid is produced by the **choroid plexus**, which is located in the **ventricles** (Figure 4–18; see Figure 2–16). It exits from the ventricular system, through foramina in the fourth ventricle, the two **foramina of Luschka** and the **foramen of Magendie**, directly into the **subarachnoid space**. Cerebrospinal fluid passes into the **dural sinuses** (Figure 4–13) through unidirectional valves termed **arachnoid villi** that are clustered in the **arachnoid granulations.** (Figures 4–15 and 4–18). ■

KEY STRUCTURES AND TERMS

cerebral angiography
anterior (carotid) circulation
posterior (vertebral-basilar)
    circulation
collateral circulation
brain stem arterial supply
    paramedian branches
    short circumferential branches
    long circumferential branches
anastomosis
circle of Willis
    anterior cerebral artery
    anterior communicating artery
    middle cerebral artery

posterior communicating artery
posterior cerebral artery
border zone infarct
superficial cerebral arteries
deep cerebral veins
great cerebral vein (of Galen)
dural sinuses
    superior sagittal sinus
    inferior sagittal sinus
    straight (or rectus) sinus
    transverse sinus
    superior petrosal sinus
    inferior petrosal sinus
blood–brain barrier

circumventricular organs
foramen of Magendie
foramina of Luschka
cisterns
    interpeduncular cistern
    quadrageminal cistern
    pontine cistern
    cisterna magna
    lumbar cistern
arachnoid villi
arachnoid granulations
(see Table 4–1 for arterial supply of
        brain structures)

Selected Readings

Davson, H., Keasley, W., and Segal, M. B. 1987. Physiology and Pathophysiology of the Cerebrospinal Fluid. Edinburgh: Churchill Livingstone.

Duvernoy, H. M. 1975. The Superficial Veins of the Human Brain. Berlin: Springer-Verlag.

Fisher, C. M. 1975. Modern concepts of cerebrovascular disease. In Meyer, J. S. (ed.), The Anatomy and Pathology of the Cerebral Vasculature. New York: Spectrum Publications, pp. 1–41.

Fishman, R. T. 1992. Cerebrospinal Fluid in Diseases of the Nervous System, 2nd ed. Philadelphia: Saunders.

Kistler, J. P., Ropper, A. H., and Martin, J. B. 1987. Cerebrovascular diseases. In Braunwald, E., Isselbacher, F. J., Peterdorf, R. G., et al. (eds.), Harrison's Principles of Internal Medicine, 11th ed. New York: McGraw-Hill, pp. 1930–1960.

McKinley, M. J., and Oldfield, B. J. 1990. Circumventricular organs. In Paxinos, G. (ed.), The Human Nervous System. San Diego: Academic Press, pp. 415–438.

Sasaki, T., and Kassell, N. F. 1990. Cerebrovascular system. In Paxinos, G. (ed.), The Human Nervous System. San Diego: Academic Press, pp. 1135–1149.

References

Carpenter, M. B., and Sutin, J. 1983. Human Neuroanatomy. Baltimore: Williams & Wilkins.

DeArmond, S. J., Fusco, M. M., and Dewey, M. M. 1976. Structure of the Human Brain. New York: Oxford University Press.

Ferner, H., and Staubestand, J. (eds.) 1983. Sobotta Atlas of Human Anatomy. Vol. 1. Head, Neck, Upper Extremities. Baltimore: Urban and Schwarzenberg.

Kuffler, S. W., and Nicholls, J. G. 1976. From Neuron to Brain. Sunderland, Mass.: Sinauer Associates Inc., Publishers.

5

The Somatic
Sensory System

THE SENSORY SYSTEMS OF THE BRAIN ARE THE FOCUS of Chapters 5 through 8. In this chapter, we consider the anatomical organization of the somatic sensory system, which mediates touch and limb position senses, as well as pain and temperature senses. This system is also critically involved in the maintenance of arousal and in the sensory regulation of movement. To carry out these functions, the somatic sensory system processes stimuli both from the body surface and from within the body—from the muscles, joints, and viscera.

The neural systems transmitting sensory information from the limbs, neck, and trunk to the cerebral cortex comprise the ascending spinal cord pathways. These pathways are distinct from the trigeminal system, which transmits somatic sensory information from the head. In this chapter, we consider the ascending spinal cord pathways; the trigeminal system is examined in Chapter 12. Even though the ascending spinal cord pathways and the trigeminal system are distinct, their general organization is similar.

In studying the functional anatomy of the somatic sensory system, we first survey its general organization, which parallels the longitudinal axis of the central nervous system. This initial examination provides an **overall view** of the functional anatomy of the somatic sensory pathways. Then we examine the anatomical organization at different levels through the nervous system, beginning with the morphology of the somatic sensory receptors and continuing to the cerebral cortex.

FUNCTIONAL ANATOMY OF THE SOMATIC
SENSORY PATHWAYS

The Dorsal Column–Medial Lemniscal System and the Anterolateral System Mediate Different Somatic Sensations

The somatic, or bodily, senses consist of four distinct **modalities**: limb position sense, touch, thermal sensation, and pain. We engage all of these submodalities during routine activity. For example, in picking up a

cup of hot coffee, limb position sense is used in identifying the shape of our hand as we grasp the handle; contact with the cup is detected by touch. Thermal sensations inform us of the temperature of the cup, and, if the cup is too hot, we experience pain. Each modality can be further subdivided into submodalities, which adds to the richness of somatic sensations and is clinically important for neurological diagnosis.

Touch and limb position sense are mediated by an ascending neural system that is separate from the system for pain and temperature senses. The **dorsal column–medial lemniscal system** (Figures 5–1B and 5–2A) mediates touch and limb position sense. (The spinal paths carrying limb position information from the upper and lower extremities have a slightly different organization, which we will consider below.) In contrast, the **anterolateral system** (Figures 5–1C and 5–2B) subserves pain and temperature sense and, to a much lesser extent, touch. Each of these neural systems consists of a neuron chain that comprises a functionally and sometimes anatomically distinct pathway. Beginning in the periphery with the sensory receptors, both systems project to the contralateral cerebral cortex of the parietal lobe. Recalling the dorsal column–medial lemniscal system introduced in Chapter 3, we will now compare it to the anterolateral system, emphasizing the four key differences in the organization of these pathways.

The Two Ascending Pathways Each Receive Inputs From Different Classes of Sensory Receptor Neurons

In Chapter 3, we saw that the dorsal root ganglion neuron is the primary sensory neuron that provides information to the somatic sensory systems. Afferent input from different functional classes of dorsal root ganglion neurons contributes information to the two systems. Sensory receptors sensitive to **mechanical** stimulation of body tissues provide the major afferent input to the dorsal column–medial lemniscal system. In contrast, sensory receptors sensitive to **noxious** (i.e., painful) and **thermal** stimuli provide the major afferent inputs to the anterolateral system.

Although the segregation of the different types of afferent input into the two ascending systems is not absolute, it is sufficiently complete to have important clinical consequences. For example, after a complete lesion of the dorsal column–medial lemniscal system, only a crude sense of touch remains. This indicates that the anterolateral system does receive an input from mechanoreceptors. Although simple tactile thresholds may not be changed, the person's discriminative capabilities are markedly reduced. An individual suffering from such a lesion, using only residual somatic sensory capabilities, may not be able to distinguish gradations of rough and smooth (e.g., grades of sandpaper), or the shapes of grasped objects (e.g., spheres vs. cubes) without actually looking at them. Moreover, this individual would not be capable of identifying the position of his or her arm without looking at it. By contrast, a lesion of the anterolateral system leaves touch and limb position senses unaffected but makes people insensitive or less sensitive to pain.

The Dorsal Column–Medial Lemniscal and Anterolateral Systems Have Different Relay Nuclei in the Spinal Cord and Brain Stem

The first major relay in the dorsal column–medial lemniscal system is in the **dorsal column nuclei**, in the medulla. Here, the first-order neurons in the pathway—the primary sensory neurons—synapse on second-order neurons in the central nervous system. In contrast, the anterolateral sys-

tem first relays in the **dorsal horn** of the spinal cord. The general anatomical organization of these two systems is presented in Figure 5–1B and C, along with schematic myelin-stained sections through key levels through the nervous system. Figure 5–2 compares the anatomy of the two systems as viewed from the dorsal brain stem.

The Two Somatic Sensory Pathways Decussate at Different Levels of the Neuraxis

We do not know why the axons of long neural pathways decussate. We do know, however, that virtually all sensory and motor pathways have a neuron whose axon crosses the midline somewhere along its course. Knowing the level of decussation is clinically important for determining where an injury to the nervous system has occurred (see section below on sensory deficits after spinal cord trauma). The dorsal column–medial lemniscal system decussates in the medulla (Figure 5–2A), whereas the anterolateral system crosses in the spinal cord (Figure 5–2B). Curiously, for both systems, the axon of the second neuron in the circuit decussates.

The Dorsal Column–Medial Lemniscal and Anterolateral Systems Synapse in Different Brain Stem and Diencephalic Regions

The dorsal column–medial lemniscal system is an anatomically discrete pathway, and all of the fibers that comprise this system have similar connections. Axons in the dorsal columns synapse primarily on neurons in the dorsal column nuclei. The second-order neurons in the dorsal column nuclei, in turn, transmit information to the ventral posterior lateral nucleus of the thalamus (Figure 5–1B). The anterolateral system, on the other hand, is spread out within the lateral and ventral spinal columns and contains ascending pathways that synapse in separate brain regions: the **spinothalamic tract**, the **spinoreticular tract**, and the **spinomesencephalic tract**.

The organization of the spinothalamic tract parallels that of the dorsal column–medial lemniscal system more closely than the two other paths of the anterolateral system. This tract carries information about painful stimuli to the ventral posterior lateral nucleus, but to a portion separate from where the axons of the medial lemniscus terminate. We think that the projection of both the spinothalamic tract and the medial lemniscus to the ventral posterior lateral nucleus is important in the discriminative aspects of somatic sensations: for example, the medial lemniscus is important for identifying the precise location of a tap on the skin; for the spinothalamic tract, pin prick localization.

In addition, a portion of the spinothalamic tract terminates more medially in the thalamus, primarily in the **intralaminar nuclei**. The spinoreticular tract transmits sensory information to neurons in the reticular formation of the pons and medulla, and many of these neurons, in turn, project to the intralaminar nuclei of the thalamus. The function of this medial thalamic projection is to mediate the emotional aspects of pain (see below). For example, you may become angry if you are burned when you pick up a hot coffee cup. The salience of the stimulus also helps you to remember not to be so careless the next time! The reticular formation and intralaminar nuclei are also important in maintaining arousal.

The component of the spinothalamic tract that terminates in the ventral posterior lateral nucleus is also termed the **neospinothalamic tract** because it is a larger tract in phylogenetically higher animals. The part that terminates in the intralaminar nuclei—together with the spinoreticular

A

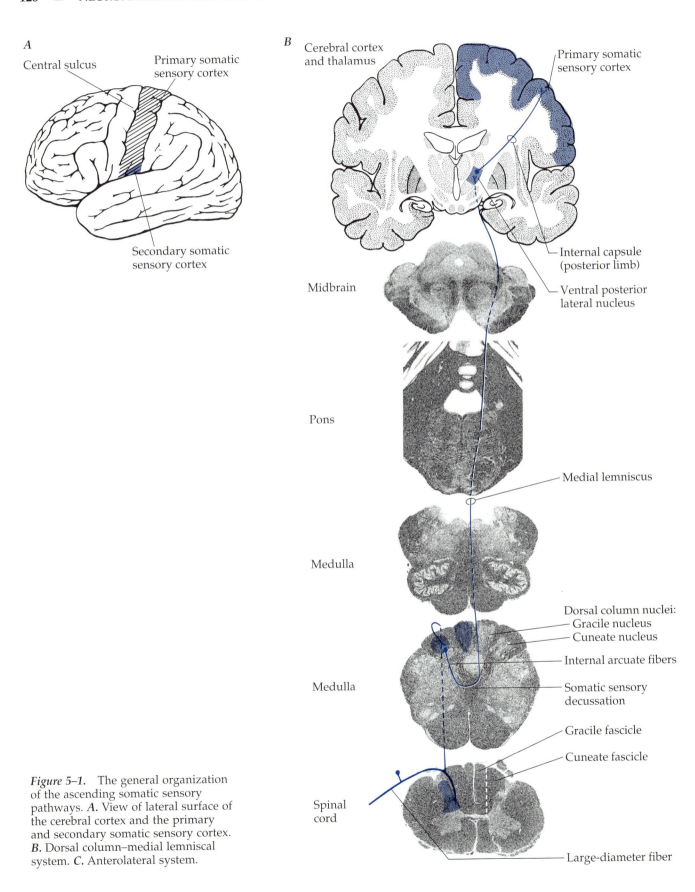

Central sulcus

Primary somatic sensory cortex

Secondary somatic sensory cortex

B

Cerebral cortex and thalamus

Primary somatic sensory cortex

Internal capsule (posterior limb)

Ventral posterior lateral nucleus

Midbrain

Pons

Medial lemniscus

Medulla

Dorsal column nuclei:
Gracile nucleus
Cuneate nucleus

Internal arcuate fibers

Somatic sensory decussation

Medulla

Gracile fascicle

Cuneate fascicle

Spinal cord

Large-diameter fiber

Figure 5–1. The general organization of the ascending somatic sensory pathways. *A.* View of lateral surface of the cerebral cortex and the primary and secondary somatic sensory cortex. *B.* Dorsal column–medial lemniscal system. *C.* Anterolateral system.

C

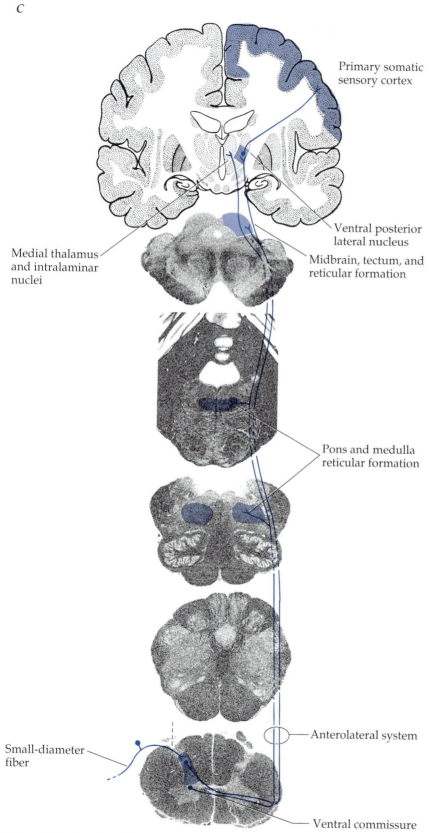

Primary somatic
sensory cortex

Ventral posterior
lateral nucleus

Medial thalamus
and intralaminar
nuclei

Midbrain, tectum, and
reticular formation

Pons and medulla
reticular formation

Anterolateral system

Small-diameter
fiber

Ventral commissure

Figure 5–1. *(continued)*

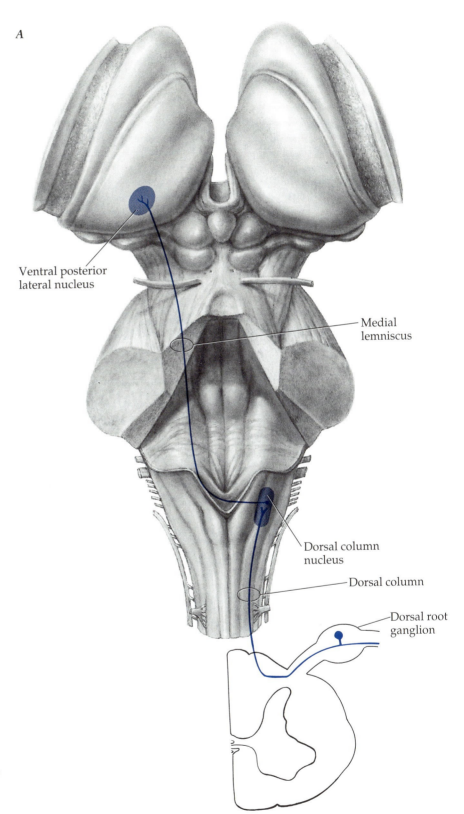

A

Ventral posterior
lateral nucleus

Medial
lemniscus

Dorsal column
nucleus

Dorsal column

Dorsal root
ganglion

Figure 5–2. Dorsal view of the brain
stem without the cerebellum, illustrating the course of the dorsal
column–medial lemniscal system
(A) and the anterolateral system *(B).*
Note that the decussating axons of the
anterolateral system (part B) cross the
midline in the ventral commissure
(see Figure 5–6).

B

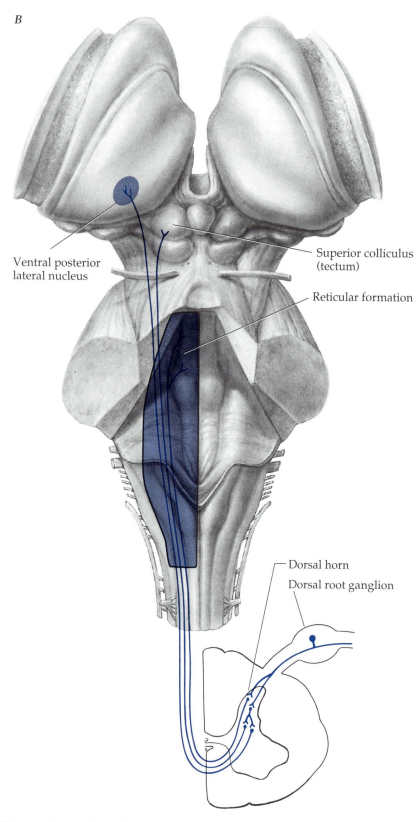

Ventral posterior
lateral nucleus

Superior colliculus
(tectum)

Reticular formation

Dorsal horn

Dorsal root ganglion

Figure 5–2.   (continued)

tract—is sometimes called the **paleospinothalamic tract**. The spinomesencephalic tract terminates in the midbrain tectum and periaqueductal gray matter. The tectum integrates visual, auditory, and somatic sensory information for orienting the head and body to salient stimuli (see Chapter 6). One somatic sensory function of the periaqueductal gray matter is in feedback regulation of pain transmission in the spinal cord.

■ REGIONAL ANATOMY

The rest of this chapter takes a regional approach to studying the somatic sensory system. Progressing in sequence from the periphery to the cerebral cortex, we examine each key component of the dorsal column–medial lemniscal system and anterolateral system. Knowing **regional anatomy** is key to understanding how injury to a discrete portion of the central nervous system affects different functional systems indiscriminately. Knowing the longitudinal organization of these systems, and their continuity between levels, helps us understand **functional organization**.

The Terminal Processes of Dorsal Root Ganglion Neurons Are the Somatic Sensory Receptors

The **dorsal root ganglion neurons** (Figure 5–3), named for the **dorsal root ganglia** in which their cell bodies are located, transduce sensory information into neural signals, and transmit these signals to the central nervous system. **Ganglia** are collections of neuronal cell bodies that are located outside the central nervous system. The dorsal root ganglia are located in the intervertebral foramina. Early in development, dorsal root ganglion neurons have a bipolar morphology: a peripheral and a central axon branch emerge from the two poles of the cell body. Later, the proximal portions of the two axonal processes fuse. Thus, late in development and in maturity, the dorsal root ganglion neurons are **pseudounipolar neurons**. A single axon emerges from the cell body and bifurcates; one axonal branch is directed toward the periphery and the other, centrally. We often call the peripheral and central axon branches of dorsal root ganglion neurons a **primary afferent fiber**.

The **peripheral** axon branch of dorsal root ganglion neurons innervates tissue, such as skin and muscle. The distal terminal of the peripheral branch is the **sensory receptor**; it is the only part of the neuron's membrane sensitive to stimulation. Here, stimulus energy is transduced into neural

Figure 5–3. The dorsal root ganglion cell and the organization of the primary afferent fiber. The sensory receptor illustrated is a mechanoreceptor, a Pacinian corpuscle.

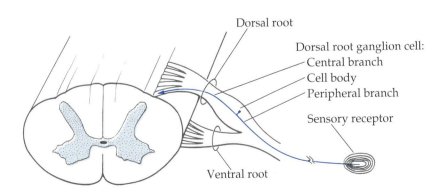

events. Sensory receptors either have a specialized non–neural tissue capsule covering the axon or are bare nerve endings. Receptors with **bare nerve endings** are **nociceptors**—which are sensitive to noxious or tissue-damaging stimuli and mediate pain—and **thermoreceptors**—which are sensitive either to cold or warmth and mediate thermal sensations. **Encapsulated receptors** are **mechanoreceptors**, which mediate the modalities of touch and limb position sense. The capsule of a mechanoreceptor does not participate directly in stimulus transduction, nor does it confer sensitivity to a particular submodality. Rather, it acts as a filter to shape the receptor's response to a stimulus.

There are five major types of encapsulated receptors located in the skin and deep tissue: Meissner's corpuscles, pacinian corpuscles, Ruffini's corpuscles, Merkel's receptors, and hair receptors (Figure 5–4). Table 5–1 lists the mechanoreceptors that mediate touch on hairless, or glabrous, skin and limb position sense. Meissner's and Pacinian corpuscles are **rapidly adapting**. They respond to a continuous and enduring stimulus by firing a burst of action potentials to mark the onset and offset of the stimulus. Ruffini's corpuscles and Merkel's receptors are **slowly adapting**, firing action potentials for the duration of the stimulus. Hair receptors may be either slowly or rapidly adapting. Each primary afferent fiber has multiple terminal branches and, therefore, has multiple sensory receptors. The **muscle spindle receptor** is a specialized encapsulated receptor located in muscle that serves position sense. This structure is innervated by multiple afferent fibers with different properties and diameters. The muscle spindle is more complicated than the other encapsulated receptors because it contains tiny muscle fibers that are controlled by the central nervous system and that regulate receptor sensitivity.

The modality sensitivity of a receptor also determines the diameter of its axon and the patterns of connections in the central nervous system. Mechanoreceptors have a **large-diameter axon covered by a thick myelin sheath**. The mechanoreceptors are the fastest conducting sensory receptors in the somatic sensory system. The dorsal column–medial lemniscal system receives afferent input principally from these mechanoreceptors with

Figure 5–4. The morphology of peripheral somatic sensory receptors on hairy skin (*left*) and hairless, or glabrous, skin (*right*). (Adapted from Light and Perl, 1984.)

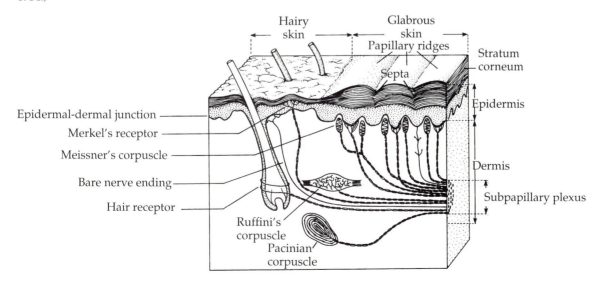

Table 5–1.   Modalities and submodalities of somatic sensation and afferent fiber classes.

Modality & Submodality	Receptor type	Fiber diameter (µm)	Class	Myelination[1]
Touch Superficial Deep Vibration	Mechanoreceptors Meissner's, Merkel's Ruffini's Pacinian	6–12	A-β (2)	Myelinated
Position Sense Static Dynamic (kinesthesia)	Mechanoreceptors Muscle stretch receptors; joint mechanoreceptors Muscle stretch receptors; joint mechanoreceptors	13–20 6–12	A-α A-β (1,2)	Myelinated
Thermal Cold Warmth	Thermoreceptors	1–5 0.2–1.5	A-δ; C (3,4)	Myelinated; unmyelinated
Pain Fast (pricking) Slow (burning)	Nociceptors	1–5 0.2–1.5	A-δ; C (3,4)	Myelinated; unmyelinated Myelinated Unmyelinated

[1]A small number of thinly myelinated and unmyelinated fibers are sensitive to mechanical stimuli. These mechanoreceptors are present in the hairy skin.

large-diameter axons. Dorsal root ganglion neurons that are sensitive to noxious or thermal stimuli have **small-diameter myelinated or unmyelinated axons**. The anterolateral system receives afferent input mostly from the receptors with small-diameter axons. The myelin sheath of peripheral axons is formed by **Schwann cells**, in contrast to oligodendrocytes, which form the myelin sheath of central axons. Physiological studies have shown that the larger the diameter of the axon, the faster it conducts action potentials. Table 5–1 lists the functional categories of primary afferent fibers, including the two afferent fiber nomenclatures based on axonal diameter: A-α (1); A-β (2); A-δ (3); and C (4).

The **central branches** of dorsal root ganglion neurons collect into the **dorsal roots** and enter the spinal cord (Figure 5–3). As they approach the spinal cord, these roots branch into numerous rootlets that enter along the dorsolateral margin of a single spinal segment (Figure 5–3; see also Figure 1–3). The area of skin innervated by the axons in a single dorsal root is termed a **dermatome**. It is clinically important that dermatomes of adjacent dorsal roots overlap extensively with those of their neighbors (Figure 5–5, inset). This explains the common clinical observation that, when a physician probes sensory capacity after injury to a single dorsal root, no anesthetic area is observed. Dorsal root injury commonly produces **radicular pain**, which is localized to the dermatome of the injured root, although patients with such damage are sometimes aware of tingling or even a diminished sensory capacity. By comparing the location of radicular pain or other sensory disturbances with a dermatomal map, such as in Figure 5–5, the clinician can localize the site of damage.

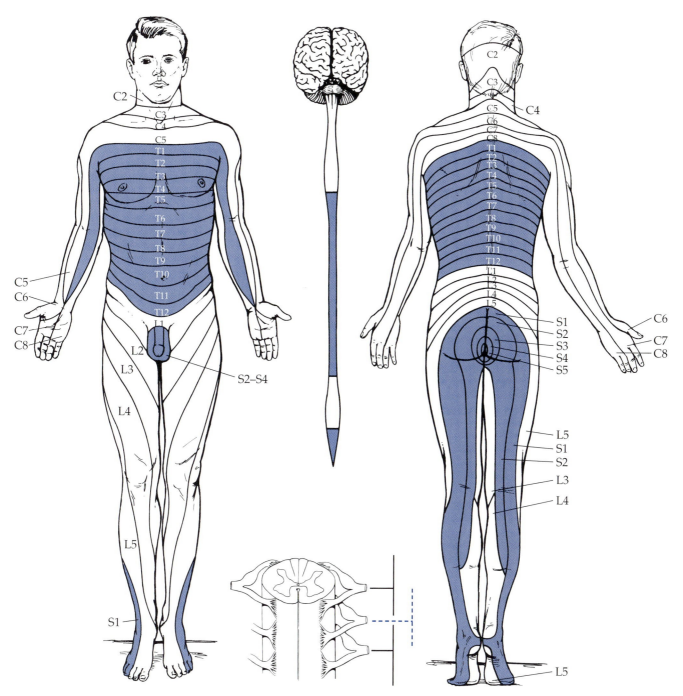

Figure 5–5. The dermatomes of the body have a segmental organization. Note the correspondence between the spinal cord divisions (shown on a ventral view of the central nervous system) and dermatome locations. The inset illustrates dermatomal overlap.

Dorsal Root Axons With Different Diameters Terminate in Different Central Nervous System Locations

The central branch of a dorsal root ganglion neuron enters the spinal cord at its dorsolateral margin (Figures 5–3 and 5–6). Even here, axons that serve different sensory functions are segregated. Large-diameter axons,

A

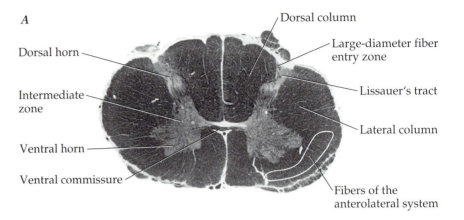

Dorsal horn

Intermediate zone

Ventral horn

Ventral commissure

Dorsal column

Large-diameter fiber entry zone

Lissauer's tract

Lateral column

Fibers of the anterolateral system

B

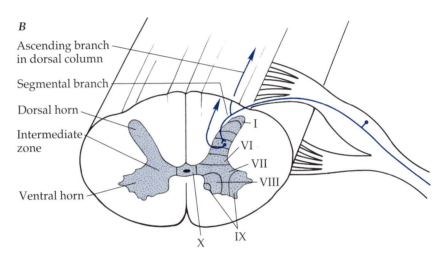

Ascending branch in dorsal column

Segmental branch

Dorsal horn

Intermediate zone

Ventral horn

I

VI

VII

VIII

X

IX

C

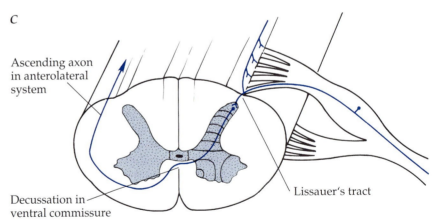

Ascending axon in anterolateral system

Decussation in ventral commissure

Lissauer's tract

Figure 5–6. *A.* Myelin-stained section through the cervical spinal cord. *B, C.* Schematic drawings based on the section in *A* and illustrating the pattern of termination of large-diameter fibers *(B)* and small-diameter fibers *(C)*. Note that small-diameter fibers also terminate in lamina 2.

which mediate touch and limb position senses, enter medial to the small-diameter axons, which mediate pain and temperature senses (Figure 5-6B and C). The locations of entry can be distinguished (Figure 5–6A): the **large-diameter fiber entry zone** (in the dorsal column) and **Lissauer's tract**, for small fibers (overlying the dorsal horn).

Once inside the spinal cord, dorsal root ganglion axons branch extensively. We can discern a general branching pattern with three broad classes of termination: segmental, ascending, and descending (Figure 5–6).

- **Segmental branches** enter the gray matter of the spinal cord and synapse on a variety of neuron types, such as interneurons and motor neurons—which are part of reflex circuits—and neurons that project to the brain (see below).
- **Ascending branches** carry sensory information rostrally to the upper spinal cord and to the brain.
- **Descending branches** synapse on spinal cord interneurons located caudal to the level of entry and contribute sensory information for intersegmental reflexes (for example, limb withdrawal).

The Spinal Gray Matter Consists of Laminar Sheets of Neurons

As we will see, the segmental branches of afferent fibers have specific termination patterns in the gray matter. To understand these patterns, however, we must first briefly consider the cytoarchitecture of the three divisions of the gray matter: dorsal horn, intermediate zone, and ventral horn (Figure 5–6A). Similar to other areas of the central nervous system, spinal cord neurons are clustered into nuclei (Table 5–2). The Swedish neuroanatomist Bror Rexed further recognized that neurons in the dorsal horn are arranged in flattened sheets that run parallel to the long axis of the spinal cord. Each sheet can be distinguished from adjacent sheets by a variety of microscopic criteria based on neuronal morphology and packing density, similar to the cytoarchitectonic characteristics of cortical laminae (see Chapter 3, Figure 3–15). Individual sheets, termed **Rexed's laminae**, contain neurons that have different anatomical connections and functions.

Rexed also parceled the intermediate zone and the ventral horn into laminae; they are, however, shaped more like rods or columns than flattened sheets. In any given spinal segment, there are ten Rexed's laminae. The dorsal horn is formed by laminae 1 through 6, the intermediate zone by the dorsal portion of lamina 7, and the ventral horn by the ventral portion of lamina 7 and laminae 8 and 9. Lamina 10 comprises the gray matter surrounding the central canal.

Some laminae also correspond to spinal cord nuclei (Table 5–2). Nuclear terminology is simply an alternate way to locate spinal cord neurons. We use the laminar nomenclature more often because there is a specific relationship between individual laminae, the pattern of termination of afferent fibers, and the location of neurons that send their axons to the brain stem or thalamus (see below).

Table 5–2. Spinal cord nuclei and laminae.

Region	Rexed's laminae	Nuclei
Dorsal horn	1	Marginal zone
Dorsal horn	2	Substantia gelatinosa
Dorsal horn	3, 4	Nucleus proprius
Intermediate zone	7	Clarke's nucleus
Intermediate zone	7	Intermediolateral nucleus
Ventral horn	9	Motor nuclei

Large-diameter Afferents Terminate in the Dorsal Column Nuclei and the Deeper Laminae of the Dorsal Horn

Ascending and descending branches of **large-diameter** dorsal root ganglion neurons course within a circumscribed region of the white matter, the **dorsal column** (Figure 5–6). The two other regions of the spinal cord white matter, the lateral and ventral columns, contain axons of central nervous system neurons and not branches of dorsal root ganglion neurons. A large-diameter fiber, on entering the spinal cord, enters medial to Lissauer's tract and skirts over the cap of the gray matter to enter the dorsal column (Figure 5–6B). The ascending branch mainly relays information to the dorsal column nuclei for perception. The segmental branches of large-diameter fibers that innervate receptors in the skin and some deep tissues terminate in specific locations in the gray matter (Figure 5–6B): in **laminae 3** through **6** in the **intermediate zone** and in the **ventral horn**. Remarkably, these fibers do not terminate in the superficial laminae of the dorsal horn. Mechanoreceptors that innervate receptors in muscle terminate in laminae 5, 6, 7, and 9.

Small-diameter Fibers Terminate in the Superficial Laminae of the Dorsal Horn

The pattern by which small-diameter axons, which subserve pain and temperature senses, enter and terminate in the spinal cord (Figure 5–5C) is quite different from that of the large-diameter axons. Once a small-diameter fiber enters the spinal cord, it branches and ascends and descends within **Lissauer's tract**, the white matter region that caps the dorsal horn (Figure 5–6). The dorsal horn terminals derive directly from these ascending and descending branches. Small-diameter myelinated and unmyelinated axons only terminate in **laminae 1** and **2**, the two laminae that do not receive input from the large-diameter fibers.

The Dorsal Columns Have Two Separate Components That Mediate Touch From the Upper and Lower Extremities

Each dorsal column transmits sensory information from the **ipsilateral side of the body** to the ipsilateral medulla. Most dorsal column axons are ascending branches of dorsal root ganglion neurons. A significant minority, though, are axons of dorsal horn neurons (approximately 15 percent) and therefore are postsynaptic to the primary afferent fibers. These neurons, located in the **deeper laminae of the dorsal horn**, receive afferent input from segmental branches of afferent fibers (Figure 5–6B). The information carried by the projection from these dorsal horn neurons reflects extra processing by the central nervous system, more so than the information carried by dorsal root ganglion fibers. For example, the corticospinal tract sends axons to these spinal laminae. It is thought that these terminals regulate dorsal horn sensory processing during voluntary movement.

There is a systematic relationship between the position of an axon in the dorsal column and the body location from which it receives input. Sensory information from the lower limb is carried by axons in the most medial portion of the dorsal column, a region termed the **gracile fascicle** (Figure 5–7). Such information from the lower trunk is transmitted rostrally by axons located lateral to the lower limb input, but still within the gracile fascicle. Sensory information from the rostral trunk, upper limb, neck, and occiput ascends in the **cuneate fascicle**, which begins approxi-

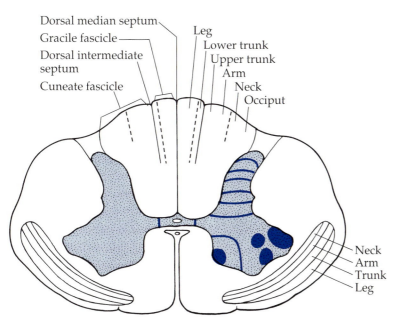

Figure 5–7. The dorsal columns and the ascending axons of the anterolateral system are somatotopically organized.

mately at the level of the sixth thoracic segment. The gracile and cuneate fascicles are separated by the **dorsal intermediate septum**, whereas the dorsal columns of the two halves of the spinal cord are separated by the **dorsal median septum** (Figure 5–7).

The organization of sensory input in the dorsal columns, termed **somatotopy**, illustrates how sensory information from the body is represented throughout the somatic sensory system. Beginning with the sequential ordering of the dorsal roots (Figure 5–5; see also Figure 1–3, inset), somatotopic organization adheres to a simple rule: **Adjacent body parts are represented in adjacent sites in the central nervous system.** This ensures that local neighborhood relations in the periphery are preserved in the central nervous system. Similar principles apply to the topographic organization of the peripheral receptive sheet in the visual system (retinotopy) and in the auditory system (tonotopy).

The somatotopic organization of the dorsal columns also can be appreciated by examining post mortem tissue from individuals who sustained trauma to the spinal cord. The sections shown in Figure 5–8A were taken from a patient whose lumbar spinal cord had been crushed. The sections are stained for myelin. Axons that have degenerated have lost their myelin sheath and are not stained (see Figure 1–16B). In the caudal thoracic spinal cord (Figure 5–8, bottom section), close to the crushed region, nearly the entire gracile fascicle is demyelinated. (Note that the cuneate fascicle is not located at this level.) At more rostral levels in the thoracic spinal cord, demyelination of the dorsal columns is restricted to a region close to the midline. This is because contingents of healthy axons continue to enter the spinal cord lateral to the degenerated axons from the lumbar cord. In the cervical enlargement and upper cervical cord (Figure 5–8, top two sections), the degenerated region is confined to a small wedge along the midline. The pattern by which axons enter and ascend in the dorsal columns is shown schematically in Figure 5–8B.

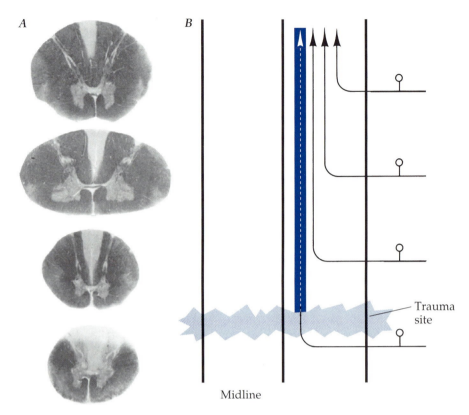

Figure 5–8. The somatotopic organization of the dorsal columns can be demonstrated by examining spinal cord sections from a patient who sustained damage to the lumbar spinal cord. *A.* Four levels through the spinal cord, rostrocaudally from top to bottom: a section rostral to the cervical enlargement, through the cervical enlargement, and two thoracic sections. *B.* The course taken by the central branches of the dorsal root fibers as they enter the spinal cord and ascend in the dorsal columns. The dashed line depicts the course of a degenerated axon transsected by the crush.

Ascending Axons of the Anterolateral System Originate in the Spinal Gray Matter

In contrast to the dorsal columns, which contain predominantly the central axons of dorsal root ganglion neurons, virtually all of the ascending axons in the anterolateral system originate from neurons in the gray matter of the spinal cord. These ascending projection neurons are widely scattered in the spinal gray matter but are concentrated in the dorsal horn. There is, however, a specific relationship between the lamina in which an ascending projection neuron is located and the termination site of its axon in the brain. The pathway to the ventral posterior lateral nucleus of the thalamus originates primarily from neurons in laminae 1 and 5. The spinal cord neurons whose axons project to the intralaminar nuclei and reticular formation of the pons and medulla are located more ventrally in the gray matter, in laminae 6 through 8. The projection to the midbrain originates from neurons in laminae 1 and 5, similar to the projection to the ventral posterior lateral nucleus.

Most axons of the anterolateral system decussate in the spinal cord before ascending to the brain stem or thalamus. This crossover occurs at a commissure, a white matter site in the central nervous system where axons decussate. In this case, the crossover occurs at the **ventral (anterior) commissure**, located ventral to the central canal (see Figures 5–6A and C).

The anterolateral system is named for its spinal axons, which ascend in the anterior portion of the lateral column (Figures 5–6 and 5–7). The location of the anterolateral system is revealed by examining the degenerated area in the lateral column in Figure 5–8A. Demyelination in the lateral column is mostly due to degeneration of anterolateral fibers (there are other degenerating axons that had terminated in the cerebellum). The anterolateral system, like the dorsal column–medial lemniscal system, is somatotopically organized: Axons transmitting sensory information from more caudal segments are located lateral to those from more rostral segments (Figure 5–7). The somatotopic organization in the anterolateral system, however, is not as precise as that for the dorsal columns. That is why only a trend is apparent in the location of degenerating axons when viewing the sections in Figure 5–8A.

Three Key Sensory Deficits That Follow Spinal Cord Injury Permit Localization of Trauma

Spinal cord injury results in deficits in somatic sensation and in the control of body musculature at the **level of, and caudal to, the lesion**. Motor deficits that follow such injury will be considered in Chapter 9. Here, we consider the somatic sensory deficits. In general, somatic sensory deficits have three major characteristics: (1) the sensory **modality** that is affected, for example, whether pain or touch is impaired; (2) the **laterality**, or side of the body where deficits are observed; and (3) the **body regions** that are affected. Damage to one half of the spinal cord, or hemisection, illustrates all three of these characteristic deficits (Figure 5–9). Spinal hemisection can occur, for example, when a tumor encroaches on the cord from one side, or when the cord is injured traumatically. The **Brown–Sequard syndrome** comprises the sensory and motor deficits that follow spinal cord hemisection. Axons in the dorsal columns are **uncrossed** in the spinal cord; hence deficits in **touch** and **limb position sense** are present ipsilateral to the spinal cord lesion (Figure 5–9). In contrast, the axons of the anterolateral system decussate in the spinal cord. Therefore, **pain** and **temperature senses** are impaired on the side of the body that is **contralateral** to the lesion.

We can determine the spinal cord level at which injury occurs by comparing the distribution of sensory loss with the sensory innervation patterns of the dorsal roots (i.e., the dermatomal maps; Figure 5–5). Because of the differences in the anatomical organization of the two systems mediating somatic sensations, a single level of spinal injury will result in different levels of sensory impairment for tactile and pain sensations. For tactile sensation, the level of injury in the spinal cord simply corresponds to the most rostral dermatome in which sensation is impaired. For pain sensation, the injured spinal cord level is about two segments higher than the most rostral dermatome in which sensation is impaired. This is because the axons of the anterolateral system decussate over a distance of one to two spinal segments before ascending to the brain stem and diencephalon.

Two pathological processes affect the dorsal column–medial lemniscal and the anterolateral systems in different ways. First, in **tabes dorsalis**, an advanced stage of neurosyphilis, dorsal root ganglion neurons with

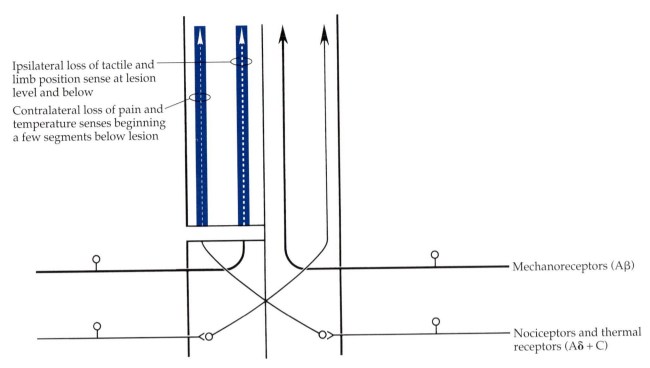

Ipsilateral loss of tactile and limb position sense at lesion level and below

Contralateral loss of pain and temperature senses beginning a few segments below lesion

Mechanoreceptors (Aβ)

Nociceptors and thermal receptors (Aδ + C)

Figure 5–9. The patterns of decussation of the dorsal column–medial lemniscal and anterolateral systems are illustrated in relation to spinal cord hemisection (Brown–Sequard syndrome).

large-diameter axons are lost. Thus, patients lose touch and limb position sense. Fortunately, tabes dorsalis is rarely seen today thanks to antibacterial therapies. At present, patients with neurological signs attributable to injury of the dorsal column–medial lemniscal system more commonly have sustained spinal cord trauma than a syphilitic infection.

Second, in **syringomyelia**, a cavity (or **syrinx**) forms in the central portion of the spinal cord (Figure 5–10A). In the early stages of this condition, the decussating axons of the anterolateral system—which are located in the ventral commissure—are damaged selectively; this results in a loss of pain and temperature sense. Because of the location of the cavity, the axons of the dorsal columns are spared, and therefore touch and limb position senses are unaffected (Figure 5–10B). Syringomyelia interrupts decussating axons from both sides of the body; hence, the sensory loss that occurs is usually bilaterally symmetrical. Cavity formation occurs most commonly in the cervical and upper thoracic spinal segments, thereby producing a capelike distribution of sensory loss on the arms, shoulder, and upper trunk. In this disease, the rostrocaudal distribution of the pain and temperature sensory loss is more limited than in spinal cord hemisection. Also, body regions below the level of injury in syringomyelia have normal sensation, whereas in spinal cord hemisection, pain and temperature sensations are lost caudal to the lesion. This loss begins one to two segments below the level of injury.

Neurosurgeons have taken advantage of the spatial separation of the anterolateral and dorsal column–medial lemniscal systems in the spinal cord. Although rarely performed today because of better analgesics, a sur-

A

Large-diameter fiber
(tactile, vibration, and
position senses)

Small-diameter fiber
(pain and temperature
senses)

Decussating axons
in ventral commissure

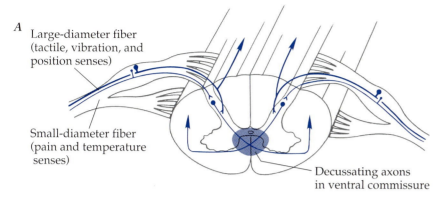

B

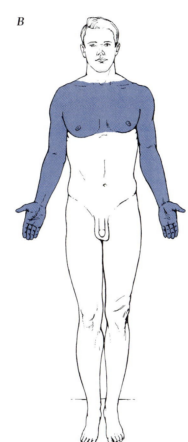

Figure 5–10. Syringomyelia disrupts the decussating fibers of the anterolateral system but usually not the ascending fibers of the dorsal column–medial lemniscal system. *A.* Spinal cord cross section showing the patterns of terminations of small- and large-diameter axons and how the components of the anterolateral system decussate and ascend. The dorsal column–medial lemniscal system ascends ipsilaterally in the spinal cord. The blue tinted region is affected by the formation of a syrinx (cavity). *B.* Distribution of loss of pain and temperature sense over body. (Adapted from Kandel, E. R., and Schwartz, J. H. 1985. Principles of Neural Science. New York: Elsevier.)

gical procedure for the relief of intractable pain, termed **anterolateral cordotomy**, transects the portion of the spinal cord in which axons carrying pain information project to the brain. With time, partial or even complete recovery of pain and temperature senses may occur. Such recovery is thought to be mediated by other sensory pathways (including the small **ipsilateral** projection of the anterolateral system), which become more important for pain function after unilateral destruction of the projection of the anterolateral system. This illustrates the remarkable plastic capabilities of the mature human central nervous system.

Somatic Sensory Decussation in the Medulla Is Located Rostral to the Pyramidal Decussation

Dorsal column axons synapse on neurons in the **dorsal column nuclei** (Figures 5–11A and B), the first major relay in the ascending pathway for touch and limb position senses. These and other relay nuclei do not simply transmit information to the next level in the sequence—or **hierarchy**—of the pathway. Rather, somatic sensory information is transformed in the dorsal column nuclei. Like fine-tuning a television channel, local inhibitory synaptic interactions in the dorsal column nuclei enhance contrast and spatial resolution so that when adjacent portions of the skin are touched, the person can discern the difference.

Axons of the gracile fascicle synapse in the **gracile nucleus**, whereas those from the cuneate fascicle synapse in the **cuneate nucleus**. The section shown in Figure 5–11A is at the level of the crossing of the corticospinal tract, or motor (pyramidal) decussation. The gracile nucleus is located within the gracile fascicle, and the cuneate nucleus is located at the base of the cuneate fascicle. At this level, the cuneate nucleus can be seen "emerging" from the deeper portion of the dorsal horn. The dorsal column nuclei are larger in the more rostral level shown in Figure 5–11B. From the dorsal column nuclei, the axons of the second-order neurons sweep ventrally through the medulla, where they are called the **internal arcuate fibers**, and decussate (Figure 5–11B). Note that the decussation of the dorsal column–medial lemniscal system, the sensory decussation (Figure 5–11B), occurs at a more rostral level than the pyramidal, or motor, decussation (Figure 5–11A).

Figure 5–11. Myelin-stained transverse sections through two levels of the medulla. *A.* Level of the decussation of the corticospinal tract in the pyramid. *B.* Level of the dorsal column nuclei. The inset indicates the approximate planes of section. Trajectories of internal arcuate fibers from the gracile and cuneate nuclei are shown in *B*. Box in right side of *B* marks the location of the axons of the anterolateral system. *Arrows* in *B* indicate planes of section in Figure 5–12.

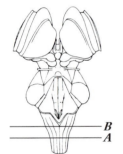

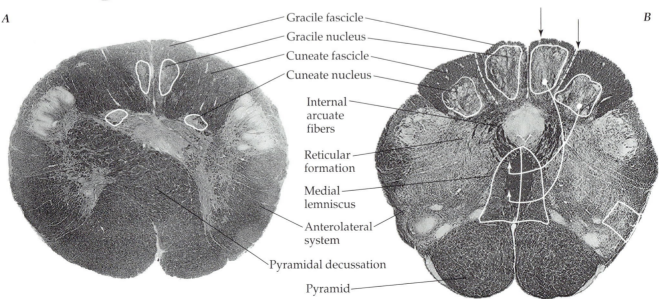

Immediately after crossing the midline, the fibers ascend to the thalamus in the **medial lemniscus**. Axons from the gracile nucleus decussate ventral to axons from the cuneate nucleus and ascend in the ventral part of the medial lemniscus, compared with axons from the cuneate nucleus (Figure 5–11B). Because of this pattern, the somatotopic organization of the medial lemniscus in the medulla resembles a person standing upright: lower limb ventral, followed by the trunk, upper limb, and back of the head (occiput) proceeding dorsally. The human form is, however, deprived of a face because tactile input from the trigeminal nerve, which innervates the face and intraoral structures, is processed by central trigeminal systems located farther rostrally in the pons.

Figure 5–12 illustrates two parasagittal sections; the planes of the sections are indicated in Figure 5–11B. In part A, the section is closer to the midline and slices through the gracile nucleus; in part B, the section is farther from the midline and cuts through the cuneate nucleus. To better under-

A

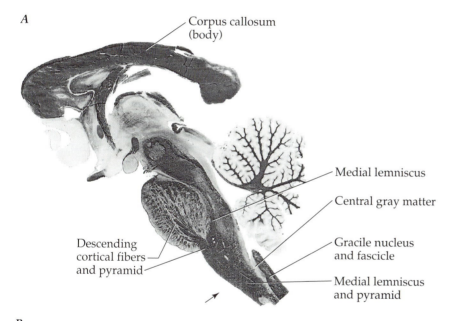

Corpus callosum
(body)

Medial lemniscus

Central gray matter

Descending
cortical fibers
and pyramid

Gracile nucleus
and fascicle

Medial lemniscus
and pyramid

Figure 5–12. Myelin-stained sagittal sections through the brain stem, close to midline (*A*) and farther from midline (*B*). The arrow in part *A* marks the approximate level of the section shown in Figure 5–11B.

B

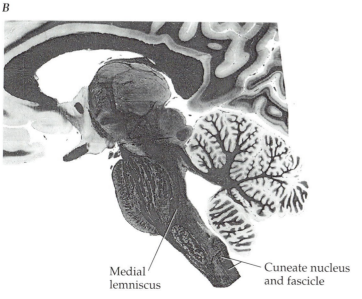

Medial
lemniscus

Cuneate nucleus
and fascicle

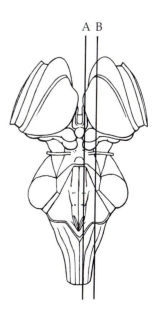

A B

stand the anatomy of the caudal medulla, we will now identify the dorsoventral sequence of structures located along the parasagittal planes in Figure 5–11B (at arrows) and on the parasagittal sections (arrow). In the more medial plane, we can identify three regions: (1) the gracile fascicle and nucleus; (2) gray matter in the central medulla (corresponding to cranial nerve and other nuclei); and (3) the homogeneous expanse of white matter in the ventral medulla corresponding to the medial lemniscus and the pyramid. Note also the three regions of the lateral section: (1) the cuneate fascicle and nucleus, (2) the reticular formation, and (3) the pyramid.

In contrast to the dorsal column–medial lemniscal system, which ascends in the medial medulla, the anterolateral system ascends along its ventrolateral margin (Figure 5–11). For the spinothalamic and spinomesencephalic tracts, the medulla simply serves as a conduit through which axons pass to reach more rostral locations. For the spinoreticular tract, the axons terminate in the reticular formation of the pons and medulla (see below).

Vascular Lesions of the Caudal Brain Stem Differentially Affect Somatic Sensory Function

As we saw in Chapter 4, the caudal brain stem receives blood from the **vertebral–basilar**, or **posterior** circulation. Small perforating branches of this arterial system supply blood to pie-shaped slices of the medulla and pons (each with the apex pointed dorsal and medial; see Figure 4–3). The areas served by the posterior inferior cerebellar artery and smaller branches of the vertebral artery are illustrated in Figure 5–13. Occlusion of the **posterior inferior cerebellar artery (PICA)**, which supplies the dorsolateral portion of the medulla, interrupts the ascending anterolateral system fibers but not the medial lemniscus. For example, a patient who experienced an infarction of the posterior inferior cerebellar artery can have diminished pain and temperature sensation on the limbs and trunk but unaffected touch sense. This sensory loss is contralateral to the side of the lesion because the axons of the anterolateral system decussate in the spinal cord (Figure 5–9) before ascending in the lateral spinal cord and medulla. (Such sensory loss is one of multiple neurological signs that comprise the **lateral medullary syndrome**, or **Wallenberg's syndrome**, which will be discussed further in Chapter 13.)

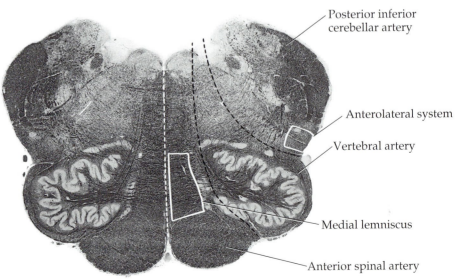

Figure 5–13. The pattern of arterial perfusion of the rostral medulla.

Posterior inferior cerebellar artery

Anterolateral system

Vertebral artery

Medial lemniscus

Anterior spinal artery

Infarction of smaller branches of the vertebral artery interrupts axons of the medial lemniscus but not those of the anterolateral system. As a consequence, touch and limb position senses are disrupted, but not pain and temperature senses. Such vertebral artery infarction produces sensory deficits that are on the contralateral side of the body, because the medial lemniscal axons decussate at a more caudal level in the medulla (Figure 5–11B). This type of infarction also destroys axons of the corticospinal tract in the pyramid. The motor deficits of vertebral artery infarction are considered later (see Chapters 9 and 13).

The Reticular Formation of the Medulla and Pons Receives a Projection From the Anterolateral System

The **spinoreticular tract** terminates in the pontomedullary reticular formation (Figures 5–11, 5–12, and 5–14). The nuclei of the reticular formation are diverse and difficult to distinguish. These projections to the

A

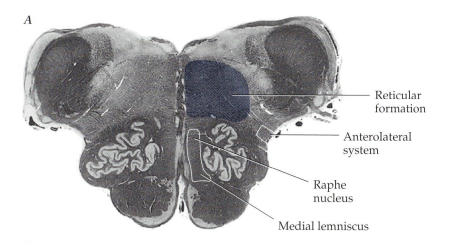

Reticular formation

Anterolateral system

Raphe nucleus

Medial lemniscus

B

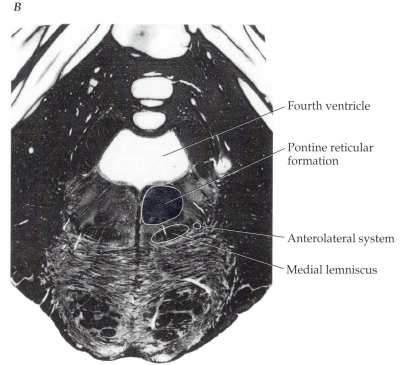

Fourth ventricle

Pontine reticular formation

Anterolateral system

Medial lemniscus

Figure 5–14. Myelin-stained transverse sections through the medulla (*A*) and pons (*B*). The inset shows the approximate plane of section.

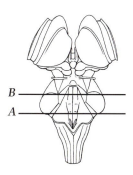

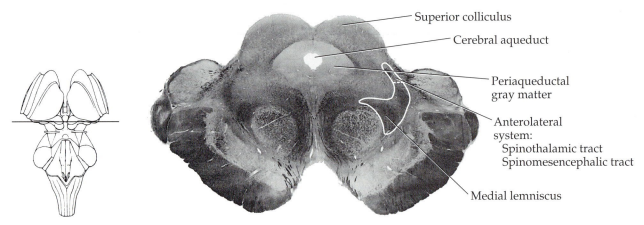

Figure 5–15. A myelin-stained transverse section through the midbrain. The inset shows the approximate plane of section.

reticular formation are thought to be important in regulating arousal—a general function of the reticular formation—and in the affective, or emotional, aspects of pain sensation. In the pons, the medial lemniscus is located more dorsally than in the medulla and is oriented from medial to lateral rather than dorsoventrally, as it is in the medulla. Thus, as the medial lemniscus ascends in the brain stem the homunculus becomes oriented differently: it is standing upright in the medulla and is somewhat reclined in the pons and midbrain.

For the dorsal column–medial lemniscal system, the midbrain serves as a conduit for the axons of the medial lemniscus, which synapse in the thalamus. The medial lemniscus lies in a horn-shaped collection of myelinated axons adjacent to the red nucleus, a nucleus that is important for movement control (Figure 5–15). Fibers of the anterolateral system are located dorsal and lateral to the medial lemniscus. The **spinothalamic tract**, like the medial lemniscus, only courses through the midbrain en route to the thalamus. However, the **spinomesencephalic tract** projects to the superior colliculus (Figure 5–15; see Chapter 6) and to the periaqueductal gray matter (see following section).

Descending Pain Suppression Pathways Originate From the Brain Stem

Neurons in the gray matter surrounding the cerebral aqueduct in the midbrain play a key role in modulating pain perception. A **descending pain inhibitory system** originates from this region. Pain suppression may be a survival mechanism that allows us to function despite pain, such as during physical combat or in childbirth. Receiving complex patterns of input from diencephalic and telencephalic structures involved in emotions (see Chapters 14 and 15), neurons of the **periaqueductal gray matter** (Figure 5–15) project to the **raphe nuclei** in the medulla (Figure 5–14A). These raphe neurons, which use **serotonin** as their neurotransmitter, project to the dorsal horn of the spinal cord. Serotonin suppresses pain transmission in the dorsal horn by: (1) directly inhibiting ascending projection neurons that transmit information about painful stimuli to the brain, and (2) exciting inhibitory interneurons in the dorsal horn which use the neurotransmitter **enkephalin**. A second region of the brain stem, located in the lateral medullary reticular formation (Figure 5–14A), gives rise to a descending noradrenergic projection that also suppresses pain transmission.

Separate Nuclei in the Medial and Lateral Thalamus Process Somatic Sensory Information

The thalamus (Figure 5–16) is a nodal point for the transmission of sensory information to the cerebral cortex. Indeed, with the exception of olfaction, information from all sensory systems is processed in the thalamus and relayed to the cerebral cortex. The dorsal column–medial lemniscal and anterolateral systems are no exceptions. There are two major thalamic regions that receive somatic sensory input. One, located laterally, contains the **ventral posterior nucleus** (Figures 5–16 and 5–17) and the **posterior nuclei**. Both the medial lemniscus and the spinothalamic tract project to these nuclei. The lateral thalamic nuclei are important in somatic sensory discriminations, such as being able to precisely localize the stimulation site on the body. The second region that receives somatic sensory input is found medially in the thalamus, in the **intralaminar nuclei**. Only the spinothalamic tract has a major projection to these nuclei. The medial nuclei are thought to be important in the affective aspects of pain sensation, such as the unpleasant feeling and suffering that painful stimuli evoke.

The ventral posterior nucleus is the principal somatic sensory relay nucleus in the thalamus. It receives the major projections of the medial lemniscus and spinothalamic tract and provides the dominant input to the primary somatic sensory cortex, the key cortical area for perceiving somatic sensory stimuli. The ventral posterior nucleus has two subdivisions. The first, the **ventral posterior medial nucleus** (Figures 5–16 and 5–17B), mediates somatic sensations of the face and perioral structures. The second, the **ventral posterior lateral nucleus** (Figures 5–16 and 5–17B), mediates sensation from the limbs and trunk. Although both the spinothalamic tract and the medial lemniscus terminate in the ventral posterior lateral nucleus, their terminal fields hardly overlap. The course of

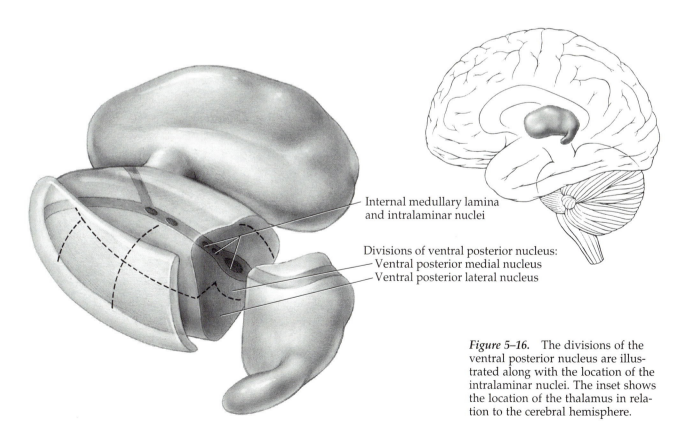

Internal medullary lamina and intralaminar nuclei

Divisions of ventral posterior nucleus:
Ventral posterior medial nucleus
Ventral posterior lateral nucleus

Figure 5–16. The divisions of the ventral posterior nucleus are illustrated along with the location of the intralaminar nuclei. The inset shows the location of the thalamus in relation to the cerebral hemisphere.

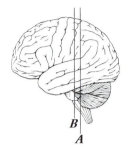

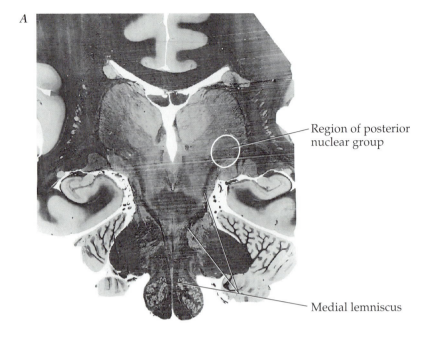

Region of posterior
nuclear group

Medial lemniscus

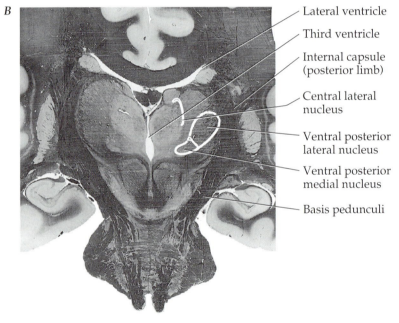

Lateral ventricle

Third ventricle

Internal capsule
(posterior limb)

Central lateral
nucleus

Ventral posterior
lateral nucleus

Ventral posterior
medial nucleus

Basis pedunculi

Figure 5–17. Myelin-stained transverse sections through the diencephalon. The section illustrated in *A* is located caudal to the section shown in *B*. The inset shows the approximate planes of section. The posterior nuclei are located in the general region defined by the oval in *A*. The central lateral nucleus consists of a thin band of neurons in the internal medullary lamina (*B*).

the medial lemniscus in the rostral brain stem, and its termination in the thalamus, is shown in the coronal section in Figure 5–17A. As the medial lemniscus approaches the thalamus, its location becomes more lateral.

The pattern of termination of medial lemniscal axons in the ventral posterior lateral nucleus has been carefully studied and compared with the physiological properties of neurons in this nucleus. Small groups of medial lemniscal axons terminate in elongated rod-shaped fields that are oriented along the rostral–caudal axis. The neurons within a given rod-shaped region form a functional unit; they all process information about a single somesthetic modality, such as touch or position sense, and from the same body location. Neurons in a rod-shaped field, in turn, project to a small group of neurons in the primary somatic sensory cortex that also constitute a functional unit, the **cortical column** (see below).

The **posterior nuclear group** is a collection of nuclei located caudal and ventral to the ventral posterior nucleus, near the junction of the midbrain and diencephalon (Figure 5–17A). These nuclei, which have long been thought to participate in pain sensation, receive input from diverse sources and are likely to be part of a variety of **functional circuits**. A portion of the **posterior nucleus**, one of the nuclei in this group, plays a selective role in somatic sensation. It receives a major input from the ascending somatic sensory pathways and projects to a cortical region within the lateral sulcus (see below). The posterior nuclear group also includes the suprageniculate and limitans nuclei, which receive input from the midbrain tectum and may participate in visuomotor function, and the magnocellular nucleus of the medial geniculate complex, which is a diffuse-projecting nucleus with a regional pattern of termination.

The **intralaminar nuclei**, including the central lateral nucleus (Figure 5–17) also receives spinothalamic input. The intralaminar nuclei also receive inputs from the reticular formation of the pons and medulla. The intralaminar nuclei are diffuse-projecting (see Chapter 3 and Table 3-1); they send their axons to large regions of the cerebral cortex rather than a restricted functional area. The cortical targets of the intralaminar nuclei in the medial thalamus that receive spinothalamic input include the somatic sensory areas of the parietal lobe (see below) as well as motor areas and the limbic association cortex (see Chapter 1).

The Primary Somatic Sensory Cortex Is Located in the Postcentral Gyrus

Located in the postcentral gyrus of the parietal lobe (Figure 5–18), the **primary somatic sensory cortex** is the principal region of the cerebral cortex to which the ventral posterior nucleus projects. Axons from the ventral posterior nucleus travel to the cerebral cortex through the **posterior limb of the internal capsule** (see Figures 11–6 and 11-7), which is bounded by

Figure 5–18. *A.* The locations of the primary and secondary somatic sensory areas are indicated on a lateral view of cerebral cortex. *B.* A schematic section cut perpendicular to the mediolateral axis of the postcentral gyrus. (Adapted from Kandel, E. R., and Schwartz, J. H. 1985. Principles of Neural Science. New York: Elsevier.)

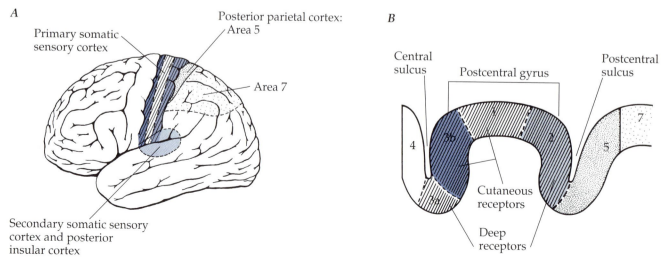

the thalamus and caudate nucleus medially and the globus pallidus and putamen laterally (Figure 5–17B; see also Figures AII–6 and AII–7). These axons provide the major subcortical input to the somatic sensory cortex.

The Somatic Sensory Cortex Has a Columnar Functional Organization

The primary somatic sensory cortex is part of the neocortex, the portion of the cerebral cortex that has six cell layers (see Figure 3–15). Neurons in local regions of the somatic sensory cortex, spanning all cortical layers, have two common properties: (1) they all receive input from the same peripheral location on the body, and (2) they receive input from the same class of peripheral sensory receptor. This is the **columnar organization**. Although originally conceived as cylindrical in shape, the cortical columns have a more irregular configuration.

The column is the fundamental processing unit of the somatic sensory cortex. The thalamocortical axons from the ventral posterior nucleus synapse on cell bodies of neurons located in the deep portion of layer 3 and throughout layer 4. These are the **input layers** of the somatic sensory cortex. The thalamic axons also synapse directly on the dendrites of some of the neurons in other cortical layers. Neurons in the input layers, in turn, distribute afferent information to neurons in layers above and below, which are the **output layers**. As we shall discover below, neurons in the output layers project their axons to other somatic sensory cortical areas.

The Somatic Sensory Cortex Has a Somatotopic Organization

The primary somatic sensory cortex receives input from receptors located on the contralateral side of the body. Similar to all other levels of the somatic sensory system, this cortex is somatotopically organized. Reflecting this somatotopy is a precise topographic relationship describing the connections between projection neurons in the ventral posterior nucleus and the primary somatic sensory cortex (Figure 5–19). The lateral portion of the ventral posterior lateral nucleus receives somatic sensory input from the leg and lower trunk, and projects to the medial portion of the postcentral gyrus. Much of the lower limb representation is on the medial surface of the parietal lobe, in the sagittal (or interhemispheric) fissure. The medial part of the ventral posterior lateral nucleus receives input from the neck, arm, and upper trunk, and projects to the postcentral gyrus on the lateral surface of the hemisphere. The ventral posterior medial nucleus, the thalamic relay nucleus for facial somatic sensory information, projects to the most lateral part of the postcentral gyrus, adjacent to and within the lateral sulcus.

In the somatic sensory cortex, the somatotopic organization is remarkably similar to a map of the surface of the body, a configuration termed the **sensory homunculus**. The representations of the various body parts on the map do not have the same proportions as the body itself. Rather, the portions of the body used in discriminative tactile tasks, such as the fingers, have a disproportionately greater representation on the map than areas that are not as important for touch discrimination, such as the leg (Figure 5–19). It was once thought that these areal differences were fixed and simply reflected the density of peripheral receptors. We now know that the body map of the brain is not static, but dynamically controlled by the pattern of use of different body parts in tactile exploration. If one body part is prevented from use in tactile discrimination (e.g., after peripheral nerve injury), its cortical representation shrinks. In contrast, if one part is used more extensively (e.g., the second through

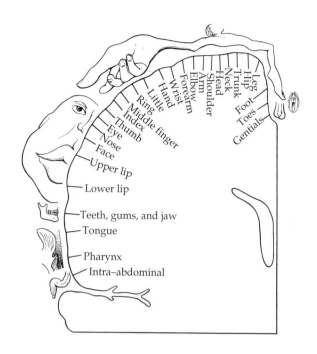

Figure 5–19. The primary somatic cortex is somatotopically organized. This figure illustrates a schematic coronal section through the postcentral gyrus. (Adapted from Penfield, W., and Rasmussen, T. 1950. The Cerebral Cortex of Man: A Clinical Study of Localization Function. New York: Macmillan.)

fifth fingers of the left hand of an accomplished violinist), its representation expands.

The Primary Somatic Sensory Cortex Has a Modality-specific Organization

In the primary somatic sensory cortex, as in other cortical areas, regions with different cytoarchitecture subserve different functions. The primary somatic sensory cortex consists of four cytoarchitectonic divisions, or **Brodmann's areas** (see Figure 3–16), numbered 1, 2, 3a, and 3b (Figure 5–18). Areas 3a and 2 receive information from receptors located in deep structures, such as the muscles and joints, and areas 3b and 1, from mechanoreceptors of the skin. In each of these areas there is a separate representation of the body. In areas 3b and 1, the representations are complete and highly detailed; in areas 3a and 2, the representations appear to be more coarse.

The cutaneous and deep projections to the different cytoarchitectonic areas arise from different portions of the ventral posterior nucleus. These differences provide important insights into the functions subserved by the four primary somatic sensory cortical areas. The contrasting ways in which the cortex receives inputs indicates that it processes each somatic sensory modality separately. Areas 3a and 2 play important roles in limb position sense and shape discrimination of grasped objects; areas 3b and 1 play a major role in touch perception. Surprisingly, neither experimental studies in animals nor the analysis of sensory changes in humans who have had parietal lobe lesions has demonstrated that the primary somatic sensory cortex plays a critical role in processing painful stimuli. Positron emission tomographic (PET) studies in humans, however, have recently suggested a role for the somatic sensory cortical areas in pain (see Box 5–1).

Box 5–1. *The Cortical Representation of Pain*

The primary and secondary somatic sensory cortical areas have a well-documented role in tactile perception and limb position senses. Moreover, much of what we know about the properties of neurons in these areas is based on their responses to mechanical stimuli. Using positron emission tomography (PET; see Figure 1–18), a noninvasive imaging technique, it has been shown that the primary and secondary somatic sensory cortical areas are also involved in processing noxious stimuli. It is thought that the primary sensory area, which receives input from the lateral thalamus, and the secondary area, which receives input from the primary area, are important for **localizing** and **discerning the intensity** of painful stimuli.

PET has also shown that two other cortical regions are activated by noxious stimulation (painful heat stimuli). One area, the **anterior insular cortex,** is selectively activated by painful stimuli, and this region is shown in the PET scans in Figure 5–20. Part A shows a three-dimensional view, reconstructed from a series of slices; an example of one slice is shown in part B. The other area involved in pain, the **anterior cingulate cortex,** is activated by both noxious and nonnoxious stimuli. This area is not shown in the PET scans. It corresponds approximately to Brodmann's area 24 (see Figure 3–16).

The cingulate and anterior insular areas, which receive input

from the medial thalamus, are thought to be important in the **affective and reactive components of pain.** The anterior insular cortex has direct projections to key limbic system structures, including the amygdaloid complex and limbic association cortex. The cingulate cortex is part of the limbic system (Chapter 15), which comprises the cortical and subcortical circuitry for emotions.

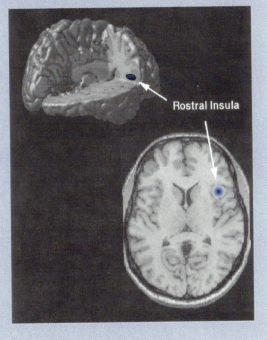

Rostral Insula

Figure 5–20. Positron emission tomography using ^{15}O (see Box 1–1) showing the distribution of selective increase in cerebral blood flow during noxious thermal stimulation. Scans reflect computed differences between activation patterns produced by noxious thermal stimulation and nonnoxious activation. *A.* A three-dimensional view, reconstructed from a series of slices. The highlighted region corresponds to the anterior insular cortex. *B.* A two-dimensional slice through the active region of anterior insular cortex. Darker blue indicates greater ^{15}O utilization by the tissue. (Coghill et al., 1994; Courtesy of Dr. Gary Duncan, Universitié de Montréal and Montreal Neurological Institute.)

Efferent Projections Arise From the Primary Somatic Sensory Cortex

The primary somatic sensory cortex, as well as other cortical regions, contains three kinds of efferent projections mediated by three separate classes of neurons: corticocortical association, callosal, and descending projection. The various classes of efferent projection neurons are located in the output layers of the cortex (layer 2, part of layer 3, and layers 5 and 6). Moreover, efferent projection neurons with different targets are located in different cortical layers.

- **Corticocortical association neurons** give rise to "ascending" projections, in much the same way as the ascending somatic sensory pathways of the spinal cord and brain stem. This is because their axonal projections are directed to higher-order sensory cortical areas and the primary motor cortex. Together, these areas process somatic sensory information for perception as well as for planning and controlling behavioral responses. Corticocortical association neurons are located predominantly in layers 2 and 3.

- **Callosal neurons** make the second type of projection, which is to the contralateral somatic sensory cortex via the body of the **corpus callosum** (Figure 5–12). One function of callosal connections in sensory systems may be to "stitch together" the representations of each half of the body in the primary somatic sensory cortex of each hemisphere. In accord with this hypothesis, only neurons located in the representation of proximal body parts, and not the hand and foot areas, are connected with the contralateral hemisphere. Like the association neurons, the callosal neurons are located in layers 2 and 3.

- **Descending projection neurons** are the third type of cortical projection neuron. There are separate classes of projection neurons whose axons descend to: (1) the striatum (the caudate nucleus and putamen); (2) the ventral posterior nucleus of the thalamus; (3) the brain stem, especially the dorsal column nuclei; or (4) the dorsal horn of the spinal cord. Descending projection neurons are found in layers 5 and 6. Those neurons in layer 5 terminate in the striatum, brain stem, and spinal cord, whereas those projecting to the thalamus are located in layer 6. Except for the projection to the striatum, whose function is poorly understood, the descending projections from the somatic sensory cortex are thought to act as "gatekeepers" that regulate the quantity of somatic sensory information that ascends through the central nervous system.

Higher-order Somatic Sensory Cortical Areas Are Located in the Parietal Lobe, Parietal Operculum, and Insular Cortex

In addition to the primary somatic sensory cortex, there are multiple regions in the parietal lobe and insular cortex that process somatic sensory information (Figure 5–18A) for perception and other higher brain functions. Each of these areas receives the major somatic sensory input from the primary somatic sensory cortex and not from the thalamus. There are two major somatic sensory cortical areas that receive input from the primary cortex: (1) the secondary somatic sensory cortex and related areas in the lateral sulcus, and (2) the posterior parietal cortex.

As its name implies, the **secondary somatic sensory cortex**, located largely on the parietal operculum, receives its major input from the primary somatic sensory cortex. Similar to the primary area, the secondary somatic sensory cortex is somatotopically organized. This part of the cortex begins a cascade of somatic sensory projections into the parietal and temporal operculum and the insular cortex. The pathway from the primary somatic sensory cortex to its secondary counterpart and then to the insular cortical areas comprises a processing sequence related to **object recognition by touch and position sense**. Similar pathways from primary to secondary and then to higher-order areas in the temporal lobe also exist for vision (see Chapter 6) and hearing (see Chapter 7).

The **posterior parietal cortex**, which includes Brodmann's areas 5 and 7, receives somatic sensory input from the other somatic sensory cortical areas, especially area 2 of the primary somatic sensory cortex. The posterior parietal cortex plays an important role in perception of body image. A lesion of this region in the nondominant hemisphere (typically the right hemisphere) produces a complex sensory syndrome in which the individual neglects the contralateral half of the body. For example, a patient may fail to dress half of her body or comb half of her hair. Other portions of the posterior parietal cortex receive visual and auditory inputs as well as somatic sensory information. These areas are involved in multi-modal perceptual mechanisms and in attention.

Thalamocortical somatic sensory processing offers a general principle of organization of sensory systems. The main thalamic sensory nucleus for a given modality (e.g., ventral posterior nucleus for somatic sensation) has a restricted projection to the primary sensory cortex. Projections from the primary sensory cortical area, in turn, distribute the sensory information to multiple, distinct cortical regions. These "upstream" sensory areas are each devoted to processing a specific aspect of the sensory experience. Although serial pathways from one region to the next can sometimes be identified, we now know that the primary and higher-order sensory areas are extensively interconnected and that the operations of any one set of connections are dependent on the operations of others. The higher-order sensory areas, in turn, typically project to cortical regions that receive inputs from the other sensory modalities termed **association areas.** One such multimodal convergent zone is the large expanse of cortex at the junction of the parietal, temporal, and occipital lobes.

Summary

Somatic Sensory Pathways

There are two major somatic sensory pathways (Figures 5–1 and 5–2; Table 5–1): the **dorsal column–medial lemniscal system**, which mediates **tactile and limb position sense**, and the **anterolateral system**, which mediates **pain and temperature sense** and a less discriminative form of tactile sense. These systems differ in four major ways: (1) modality sensitivity of input from dorsal root ganglion neurons, (2) location of first relay site, (3) level of decussation, and (4) functional and anatomical homogeneity of the pathway.

Receptor Neurons

Dorsal root ganglion neurons are **pseudounipolar neurons** (Figure 5–3). They receive somatic sensory information and transmit it from the periphery to the spinal cord. The distal terminal of dorsal root ganglion neurons is the **sensory receptor**. Receptors sensitive to **noxious** and **thermal stimuli** have **bare nerve endings** and have **small-diameter axons** (A-δ; C). Those sensitive to **mechanical** stimuli have encapsulated endings and have **large-diameter axons** (A-α; A-β). There are four major mechanoreceptors that innervate glabrous skin and subcutaneous tissue (Figure 5–4): **Meissner's corpuscles**, **pacinian corpuscles**, **Merkel's receptors**, and **Ruffini's corpuscles.** The **muscle spindle** is the key receptor for muscle stretch.

Spinal Cord

The axons of dorsal root ganglion neurons enter the spinal cord via the **dorsal root**. A **dermatome** is the area of skin innervated by a single

dorsal root (Figure 5–5). The afferent information carried by adjacent dorsal roots overlaps nearly completely on the body surface. Once in the spinal cord, dorsal root ganglion neurons have three major branches: **segmental**, **ascending**, and **descending** (Figure 5–6). The principal branching pattern of large-diameter fibers is to ascend to the brain stem in the dorsal columns. Whereas small-diameter fibers ascend and descend in **Lissauer's tract**, they eventually terminate in the gray matter of the spinal cord.

The ascending somatic sensory pathways course in two locations in the spinal cord. The dorsal column–medial lemniscal system ascends in the **dorsal columns**. The dorsal columns have two fascicles (Figures 5–7 and 5–8). The **gracile fascicle** carries axons from the leg and lower trunk, and the **cuneate fascicle** carries axons from the upper trunk, arm, neck, and back of the head. The majority of the axons in the dorsal columns are central branches of dorsal root ganglion neurons. The axons of the anterolateral system derive from dorsal horn neurons, and decussate in the **ventral commissure** (Figure 5–6). The anterolateral system ascends in the lateral column (Figures 5–6 and 5–7). Spinal cord hemisection has a differential effect on the somatic sensory modalities caudal to the lesion, producing loss of touch and position senses on the side of the lesion, and pain and temperature senses on the opposite side (Figure 5–9). Central spinal lesions can selectively disrupt the decussating axons of the anterolateral system (Figure 5–10).

Brain Stem

Dorsal column axons terminate in the **dorsal column nuclei** in the caudal medulla (Figures 5–11 and 5–12). Axons of neurons in the dorsal column nuclei decussate and ascend in the **medial lemniscus** (Figures 5–11 through 5–15, 5–17A) and terminate in the thalamus. Fibers of the anterolateral system terminate in the **reticular formation** (Figures 5–11 and 5–14) (**spinoreticular tract**), **midbrain tectum** (Figure 5–15) (**spinomesencephalic tract**), and **thalamus (spinothalamic tract)** (Figures 5–16 and 5–17).

Thalamus

The axons of the medial lemniscus and the spinothalamic tract synapse in the thalamus. Both brain stem pathways synapse in the lateral division of the ventral posterior nucleus of the thalamus (**ventral posterior lateral nucleus**) (Figures 5–16 and 5–17B) and the posterior nuclei (Figure 5–17A). In addition, the spinothalamic tract terminates in the **intralaminar nuclei**.

Somatic Sensory Cortical Regions

There are three major somatic sensory cortical areas. The **primary somatic sensory cortex** (1) (Figure 5–18) receives the direct projection from the ventral posterior lateral nucleus, via the **posterior limb of the internal capsule**. The primary somatic sensory cortex has a **columnar** functional organization. The **secondary somatic sensory cortex** (2), and **posterior parietal cortex** (3) receive input from the primary somatic sensory cortex. Each of these cortical areas are somatotopically organized.

Efferent projections from the somatic sensory cortical areas arise from specific cortical layers. **Corticocortical association** connections (with other cortical areas on the same side of the cerebral cortex) are made by neurons in layers 2 and 3. **Callosal** connections (with the other side of the cerebral cortex) are also made by neurons in layers 2 and 3. **Descending**

projections to the striatum, brain stem, and spinal cord originate from neurons located in layer 5, whereas the projection to the thalamus originates from neurons located in layer 6. ■

KEY STRUCTURES AND TERMS

dorsal column–medial lemniscal
    system
  gracile fascicle
  cuneate fascicle
  gracile nucleus
  cuneate nucleus
  internal arcuate fibers
  medial lemniscus
anterolateral system
  spinothalamic tract
    neospinothalamic tract
    paleospinothalamic tract
  spinoreticular tract
  spinomesencephalic tract
dorsal root ganglion neurons
dorsal root ganglia
pseudounipolar neurons
bare nerve endings
mechanoreceptors
  Meissner's corpuscle
  Pacinian corpuscle
  Ruffini's corpuscle

Merkel's receptor
muscle spindle
dorsal roots
dermatome
radicular pain
spinal cord regions
  dorsal horn
    ascending projection neuron
  intermediate zone
  ventral horn
  dorsal column
  lateral column
  ventral column
ventral (anterior) commissure
large-diameter fiber entry zone
Lissauer's tract
Rexed's laminae
dorsal intermediate septum
dorsal median septum
Brown–Sequard syndrome
tabes dorsalis
syringomyelia

posterior inferior cerebellar artery
lateral medullary syndrome
periaqueductal gray matter
raphe nuclei
serotonin
enkephalin
ventral posterior nucleus
  ventral posterior medial nucleus
  ventral posterior lateral nucleus
posterior nuclear group
intralaminar nuclei
internal capsule—posterior limb
cortical column
primary somatic sensory cortex
  Brodmann's areas (1, 2, 3a,
    and 3b)
secondary somatic sensory cortex
posterior parietal cortex
corpus callosum
corticocortical association neurons
callosal neurons
descending projection neuron

Selected Readings

Brown, A. G. 1981. Organization in the Spinal Cord: The Anatomy and Physiology of Identified Neurons. New York: Springer.

Brown, A. G. 1981. The terminations of cutaneous nerve fibers in the spinal cord. Trends in Neuroscience 4:64–67.

Dubner, R., and Bennett, G. J. 1983. Spinal and trigeminal mechanisms of nociception. Ann. Rev. Neurosci. 6:381–418.

Fields, H. L. 1987. Pain. New York: McGraw-Hill.

Kandel, E. R., and Jessell, T. M. 1991. Touch. In Kandel, E. R., Schwartz, J. H., and Jessell, T. M. (eds.), Principles of Neural Science, 3rd ed. New York: Elsevier, pp. 366–384.

Jessell, T. M., and Kelly, D. D. 1991. Pain and analgesia. In Kandel, E. R., Schwartz, J. H., and Jessell, T. M. (eds.), Principles of Neural Science, 3rd ed. New York: Elsevier, pp. 385–399.

Martin, J. H., and Jessell, T. M. 1991. Modality coding in the somatic sensory system. In Kandel, E. R., Schwartz, J. H., and Jessell, T. M. (eds.), Principles of Neural Science, 3rd ed. New York: Elsevier, pp. 341–352.

Martin, J. H., and Jessell, T. M. 1991. Anatomy of the somatic sensory system. In Kandel, E. R., Schwartz, J. H., and Jessell, T. M. (eds.), Principles of Neural Science, 3rd ed. New York: Elsevier, pp. 353–366.

Mountcastle, V. B. 1984. Central nervous mechanisms in mechanoreceptive sensibility. In Darian-Smith, I. (ed.), Handbook of Physiology, Section 1: The Nervous System, Vol. III. Sensory Processes. Bethesda, Md.: American Physiological Society, pp. 789–878.

Rustioni, A., Weinberg, R. J. 1989. The somatosensory system. In Bjumörklund, A., Hókfelt, T., and Swanson, L. W. (eds.), Handbook of Chemical Neuroanatomy. Vol. 7. Integrated Systems of the CNS, Part II. Central Visual, Auditory, Somatosensory, Gustatory. Amsterdam: Elsevier, pp. 219–321.

Willis, W. D. 1985. Nociceptive pathways: Anatomy and physiology of nociceptive ascending pathways. Phil. Trans. Soc. Lond. B 308:253–268.

Willis, W. D., Jr. 1985. The Pain System: The Neural Basis of Nociceptive Transmission in the Mammalian Nervous System. Basel: Karger.

Willis, W. D., and Coggeshall, R. E. 1978. Sensory Mechanisms of the Spinal Cord. New York: Plenum.

References

Appelberg, A. E., Leonard, R. B., Kenshalo, D. R., Jr., et al. 1979. Nuclei in which functionally identified spinothalamic tract neurons terminate. J. Comp. Neurol. 188:575–586.

Burton, H., and Jones, E. G. 1976. The posterior thalamic region and its cortical projection in new world and old world monkeys. J. Comp. Neurol. 168:249–302.

Coghill, R. C., Talbot, J. D., Evans, A. C., et al. 1994. Distributed processing of pain and vibration by the human brain. J. Neurosci. 14:4095–4108.

Collins, R. D. 1962. Illustrated Manual of Neurologic Diagnosis. Philadelphia: Lippincott.

Craig, A. D., Jr., and Burton, H. 1981. Spinal and medullary laminal projection to nucleus submedius in medial thalamus: A possible pain center. J. Neurophysiol. 45:443–466.

Friedman, D. P., Murray, E. A., O'Neil, J. B., and Mishkin, M. 1986. Cortical connections of the somatosensory fields of the lateral sulcus of macaques: Evidence for a corticolimbic pathway for touch. J. Comp. Neurol. 252:323–347.

Gobel, S. 1979. Neural circuitry in the substantia gelatinosa of Rolando: Anatomical insights. In Bonica, J. J. (ed.), Advances in Pain Research and Therapy, Vol. 3. New York: Raven Press, pp. 175–195.

Jones, A. K. P., Brown, W. D., Firston, K. J., et al. 1991. Cortical and subcortical localization of response to pain in man using positron emission tomography. Proc. R. Soc. Lond. B 244:39–44.

Jones, E. G. 1984. Organization of the thalamocortical complex and its relation to sensory processes. In Darian-Smith, I. (ed.), Handbook of Physiology, Section 1: The Nervous System, Vol. III. Sensory Processes. Bethesda, Md.: American Physiological Society, pp. 149–212.

Jones, E. G., and Friedman, D. P. 1982. Projection pattern of functional components of thalamic ventrobasal complex on monkey somatosensory cortex. J. Neurophysiol. 48:521–544.

Jones, E. G., and Leavitt, R. Y. 1974. Retrograde axonal transport and the demonstration of non-specific projections to the cerebral cortex and striatum from thalamic intralaminar nuclei in the rat, cat and monkey. J. Comp. Neurol. 154:349–378.

Jones, E. G., and Powell, T. P. S. 1971. An analysis of the posterior group of thalamic nuclei on the basis of its afferent connections. J. Comp. Neurol. 143:185–216.

Light, A. R., and Perl, E. R. 1984. Peripheral sensory systems. In Dyck, P. J., Thomas, P. K., Lambert, E. H., and Bruge, R. (eds.) Peripheral Neuropathy, 2nd ed. Vol. 1. Philadelphia: Saunders, pp. 210–230.

Mantyh, P. W. 1983. The spinothalamic tract in the primate: A reexamination using wheat germ agglutinin conjugated to horseradish peroxidase. Neurosci. 9:847–862.

Ralston, H. J., III, and Ralston, D. D. 1982. The distribution of dorsal root axons to laminae IV, V, and VI of the macaque spinal cord: A quantitative electron microscopic study. J. Comp. Neurol. 212:435–448.

Talbot, J. D., Marrett, S., Evans, A. C., et al. 1991. Multiple representations of pain in human cerebral cortex. Science 251:1355–1358.

Willis, W. D., Kenshalo, D. R., Jr., and Leonard, R. B. 1979. The cells of origin of the primate spinothalamic tract. J. Comp. Neurol. 188:543–574.

6

The Visual System

IN MANY WAYS THE VISUAL SYSTEM IS ORGANIZED like the systems for touch and pain, considered in the previous chapter. For instance, the topography of connections in the visual system is determined largely by how the receptive sheet is organized. In fact, these connections are so systematized and predictable that often the clinician can use a visual sensory defect to pinpoint the location of central nervous system damage with remarkable precision. Another similarity is that all three systems have a **hierarchical** and **parallel** organization. In a hierarchically organized system, we can discern **distinct functional levels with respect to one another**, each with clear anatomical substrates. In vision, as in somatic sensation, multiple hierarchically organized pathways carry information from the receptors to structures in the central nervous system. Each of these pathways process visual information for a different purpose. For example, separate systems participate in perception of visual form, motion, and color.

Visual perception, like perception for the other senses, is not a passive process; our eyes do not simply receive visual stimulation. Rather, the position of the eyes is precisely controlled to scan the environment and to attend selectively and orient to specific visual stimuli. In addition to the pathways for visual perception, there is also an anatomically separate pathway for controlling eye movements. We begin this chapter with an overview of the separate visual pathways for perception and eye movement control. Next, we consider the structure and anatomical connections of their components. Finally, we examine how the physician can use knowledge of the organization of the visual system to localize disturbances of brain function with precision.

THE FUNCTIONAL ANATOMY OF THE VISUAL SYSTEM

Anatomically Separate Visual Paths Mediate Perception and Ocular Reflex Function

Both the visual pathway that subserves perception and the pathway that controls eye movement originate in the retina. Here, the photoreceptors—which transduce visual stimuli into neural signals—are located

(Figure 6–1A, inset). Photoreceptors synapse on retinal interneurons which, in turn, synapse on ganglion cells. **Ganglion cells** are the retinal neurons that project to the brain stem and thalamus. The axons of ganglion cells travel in the **optic nerve** (cranial nerve II), with ganglion cells from each eye contributing axons to the optic nerve on the same side. Some optic nerve axons decussate in the **optic chiasm** en route to the thalamus and brain stem (Figure 6–1A; see below), whereas other axons in the nerve remain uncrossed. Together the crossed and uncrossed fibers of the optic nerves, reordered according to a precise plan (see below), course in the **optic tract**.

Figure 6–1. Organization of the two visual pathways, the retinal–geniculate–calcarine pathway *(A)* and the pathway to the midbrain *(B).* The inset on the left shows the general organization of the retina. The photoreceptor transduces visual stimuli and transmits the sensory information, encoded in the form of nonpropagated potentials, to retinal interneurons. The interneurons transmit the visual information to the ganglion cells. Ganglion cell axons form the optic nerve once they exit the eyeball. The inset on the right shows the medial surface of the occipital lobe and the primary visual cortex, which is tinted blue.

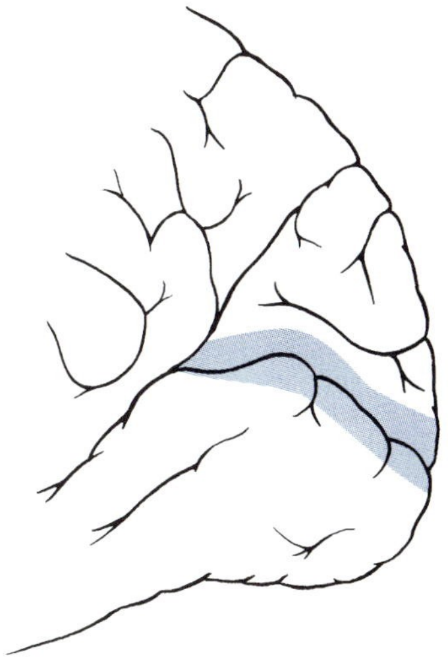

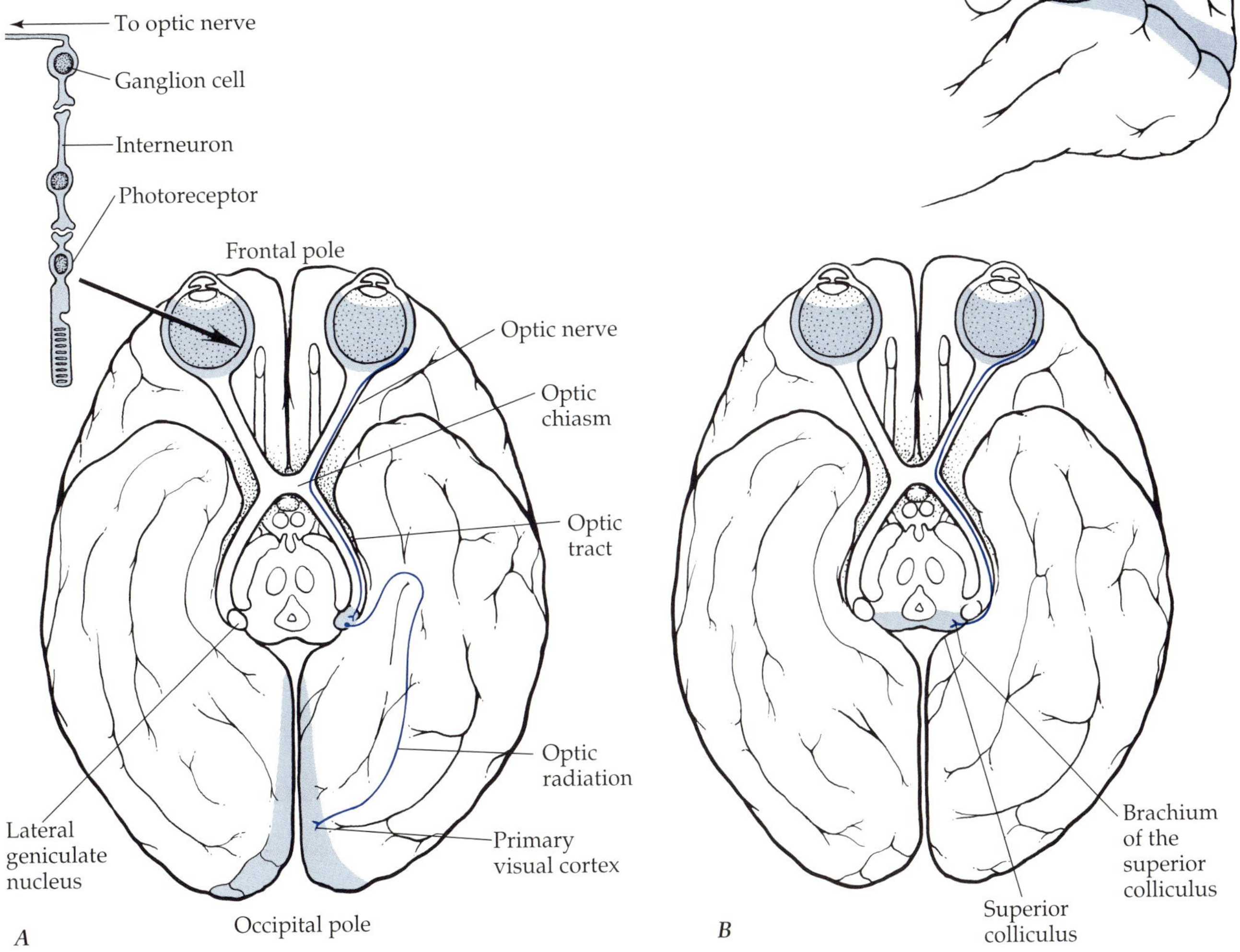

To optic nerve

Ganglion cell

Interneuron

Photoreceptor

Frontal pole

Optic nerve

Optic chiasm

Optic tract

Optic radiation

Lateral geniculate nucleus

Primary visual cortex

Occipital pole

A

Brachium of the superior colliculus

Superior colliculus

B

*The Pathway to the Primary Visual Cortex Mediates
the Perception of Visual Form, Color, and Movement*

The principal thalamic target for ganglion cells is the **lateral geniculate nucleus**. This thalamic relay nucleus for vision is analogous to the ventral posterior nucleus, the somatic sensory relay nucleus. The lateral geniculate nucleus, in turn, projects to the **primary visual cortex** via a pathway called the **optic radiations**. The primary visual cortex is located in the occipital lobe, along the banks and within the depths of the **calcarine fissure** (Figure 6–1, see inset showing medial surface of cortex; see also Figure 6–11B). The function of the primary visual cortex was considered briefly in Chapter 1 (see Box 1–1 and Figure 1–18). The primary visual cortex is also referred to as the **striate cortex** because myelinated axons form a prominent striation, termed the **stripe of Gennari**. This stripe is so distinct that it actually can be observed in unstained dissected tissue.

Efferent projections from the primary visual cortex follow one of three principal paths. One path "ascends" to the **secondary** and **higher-order visual cortical areas** in the occipital lobe. Whereas the primary visual cortex is important in basic visual signal processing, fundamental to all aspects of visual perception, the different higher-order cortical areas are each thought to be important in a different aspect of vision. For example, one area is important in color vision and another in perceiving visual motion. The ascending path is also important in guiding our movements to visual targets. The axons of the second path decussate in the corpus callosum and terminate in the contralateral primary visual cortex. This projection helps to unify the images from the two eyes into a perception of a single visual world. Finally, the third path from the primary visual cortex descends to oculomotor centers in the midbrain. One important role of this descending path is in focusing the visual image on the retina.

*The Pathway to the Midbrain Is Important in
Voluntary and Reflexive Control of the Eyes*

Certain ganglion cells project to the midbrain (Figure 6–1B), principally to two structures: (1) the **superior colliculus** and (2) the **pretectal nuclei**. The superior colliculus, found in the **tectum** of the midbrain, is located dorsal to the cerebral aqueduct (Figure 6–1B; see Figure 3–8). In lower vertebrates, such as amphibians and birds, the superior colliculus is termed the **optic tectum** and is the principal brain structure for vision, in lieu of a visual cortex. In mammals and especially humans, the superior colliculus has a minimal role in perception but an important role in voluntary control of **saccades**. These rapid eye movements are quick shifts in visual gaze that we use to look from one object to another. We will examine the neural circuits for controlling saccades and other eye movements in Chapter 13 (see Box 13–1). The optic tract axons traveling to the superior colliculus skirt the lateral geniculate nucleus and enter the superior colliculus through the **brachium of the superior colliculus** (Figures 6–1B and 6–6). The projections of the superior colliculus are organized to control rapid eye movements to salient stimuli and to coordinate movement of the head with eye movements.

The pretectal nuclei, the other major brain stem target of the optic tract, are located rostral to the tectum, at the midbrain–diencephalic junction (see Figure 6–8B). Similar to the projection to the colliculus, the visual axons coursing to the pretectum travel in the brachium of the superior colliculus. The pretectal nuclei participate in **pupillary reflexes**, which regulate the amount of light reaching the retina, as well as other visual reflexes.

There are other diencephalic and brain stem projections of the optic tract that subserve particular functions. The projection to the hypothalamus is important for diurnal regulation of hormone secretion (see Chapter 14). There is also a projection to midbrain nuclei that are important in the reflexive control of eye position to stabilize images on the retina during motion of the head. These nuclei comprise the **accessory optic system**. The neural structures that mediate pupillary and other visual reflexes will be covered in Chapter 13 because the efferent axons of the reflexes are carried by motor cranial nerves.

Next, we turn to the detailed anatomy of each major visual system component. We begin with the optical properties of the eye and the retina and then examine retinal projections to the brain stem. Finally, we trace the pathway from the thalamus to the cerebral cortex and discuss the clinical consequences of damage to this pathway.

■ REGIONAL ANATOMY

The Optical Properties of the Eye Transform Visual Stimuli

After light enters the eye through the cornea, the transparent avascular portion of the sclera, it is focused onto the retinal surface by the lens. The area seen by both eyes when their position remains fixed is called the **visual field** (Figure 6–2; see also Figure 6–20). The field of view of each eye is not simply half of the total visual field. Just as when we look through binoculars, the visual field of each eye overlaps extensively (Figure 6–2A) to form the total visual field. However, this is where the comparison with binoculars ends. The total visual field (or simply the visual field) is the sum of the right and left hemifields and consists of a central overlap (binocular) zone, where we have stereoscopic vision, and two monocular zones. The visual field is divided into symmetrical right and left halves. The retina is also divided in half by a vertical line passing through the **fovea**, a specialized high-resolution portion of the retina, into a **nasal hemiretina** and a **temporal hemiretina**. Each hemiretina includes half of the fovea and the remaining perifoveal and peripheral retina.

Because of the lens, the visual image becomes inverted and reversed when projected on the retina (Figure 6–2B). This image reversal causes the right half of a visual image to fall on the left half of the retina of each eye— the left temporal hemiretina and the right nasal hemiretina. Conversely, the left half of the image falls on the right temporal hemiretina and the left nasal hemiretina.

The Retina Contains Five Major Layers

The retina—a thin sheet of neurons and glial cells—is apposed to the posterior inner surface of the eyeball. Although located in the periphery of the body, the retina is not part of the peripheral nervous system; it is actually a displaced portion of the central nervous system. It develops from an outpouching of the diencephalon (see Figure 2–3) and not the **neural crest,** from which the somatic sensory receptors derive.

The retina is not uniform; it has two morphologically distinct portions. The first is the **optic disk,** where retinal axons leave the eyeball

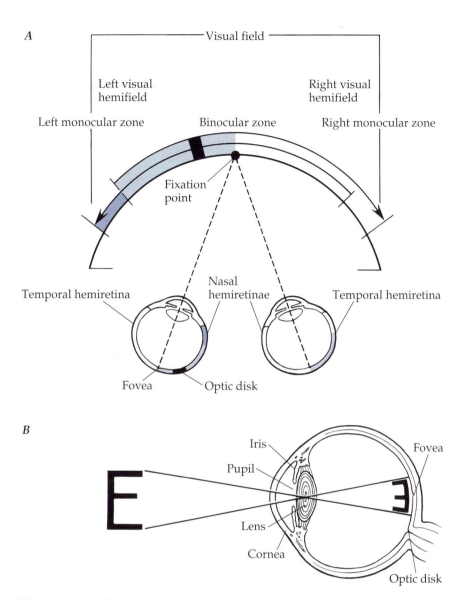

Figure 6–2. **A.** Horizontal view of the relationship between the location of the visual fields for each eye, an image in space, and how the image falls on the retina. **B.** Sagittal view shows the key features of the optical properties of the eye. Note that the blind spot is shown only for the left visual field. (Adapted from Kandel, E. R., and Schwartz, J. H. 1985. Principles of Neural Science. New York: Elsevier.)

and the blood vessels serving a part of the retina enter and leave the eye (see below). This corresponds to the blind spot because there are no photoreceptors in the optic disk. Interestingly, we are not aware of our own visual blind spot until it is demonstrated (see later). The **fovea** is the central portion of the second morphologically distinct region of the retina, the **macula lutea**. The brain precisely controls the position of the eyes to ensure that the principal portion of an image falls on the fovea of each eye, where visual acuity is greatest. Indeed, the functions of many brain stem visual nuclei are devoted largely to positioning the eyes for this purpose. Visual acuity decreases continuously from the fovea to the peripheral retina.

The retina is a laminated structure, as revealed in a section oriented at a right angle to its surface (Figure 6–3B). We will see that other compo-

A

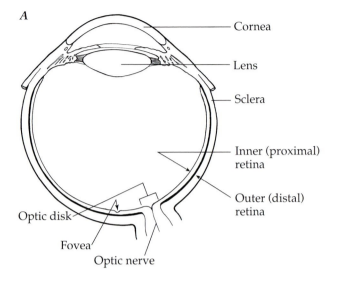

Cornea

Lens

Sclera

Inner (proximal) retina

Outer (distal) retina

Optic disk

Fovea

Optic nerve

B

Pigment epithelium

Rod and cone segments

Outer limiting membrane

Outer nuclear layer

Rod and cone terminals

Outer synaptic layer

Inner nuclear layer

Inner synaptic layer

Ganglion cell layer

Optic nerve fibers

Inner limiting membrane

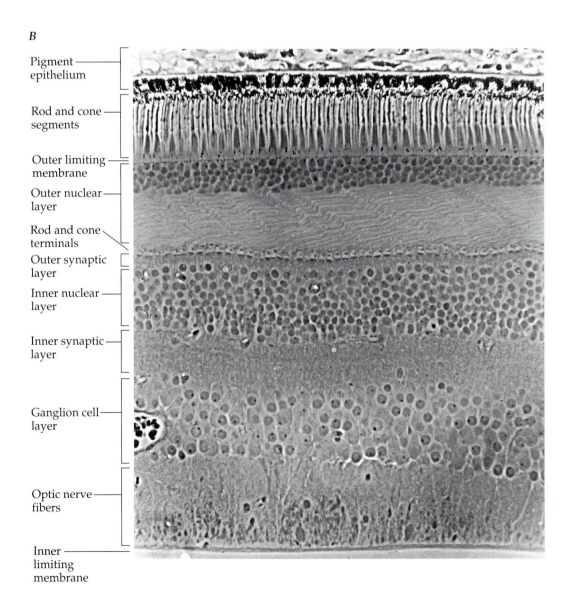

nents of the visual system also have a laminar organization. Lamination is one way the nervous system packs together neurons with similar functions and patterns of connections. Our spatial reference point for describing the location of the different layers is the **three-dimensional center** of the eye. The **inner,** or proximal, retinal layers are close to the center of the eye; the **outer,** or distal, layers are farther from the center (Figure 6–3A).

The retina contains five principal layers; cell bodies are located in three and synapses are present in two (Figure 6–3C): (1) outer nuclear layer, (2) outer synaptic (or plexiform) layer, (3) inner nuclear layer, (4)

Figure 6–3. Histology of the retina. *A.* Schematic diagram of eyeball indicating the inner and outer portions of the retina. *B.* A transverse section of the retina. *C.* Wiring diagram of the generalized vertebrate retina. The interplexiform cell, identified in numerous species, feeds processed visual information from amacrine cells in the inner retina back to horizontal cells in the outer retina. It should be noted that in the mammalian retina, horizontal cells do not synapse on cones. (*A,* Courtesy of Dr. John E. Dowling, Harvard University; adapted from Boycott, B. B., and Dowling, J. E. 1969. Organization of the primate retina: Light microscopy. Proc. Trans. R. Soc. Lond. B 255:109–194; *C,* Adapted from Dowling, J. E., and Boycott, B. B. 1966. Organization of the primate retina: Electron microscopy. Proc. R. Soc. Lond. B 166:80–111.)

C

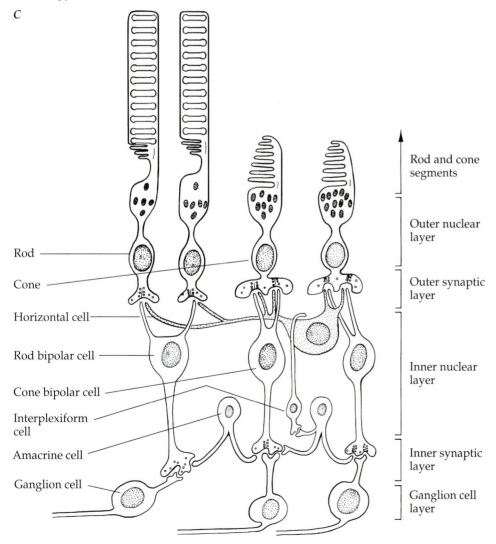

Rod and cone segments

Outer nuclear layer

Outer synaptic layer

Rod

Cone

Horizontal cell

Rod bipolar cell

Inner nuclear layer

Cone bipolar cell

Interplexiform cell

Amacrine cell

Inner synaptic layer

Ganglion cell

Ganglion cell layer

inner synaptic (or plexiform) layer, and (5) ganglion cell layer. In addition to the five principal layers, there are numerous strata that contain processes of particular retinal cells.

The **outer nuclear layer** contains the cell bodies of the two classes of photoreceptors: rods, which are for night vision, and **cones,** for daylight vision. Cones mediate the most discriminative aspects of visual perception and they are densest in the fovea, where they number approximately 200,000 per square mm. Cone density decreases continuously by about one order of magnitude 1 mm from the fovea (Figure 6–4). Cones contain the photopigments for color vision and come in three different classes according to their absorption spectra: red, green, or blue.

By contrast, rods are absent in the fovea (Figure 6–4) and are densest along an elliptical ring in the perifoveal region passing through the optic disc. Along this ring, there is a site of maximal density ("hot spot") of approximately 175,000 per square mm. These photoreceptors contain the photopigment **rhodopsin** and are optimally suited for detecting low levels of illumination, such as at dusk or at night. In fact, a single photon can activate a rod cell! In contrast, cones are relatively insensitive to light and they mediate daylight vision. The location of maximal rod density, along the parafoveal elliptical ring, corresponds approximately to the location of maximal light sensitivity. This is one factor that helps to explain why, when discerning a faint object at night, we do not look directly at it but rather off to one side.

Figure 6–4. Distribution of rods *(A)* and cones *(B)* in the human retina. The density of photoreceptors is indicated by a gray scale: retinal regions containing a higher density of photoreceptors are shaded darker than regions with a low photoreceptor density. The white spot to the left of center in both *A* and *B* corresponds to the optic disk, where no photoreceptors are located. (Courtesy of Dr. Christine Curcio J. Comp. Neurol. 292:497, 1990; Figure 5.)

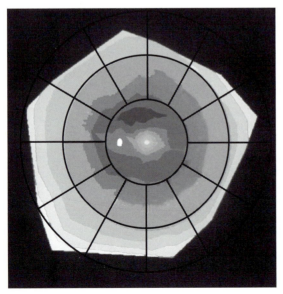

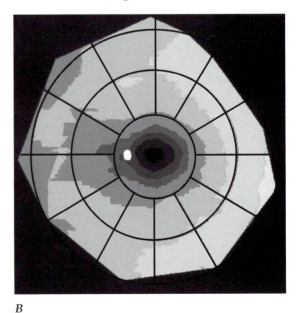

A   *B*

Connections between photoreceptors and retinal interneurons are made in the **outer synaptic (or plexiform) layer**. The **inner nuclear layer** contains the cell bodies and proximal processes of the retinal interneurons—bipolar, horizontal, and amacrine cells (Figure 6–3C).

- **Bipolar cells** link photoreceptors directly with the retinal projection neurons, ganglion cells. Of the two principal classes of bipolar cells, **cone bipolar cells** and **rod bipolar cells**, the former receive synaptic input from a small number of cone cells to give us high visual acuity and color vision. By contrast, rod bipolar cells receive convergent input from many rods for less visual acuity but increased sensitivity to **low levels of illumination**.
- The actions of **horizontal cells** and **amacrine cells** enhance visual contrast through interactions between laterally located photoreceptors and bipolar cells. Horizontal cells are located in the outer part of the inner nuclear layer, whereas amacrine cells are found in the inner portion. Many amacrine cells contain **dopamine** and are thought to help adapt retinal synaptic activity to the dark.

The **inner synaptic (or plexiform) layer** is where synaptic connections between the bipolar cells and the ganglion cells are made. The innermost retinal cell layer, the **ganglion cell layer**, is named after the retinal output cells. Ganglion cell axons collect along the inner retinal surface (Figures 6–3B and 6–5A). These axons are unmyelinated, which increases the transparency of the retina and facilitates light transmission to the photoreceptor layer in the outer retina. Ganglion cell axons leave the eye at the **optic disk** (Figure 6–5A) where they become myelinated and form the **optic nerve**. The cellular organization of the retina might seem unexpected because light must travel through retinal layers that contain projection neurons and interneurons to reach the photoreceptors. At the fovea, however, the retinal interneurons and ganglion cells are displaced, exposing the photoreceptors directly to visual stimuli and optimizing the optical quality of the image.

Müller cells are the principal retinal neuroglial cell, and their nuclei are located in the inner nuclear layer. These cells have important structural and metabolic functions. An individual Müller cell stretches vertically from the inner surface of the retina (the inner limiting membrane) to the distal margin of the optic nerve fibers (outer limiting membrane) (Figure 6–3B).

The other nonneural elements associated with the retina are clinically important. The **pigment epithelium** is external to the photoreceptor layer (Figure 6–3B). It serves a phagocytic role, removing rod outer segment disks that are discarded as part of a normal renewal process. In the retinal disease **retinitus pigmentosa**, this phagocytic process becomes defective. Because the retina does not tightly adhere to the pigment epithelium, it can become detached following a blow to the head or eye. This results in a partially detached retina and loss of vision in the detached portion.

The circulation of the retina has a dual organization. The arterial supply of the inner retina is provided by branches of the ophthalmic artery, which is a branch of the internal carotid. The outer retina is devoid of blood vessels. Its nourishment derives from the choroidal circulation.

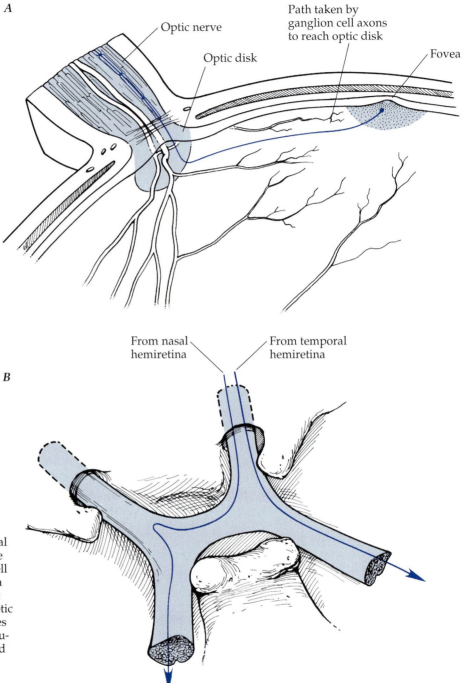

A

Optic nerve

Optic disk

Path taken by
ganglion cell axons
to reach optic disk

Fovea

From nasal
hemiretina

From temporal
hemiretina

B

Figure 6–5. The path that the retinal ganglion cell axons take to reach the optic tract. *A.* Course of ganglion cell axons along the surface of the retina and into the optic nerve at the optic disk. *B.* Regional anatomy of the optic chiasm. Direction of arrows indicates axon trajectory toward lateral geniculate nucleus and midbrain. (Adapted from Patten, H. 1977. Neurological Differential Diagnosis. New York: Springer-Verlag.)

Each Optic Nerve Contains All of the Axons of Ganglion Cells in the Ipsilateral Retina

The optic nerve is the **second cranial nerve**, but because the retina develops from the diencephalon it is actually a central nervous system pathway rather than a peripheral nerve. The optic nerves from both eyes converge at the **optic chiasm** (Figures 6–1 and 6–5B). The axons of ganglion cells of each **nasal hemiretina** decussate in the optic chiasm and enter the contralateral optic tract whereas those of each **temporal**

hemiretina remain on the same side and enter the ipsilateral optic tract. Thus, each optic tract contains axons from the contralateral nasal hemiretina and the ipsilateral temporal hemiretina. Despite the incomplete decussation of the optic nerves in the chiasm, there is a complete crossover of **visual information**: visual stimuli from **one half of the visual field** are processed within the **contralateral thalamus, cerebral cortex, and midbrain**. This is because the uncrossed axonal contingent in the optic tract arises from ganglion cells of the ipsilateral temporal retina, the hemiretina that receives stimuli from the **contralateral** visual field (Figure 6–2A).

The Superior Colliculus Is Important in Oculomotor Control and Orientation

The optic tract splits on the ventral diencephalic surface. The major contingent of axons terminates in the lateral geniculate nucleus and gives rise to the pathway for visual perception (see below). A smaller contingent skirts the lateral geniculate nucleus and passes over the surface of the medial geniculate nucleus, which is the thalamic auditory nucleus (see Chapter 7). These axons collectively are termed the **brachium of the superior colliculus** (Figures 6–6 and 6–7) because their major site of termination is the superior colliculus.

The superior colliculus is laminated, consisting of seven alternating layers of neuronal cell bodies and of axons. Some of these layers are clearly visible in the myelin-stained section in Figure 6–7A. A schematic diagram of the lamination pattern in the superior colliculus and the connections of the various layers is shown in Figure 6–7B. Visual information is processed by the dorsal three layers. Layer 1 receives a **direct** retinal projection from axons in the brachium of the superior colliculus, whereas layers 2 and 3 receive visual input **indirectly** from layer 1 via interneurons and from a descending projection from the primary visual cortex. Neurons in these layers are **retinotopically organized**. The ventral four layers receive somatic sensory and auditory information, in addition to projections from other sources. The **spinotectal tract,** one component of the anterolateral system (see Chapter 5), brings somatic sensory information to the superior colliculus.

The superior colliculus helps to orient the eyes and head to salient stimuli in the environment. It does this by combining sensory information from the different modalities in a unique way: the representations of somatic sensory and auditory information in deeper collicular layers are aligned with the visual representation in superficial layers according to a **spatial map** of the external world. Aggregates of neurons in the superior colliculus that are located above one another, but in different layers, all respond to stimuli that have a common spatial location. For example, neurons that respond to visual information from the superior visual field are located dorsal to neurons that respond to sounds from in front of and above the head and neurons that respond to tactile stimulation of the forehead. Such a collection of neurons in the superior colliculus might be important in orienting us to a buzzing insect that lands on the forehead!

The superior colliculus also contains part of the neural apparatus for affecting eye and neck muscle control. There are two major projections of the superior colliculus, one to the regions of the reticular formation that specifically control vertical or horizontal eye movements and the other to the cervical spinal cord to control neck muscles. The systems for controlling neck and eye movements will be discussed in Chapters 9 and 13.

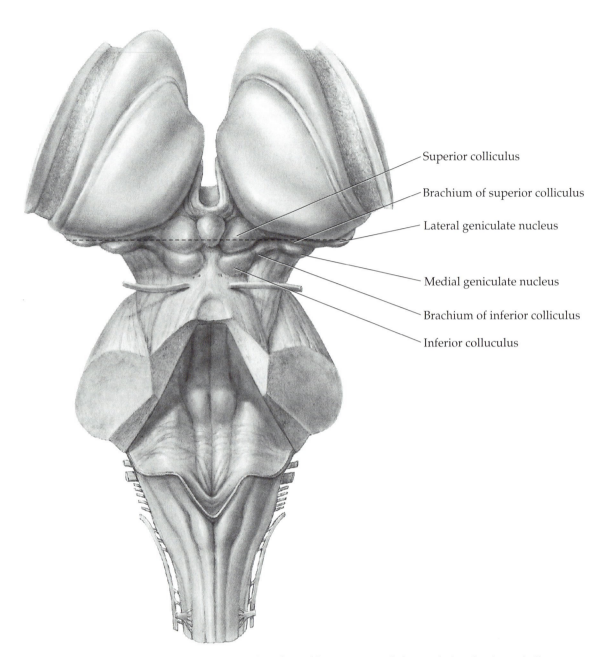

Figure 6–6. Dorsal surface of brain stem and diencephalon (with cerebellum removed) showing the locations of components of the visual system in the diencephalon and midbrain.

The neural systems for visuomotor function and visual perception appear to converge in the cerebral cortex. Certain superior colliculus neurons have an axon that ascends to the **lateral posterior** and **pulvinar** nuclei of the thalamus (see Figure 3–10). In turn, these thalamic nuclei project primarily to **higher-order visual areas and to association areas of the parietal, temporal, and occipital lobes**. One function of this ascending projection from the superior colliculus may be to inform cortical areas important for visual perception about the speed and direction of eye movements. This information is important for distinguishing between movement of a stimulus and movement of the eyes.

A

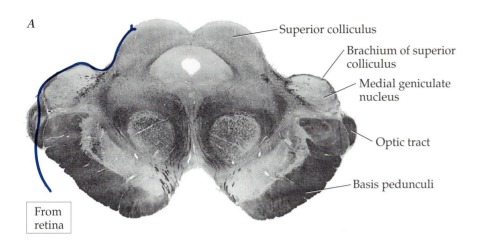

Superior colliculus

Brachium of superior colliculus

Medial geniculate nucleus

Optic tract

Basis pedunculi

From retina

B

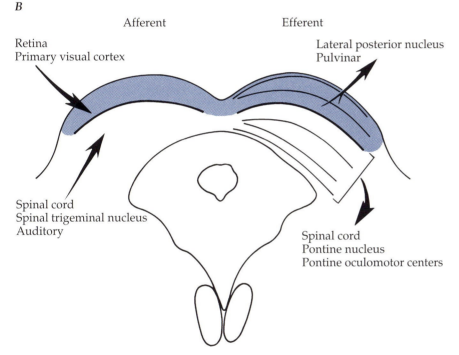

Afferent

Efferent

Retina
Primary visual cortex

Lateral posterior nucleus
Pulvinar

Spinal cord
Spinal trigeminal nucleus
Auditory

Spinal cord
Pontine nucleus
Pontine oculomotor centers

Figure 6–7. *A.* Myelin-stained transverse section through the rostral midbrain (superior colliculus). The path of a ganglion cell axon to the superior colliculus is shown in blue. The dashed line in Figure 6–6 indicates the plane of section in *A.* *B.* Schematic diagram illustrating the seven layers of the superior colliculus and their major input and output connections. The layers of the superior colliculus receiving visual information are tinted blue.

Ganglion Cell Axons From the Ipsilateral and Contralateral Halves of the Retina Terminate in Different Layers of the Lateral Geniculate Nucleus

The major retinal projection is to the **lateral geniculate nucleus** of the thalamus (Figures 6–6 and 6–8). This nucleus contains two divisions—dorsal and ventral. The dorsal division is larger and projects to the primary visual cortex; this division serves **visual perception**. The ventral division is a diffuse-projecting thalamic nucleus (see Chapter 3). Here, we focus on the dorsal division of the lateral geniculate nucleus and refer to it simply as the lateral geniculate nucleus. This nucleus forms a surface landmark on the ventral diencephalon sometimes called the lateral geniculate body.

A coronal section through the lateral geniculate nucleus is shown in Figure 6–8A. In Figure 6–8B, which is a section sliced in a plane approximately orthogonal to the one in Figure 6–8A, we see how the main portion of the optic tract terminates in the lateral geniculate nucleus.

The lateral geniculate nucleus contains six major cell layers. Whereas all of these cell layers process input from the **contralateral visual field**, each layer receives projections exclusively from either the **ipsilateral** or the **contralateral retina**. This pattern of connections is demonstrated in Figure 6–9A, an autoradiograph of the lateral geniculate nucleus of a rhesus monkey. To obtain this image, tritiated fucose was injected into one

Figure 6–8. *A.* Myelin-stained coronal section through the lateral geniculate nucleus. *B.* Transverse section through the midbrain–diencephalic juncture. The inset shows the planes of section.

A

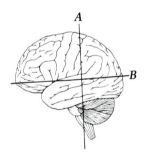

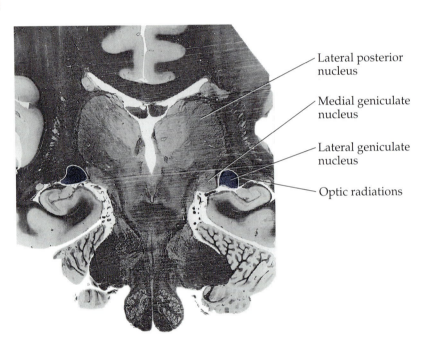

Lateral posterior nucleus

Medial geniculate nucleus

Lateral geniculate nucleus

Optic radiations

B

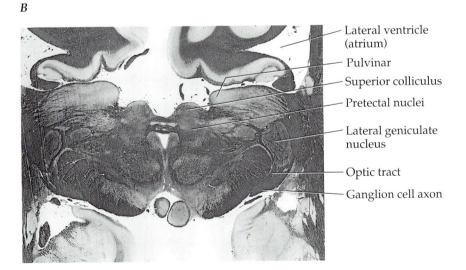

Lateral ventricle (atrium)

Pulvinar

Superior colliculus

Pretectal nuclei

Lateral geniculate nucleus

Optic tract

Ganglion cell axon

A

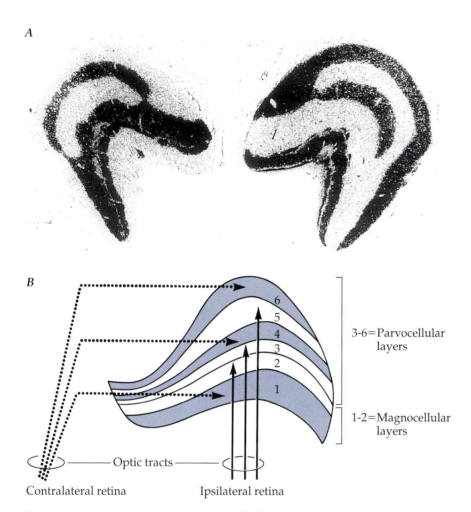

B

6
5
4
3
2
1

3-6 = Parvocellular
layers

1-2 = Magnocellular
layers

——— Optic tracts ———

Contralateral retina   Ipsilateral retina

Figure 6–9. Each of the six cell layers of the lateral geniculate nucleus receives afferent input from either the ipsilateral or the contralateral eye. *A.* Autoradiograph of the monkey lateral geniculate nucleus. The left eye was injected with ³H fucose. Labeled regions are dark. The six principal layers of the lateral geniculate nucleus are labeled. For example, layers 1, 4, and 6 are labeled on the section of the lateral geniculate nucleus shown on right. In addition, there are thin sublaminae that also receive retinal input. *B.* Schematic diagram of input connections of the human lateral geniculate nucleus. (*A*, Courtesy of Drs. David H. Hubel and Torsten N. Wiesel; from Hubel, D. H., and Wiesel, T. N. 1977. Ferrier lecture: Functional architecture of macaque monkey visual cortex. Proc. R. Soc. Lond. B 198:1–59.)

eye of an anesthetized animal. The ganglion cells incorporated this radiolabeled material into glycoproteins, which were then carried to their terminals in the lateral geniculate nucleus by anterograde axonal transport. Exposing the tissue to photographic emulsion produced an autoradiograph that revealed the distribution of radiolabeled material.

Each layer of the lateral geniculate nucleus contains a complete and orderly representation of the contralateral visual field. It is important to note that the visual representations are in spatial register: **cells oriented along an axis orthogonal to the plane of the layers receive input from the same portion of the contralateral visual field**. We will see below that neurons in the dorsal and ventral layers have different functions and a different morphology.

The Primary Visual Cortex Is the Target of Projections From the Lateral Geniculate Nucleus

Projection neurons in all six layers of the lateral geniculate nucleus send their axons to the primary visual cortex (Figure 6–10). This path—the **optic radiations**—is occasionally referred to as the geniculocalcarine tract. This is because the axons connect the lateral geniculate nucleus with the primary visual cortex, located along the **calcarine fissure** predominantly on the medial brain surface (Figure 6–11). The optic radiations take an indirect course around the lateral ventricle to reach their cortical target (Figure 6–10). A portion of the optic radiations subserving vision from the superior visual field courses rostrally within the temporal lobe (termed **Meyer's loop**), before heading caudally to the primary visual cortex (Figure 6–10).

The primary visual cortex (Figure 6–11), which is located on the medial brain surface, corresponds to Brodmann's cytoarchitectonic **area 17** (Figure 6–12; also see Figure 3–16). It has six principal layers, with layer 4 further subdivided into sublaminae (Figure 6–12C). One layer 4 sublamina contains the **stripe of Gennari**, a dense plexus of myelinated fibers that are axon collaterals of primary visual cortex neurons. Similar to the primary somatic sensory cortex, neurons in different layers of the primary visual cortex have different patterns of input and output connections. The higher-order visual areas are located in Brodmann's areas 18 and 19 (Figure 6–11), which encircle area 17. The boundary between areas 17 and 18 is distinct because it is where the stripe of Gennari ends (Figure 6–12A).

The Magnocellular and Parvocellular Systems Have Differential Laminar Projections in the Primary Visual Cortex

The different layers of the lateral geniculate nucleus, in addition to receiving input from either the ipsilateral or the contralateral retina, also

Figure 6–10. Course of the axons of the optic radiations from the lateral geniculate nucleus, over the lateral ventricle to reach the primary visual cortex. (Adapted from Brodal, A. 1981. Neurological Anatomy. New York: Oxford University Press.)

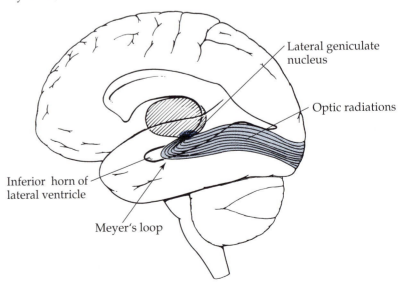

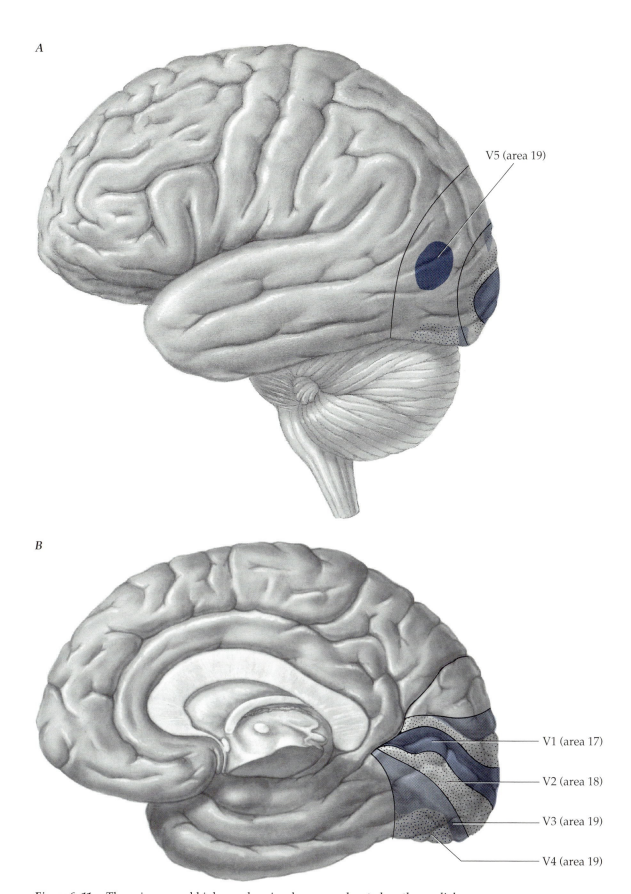

A

V5 (area 19)

B

V1 (area 17)

V2 (area 18)

V3 (area 19)

V4 (area 19)

Figure 6–11. The primary and higher-order visual areas are located on the medial and lateral surfaces of the occipital lobe. *A.* Lateral view of the brain. *B.* Medial view of the brain. Lines correspond to cytoarchitectonic boundaries. V3, V4, and V5 comprise part of cytoarchitectonic area 19. The borders of V1 and V2 are better established, whereas those of V4 and V5 are very approximate. (Adapted, with permission, from Clarke and Miklossy, 1990, and Sereno et al., 1995.)

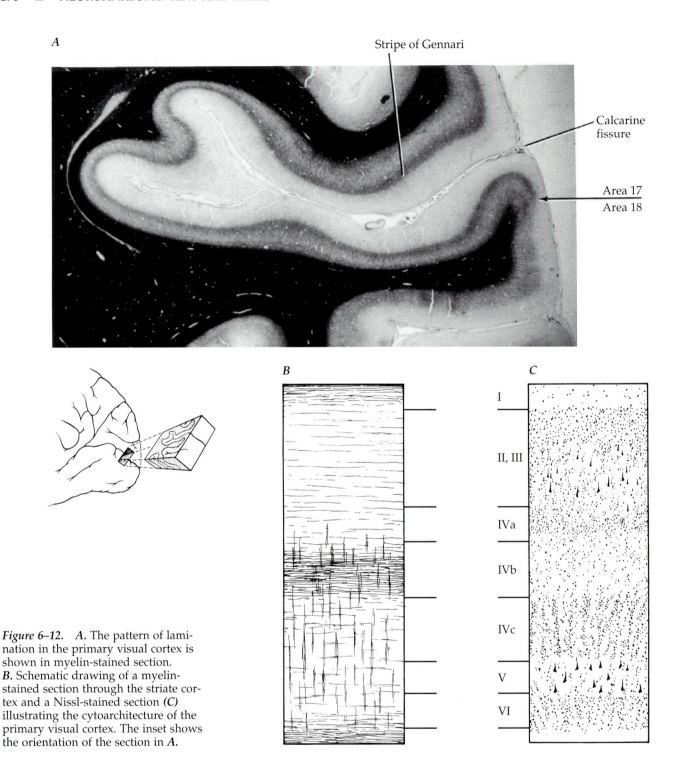

Figure 6–12. **A.** The pattern of lamination in the primary visual cortex is shown in myelin-stained section. **B.** Schematic drawing of a myelin-stained section through the striate cortex and a Nissl-stained section **(C)** illustrating the cytoarchitecture of the primary visual cortex. The inset shows the orientation of the section in **A.**

receive input from a distinct class of retinal ganglion cells, either M cells or P cells (Figure 6–13). The M and P cells give rise to two visual information channels, the **magnocellular** and **parvocellular** systems, which process distinct features of a visual stimulus (Figure 6–13).

The **M cell** has a large dendritic arbor, enabling it to integrate visual information from a wide portion of the retina. We believe that M cells play a key role in the analysis of stimulus motion as well as gross spatial features of a stimulus. The ventral two layers of the lateral geniculate nucleus

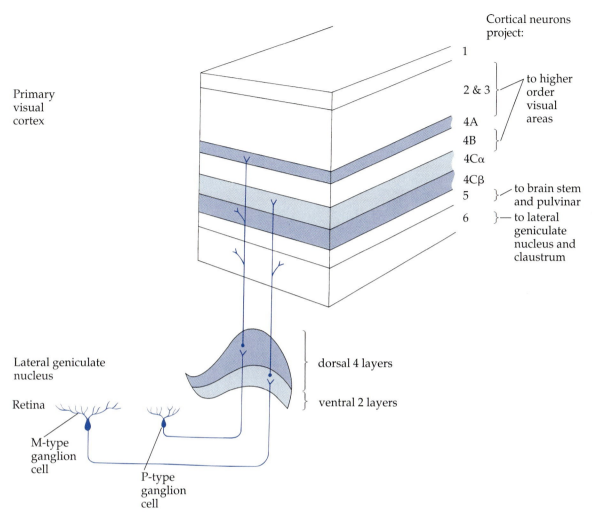

Cortical neurons
project:

1

2 & 3   to higher
order
4A   visual
4B   areas
4Cα
4Cβ
5   to brain stem
and pulvinar
6   to lateral
geniculate
nucleus and
claustrum

Primary
visual
cortex

Lateral geniculate
nucleus

dorsal 4 layers

ventral 2 layers

Retina

M-type
ganglion
cell

P-type
ganglion
cell

Figure 6–13. Projections of the parvocellular and magnocellular visual systems
to the primary visual cortex. The magnocellular projection from the lateral geniculate nucleus terminates primarily in layer 4Cα, whereas the parvocellular projection terminates primarily in layers 4A and 4Cβ. In addition, both terminate in
layer 6, which contains neurons that project back to the thalamus. (Only laminae
receiving major thalamic projections are tinted blue.)

receive input from the M cells. Because the thalamocortical neurons
located in these two layers are larger than those in the other layers, we call
them magnocellular neurons. The **P cell**, with its small dendritic arbor,
processes visual information from a small portion of the retina (Figure
6–13). These cells are color-sensitive; they are important for discriminative
aspects of vision, such as distinguishing form and color. The P-type ganglion cells terminate in the dorsal four layers of the lateral geniculate
nucleus. Here the thalamocortical neurons are small, hence the name parvocellular neurons.

Whereas neurons in the lateral geniculate nucleus have a relatively
light projection to many layers in the primary visual cortex, the densest
projections—and presumably those with the strongest postsynaptic
actions—are to **layer 4**. Neurons in the magnocellular and parvocellular
layers project to different sublaminae in layer 4. The magnocellular system
projects primarily to layer 4Cα, whereas the parvocellular system projects
primarily to layers 4A and 4Cβ.

Interneurons in the layer 4 sublaminae (Figure 6–12C) connect with neurons in superficial and deeper cortical layers which, in turn, distribute visual information to other cortical and subcortical regions (Figure 6–13). The differential laminar projections of the magnocellular and parvocellular systems set the stage for distinct visual processing channels that distribute information about different aspects of a stimulus to the secondary and higher-order visual cortical areas (see below).

The Primary Visual Cortex Has a Columnar Organization

Different areas of the cerebral cortex share a similar functional organization: The properties of neurons located above and below one another—yet in different layers—have similar properties. This is the **columnar organization** of the cerebral cortex. In the primary somatic sensory cortex (see Chapter 5), neurons in a cortical column all process sensory information from the same **peripheral location** and the same **submodality**. The primary visual cortex also has a columnar organization. This organization was first revealed by recording the electrical

Figure 6–14. The primary visual cortex has a columnar organization. *A.* Ocular dominance columns. *B.* Orientation columns. *C.* Color sensitive neurons. Whereas the ocular dominance and orientation columns extend throughout all cortical layers, the color blobs are present only in layers 2 and 3. Both the magnocellular and parvocellular systems contribute to the ocular dominance and orientation columns. The color blobs receive a major input from the parvocellular system.

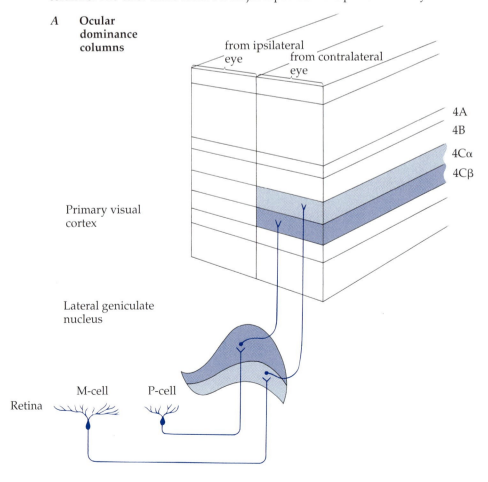

A **Ocular dominance columns**

from ipsilateral eye

from contralateral eye

4A
4B
4Cα
4Cβ

Primary visual cortex

Lateral geniculate nucleus

M-cell   P-cell

Retina

B   Orientation columns

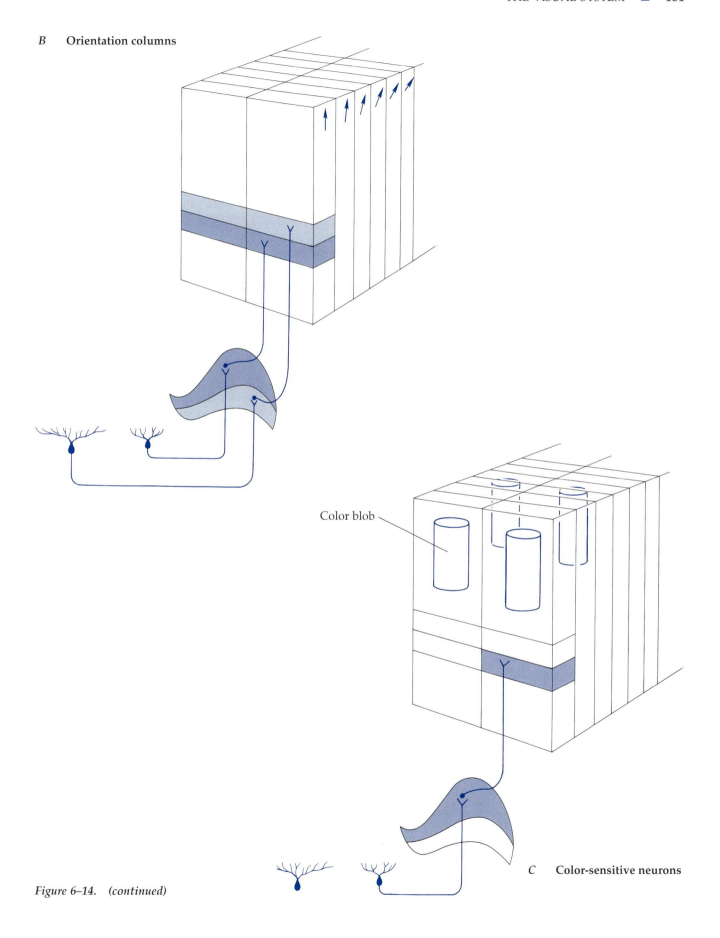

Color blob

C   Color-sensitive neurons

Figure 6–14.   (continued)

responses of neurons to simple visual stimuli presented to one or the other eye. Neurons in a cortical column have similar functions because local connections primarily distribute the thalamic input vertically, from layer 4 to superficial and deeper layers, rather than horizontally within the same layer. Horizontal connections do exist; however, they mediate other kinds of functions, such as enhancing contrast and binding together visual information from different parts of a scene to form perceptions.

There are at least two types of columns in the primary visual cortex: (1) **ocular dominance columns** (Figure 6–14A), where neurons receive visual input primarily from the ipsilateral or the contralateral eye, and (2) **orientation columns** (Figure 6–14B), where neurons are maximally sensitive to simple visual stimuli with similar spatial orientations. In addition, there are also vertically oriented **aggregates of neurons in layers 2 and 3 that are sensitive to the color** of visual stimuli (Figure 6–14C). These aggregates are not considered to be columns because they are located only in superficial layers.

Input From the Lateral Geniculate Nucleus Is Segregated Into Separate Ocular Dominance Columns in the Primary Visual Cortex

The axon terminals of lateral geniculate neurons that receive input from the ipsilateral retina remain segregated from the terminals of neurons that receive their input from the contralateral retina. The lateral geniculate terminals carrying input from one eye form bands in layer 4 that alternate with terminals transmitting input from the other eye. This means that neurons in layer 4 are monocular; they receive visual input either from one or the other eye.

Researchers can visualize the projections from one eye to layer 4 in the primary visual cortex using transneuronal transport of a tracer substance (Figure 6–15). Similar to the demonstration cited earlier, tritiated fucose is injected into the eye. At the ganglion cell synapse in the lateral geniculate nucleus, we think that a small amount of fucose is released along with the neurotransmitter. Next, labeled fucose is taken up by projection neurons in the lateral geniculate nucleus and transported to their terminals in the primary visual cortex. On autoradiographs of sections orthogonal to the pial surface of the cortex, labeled patches corresponding to the projections of the injected eye can be seen (Figure 6–15A). Portions of layer 4 receiving input from the uninjected eye are unlabeled and alternate with the labeled regions. The labeled patches in layer 4 form stripes when viewed in a plane tangential to the cortical surface. This is shown in Figure 6–15B, which presents a photographic montage through layer 4 (the inset indicates the plane of section in A and montage sections in B).

Mixing of information from both eyes, giving rise to binocular inputs, occurs in neurons located above and below layer 4. These binocular interactions are mediated by cortical interneurons. The binocular neurons receive a stronger synaptic input from the same eye that projected information to the monocular neurons in layer 4, and a weaker input from the other eye. This pattern of lateral geniculate axon terminations in layer 4 and blending of connections above and below layer 4 forms the anatomical basis of the **ocular dominance columns** (Figure 6–14A). A given retinal location in each eye is represented in the cortex by a pair of adjacent ocular dominance columns. It is thought that horizontal connections between neurons in adjacent ocular dominance columns are important for depth perception.

A

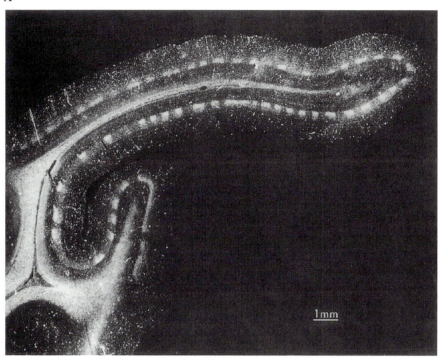

B

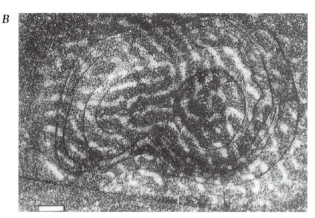

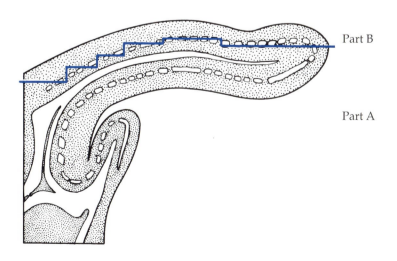

Part B

Part A

Figure 6–15. Projections from the retina, through the lateral geniculate nucleus, to the primary visual cortex can be demonstrated using autoradiography. *A.* The section was cut orthogonal to pial surface. *B.* A montage approximating a plane parallel to the pial surface. The inset is a schematic drawing of the section shown in *A* showing the composite plane of the montage in *B.* (*A*, From Hubel, D. H., and Wiesel, T. N. 1977. Ferrier lecture: Functional architecture of macaque monkey visual cortex. Proc. R. Soc. Lond. B 198:1–59. *B*, From Hubel, D. H., Wiesel, T. N., and LeVay S. 1977. Plasticity of ocular dominance columns in monkey striate cortex. Philos. Trans. R. Soc. Lond. B 278:377–409.)

*Orientation Columns Are Revealed by an Autoradiographic
Mapping Technique That Images Functional Organization*

Physiological studies have shown that most neurons in the primary visual cortex respond to simple bar-shaped stimuli with a particular orientation. However, unlike ocular dominance, which is an attribute based on anatomical connections from one eye or the other, orientation specificity of neurons in a column in the primary visual cortex (Figure 6–14B) is a property produced by connections between local cortical neurons. Standard, and even sophisticated, anatomical staining techniques do not reveal these functional sets of connections and thus do not reveal orientation columns (Figure 6–14B). How do we overcome this problem? Scientists turn to a technique that produces an image of the distribution of neuronal activity in response to a visual stimulus with a particular orientation, similar to positron emission tomography (PET) (see Box 1–1). One such method uses a radiolabeled glucose analog, 2-deoxyglucose, to produce an image that reflects neuronal glucose utilization. Utilization of glucose is proportional to neural activity because this sugar is the energy source for the brain. Although active neurons incorporate 2-deoxyglucose as if it were glucose, the analog becomes trapped within the neuron because cells lack the enzyme to further metabolize it. Because the 2-deoxyglucose is radiolabeled, we can determine its location using autoradiographic methods.

Orientation columns in the primary visual cortex of the rhesus monkey are illustrated in Figure 6–16, which is an autoradiograph obtained after visual stimulation at one stimulus orientation. Similar to the montage in Figure 6–15B, the plane of section is parallel to that of the cortex surface. Cells selective for stimulus orientation (and therefore the orientation columns themselves), are located from layer 2 to layer 6, and spare a portion of layer 4, which contains neurons that are insensitive to stimulus orientation.

*High Levels of Cytochrome Oxidase Activity Distinguish
Clusters of Color-sensitive Neurons in Layers 2 and 3*

Parvocellular color-sensitive neurons project to layer 4Cβ. In addition, they also have a small projection more superficially, to layers 2 and 3. Centered within the ocular dominance columns are aggregates of neurons sensitive to the wavelength of the visual stimulus (Figure 6–14C). These color-sensitive neurons are assembled into clusters in layers 2 and 3. The locations of these color-sensitive cells correspond to regions of primary visual cortex that have high levels of activity of the mitochondrial metabolic enzyme **cytochrome oxidase** (Figure 6–17). Thus, their distribution can be determined using a method for **histochemical localization of cytochrome oxidase activity**. The regions of increased enzyme activity, which correspond to the clusters of color-sensitive neurons, are termed **blobs**. Figure 6–17 illustrates a tangential section, stained for cytochrome oxidase, through layers 2 and 3 of the primary visual cortex of the rhesus monkey. The small dots in the primary visual cortex correspond to the color blobs. In the secondary visual cortex (V2), there are alternating stripes of increased (the thick and thin stripes) or decreased (the pale interstripe) cytochrome oxidase activity. We will discover how neurons in the thick stripe, thin stripe, and pale interstripe are part of distinct visual processing channels.

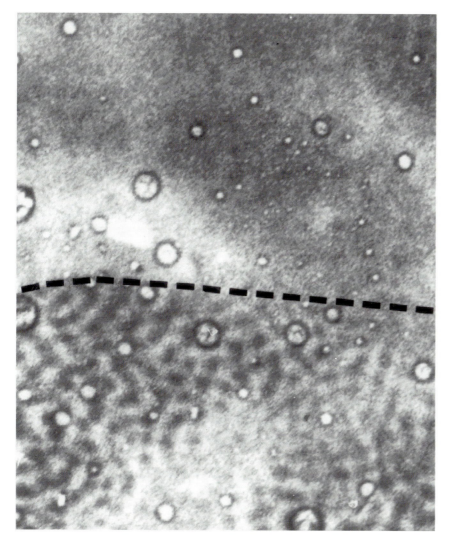

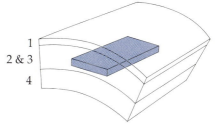

Figure 6–16. This 2-deoxyglucose autoradiograph illustrates the orientation columns in the primary visual cortex of the rhesus monkey. Vertical black and white stripes were presented to one portion of the visual field (upper field) and stripes of all orientations to an adjacent portion (lower field). This resulted in deoxyglucose-labeled orientation columns in the cortical representation of the upper visual field, which is in the region of autoradiograph below the dashed line, and no orientation columns in the lower visual field representation, above the dashed line. The inset shows the plane of section. (Autoradiograph courtesy of Dr. Roger Tootell, Harvard University.)

Higher-order Visual Cortical Areas Analyze Distinct Aspects of Visual Stimuli

Also located in the occipital lobe are the higher-order visual areas (Figure 6–11). Each area contains a partial or complete representation of the retina. Higher-order visual areas are collectively termed the **extrastriate cortex** because they lack the stripe of Gennari that characterizes the primary visual area (see Figure 6–12A). Extrastriate areas receive input directly or indirectly from the primary visual area. Many of the extrastriate areas also receive input from the pulvinar and the lateral posterior

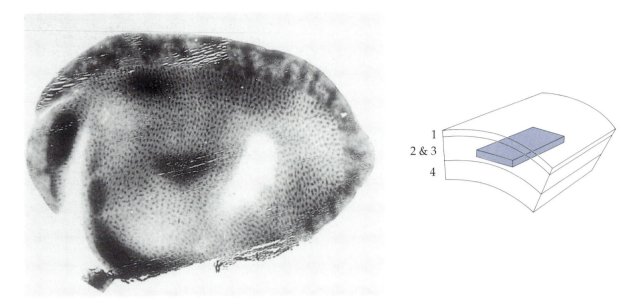

Figure 6–17. Clusters of neurons that are involved in color vision are identified by histochemical localization of cytochrome oxidase. The section was cut parallel to the pial surface and predominantly through layers 2 and 3 of the occipital lobe of the visual cortex in a rhesus monkey (inset). Cytochrome oxidase activity is greater in the dark regions than in the lighter regions. In area 17 (primary visual cortex), regions that have high cytochrome oxidase activity have a spherical shape in cross section and are cylindrical in three dimensions. Cytochrome oxidase staining in area 18 (secondary visual cortex) reveals stripes rather than the polka-dot pattern. (Courtesy of Drs. Margaret Livingstone and David Hubel, Harvard University.)

Figure 6–18. Forward (*A*) projections of the primary visual cortex to higher visual areas and feedback projections from higher visual areas to the primary visual cortex (*B*). In both *A* and *B*, primary visual cortex is shown on the left and a higher-order area is shown on the right. (Adapted from Maunsell, J. H. R., and Van Essen, D. C. 1983. The connections of the middle temporal visual area (MT) and their relationship to a cortical hierarchy in the macaque monkey. J. Neurosci. 3:2563–2568.)

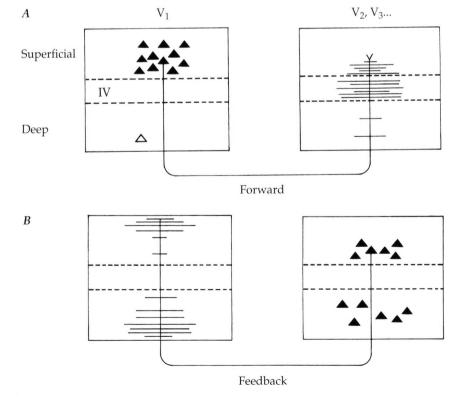

nucleus. Recently, it has been proposed that the **pulvinar** is important in distinguishing relevant from irrelevant visual stimuli, or **visual salience**. The lateral geniculate nucleus has little projection to the extrastriate areas.

Some of the most exciting insights into the biological basis of vision have been obtained by studying the extrastriate areas. We have learned that the intracortical connections between the visual areas are both hierarchical and parallel. For example, V1 projects to V2, which in turn projects to V3. This is a hierarchically organized projection to V3. In contrast, the parallel projection to V3 is a direct one from V1, skipping V2. Although we can deduce that there is less information processing in the parallel projection, it is not yet clear how the parallel and hierarchical paths differ functionally.

Lower-order visual areas project axons to higher-order areas in a characteristic way (Figure 6–18A). This projection originates from neurons in the superficial cortical layers, and is directed to neurons and processes in layer 4 (i.e., the input layer) of the next higher level. Because this projection transmits visual information in an "upstream" flow, it is termed **feedforward**. Each of the visual cortical areas also receives a "backward"—or a **feedback**—projection from the next higher level (Figure 6–18B). The feedback path originates from neurons mostly in the superficial layers and is directed to neurons in both superficial and deeper layers in the next lower level in the hierarchy. Most of the higher-order visual areas receive a projection from the next lower level as well as from V1 directly.

Research analyzing connections of the monkey visual system suggest that, out of the myriad corticocortical projections from the primary and higher-order visual areas, we can distinguish different pathways predominantly involved in perceiving motion, color, and form (Figure 6–19A).

- The **motion pathway** derives from the M-type ganglion cells. Information passes through the magnocellular layers of the lateral geniculate nucleus, to neurons in layer 4Cα of the primary visual cortex, and from there to neurons in layer 4B (Figure 6–19A, dark blue). Neurons in layer 4B, in turn, project directly to V5, and indirectly via neurons in the thick cytochrome oxidase stripes of V2 (Figure 6–19A, dark blue). There also is a small projection to more superficial layers in V1, whose function is unclear. In the rhesus monkey, V5 corresponds to a region named MT, for middle temporal area. This region is important not only for motion detection but also for regulating slow eye movements (see Box 13–1). The path from V1 (and V2) to V3 may be important for analyzing aspects of visual **form in motion**. A region that is thought to be analogous to V5 in the human can be imaged using PET (Box 6–1).

- The **pathway for color** derives from the P-type ganglion cells, which terminate in the parvocellular layers of the lateral geniculate nucleus. From there, the geniculocalcarine projection is, via neurons in layer 4Cβ, to neurons in the color blobs (layers 2 and 3), next to the thin stripes in V2 (Figure 6–19A, medium blue), and then to V4. The region that may be equivalent to V4 in the human cortex has been described using PET (Box 6–1).

- The third pathway, for **form vision**, also derives primarily from the P-type ganglion cells and the parvocellular layers of the lateral geniculate nucleus. In V1, neurons in layer 4Cβ project to the interblob regions of layers 2 and 3, and from there, to the pale interstripe por-

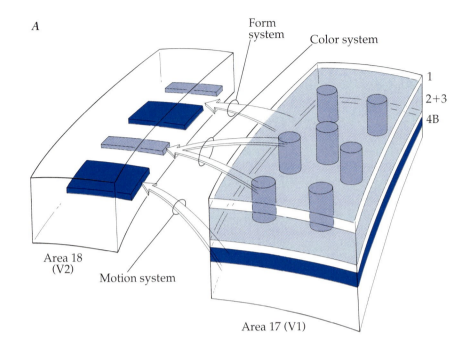

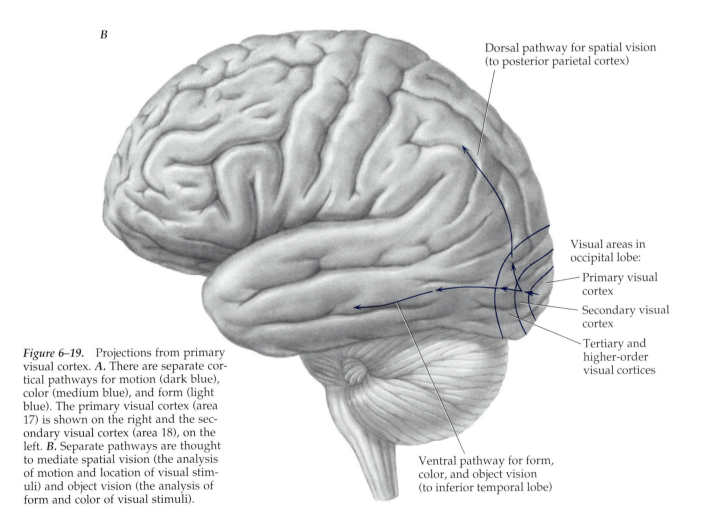

Figure 6–19. Projections from primary visual cortex. *A.* There are separate cortical pathways for motion (dark blue), color (medium blue), and form (light blue). The primary visual cortex (area 17) is shown on the right and the secondary visual cortex (area 18), on the left. *B.* Separate pathways are thought to mediate spatial vision (the analysis of motion and location of visual stimuli) and object vision (the analysis of form and color of visual stimuli).

Box 6–1. *Positron Emission Tomography of the Extrastriate Areas Important For Motion and Color Vision.*

The visual cortical areas in the human brain that are important for motion detection and color vision can be revealed by positron emission tomography (PET). The primary and secondary visual areas become active irrespective of whether an individual views a monochromatic scene in motion or a stationary colorful scene. Distinctions are revealed in the higher visual areas. An area on the lateral surface of the occipital lobe, which may correspond to V5, becomes selectively activated by visual motion (Figure 6–20A). A region on the medial brain surface near the fusiform gyrus, which may correspond to V4, becomes active when the subject views the colorful scene (Figure 6–20B).

Damage to a lateral corti region in one patient produced a remarkable visual disorder, motion blindness (hemiakinetopia) in the contralateral visual field. In this patient with motion blindness, moving objects appear frozen. An approaching form seems to be at one time in the distance and next, close by. Although quite rare, motion blindness provides remarkable support for the idea that motion detection is localized to a discrete cortical region.

In contrast to a lateral cortical region, which produced motion blindness, a lesion of the caudal portion of the fusiform gyrus located medially (Figure 6–20B), can produce cortical color blindness (hemiachromatopia) in the contralateral visual field. Individuals with such damage may not experience severe loss of form vision presumably because of the residual capabilities of the intact lower-order visual areas. Whereas color blindness due to the absence of certain photopigments is a common condition, color blindness due to a cortical lesion is extraordinarily rare.

A
B
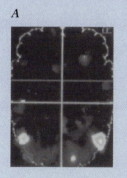
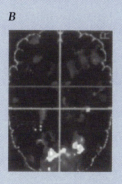
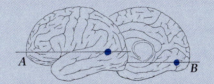

Figure 6–20. Positron emission tomographic (PET) scans through the human brain showing increases in cerebral blood flow in a cortical region thought to be V5, while the subject views a monochromatic scene in motion *(A)*, and in a cortical region thought to be V4, while a stationary colorful scene is viewed *(B)*. (Courtesy of Professor S. Zeki.)

tion of V2 (Figure 6–19A, light blue). Next, V2 neurons project to V4. Whereas both the motion and form systems are thought to contribute to depth perception, the color system does not.

The notion of functionally distinct paths for different visual stimulus attributes helps to explain the remarkable perceptual defects that occur in humans following damage to the temporal and parietal lobes. Damage to the inferior temporal lobe produces a selective defect in *object recognition.* Patients with a lesion of the medial portion of the inferior temporal lobe can have the bizarre condition termed prosopagnosia, in which they lose the ability to recognize faces, even of persons very familiar to them. On the other hand, damage to the posterior parietal lobe impairs the patient's capacity to *localize* objects in the environment but spares the ability to recognize. These findings suggest that there are two "streams" of visual processing in the cortex (Figure 6–19B): the ventral stream carries information about specific features of objects and scenes to the inferior temporal lobe, and the dorsal stream carries spatial information. Thus, the ventral stream is concerned with seeing *what* as opposed to *where*, which is the function of the dorsal stream. While there are extensive interconnections, it has been suggested that the ventral stream for object recognition receives a preferential input from the parvocellular, or form and color, system. On the other hand, the dorsal stream for localization receives input primarily from the magnocellular system. Using noninvasive techniques for examining the function of the human visual system (see Box 6–1) should help to elucidate the relationship between the paths for form, color, and motion, identified in monkeys, and the paths for seeing what and where, in humans.

A lesion of the posterior parietal association cortex alters complex aspects of perception that involve more than one sensory modality, because this region receives convergent inputs from the somatic sensory, visual, and auditory cortical areas. The effects of posterior parietal lesions frequently differ for the two hemispheres. As we saw in Chapter 5, a particularly intriguing deficit is called **sensory neglect**, which accompanies lesions of the posterior parietal lobe in the nondominant hemisphere (typically the right side). In this condition, a patient ignores sensory information from the side contralateral to the lesion. Other visual perceptual deficits involving the association areas of the parietal, temporal, and occipital lobes may result in spatial distortions or failure to recognize objects.

The Visual Field Changes in Characteristic Ways After Damage to the Visual System

The pattern of projection of retinal ganglion cells to the lateral geniculate nucleus and then to the cerebral cortex is remarkably precise. Therefore, damage at specific locations in the visual path produces characteristic changes in visual perception. In this section, we examine how clinicians can apply knowledge of the topography of retinal projections to localize central nervous system damage.

We come to understand functional connections in the visual system by delineating the visual field. Recall that the **visual field** corresponds to the total field of view of both eyes when their position remains fixed (Figure 6–21). The visual field of each eye overlaps extensively with that of the other (Figures 6–2 and 6–21A). The visual field of each eye can be determined by having the patient fix his or her gaze at a site on a tangent screen with one eye closed (Figure 6–21). In doing so, the patient positions the eyes in such a way that the fixation point falls on the fovea, the high-resolution portion of the retina (Figure 6–2A). We can identify the **blind spot** (Figure 6–21B) by moving a small visual target horizontally and laterally from the fixation point. We define the perimeter of the visual field of the eye by moving the visual target from outside the field to inside. The extreme temporal portions of the visual fields, called the **temporal crescents**, are viewed **monocularly** by the ipsilateral eye. The nose prevents images in this portion of the visual field from reaching the contralateral retina. The visual field has an irregular

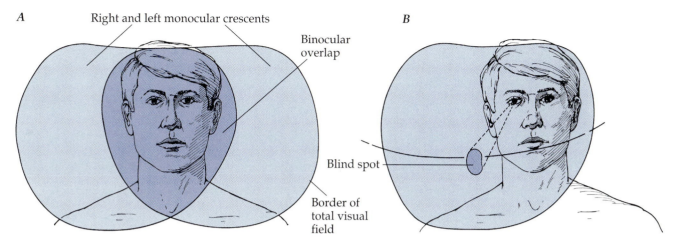

A Right and left monocular crescents

Binocular overlap

B

Blind spot

Border of total visual field

Figure 6–21. Schematic diagram of the visual field. *A.* Overlap of the visual fields of both eyes. *B.* Visual field for the right eye with the projection of the blind spot indicated. (Adapted from Patten, H. 1977. Neurological Differential Diagnosis. New York: Springer-Verlag.)

rather than a circular shape because other facial structures (infraorbital ridge and eyebrow), in addition to the nose, block portions of the light path.

A change in the size and shape of the visual field—a **visual field defect**—often points to specific pathological processes in the central nervous system (Table 6–1). Such defects may reflect damage to any of six key visual system components: (1) the optic nerve, (2) the optic chiasm, (3) the optic tract or the lateral geniculate nucleus, (4) the optic radiation in the temporal lobe (Meyer's loop), (5) the optic radiations in the parietal and occipital lobes, (6) the primary visual cortex (Figure 6–22).

OPTIC NERVE. Complete destruction of the optic nerve produces blindness in one eye (Figure 6–22A, Table 6–1); partial damage often produces a **scotoma**, a small blind spot. Ganglion cells in the various portions of the retina have a specific pattern of projection into the optic nerve. This enables localization of optic nerve damage, because a specific diminution of the visual field occurs. When a scotoma occurs in the central field of vision, for example the fovea, the patient notices reduced visual acuity. Remarkably, a peripheral scotoma is often unnoticed. This emphasizes the importance of foveal vision in our day-to-day activities (see below). Optic nerve damage also produces characteristic changes in the appearance of the optic disk (Figure 6–5A) because the damaged ganglion cell axons degenerate. Tumors and vascular disease commonly cause optic nerve damage.

OPTIC CHIASM. Ganglion cell axons from the nasal halves of the retina decussate in the optic chiasm (Figures 6–1 and 6–5B). These fibers transmit visual information from the temporal visual fields. The importance of knowing regional anatomy of the brain is clearly illustrated when we consider injury to the optic chiasm. For example, a common cause for chiasmal damage is a **pituitary tumor**. The pituitary gland is located ventral to the optic chiasm. As the tumor grows it expands dorsally, because the bony floor of the sella is located ventral to the pituitary gland (Figure 6–5B). The mass encroaches on the optic chiasm from its ventral surface. This results in damage of the decussating fibers and produces a **bilateral**

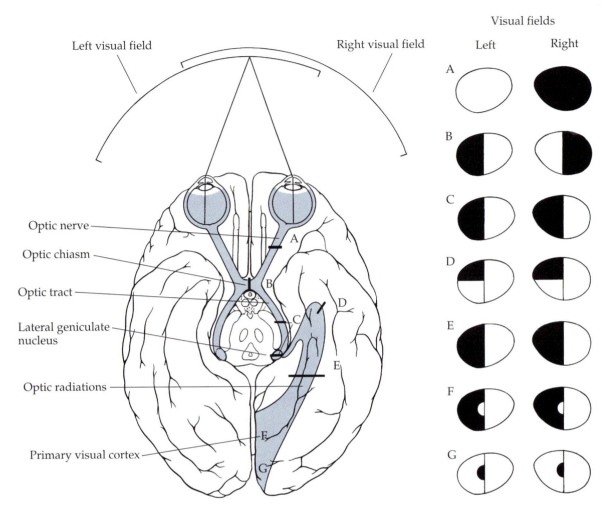

Visual fields

Left visual field   Right visual field   Left   Right

Optic nerve

Optic chiasm

Optic tract

Lateral geniculate
nucleus

Optic radiations

Primary visual cortex

Figure 6–22. Visual field defects. The left portion of the figure illustrates schematically a horizontal view of the visual system. Visual field defects are shown to the right and are listed in Table 6–1. For each defect, the visual fields of the right and left eyes are separated. All defects are presented schematically. Rarely do such defects present as bilaterally symmetrical. **A,** optic nerve; **B,** optic chiasm; **C,** optic tract (which is similar to lateral geniculate nucleus); **D,** Meyer's loop component of optic radiations; **E,** main component of optic radiations; **F** and **G,** primary visual cortex (F–infarction producing macular sparing, G–direct trauma to the occipital pole). (Adapted from Patten, H. 1977. Neurological Differential Diagnosis. New York: Springer-Verlag.)

temporal visual field defect (bitemporal hemianopia; Figure 6–22B, Table 6–1). Patients may not notice such a defect when it occurs in their peripheral vision. They commonly come to a physician following an accident caused by peripheral visual loss, for example, a traumatic injury incurred from the side, such as being hit by an automobile.

OPTIC TRACT OR THE LATERAL GENICULATE NUCLEUS.   Damage to the optic tract or the lateral geniculate nucleus, also due to tumors or a vascular accident, produces a defect in the **contralateral visual field** (homonymous hemianopia; Figure 6–22C, Table 6–1).

Table 6–1. Visual field defects.[1]

Site of lesion	Location in Figure 6–22	Deficit
Optic nerve	A	Unilateral
Optic chiasm	B	Bitemporal heteronymous hemianopia
Contralateral Defects		
Optic tract	C	Homonymous hemianopia
Lateral geniculate nucleus	C	Homonymous hemianopia
Optic radiations		
Meyer's loop	D	Upper visual quadrant homonymous hemianopia (quadrantanopia)
Main radiations	E	Homonymous hemianopia
Visual cortex		
Rostral	F	Homonymous hemianopia with macular sparing
Caudal	G	Homonymous hemianopia of the macular region

[1]Visual field defects are termed *homonymous* (or congruous) if they affect similar locations for the two eyes and are termed *heteronymous* (or incongruous) if they are different. Hemianopia is loss of half of the visual field in each eye.

OPTIC RADIATIONS. Axons of lateral geniculate neurons course around the rostral and lateral surfaces of the lateral ventricle (Figure 6–10) en route to the primary visual cortex at the occipital pole. Neurons in the medial portion of the lateral geniculate nucleus, which subserve vision from the **superior visual fields**, have axons that course rostrally into the **temporal lobe (Meyer's loop)** before they course caudally to the primary visual cortex. Temporal lobe lesions can produce a visual field defect limited to the **contralateral upper quadrant** of each visual field (quadrantinopia; Figure 6–22D, Table 6–1). This is sometimes referred to as a "pie in the sky" defect because it is often wedge-shaped. Neurons in the intermediate and lateral portions of the lateral geniculate nucleus subserve the macular region and the lower field respectively. Their axons have a more direct course around the ventricle and through the white matter underlying the parietal cortex. On rare occasions, a lesion of the white matter within the parietal lobe can affect the optic radiations and produce visual field defects (homonymous hemianopia; Figure 6–22E, Table 6–1).

PRIMARY VISUAL CORTEX. Visual space is precisely represented in the primary visual cortex (Figure 6–23). The representation of the macula lutea region of the retina (commonly termed the macular region) is caudal to the perimacular and peripheral portions. The upper visual field is represented in the inferior bank of the calcarine fissure, and the lower visual field, in the superior bank. Although the macular region is a small portion of the retina, the area of primary visual cortex devoted to it is greatly expanded with respect to the rest of the retina. This organization is similar to the large representation of the fingertips in the primary somatic sensory cortex (see Figure 5–19).

The retinotopic organization of the primary visual cortex in humans can be examined using PET. Figure 6–24 illustrates three PET scans

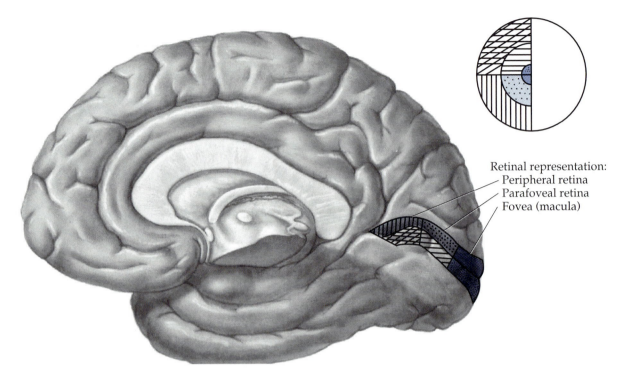

Retinal representation:
Peripheral retina
Parafoveal retina
Fovea (macula)

Figure 6–23. The primary visual cortex has a retinotopic organization with the macula located caudally and the perimacular and peripheral parts of the retina represented rostrally. The portions of the left visual field (inset) are coded to match the corresponding representations in the right primary visual cortex.

obtained in sequence in the same individual. When presented with a stimulus to the macular portion of the retina (Figure 6–24A), there is increased emission of radioactive particles from the caudal portion of the subject's visual cortex (Figure 6–23). The perimacular and peripheral stimuli resulted in emission of radioactive particles from progressively more rostral locations (Figure 6–24B and C). This remarkable example illustrates how the functional organization of the human cerebral cortex can be mapped noninvasively.

Damage to the primary visual cortex, which commonly occurs after an infarction of the **posterior cerebral artery**, produces a contralateral visual field deficit that often spares the macular region of the visual field (homonymous hemianopia with macular sparing; Figure 6–22F, Table 6–1). Two factors contribute to macular sparing. First, the area of cortex that subserves central vision is so large that a single infarction, or other pathological process, rarely destroys it entirely. Second, in the case of infarctions, the arterial supply to the cortical area that serves the macular region is provided primarily by the **posterior cerebral artery**, with a collateral supply coming from the **middle cerebral artery**. After occlusion of the posterior cerebral artery, the middle cerebral artery can rescue the macular representation. Although rare, a traumatic injury to the occipital pole can produce a deficit involving only the macular region (Figure 6–22G, Table 6–1).

A   B   C

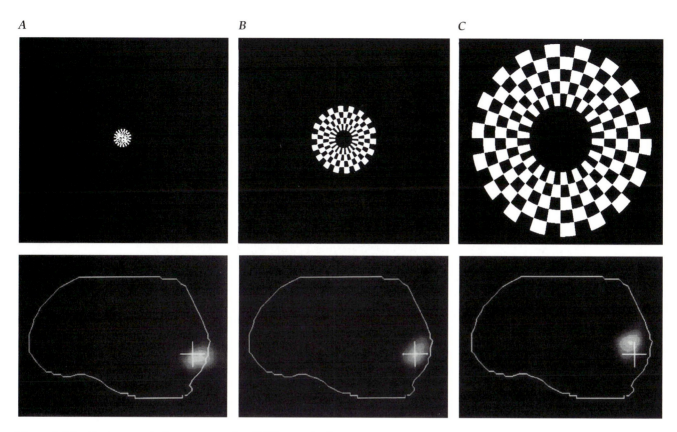

Figure 6–24. Positron emission tomography (PET) reveals the retinotopic organization of the human primary visual cortex. The top part of each panel illustrates the particular stimulus the subject viewed while the scan (shown below) was obtained. The bottom part of each panel is an ^{15}O-labeled water PET scan of a midsagittal slice. Each scan reflects the calculated difference between emission at rest and during visual stimulation. *A.* Macular stimulation. *B.* Perimacular stimulation. *C.* Peripheral stimulation. (Courtesy of Dr. Peter Fox, University of Texas.)

Retina

The retina is the peripheral portion of the visual system (Figures 6–1 and 6–3). Retinal neurons and their synaptic connections are organized into five layers. The cell bodies of photoreceptors are located in the **outer nuclear layer** (1): **cones** are the photoreceptors for **color vision and high-acuity vision, rods** are for **night vision**. Photoreceptors synapse on **bipolar cells** in the **outer synaptic (or plexiform) layer** (2), but their cell bodies are located in the **inner nuclear layer** (3). Bipolar cells, in turn, synapse on the **ganglion cells**—the output neurons of the retina—in the **inner synaptic (or plexiform) layer** (4). Amacrine cells and horizontal cells are the retinal interneurons that mediate lateral interactions among populations of photoreceptors, bipolar cells, and ganglion cells. Ganglion cells are located in the **ganglion cell layer** (5) (Figure 6–3). Light must pass through the ganglion cells and interneurons before reaching the photoreceptors. Müller cells are the principal retinal neuroglia.

Summary

Visual Field and Optic Nerves

The retina receives a visual image that is transformed by the optical elements of the eye (Figure 6–2): the image becomes inverted and reversed. Images from one half of the **visual field** (Figures 6–2 and 6–21) are projected on the **ipsilateral nasal hemiretina** and the **contralateral temporal hemiretina**. The axons from ganglion cells exit from the eye at the optic disk (Figure 6–5). Axons from ganglion cells in the temporal hemiretina project into the **ipsilateral optic nerve** and **ipsilateral optic tract** (Figure 6–1A). Ganglion cell axons from the nasal hemiretina project into the ipsilateral optic nerve, **decussate in the optic chiasm**, and course through the **contralateral optic tract** (Figure 6–1A).

Midbrain

Ganglion cell axons destined for the midbrain leave the optic tract and course in the **brachium of the superior colliculus** (Figures 6–1 and 6–6). A key midbrain site for the ganglion cell axon terminals is the **superior colliculus** (Figures 6–6 and 6–7), a laminated structure. The **superficial layers** of the superior colliculus subserve **visuomotor and visual reflex function**, and the **deeper layers subserve orientation of the eyes and head to salient stimuli**. The **pretectal nuclei** (Figure 6–8B), where interneurons for the pupillary light reflex are located, also receive retinal input.

Thalamus

The **lateral geniculate nucleus (dorsal division)** is the thalamic nucleus that receives the principal projection from the retina (Figures 6–6 and 6–8). Like other structures in the visual system, it too is laminated, and each of the **six layers** receives input from either the **ipsilateral or contralateral retina** (Figure 6–9), but visual information from the **contralateral visual hemifield**. The **pulvinar** and **lateral posterior** nuclei receive an ascending projection from the superior colliculus that may be important in determining visual salience.

Visual Cortical Areas

The lateral geniculate nucleus projects to the **primary visual cortex** (Figure 6–11) via the **optic radiations** (Figure 6–10), which course through the white matter of the temporal, parietal, and occipital lobes. Thalamic input terminates principally in **layer 4** (Figure 6–12), in sublaminae A and C (Figure 6–13)—of the primary visual cortex. Input from the ipsilateral and contralateral eyes remains segregated in this layer (Figure 6–15). This is the anatomical substrate of the **ocular dominance columns** (Figure 6–14A). The other type of column is the **orientation column** (Figures 6–14B and 6–16). Vertically oriented aggregates of neurons in layers 2 and 3, centered in the ocular dominance columns, are color-sensitive **color blobs** (Figures 6–14C and 6–17).

The primary visual cortex is retinotopically organized (Figures 6–23 and 6–24). The primary area projects to the higher-order visual areas of the occipital, parietal, and temporal lobes (Figures 6–11, 6–19, and 6–20). There are at least three functional paths from the primary visual cortex to higher-order visual areas: one for **perception of stimulus form**, one for **color** (form and color together are important for object recognition), both of which project ventrally, and the third for **perception of stimulus motion,** which projects dorsally.

Visual Field Defects

Damage to the visual pathway produces characteristic changes in visual perception (Figure 6–21, Table 6–1): (1) complete transection of the optic nerve, **total blindness in the ipsilateral eye,** (2) optic chiasm, **bitemporal heteronymous hemianopia,** (3) optic tract and lateral geniculate nucleus, **contralateral homonymous hemianopia,** (4) optic radiation in temporal lobe (Meyer's loop), **contralateral upper quadrant homonymous hemianopia,** (5) optic radiations in parietal and occipital lobes, **contralateral homonymous hemianopia,** (6) primary visual cortex, **contralateral homonymous hemianopia with macular sparing.** ■

KEY STRUCTURES AND TERMS

magnocellular system
  motion pathway
parvocellular systems
  color
  form vision
retina
  optic disk
  blind spot
  pigment epithelium
  fovea
  macula lutea
  Müller cells
  outer nuclear layer
    rods
    cones
  outer synaptic (or plexiform) layer
  inner nuclear layer
    horizontal cells and amacrine
      cells
    bipolar cells

inner synaptic (or plexiform) layer
ganglion cell layer
  ganglion cells
optic nerve (cranial nerve II)
optic chiasm
optic tract
lateral geniculate nucleus
lateral posterior nucleus
pulvinar
optic radiations
Meyer's loop
primary visual cortex (area 17)
  calcarine fissure
  stripe of Gennari
  columnar organization
    ocular dominance columns
    orientation columns
    color blobs
secondary and higher-order visual
      cortical areas

inferior temporal lobe
posterior parietal cortex
superior colliculus
  brachium of the superior
      colliculus
  spinotectal tract
saccades
pretectal nuclei
  pupillary reflexes
visual fields
  nasal hemiretina
  temporal hemiretina
  temporal crescents
visual field defect
  bitemporal hemianopia
  homonymous hemianopia
  quadrantanopia
  macular sparing
posterior cerebral artery

Selected Readings

DeYoe, E. A., and Van Essen, D. C. 1988. Concurrent processing streams in monkey visual cortex. Trends in Neurosci. 11:219–226.

Dowling, J. E. 1987. The Retina: An Approachable Part of the Brain. Cambridge, Mass.: Harvard University Press.

Hendrickson, A. 1985. Dots, stripes and columns in monkey visual cortex. Trends in Neurosci. 8:406–410.

Huerta, M. F., and Harting, J. K. 1984. Connectional organization of the superior colliculus. Trends in Neurosci. 7:286–289.

Merigan, W. H. 1993. Human V4? Current Biology 3:226–229.

Mishkin, M., Ungerleider, L. G., and Macko, K. A. 1983. Object vision: Two cortical pathways. Trends in Neurosci. 6:414–416.

Patten, H. 1977. Neurological Differential Diagnosis. New York: Springer-Verlag.

Robinson, D. L., and Petersen, S. E. 1992. The pulvinar and visual salience. Trends Neurosci. 15:127–132.

Sereno, M. I., Dale, A.M., Reppas, J. B., Kwong, K. K., Belliveau, J. W., Brady, T. J., Rosen, B. R., and Tootell, R. B. H. 1995. Borders of multiple visual areas in humans revealed by functional magnetic resonance imaging. Science 268:889–893.

Stein, B. E. 1984. Development of the superior colliculus. Ann. Rev. Neurosci. 7:95–125.

Tessier-Lavigne, M. 1991. Phototransduction and information processing in the retina. In Kandel, E. R., Schwartz, J. H., and Jessell, T. M. (eds.), Principles of Neural Science, 2nd ed. New York: Elsevier, pp. 400-417.

Van Essen, D. C. 1979. Visual areas of the mammalian cerebral cortex. Ann. Rev. Neurosci. 2:227–263.

Van Essen, D. C., and Maunsell, J. H. R. 1983. Hierarchical organization and functional streams in the visual cortex. Trends in Neurosci. 6:370–375.

Zeki, S. 1993. A Vision of the Brain. Oxford: Blackwell Scientific Publications.

References

Berne, R. M., and Levy, M. N. 1983. Physiology. St. Louis: Mosby.

Bishop, P. O. 1984. Processing of visual information within the retinostriate system. In Darian-Smith, I. (ed.), Handbook of Physiology, Section 1: The Nervous System, Vol. III. Sensory Processes. Bethesda, Md.: American Physiological Society, pp. 341–424.

Brodal, A. 1981. Neurological Anatomy. New York: Oxford University Press.

Clarke, S., and Miklossy, J. 1990. Occipital cortex in man: Organization of callosal connections, related myelo and cytoarchitecture, and putative boundaries of functional visual areas. J. Comp. Neurol. 298:188–214.

Curcio, C. A., Sloan, K. R., Kalina, R. E., and Hendrickson, A. E. 1990. Human photoreceptor topography. J. Comp. Neurol. 292:497–523.

Dowling, J. E., and Boycott, B. B. 1966. Organization of the primate retina: Electron microscopy. Proc. R. Soc. Lond. B 166:80–111.

Fox, P. T., Miezin, F. M., Allman, J. M., et al. 1987. Retinotopic organization of human visual cortex mapped with positron emission tomography. J. Neurosci. 7:913–922.

Gouras, P. 1991. Color vision. In Kandel, E. R., Schwartz, J. H., and Jessell, T. M. (eds.), Principles of Neural Science, 3rd ed. New York: Elsevier, pp. 467–480.

Horton, J. C., and Hedley-Whyte, E. T. 1984. Mapping of cytochrome oxidase patches and ocular dominance columns in human visual cortex. Phil. Trans. R. Soc. Lond. B 304:255–272.

Hubel, D. H., and Wiesel, T. N. 1977. Ferrier lecture: Functional architecture of macaque monkey visual cortex. Proc. R. Soc. Lond. B 198:1–59.

Kandel, E. R. 1991. Perception of motion, depths, and form. In Kandel, E. R., Schwartz, J. H., and Jessell, T. M. (eds.), Principles of Neural Science, 3rd ed. New York: Elsevier, pp. 440-465.

Livingstone, M. S., and Hubel, D. H. 1984. Anatomy and physiology of a color system in the primate visual cortex. J. Neurosci. 4:309–356.

Mason, C., and Kandel, E. R. 1991. Central visual pathways. In Kandel, E. R., Schwartz, J. H., and Jessell, T. M. (eds.), Principles of Neural Science, 3rd ed. New York: Elsevier, pp. 420–439.

Merigan, W. H., and Maunsell, J. H. R. 1993. How parallel are the primate visual pathways? Ann. Rev. Neurosci. 16:369–402.

Schiller, P. H. 1984. The superior colliculus and visual function. In Darian-Smith, I. (ed.), Handbook of Physiology, Section 1: The Nervous System, Vol. III. Sensory Processes. Bethesda, Md.: American Physiological Society, pp. 457–506.

Zeki, S., Watson, J. D. G., Lueck, C. J., et al. 1991. A direct demonstration of functional specialization in human visual cortex. J. Neurosci. 11:641–649.

Zilles, K. 1990. Cortex. In Paxinos, G. (ed.), The Human Nervous System. San Diego: Academic Press, pp. 757–802.

7

The Auditory and Vestibular Systems

T*HE AUDITORY SYSTEM MEDIATES THE SENSE OF HEARING.* This system, like the somatic sensory and visual systems, has a topographic organization determined by the peripheral receptive sheet. Similarly, the auditory system consists of multiple parallel pathways. Each component of the pathway is hierarchically organized and is thought to subserve different aspects of hearing. However, unlike the other sensory systems we examined, the connections of the auditory system reflect a key computational requirement related to the temporal analysis of sounds.

The vestibular system contributes to the sense of balance by detecting motion of the head. It is a modality that is perceived only during special circumstances. However, the vestibular system plays an ongoing role in maintaining balance and the reflex control of the position of our head and eyes. The major connections of the vestibular system reflect this motor function. We consider balance together with hearing because the vestibulocochlear nerve (cranial nerve VIII) carries afferent information from the peripheral components of both vestibular and auditory systems, via separate vestibular and cochlear divisions, to the central nervous system.

In this chapter, we first consider the general organization of the auditory and vestibular systems. Then we examine key levels through the brain stem, levels in which structures that process auditory and vestibular information are located. Finally, the connections of the auditory system with the thalamus and cerebral cortex are examined. Because important motor pathways originate from the vestibular nuclei (the vestibulospinal tracts and the medial longitudinal fasciculus), we will reexamine the central vestibular connections in greater detail in Chapter 9, from the perspective of the motor functions of vestibular system.

FUNCTIONAL ANATOMY OF THE AUDITORY AND VESTIBULAR SYSTEMS

Parallel Ascending Auditory Pathways May Be Involved in Different Aspects of Hearing

The process of hearing begins on the body surface, as sounds are conducted by the pinna and external auditory meatus to the tympanic

A

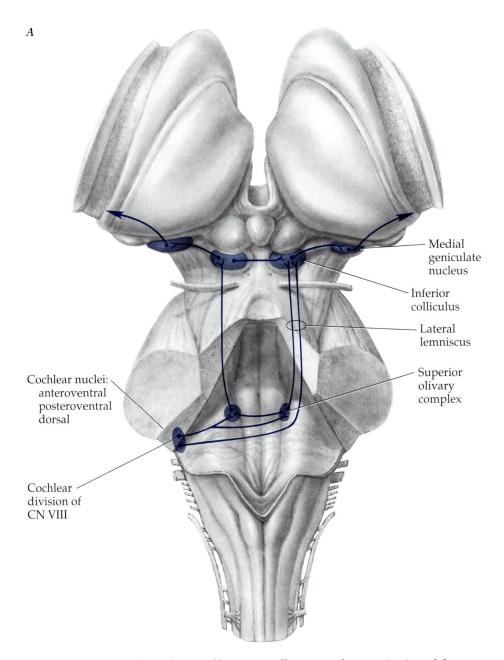

Medial
geniculate
nucleus

Inferior
colliculus

Lateral
lemniscus

Superior
olivary
complex

Cochlear nuclei:
anteroventral
posteroventral
dorsal

Cochlear
division of
CN VIII

Figure 7–1. *A.* Dorsal view of brain stem illustrating the organization of the auditory system. *B.* General organization of the auditory system revealed in cross section at different levels through the brain stem and coronal section through the diencephalon and cerebral hemispheres.

membrane. Mechanical displacement of the tympanic membrane, produced by changes in sound pressure waves, is transmitted by the middle ear ossicles, the **malleus**, **incus**, and **stapes**, to the inner ear. The inner ear transductive machinery is located in a structure in the temporal bone called the **cochlea** (see Figure 7–3). This is where the auditory receptors are located. Each auditory receptor, termed a **hair cell** because it has stereocilia on its apical surface, is sensitive to a limited frequency range of sounds.

B

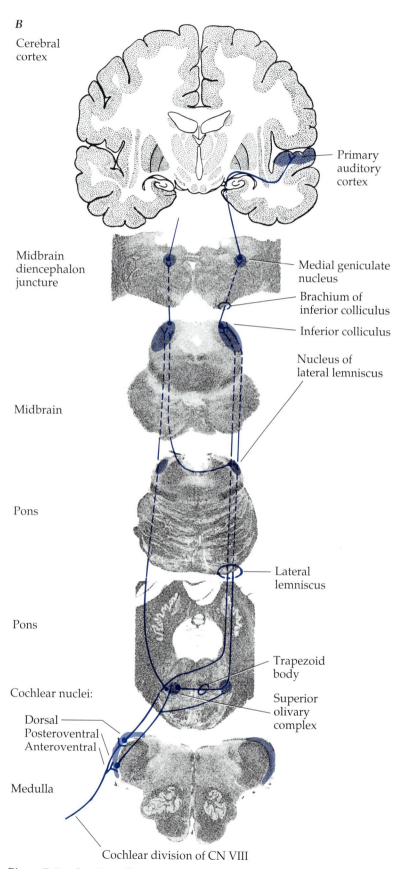

Cerebral
cortex

Primary
auditory
cortex

Midbrain
diencephalon
juncture

Medial geniculate
nucleus

Brachium of
inferior colliculus

Inferior colliculus

Nucleus of
lateral lemniscus

Midbrain

Pons

Pons

Lateral
lemniscus

Trapezoid
body

Cochlear nuclei:

Superior
olivary
complex

Dorsal
Posteroventral
Anteroventral

Medulla

Cochlear division of CN VIII

Figure 7–1. *(continued)*

There is a spatial relationship between the location of a hair cell in the cochlea and the frequency to which the receptor is most sensitive. As we will see below, from the base of the cochlea to the apex, the frequency to which a hair cell is maximally sensitive changes systematically from high frequencies to low frequencies. This differential frequency sensitivity of hair cells along the length of the cochlea is the basis of the **tonotopic organization** of the auditory receptive sheet. This is similar to the somatic sensory and visual systems, where the nuclei and cortical areas have a somatotopic and retinotopic organization. In each of these cases, the topographic organization of the central representations is determined by the spatial organization of the peripheral receptive sheet. Many of the components of the auditory system are tonotopically organized.

Hair cells are innervated by the distal processes of bipolar primary sensory neurons located in the **spiral ganglion**. The central processes of the bipolar neurons form the **cochlear division** of the **vestibulocochlear (eighth cranial) nerve**. These axons project to the ipsilateral **cochlear nuclei** (Figure 7–1A), which are located in the rostral medulla.

The cochlear nuclei are comprised of three anatomical divisions. Ascending projection neurons in each division have distinct connections with the rest of the auditory system and give rise to parallel auditory pathways that are thought to serve different aspects of hearing. The auditory projection that originates from one division of the cochlear nuclei, the anteroventral cochlear nucleus, is important in the **horizontal localization of sounds**. This nucleus projects bilaterally to the **superior olivary complex**, a cluster of nuclei in the caudal pons. Neurons in the superior olivary complex, in turn, project via an ascending pathway called the **lateral lemniscus** to the **inferior colliculus**, located in the midbrain tectum.

We can only infer the functions of the two other components of the cochlear nuclei, the posteroventral and dorsal cochlear nuclei, based on our understanding of the physiological properties of neurons in these nuclei or their projections. The dorsal cochlear nucleus projects directly to the contralateral **inferior colliculus** also via the lateral lemniscus. Neurons in the dorsal cochlear nucleus appear to have more complex physiological properties than those in the other divisions of the nucleus. It has been suggested that this projection may be important in aspects of auditory perception other than localization, for example, for recognizing temporal patterns of sound. Neurons in the posteroventral cochlear nucleus not only send their axons directly to the contralateral inferior colliculus, but also to components of the superior olivary complex that project back to the cochlea rather than to other brain regions. This **olivocochlear projection** is thought to regulate hair cell sensitivity.

One way that auditory pathways differ from somatic sensory and visual pathways is in the multiple levels at which auditory information crosses the midline through decussations and commissures. Thus, the ascending auditory paths on each side of the brain stem carry information from both ears. What is the clinical significance of this bilateral organization of central auditory connections? Unilateral brain stem damage does not cause deafness in one ear unless the injury destroys the cochlear nuclei or the entering fascicles of the cochlear nerve. Unilateral deafness is thus a sign of injury to the peripheral auditory organ or the cochlear nerve.

Although important clinically, the bilateral representation of sounds has a more general significance in providing a mechanism for sound localization (see below) and serving to enhance the detection of sounds through summation of converging inputs.

In sequence, the next segment of the ascending auditory pathway is from the inferior colliculus to the thalamic auditory nucleus, called the **medial geniculate nucleus**. The projection from the medial geniculate nucleus to the primary auditory cortex, which is called the **auditory radiation**, terminates within the lateral sulcus (also called the Sylvian fissure) on the superior surface of the temporal lobe. The primary auditory cortex is located on **Heschl's gyri** (see Figure 7–10) and is surrounded by **higher-order auditory areas**, located on both the superior and the lateral surfaces of the temporal lobe in the **superior temporal gyrus**.

The Vestibular Nuclei Receive Monosynaptic Input From the Vestibular Division of the Eighth Cranial Nerve

Head motion, both linear (such as that experienced during a fast acceleration in a car) and angular (such as during turning), is sensed by the vestibular receptors. Like their auditory counterparts, vestibular receptors are also hair cells. Vestibular receptors are located in the peripheral vestibular apparatus, which consists of the **semicircular canals**, the **utricle**, and the **saccule** (see Figure 7–3A). Vestibular hair cells are innervated by the peripheral processes of vestibular bipolar neurons, the cell bodies of which are located in the **vestibular ganglion** (or Scarpa's ganglion). The central processes of these bipolar neurons, which form the **vestibular division** of the **eighth cranial nerve**, course with the cochlear division and enter the brain stem at the lateral pontomedullary junction. Axons in the vestibular division terminate in the four **vestibular nuclei,** located in the rostral medulla and caudal pons (Figure 7–2).

There are three functionally distinct efferent projections from the vestibular nuclei.

- **Vestibulospinal tracts**, major projections to the spinal cord for controlling limb and axial muscles (see Chapter 9).
- Connections to brain stem nuclei involved in the control of **extraocular muscles** (see Chapter 13).
- A small ascending thalamocortical projection that is important in the **conscious awareness** of orientation and motion of the head and balance.

Although the pathway for perception of signals from the vestibular nuclei is not as well understood as the auditory pathways, we know that the thalamic relay nucleus for transmitting vestibular information to the cortex is a portion of the **ventral posterior nucleus**. The vestibular cortex is located in the parietal lobe (see Figure 7–10A) directly behind the primary somatic sensory cortex in cytoarchitectonic area 5 (see Figure 5–18). One function of the vestibular projection to the parietal lobe may be to integrate information about head motion with information from somatic sensory receptors in the muscles and joints. This information contributes to the perception of the position of the body in space as well as the control of body movements. This ascending vestibular pathway may also be important in the perception of body acceleration and in vertigo.

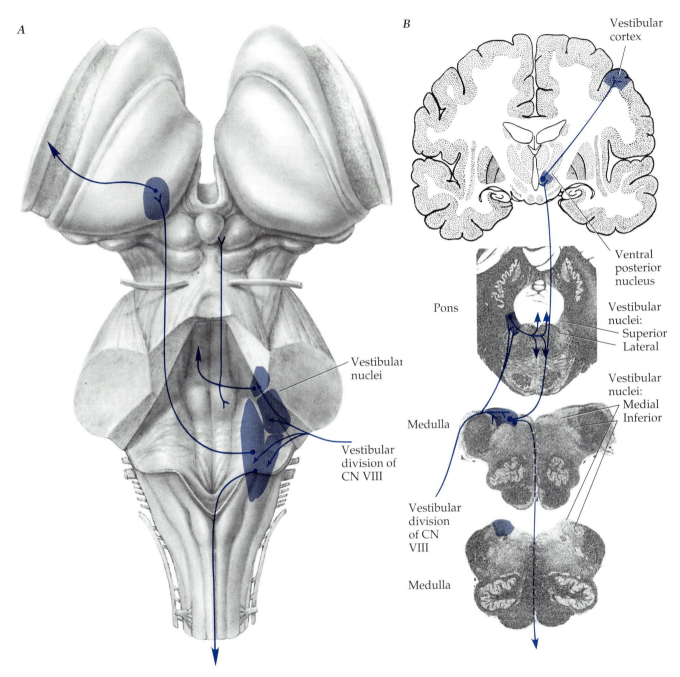

A

B

Figure 7–2. **A.** Dorsal view of brain stem illustrating the organization of the vestibular system. **B.** General organization of the vestibular system revealed in cross section at different levels through the brain stem and coronal section through the diencephalon and cerebral hemispheres.

■ REGIONAL ANATOMY

The Auditory and Vestibular Sensory Organs Are Located Within the Membranous Labyrinth

The **membranous labyrinth** is a complex sac within the **bony labyrinth**, cavities in the petrous portion of the temporal bone (Figure 7–3A). The membranous labyrinth consists of the cochlear duct—the audi-

tory sensory organ—as well as the three semicircular canals and the saccule and utricle—the vestibular sensory organs (Figure 7–3A). (Another name for the semicircular canals, utricle, and saccule is the **vestibular labyrinth**.) The morphological complexity of the auditory and vestibular sensory organs rivals that of the eyeball. Much of the membranous labyrinth is filled with **endolymph**, an extracellular fluid resembling intracellular fluid in its ionic constituents. Endolymph has a high K^+ concentration and low Na^+ concentration. In contrast, **perilymph**, a fluid resembling extracellular fluid and cerebrospinal fluid, fills the space between the membranous labyrinth and the temporal bone.

The Auditory Receptor Cells Are Located in the Organ of Corti

The cochlear duct is a coiled structure (Figure 7–3A); it is drawn uncoiled in Figure 7–3B. The hair cells are located in the **organ of Corti**, a specialized portion of the cochlear duct (Figure 7–3C) that rests on the **basilar membrane** and is covered by the **tectorial membrane** (see below). There are two kinds of hair cells in the organ of Corti, and their names reflect their position with respect to the axis of the coiled cochlea: **inner** and **outer hair cells**. Inner hair cells are arranged in a single row, whereas outer hair cells are arranged in three or four rows. Although there are fewer inner than outer hair cells (approximately 3500 versus 12,000), the inner hair cells are thought to play a key role in frequency and other fine discriminations in hearing. The function of the outer hair cells is not yet known.

Most of the axons in the cochlear division of the eighth cranial nerve innervate the inner hair cells, each of which may receive convergent input from as many as ten fibers. Moreover, each of the primary auditory fibers contacts a single, or at most, a few inner hair cells. In contrast, the outer hair cells are innervated by a minority of afferent nerve fibers and each of these fibers branch to contact multiple outer hair cells.

The organ of Corti transduces sounds into neural signals. This organ is mechanically coupled to the external environment by the tympanic membrane, the middle ear ossicles, and the oval window (Figure 7–3). Pressure changes in the external auditory meatus, resulting from sound waves, cause the **tympanic membrane** to vibrate. The **middle ear ossicles** conduct the external pressure changes from the tympanic membrane to the **scala vestibuli** of the inner ear (Figure 7–3B). Because the entire cochlear duct is filled with fluid, these pressure changes are conducted from the scala vestibuli through the fluid to the other compartments of the cochlea, the **scala media** to the **scala tympani** (Figure 7–3B). Pressure changes resulting from sounds set up a traveling wave along the compliant **basilar membrane** (Figure 7–3C), on which the hair cells and their support structures rest. The traveling wave results in shearing forces between the basilar membrane and the less compliant **tectorial membrane**. Because the hair cells have stereocilia that are embedded in the tectorial membrane, the shearing forces cause the stereocilia to bend. This results in a membrane conductance change in the hair cells.

The traveling wave on the basilar membrane, established by changes in pressure impinging on the ear resulting from sounds, is extraordinarily complex. High-frequency sounds generate a wave on the basilar membrane with a peak amplitude close to the base of the cochlea; consequently these sounds preferentially activate the **basal** hair cells. As the frequency of the sound source decreases, the location of the peak amplitude of the wave on the basilar membrane shifts continuously toward the cochlear apex. This results in the preferential activation of hair cells that are located

A

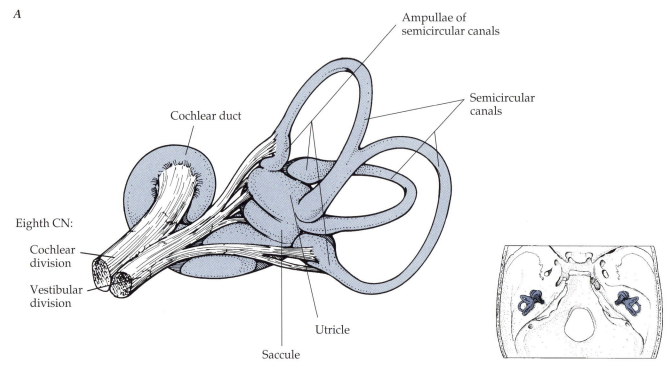

Ampullae of
semicircular canals

Semicircular
canals

Cochlear duct

Eighth CN:

Cochlear
division

Vestibular
division

Utricle

Saccule

Figure 7–3. ***A.*** The peripheral auditory and vestibular structures and innervation by the cochlear and vestibular divisions of cranial nerve VIII. The inset shows the orientation of the three semicircular canals in relation to the cranium. ***B.*** The middle ear and inner ear. An uncoiled and schematic view of the cochlea is depicted with innervation by the cochlear nerve. The upper inset in part B shows the coiled cochlea, and the line indicates the plane of the section shown in the inset in the lower portion of part B. ***C.*** Expanded view of a section through the cochlear duct illustrating the organ of Corti. (Inset in *A* adapted from Kelly, 1991; *C*, Adapted from Dallos, P. 1984. Peripheral mechanisms of hearing. In Darian-Smith, I. (ed.), Handbook of Physiology, Section 1: The Nervous System, Vol. 3. Sensory Processes. Bethesda, Md.: American Physiological Society, pp. 595–637.)

closer to the **apex of the cochlea**. Although the mechanical properties of the basilar membrane are a major determinant of the auditory tuning of hair cells, as well as the tonotopic organization of the organ of Corti, the electrical membrane characteristics of hair cells also contribute. We will see that the tonotopic organization underlies the topography of connections in the central auditory pathways.

Vestibular Hair Cells Are Located in the Ampullae of the Semicircular Canals and Maculae of the Utricle and Saccule

Receptor cells are also located in specialized regions of the semicircular canals (termed ampullae) and the saccule and utricle (termed maculae). Like the auditory receptor cells, the vestibular receptors are also hair cells and are activated by displacement of stereocilia on their apical surfaces. However, the mechanical properties of the vestibular labyrinth confer motion sensitivity to the receptors. Hair cells in the semicircular canals signal angular head motion (angular acceleration), whereas those in the utricle and saccule signal linear motion (linear acceleration).

The mechanism that activates vestibular receptors is different from that of the auditory receptors. The hair cells of the semicircular canals are covered by a gelatinous mass (termed the cupula) into which the stereocilia

B

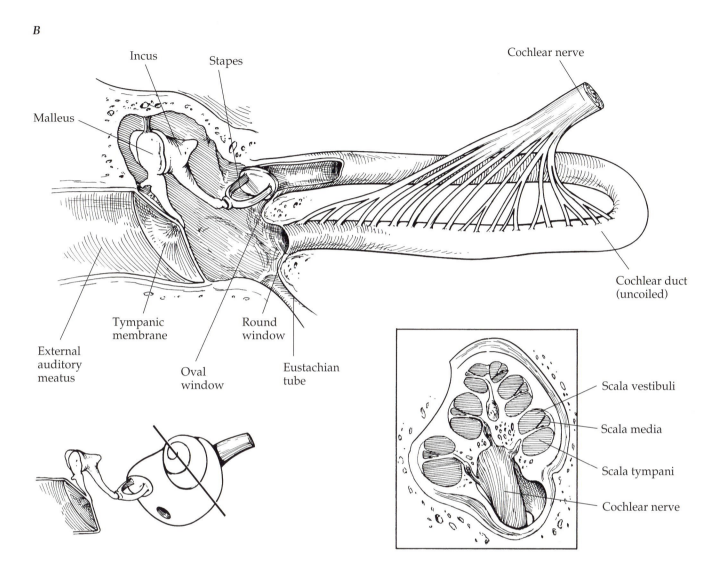

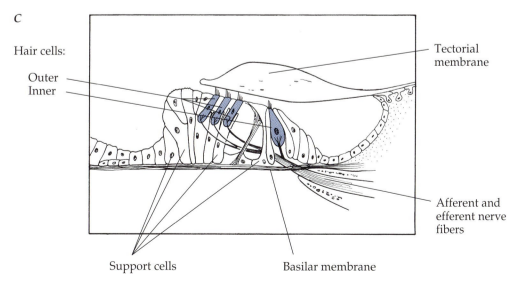

Figure 7–3. *(continued)*

embed. Angular head movement induces the endolymph within the canals to flow, displacing the gelatinous mass, which in turn deflects the hair cell stereocilia. The utricle and saccule also have a gelatinous covering over hair cells in their maculae. Calcium carbonate crystals, embedded in the gelatin, rest on the stereocilia of the hair cells. Head movement causes the crystals to deform the gelatinous mass, thereby deflecting the stereocilia. The saccule and utricle are sometimes called the **otolith organs** because otolith is the term for the calcium carbonate crystals. The semicircular canals, utricle, and saccule each have a different orientation with respect to the head, thereby conferring selective sensitivity to head movement in different directions. In the following sections, we examine the central connections of the vestibular and cochlear divisions of the eighth cranial nerve.

The Vestibular Nuclei Have Functionally Diverse Projections

Primary vestibular sensory neurons project their axons into the vestibular nuclei, which occupy the floor of the fourth ventricle in the dorsolateral medulla and pons (Figure 7–2A). There are four separate vestibular nuclei: (1) inferior, (2) medial, (3) lateral, and (4) superior (Figures 7–2 and 7–4). Within the nuclear complex, the medial vestibular nucleus is present throughout most of the rostrocaudal extent, absent only at the rostral pole where the superior vestibular nucleus is located (Figures 7–2 and 7–4). The inferior and lateral nuclei occupy portions in the lateral medulla and pons. The sulcus limitans (see Chapter 2) marks the medial boundary of the vestibular nuclei (Figure 7–4). Laterally, the vestibular nuclei are bordered by the inferior and middle cerebellar peduncles (Figure 7–4), components of the cerebellum. The region in which the vestibular nuclei are located is termed the **cerebellopontine angle**. Because various cranial nerves and the cerebellum are clustered in this region, the growth of a tumor in the cerebellopontine angle produces a characteristic set of neurological signs (see Chapter 13).

The different vestibular nuclei have extensive interconnections with components of the nuclear complex on the same side (intrinsic connections) and on the opposite side (commissural connections). These connections are important in the basic processing of the vestibular signal. The extrinsic projections of the vestibular nuclei are complex and serve diverse functions. There is an ascending projection to the **ventral posterior nucleus**. As we saw in Chapter 5, most of the neurons in this nucleus send their axons to the primary somatic sensory cortex in the parietal lobe (see Figure 5–18). The vestibular projection to the parietal lobe is located caudal to the somatic sensory cortex and is thought to be important in conscious awareness of information sent from the vestibular labyrinth.

The vestibular projections to the spinal cord originate from neurons located primarily in the lateral and medial vestibular nuclei (see Chapter 9). These spinal projections play an important role in balance and in maintaining posture, by controlling axial and limb musculature (see Chapter 9). All of the vestibular nuclei project axons into the medial longitudinal fasciculus (MLF), a projection important in eye movement control (see Chapter 13). The MLF is one of the most important brain stem tracts. It contains axons from numerous brain stem nuclei that together are important in coordinating movement of the two eyes.

The vestibular primary sensory neurons project directly to the cerebellum (see Chapter 10). In fact, the vestibular sensory neurons are the only primary sensory neurons that have this privileged access to the cere-

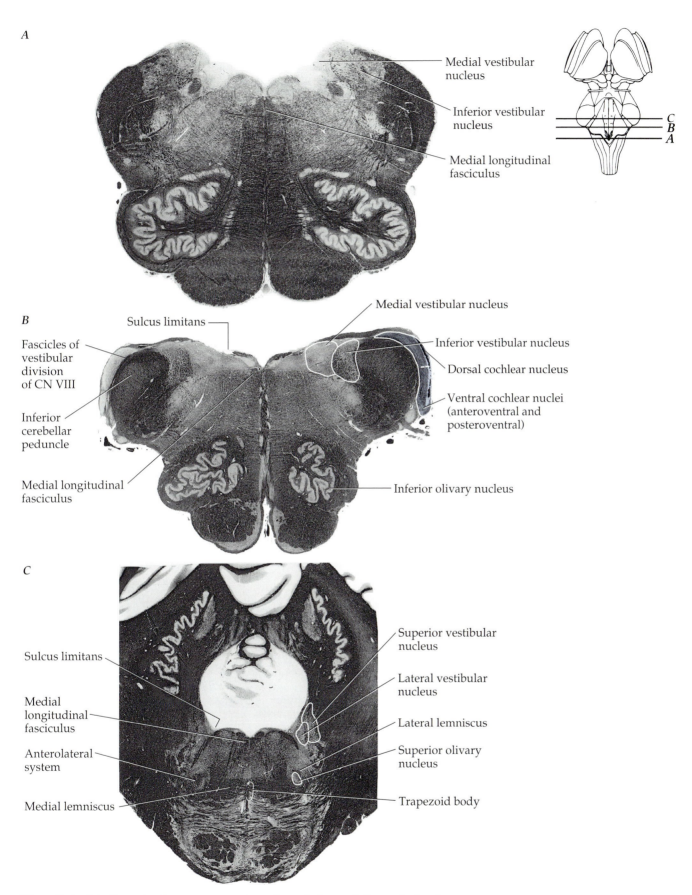

A

Medial vestibular nucleus

Inferior vestibular nucleus

Medial longitudinal fasciculus

B

Sulcus limitans

Fascicles of vestibular division of CN VIII

Inferior cerebellar peduncle

Medial longitudinal fasciculus

Medial vestibular nucleus

Inferior vestibular nucleus

Dorsal cochlear nucleus

Ventral cochlear nuclei (anteroventral and posteroventral)

Inferior olivary nucleus

C

Sulcus limitans

Medial longitudinal fasciculus

Anterolateral system

Medial lemniscus

Superior vestibular nucleus

Lateral vestibular nucleus

Lateral lemniscus

Superior olivary nucleus

Trapezoid body

Figure 7–4. Myelin-stained transverse sections through the medulla, at the level of the inferior and medial vestibular nuclei *(A)*, cochlear nuclei *(B)* and caudal pons *(C)*. The inset shows planes of sections.

209

bellum. In addition, secondary vestibular neurons in the vestibular nuclei project to the cerebellum. Together, the cerebellar projections of the primary and secondary vestibular neurons are essential for normal eye–head coordination and balance.

The Topography of Connections Between Brain Stem Auditory Nuclei Provides Insight Into the Functions of Parallel Ascending Auditory Pathways

There are three major auditory relay nuclei in the brain stem: the **cochlear nuclei**, where the auditory nerve from the ipsilateral ear terminates, as well as the **superior olivary nuclear complex** and the **inferior colliculus**, where information from both ears is integrated. Each of these nuclei is located in a different brain stem division: the cochlear nuclei are located in the medulla, the superior olivary nuclei in the pons, and the inferior colliculus in the midbrain. Knowing the connections among auditory relay nuclei is an essential first step toward understanding the anatomical substrates of hearing.

The Cochlear Nuclei Are the First Central Nervous System Relays For Auditory Information

The three divisions of the cochlear nuclei—the dorsal, anteroventral, and posteroventral (Figure 7–4B)—each have a tonotopic organization. They also have different patterns of efferent connections. Many neurons in the anteroventral cochlear nucleus project to the **superior olivary complex** (Figure 7–4C), the first site in the auditory pathway for **binaural convergence**. Other neurons in both of the posteroventral and the dorsal divisions project directly to the contralateral **inferior colliculus**, bypassing the superior olivary complex. The various divisions of the cochlear nuclei (as well as the vestibular nuclei) are supplied by the posterior inferior cerebellar artery (see Figures 4–1 and 4–3B).

The cochlear nucleus is the most central site in which a lesion can produce deafness in the **ipsilateral ear**. This is because it receives a projection from only the ipsilateral ear. Lesions of the other central auditory nuclei do not produce deafness, because at each of these sites there is convergence of auditory inputs from both ears. Such lesions do, however, produce other auditory perceptual deficits, such as impaired localization of sounds, tinnitus, and sometimes partial hearing loss.

The Superior Olivary Complex Processes Stimuli From Both Ears For Spatial Localization

The **superior olivary complex** is located in the caudal pons, lateral to the medial lemniscus and dorsal to the spinal anterolateral fibers (Figure 7–4C). The nuclear complex contains three major components: the medial superior olivary nucleus, the lateral superior olivary nucleus, and the nucleus of the trapezoid body. The superior olivary nuclei should be distinguished from the inferior olivary nucleus (Figure 7–4A), which contains neurons that project to the cerebellum.

The superior olivary complex receives input primarily from the anteroventral cochlear nucleus, and together these structures give rise to the pathway for **sound localization**. To understand how the anatomical connections between the anteroventral cochlear nucleus and the superior olivary complex contribute to this function, we must first briefly consider how sounds are localized. We recognize a sound as coming from one side

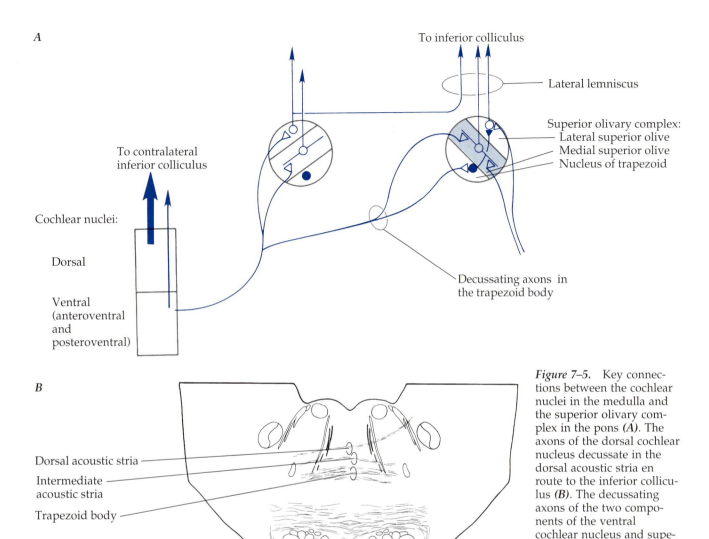

Figure 7–5. Key connections between the cochlear nuclei in the medulla and the superior olivary complex in the pons *(A)*. The axons of the dorsal cochlear nucleus decussate in the dorsal acoustic stria en route to the inferior colliculus *(B)*. The decussating axons of the two components of the ventral cochlear nucleus and superior olivary complex course in the intermediate acoustic stria and the trapezoid body.

of the head or the other by two means depending on its frequency. **Low-frequency** sounds activate the two ears at slightly different times producing a characteristic **interaural time difference**. The farther a sound source is located from the midline, the greater the interaural time difference (reaching a value of approximately 100 μs). At **high frequencies**, the interaural timing difference is an ambiguous cue. However, the head acts as a shield and attenuates these sounds. Thus, a high-frequency sound arriving at the two ears results in an **interaural intensity difference**. This is the "duplex theory" of sound localization.

There is a correspondence between the duplex theory and the neuroanatomical substrates of sound localization. Neurons in the **medial superior olivary nucleus** are sensitive to **interaural time differences** and, in accord with the duplex theory, they respond selectively to low-frequency tones. Individual neurons in the medial superior olive receive monosynaptic connections from the anteroventral cochlear nuclei on both sides, but these inputs are **spatially segregated on their medial and lateral dendrites** (Figure 7–5A). This segregation of inputs is thought to underlie the sensitivity to interaural time differences. In contrast, neurons in the **lateral superior olivary nucleus** are sensitive to **interaural intensity differences**, and they are tuned to high-frequency stimuli. Sensitivity to interaural intensity differences is thought to be determined by convergence of a monosynaptic excitatory input from the ipsilateral anteroventral cochlear nucleus and a disynaptic inhibitory connection from the contralateral anteroventral cochlear nucleus, relayed through the **nucleus of the trapezoid body** (Figure 7–5A).

Many of the projections of the posteroventral and dorsal cochlear nuclei bypass the superior olivary complex to reach the inferior colliculus directly. This ascending projection does not seem to play a role in sound localization, but rather may contribute to perception of sound quality, including pitch and loudness. This path may also participate in acoustic reflexes, such as orientation and startle reactions.

Most of the axons from each division of the cochlear nucleus decussate and reach the superior olivary complex or the inferior colliculus by a different path. Axons from the dorsal cochlear nucleus course in the dorsal acoustic stria. Axons from the posteroventral cochlear nucleus decussate in both the intermediate acoustic stria and the **trapezoid body** (or ventral acoustic stria), whereas those from the anteroventral cochlear nucleus cross over only in the trapezoid body. Of the three auditory decussations, only the trapezoid body can be readily discerned. It is present on the myelin-stained section through the caudal pons (Figure 7–4C). The medial lemniscus is difficult to see at this level, obscured by the trapezoid body. Axons in the dorsal and intermediate acoustic striae and the trapezoid body converge to form the **lateral lemniscus**, a pathway that runs from the caudal pons (Figure 7–4C) to the midbrain (Figure 7–6).

Stimulation of the Olivocochlear Bundle Suppresses Auditory Responses in the Cochlear Nerve

There are neurons in the superior olivary complex that do not appear to be directly involved in processing the horizontal location of the source of sounds. These neurons give rise to axons that project back to the

Figure 7–6. Myelin-stained transverse section through the rostral pons. The inset shows the plane of section.

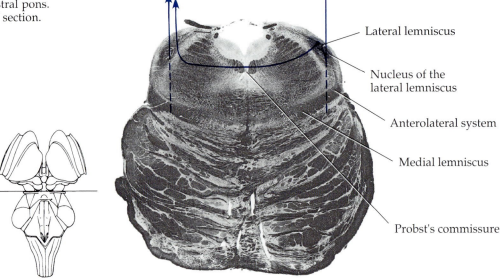

Lateral lemniscus

Nucleus of the lateral lemniscus

Anterolateral system

Medial lemniscus

Probst's commissure

cochlea, via the vestibulocochlear nerve. This efferent pathway is called the **olivocochlear bundle**. The neurons that contribute to this efferent path are located in the superior olivary complex on both the **ipsilateral** and **contralateral** sides with respect to the cochlea, to which these axons project. The neurons contributing axons to the olivocochlear bundle receive auditory input directly from the cochlear nuclei, as well as auditory information relayed from higher levels of the auditory pathway. The olivocochlear bundle is thought to regulate the flow of auditory information into the brain, similar to how inhibitory mechanisms in the dorsal horn regulate somatic sensory input to the spinal cord.

The olivocochlear control system affects the outer and inner hair cells differently. The outer hair cells receive a synaptic connection directly from the axons of the olivocochlear bundle. *In vitro* studies have shown that outer hair cells contract when acetylcholine, which is one of the neurotransmitters of the olivocochlear bundle, is directly applied to the receptor. This mechanical change, if it also occurs *in vivo*, would likely cause the stereocilia to withdraw somewhat from the tectorial membrane and thereby reduce the mechanical sensitivity of the receptors. The inner hair cells, on the other hand, do not receive a direct synaptic connection from the olivocochlear bundle. Rather, the olivocochlear axons form inhibitory synapses on the terminals of auditory nerve fibers that innervate the inner hair cells. It seems that the olivocochlear bundle could regulate both auditory transduction by the outer hair cells and auditory afferent nerve fiber transmission from the inner hair cells. The vestibular receptors also have an efferent connection from the central nervous system, although much less is known about this system. The neurons that project their axons to the vestibular labyrinth, via the vestibulocochlear nerve, are located near the medial vestibular nucleus.

Auditory Brain Stem Axons Ascend in the Lateral Lemniscus

The lateral lemniscus is a discrete bundle of axons in the caudal pons (Figure 7–4C) but it is clearly visualized as a separate tract only in the rostral pons (Figure 7–6) and midbrain (Figure 7–7B). (The lateral lemniscus should be distinguished from the medial lemniscus [Figure 7–6], which relays somatic sensory information to the thalamus.) Virtually all of the fibers in the lateral lemniscus terminate in the inferior colliculus. Many of the axons also send collateral branches into the **nucleus of the lateral lemniscus**, which is centered within the structure for which it is named (Figure 7–6). The nucleus of the lateral lemniscus contains many neurons that project their axons to the contralateral inferior colliculus via Probst's commissure. This is another site in the auditory pathway where information crosses the midline.

As we saw above, decussation of auditory information has an important clinical implication: Damage to the central auditory pathway rostral to the cochlear nuclei does not produce a unilateral hearing loss. In the rostral pons (Figure 7–6)—the lateral lemniscus together with the ascending somatic sensory pathways, the medial lemniscus and the anterolateral system—form a continuous band of myelinated axons that roughly divides the pontine **tegmentum** from the **base**. Recall that the **tectum** of the brain stem is the component located dorsal to the cerebral aqueduct and is well developed only in the midbrain.

A

See Fig 7–8

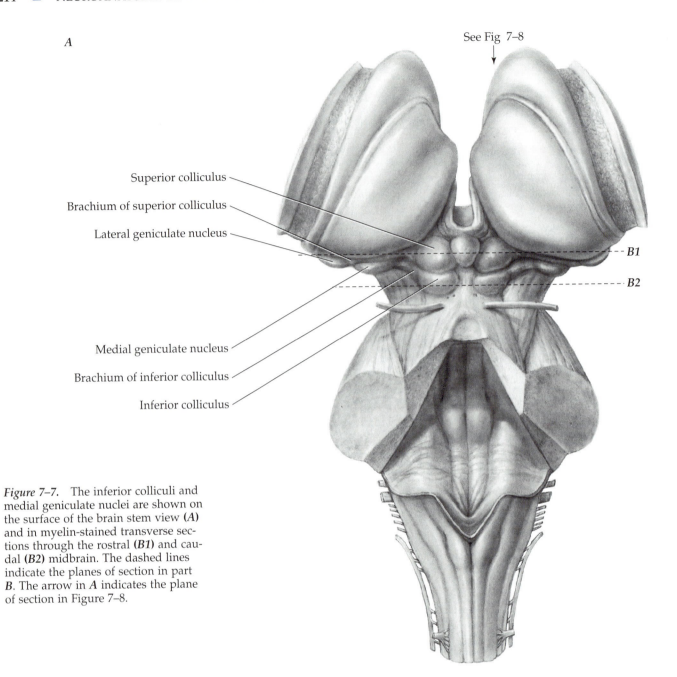

Superior colliculus

Brachium of superior colliculus

Lateral geniculate nucleus

- - - B1

- - - B2

Medial geniculate nucleus

Brachium of inferior colliculus

Inferior colliculus

Figure 7–7. The inferior colliculi and medial geniculate nuclei are shown on the surface of the brain stem view (*A*) and in myelin-stained transverse sections through the rostral (*B1*) and caudal (*B2*) midbrain. The dashed lines indicate the planes of section in part *B*. The arrow in *A* indicates the plane of section in Figure 7–8.

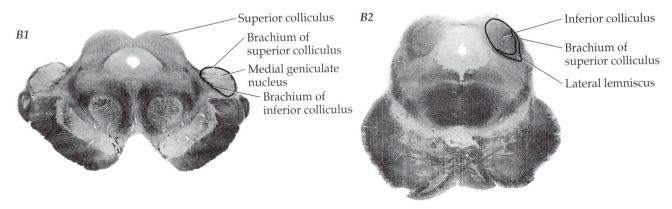

B1

Superior colliculus

Brachium of superior colliculus

Medial geniculate nucleus

Brachium of inferior colliculus

B2

Inferior colliculus

Brachium of superior colliculus

Lateral lemniscus

The Inferior Colliculus Is Located in the Midbrain Tectum

The inferior colliculus is located on the dorsal surface of the midbrain, caudal to the superior colliculus (Figure 7–7A). Even though both colliculi are located in the midbrain tectum, their roles in stimulus processing are different. The superior colliculus is part of the visual system (see Chapter 6). It receives visual input in parallel with the lateral geniculate nucleus and functions in visuomotor control. In contrast, the inferior colliculus is an auditory nucleus where virtually all ascending fibers in the lateral lemniscus synapse.

The internal structure of the rostral and caudal portions of the midbrain is easier to distinguish than that of the various levels of the medulla or pons because of two landmarks in the tegmentum: the **decussation of the superior cerebellar** peduncle and the **red nuclei** (Figure 7–7B). Both of these structures are key components of the motor system (see Chapters 9 and 10). The decussation of the superior cerebellar peduncle is a white matter structure centered over the midline and clearly distinguishable from the two red nuclei, which are roughly spherical in cross section. We see that the decussation of the superior cerebellar peduncle marks the level at which the inferior colliculus is located, whereas the red nuclei mark the level of the superior colliculus. Ventrally, these two levels of the midbrain each contain the substantia nigra and the basis pedunculi. The superior and inferior colliculi are cut parasagittally in Figure 7–8; the plane of section is indicated in Figure 7–7A by the arrow.

Three component nuclei comprise the inferior colliculus: the central and external nuclei, and the dorsal cortex. The **central nucleus** of the inferior colliculus, which is the principal site of termination of the auditory paths from the pons and medulla, gives rise to an ascending auditory "lemniscal" pathway to the thalamus that continues to the primary auditory cortex. At each level, this pathway has a precise tonotopic organization. In contrast, the **external nucleus** and **dorsal cortex** give rise to "extralemniscal" or diffuse pathways in which tonotopy is either not present or is less precise.

The central nucleus receives convergent input from three sources: (1) pathways originating from the ipsilateral and contralateral **superior olivary nuclei**, (2) axons from the ipsilateral and contralateral **nucleus of the lateral lemniscus**, and (3) the direct pathway from the contralateral **dorsal and posteroventral cochlear nuclei**. All of the axons that project into the central nucleus of the inferior colliculus from the medulla and pons are located in the lateral lemniscus. The function of this nucleus is to process sounds for auditory perception and reflex adjustments, such as the acoustic startle response.

The central nucleus is **laminated** (although not apparent on myelin-stained sections): neurons in a single lamina are maximally sensitive to **similar tonal frequencies**. Lamination of neurons and the presynaptic terminals of ascending auditory fibers is the structural basis for tonotopy in the central nucleus. We have seen for the somatic sensory and visual systems that lamination is also used for packaging neurons with similar functional attributes or connections.

The function of the other nuclei in the inferior colliculus is much less clear. Studies in which lesions are placed in the **external nucleus** of the inferior colliculus of experimental animals suggest that it plays a role in **acousticomotor function**, such as the orientation of the head and body axis to auditory stimuli. This function of the external nucleus may utilize

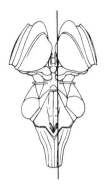

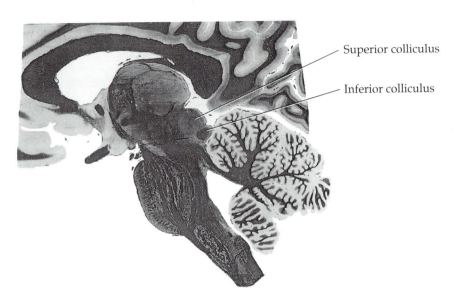

Superior colliculus

Inferior colliculus

Figure 7–8. The superior and inferior colliculi can be identified on this sagittal section through the brain stem. The plane of section is indicated by the arrow in Figure 7–7.

somatic sensory information, which is also projected to this nucleus from the spinal cord and medulla. The functions of the **dorsal cortex** are not known.

The inferior colliculus projects to the thalamus via a tract that is located just beneath the dorsal surface of the midbrain, the **brachium of the inferior colliculus** (Figure 7–7A). As different as the superior and inferior colliculi are, so too are their brachia. The brachium of the superior colliculus brings afferent information to the superior colliculus, whereas that of the inferior colliculus is an efferent pathway carrying axons away from the inferior colliculus to the medial geniculate nucleus (see next section).

The Medial Geniculate Nucleus Contains a Division That Is Tonotopically Organized

The medial geniculate nucleus is the thalamic auditory relay nucleus. It is located on the inferior surface of the thalamus, medial to the thalamic visual relay nucleus, the lateral geniculate nucleus, and rostral to the superior colliculus (Figure 7–7A). The spatial relationships between the medial and lateral geniculate nuclei and the superior colliculus can be further appreciated by comparing the dorsal view of the brain stem (Figure 7–7A) with coronal and transverse sections through the rostral midbrain and diencephalon (Figures 7–9A and 7–9B). The medial geniculate nucleus is interposed between the lateral geniculate nucleus and the main portion of the ventral thalamus.

The medial geniculate nucleus is composed of several divisions. The principal auditory relay nucleus is the ventral division of the medial geniculate nucleus (Figures 7–7B1 and 7–9). This component, often referred to simply as the medial geniculate nucleus, is the only portion that is tonotopically organized. It receives the major ascending auditory projection from the **central nucleus of the inferior colliculus**, which also is tonotopically organized.

across a
produc
cessing
primary
the ton
medial
domina

Th
to be su
cortex. (
as we s
a high-i
in the p
sensitiv
neurons
olivary
to the is
may no
ize sour

*Interpre
of the H*

Th
and 22)
lateral :
areas ai
only the
primary

Ou
human
anatomi
hemispl
nation p
left side
anatomi
importa
hemispl

Lo
and exte
tempora
importa
tempora
preting
in a per
motor s
associati
courses
This pat
pretatioi
(Broca's
spondin
gyrus (s

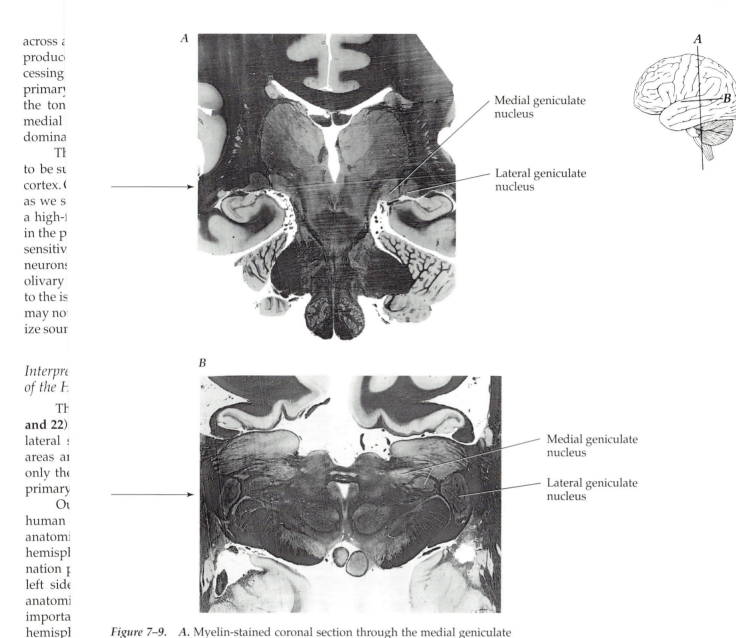

Figure 7–9. **A.** Myelin-stained coronal section through the medial geniculate nucleus. Arrow indicates level of section in part **B. B.** Transverse section through the midbrain–diencephalic juncture. Arrow shows level of section in part **A.** The inset shows the planes of section.

Although not observable on the myelin-stained sections, the ventral division of the medial geniculate nucleus is laminated, similar to the central nucleus of the inferior colliculus. For both structures, individual laminae contain neurons that are maximally sensitive to similar frequencies. In contrast, the other divisions of the medial geniculate nucleus (dorsal and medial) are organized in a different way. These divisions receive their major inputs from all of the divisions of the inferior colliculus, including the parts that are not tonotopically organized. They also receive somatic sensory and visual information and seem to serve more integrated functions, such as participating in arousal mechanisms. Moreover, these divisions of the medial geniculate nucleus are not laminated.

Summary

■ **AUDITORY SYSTEM**

Peripheral Auditory Apparatus

The auditory transductive apparatus, the **organ of Corti**, is located in the **cochlea**, a coiled structure within the temporal bone (Figure 7–3). The **hair cells** (Figure 7–3C) are the auditory receptors. They are organized into a sheet within the cochlea. This receptive sheet has a precise **tonotopic organization**: receptors sensitive to high frequencies are located near the cochlear base and those sensitive to low frequencies, near the apex. The hair cells are innervated by the peripheral processes of **bipolar cells**, whose cell bodies are located in the **spiral ganglion**. The central processes of the bipolar cells collect into the **cochlear division** of the **vestibulo-cochlear (eighth cranial) nerve** (Figure 7–1).

Medulla and Pons

Vestibulocochlear nerve fibers synapse in the **cochlear nuclei**. The cochlear nuclei (Figure 7–4B), which are located in the **rostral medulla**, have three main divisions: (1) the **dorsal cochlear nucleus**, (2) the **anteroventral cochlear nucleus**, and (3) **posteroventral cochlear nucleus**. Most of the neurons in the dorsal and posteroventral cochlear nuclei (Figure 7–4B) give rise to axons that decussate (Figure 7–5) and then ascend in the **lateral lemniscus** (Figures 7–4C and 7–6) to terminate in the **inferior colliculus** (Figures 7–7 and 7–8).

Many neurons in the anteroventral cochlear nucleus project to the **superior olivary complex** in the pons (Figures 7–4C and 7–5), on either the ipsilateral or the contralateral side (Figure 7–5). Neurons in the superior olivary complex project to either the ipsilateral or the contralateral inferior colliculus via the lateral lemniscus. Certain of these decussating axons form a discrete commissure, the **trapezoid body** (Figures 7–5 and 7–4C). The function of this pathway is in localizing sounds.

Midbrain and Thalamus

The inferior colliculus (Figures 7–7 and 7–8) contains three main nuclei. The **central nucleus** (1), the principal auditory relay nucleus in the inferior colliculus, is **laminated** and has a **precise tonotopic organization**. It projects to the **laminated portion** of the medial geniculate nucleus (Figure 7–9), which in turn projects to the **primary auditory cortex** (cytoarchitectonic area 41) (Figure 7–10). The **external nucleus** (2) and the **dorsal cortex** (3) of the inferior colliculus project to the **nonlaminated** portions of the medial geniculate nucleus, which in turn projects to **higher-order auditory areas** (Figure 7–10).

Cerebral Cortex

The primary auditory cortex is located largely on the superior surface of the temporal lobe, in **Heschl's gyri** (Figure 7–10). The higher-order auditory areas encircle the primary area (Figure 7–10). The temporal lobes on the right and left cerebral hemispheres are not symmetrical. The higher-

A

Summary

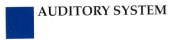

AUDITORY SYSTEM

Peripheral Auditory Apparatus

The auditory transductive apparatus, the **organ of Corti**, is located in the **cochlea**, a coiled structure within the temporal bone (Figure 7–3). The **hair cells** (Figure 7–3C) are the auditory receptors. They are organized into a sheet within the cochlea. This receptive sheet has a precise **tonotopic organization**: receptors sensitive to high frequencies are located near the cochlear base and those sensitive to low frequencies, near the apex. The hair cells are innervated by the peripheral processes of **bipolar cells**, whose cell bodies are located in the **spiral ganglion**. The central processes of the bipolar cells collect into the **cochlear division** of the **vestibulocochlear (eighth cranial) nerve** (Figure 7–1).

Medulla and Pons

Vestibulocochlear nerve fibers synapse in the **cochlear nuclei**. The cochlear nuclei (Figure 7–4B), which are located in the **rostral medulla**, have three main divisions: (1) the **dorsal cochlear nucleus**, (2) the **anteroventral cochlear nucleus**, and (3) **posteroventral cochlear nucleus**. Most of the neurons in the dorsal and posteroventral cochlear nuclei (Figure 7–4B) give rise to axons that decussate (Figure 7–5) and then ascend in the **lateral lemniscus** (Figures 7–4C and 7–6) to terminate in the **inferior colliculus** (Figures 7–7 and 7–8).

Many neurons in the anteroventral cochlear nucleus project to the **superior olivary complex** in the pons (Figures 7–4C and 7–5), on either the ipsilateral or the contralateral side (Figure 7–5). Neurons in the superior olivary complex project to either the ipsilateral or the contralateral inferior colliculus via the lateral lemniscus. Certain of these decussating axons form a discrete commissure, the **trapezoid body** (Figures 7–5 and 7–4C). The function of this pathway is in localizing sounds.

Midbrain and Thalamus

The inferior colliculus (Figures 7–7 and 7–8) contains three main nuclei. The **central nucleus** (1), the principal auditory relay nucleus in the inferior colliculus, is **laminated** and has a **precise tonotopic organization**. It projects to the **laminated portion** of the medial geniculate nucleus (Figure 7–9), which in turn projects to the **primary auditory cortex** (cytoarchitectonic area 41) (Figure 7–10). The **external nucleus** (2) and the **dorsal cortex** (3) of the inferior colliculus project to the **nonlaminated** portions of the medial geniculate nucleus, which in turn projects to **higher-order auditory areas** (Figure 7–10).

Cerebral Cortex

The primary auditory cortex is located largely on the superior surface of the temporal lobe, in **Heschl's gyri** (Figure 7–10). The higher-order auditory areas encircle the primary area (Figure 7–10). The temporal lobes on the right and left cerebral hemispheres are not symmetrical. The higher-

across all six layers in a strip of cortex, the **isofrequency columns**. A tone produces motion of a discrete point on the basilar membrane and, by processing in the ascending auditory path, activates a strip of neurons in the primary auditory cortex. The anatomical basis of the isofrequency strips is the tonotopically organized projection from the ventral division of the medial geniculate nucleus. This is a dense projection and is directed predominantly to layers 3 and 4.

The cortical representation of other attributes of sound are thought to be superimposed on the tonotopic organization of the primary auditory cortex. One important attribute is the **interaural intensity difference**, which, as we saw earlier, is the major cue for detecting the horizontal location of a high-frequency sound. Within the representation of high-frequency tones in the primary auditory cortex are **binaural columns**, in which neurons are sensitive to similar interaural intensity differences. The properties of these neurons are remarkably similar to those of neurons in the lateral superior olivary nucleus. Aggregates of binaural columns are oriented at right angles to the isofrequency strips. Although a lesion of the primary auditory cortex may not produce a unilateral hearing loss, it does impair the ability to localize sounds originating from auditory space contralateral to the lesion.

Interpretation of Speech Is One Function of the Higher-order Auditory Cortex

The higher-order auditory cortical areas (**cytoarchitectonic areas 42 and 22**) partially encircle the primary auditory cortex on the superior and lateral surfaces of the temporal lobe (Figure 7–10). These higher-order areas are distinguished morphologically from the primary area because only the primary area has a prominent layer 4, a characteristic feature of primary sensory areas (see Figure 3–16).

Our knowledge of how the auditory cortical areas are organized in human beings has provided insight into general principles governing the anatomical substrates of higher brain function. Although the two cerebral hemispheres appear to have a symmetrical gross anatomy, closer examination proves otherwise. The lateral sulcus, for example, is longer on the left side of the cerebral hemisphere than on the right side. This gross anatomical difference in the two cerebral hemispheres is paralleled by important functional differences. In most human brains, the left cerebral hemisphere is specialized for **linguistic function**.

Located within the caudal portion of the lateral sulcus on the left side and extending onto the lateral surface of the hemisphere on the **superior temporal gyrus**, is **Wernicke's area** (cytoarchitectonic area 22), which is important in **interpretive** (i.e., **sensory**) **speech mechanisms**. In the right temporal lobe, this area is a higher-order auditory area involved in interpreting the emotional content of language, for instance, noting the anger in a person's voice. An important projection of Wernicke's area is to the motor speech area, **Broca's area**, in the frontal lobe via a corticocortical association pathway called the **arcuate fasciculus**. The arcuate fasciculus courses in the white matter of the temporal, parietal, and frontal lobes. This pathway provides the connection between the cortical locus for interpretation of spoken language (Wernicke's area) and the motor speech area (Broca's area). Broca's area is located on the frontal operculum, corresponding approximately to cytoarchitectonic area 44 of the inferior frontal gyrus (see Figures 3–16 and AI–1].

The Auditory Cortical Areas Are Located on the Superior Surface of the Temporal Lobe

We can distinguish two parallel thalamocortical projections from the medial geniculate to the temporal lobe. One path is a tonotopically organized projection from the ventral division to the primary auditory cortex in Heschl's gyri. The other projection has a more complicated organization. It originates from the other divisions of the medial geniculate nucleus and is directed to the secondary auditory areas that surround the primary cortex. The thalamocortical auditory projections are termed the **auditory radiations**. The thalamocortical fibers course laterally from the medial geniculate nucleus and beneath the lenticular nucleus, in the **sublenticular** portion of the internal capsule (see Figure 11–7). (The projection of the lateral geniculate nucleus to the visual cortex, the optic radiations, courses in the retrolenticular portion of the internal capsule.)

The Primary Auditory Cortex Has a Tonotopic Organization

The primary auditory cortex (area 41) is located on two gyri within the lateral sulcus in the temporal lobe, **Heschl's gyri** (Figure 7–10). These gyri run from the lateral surface of the cortex medially to the insular region. The orientation of Heschl's gyri are approximately orthogonal to the superior, middle, and inferior gyri on the lateral surface of the temporal lobe. The primary auditory cortex, which corresponds to cytoarchitectonic area 41, is cytoarchitectually distinct from surrounding cortical auditory areas. The primary auditory cortex, similar to other areas of the cerebral cortex, has a columnar organization. In the primary auditory cortex, neurons that are sensitive to tones of similar frequencies are arranged

Figure 7–10. The locations of the primary and higher-order auditory cortical areas are shown on the lateral cerebral hemisphere view *(A)* and in a schematic horizontal cut through the cerebral hemisphere *(B)*. The primary auditory cortex corresponds approximately to the dark blue region; the higher-order auditory areas are shown in light blue. Wernicke's area is located caudal to the primary auditory cortex on the left side in most individuals. The plane of section for the cut illustrated in *B* is indicated by the arrows in *A*. The vestibular cortex is shown in *A*. It is located at the intersection of the postcentral and intraparietal sulci. (*B*, Adapted from Geschwind, N., and Levitsky, W. 1968. Human brain: Left–right asymmetries in temporal speech region. Science 161:186–187.)

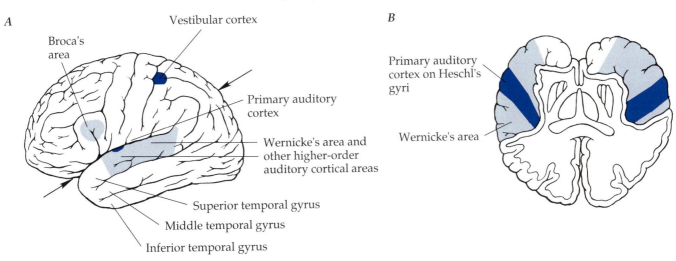

A

Broca's area

Vestibular cortex

Primary auditory cortex

Wernicke's area and other higher-order auditory cortical areas

Superior temporal gyrus

Middle temporal gyrus

Inferior temporal gyrus

B

Primary auditory cortex on Heschl's gyri

Wernicke's area

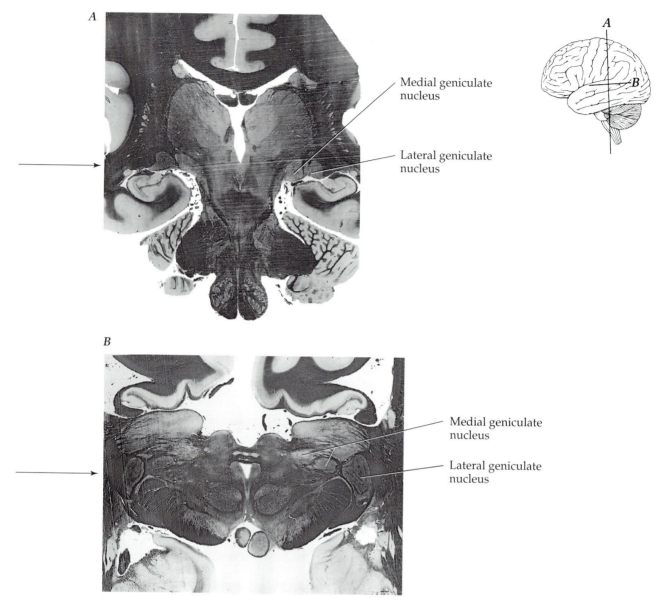

Figure 7–9. **A.** Myelin-stained coronal section through the medial geniculate nucleus. Arrow indicates level of section in part **B. B.** Transverse section through the midbrain–diencephalic juncture. Arrow shows level of section in part **A.** The inset shows the planes of section.

Although not observable on the myelin-stained sections, the ventral division of the medial geniculate nucleus is laminated, similar to the central nucleus of the inferior colliculus. For both structures, individual laminae contain neurons that are maximally sensitive to similar frequencies. In contrast, the other divisions of the medial geniculate nucleus (dorsal and medial) are organized in a different way. These divisions receive their major inputs from all of the divisions of the inferior colliculus, including the parts that are not tonotopically organized. They also receive somatic sensory and visual information and seem to serve more integrated functions, such as participating in arousal mechanisms. Moreover, these divisions of the medial geniculate nucleus are not laminated.

order auditory cortex located caudal to the primary auditory cortex of the left hemisphere is **Wernicke's area** (Figure 7–10), which is specialized for the interpretation of language.

VESTIBULAR SYSTEM

Peripheral Vestibular Sensory Organs

The vestibular sensory organs includes the **semicircular canals**, **utricle**, and **saccule** (Figure 7–3). Receptor cells, located in specialized regions of the vestibular apparatus, are innervated by the distal processes of bipolar neurons located in **Scarpa's ganglion**. The central processes of these bipolar neurons form the **vestibular division** of the eighth cranial nerve (Figure 7–3A). These fibers terminate in the vestibular nuclei, located beneath the floor of the fourth ventricle in the rostral medulla and caudal pons (Figure 7–2).

Vestibular Nuclei and Ascending Vestibular Projection

There are four separate nuclei: (1) **inferior vestibular nucleus**, (2) **medial vestibular nucleus**, (3) **lateral vestibular nucleus**, and (4) **superior vestibular nucleus** (Figure 7–2A and 7–4A, B). Most of the efferent projections of the vestibular nuclei form major motor pathways for controlling axial, limb, and extraocular muscles (Figure 7–2B). The ascending "sensory" pathway from the vestibular nuclei terminates in a portion of the **ventral posterior nucleus**, which, in turn, projects to the parietal lobe. The **vestibular cortex** is located caudal to the primary somatic sensory cortex, in cytoarchitectonic area 5 (Figure 7–10A; see Figure 5–18). This pathway may be important in the perception of vestibular information. ■

KEY STRUCTURES AND TERMS

tonotopic organization
tympanic membrane
middle ear ossicles
    malleus
    incus
    stapes
membranous labyrinth
bony labyrinth
vestibular labyrinth
    semicircular canals
    utricle
    saccule
vestibular ganglion
vestibular division of the eighth
        cranial nerve
vestibular nuclei
cochlea
    scala vestibuli
    scala media

scala tympani
organ of Corti
basilar membrane
tectorial membrane
inner hair cells
outer hair cells
spiral ganglion
vestibulocochlear (eighth cranial)
        nerve
cochlear nuclei
    anteroventral
    dorsal
    posteroventral
superior olivary complex
trapezoid body
olivocochlear projection
lateral lemniscus
inferior colliculus
    external nucleus

dorsal cortex
central nucleus of the inferior
    colliculus
brachium of the inferior colliculus
medial geniculate nucleus
auditory radiations
    sublenticular portion of the
        internal capsule
Heschl's gyri (area 41)
    isofrequency columns
    interaural intensity difference
    binaural columns
higher-order cortical auditory areas
    (areas 42 and 22)
    Wernicke's area
    arcuate fasciculus
    superior temporal gyrus

standard

Selected Readings

Aitkin, L. M., Irvine, D. R. F., and Webster, W. R. 1984. Central neural mechanisms of hearing. In Darian-Smith, I. (ed.), Handbook of Physiology, Section 1: The Nervous System, Vol. III. Sensory Processes. Bethesda, Md.: American Physiological Society, pp. 675–737.

Dallos, P. 1984. Peripheral mechanisms of hearing. In Darian-Smith, I. (ed.), Handbook of Physiology, Section 1: The Nervous System, Vol. III. Sensory Processes. Bethesda, Md.: American Physiological Society, pp. 595–637.

Fredrickson, J. M., and Rubin, A. M. 1984. Vestibular cortex. In Jones, E. G., and Peters, A. (eds.), Cerebral Cortex. Vol. 5. Sensory-Motor Areas and Aspects of Cortical Connectivity. New York: Plenum Press, pp. 99–111.

Imig, T. H., and Morel, A. 1983. Organization of the thalamocortical auditory system in the cat. Ann. Rev. Neurosci. 6:95–120.

Morest, D. K. 1993. The cellular basis for signal processing in the mammalian cochlear nuclei. In Merchán, M. A. (ed.), The Mammalian Cochlear Nuclei: Organization and Function. New York: Plenum Press, pp. 1–18.

Ojemann, G. A. 1991. Cortical organization of language. J. Neurosci. 11:2281–2287.

References

Brugge, J. F. 1994. An overview of central auditory processing. In Popper, A. N., and Fay, R. R. (eds.), The Mammalian Auditory Pathway: Neurophysiology. New York: Springer-Verlag, pp. 1–33.

Economo, C. von, and Horn, J. 1930. Über Windungsrelief, Masse und Rinderarchitektonik der Supratemporalfläche, ihre Individuellen und ihre Seitenunterschiede. Z. ges Neurol. Psychiat. 130:678–757.

Geniec, P., and Morest, D. K. 1971. The neuronal architecture of the human posterior colliculus. Acta Oto-Laryngologia. Suppl. 295:1–33.

Geschwind, N., and Levitsky, W. 1968. Human brain: Left–right asymmetries in temporal speech region. Science 161:186–187.

Imig, T. J., Ruggero, M. A., Kitzes, L. M., et al. 1977. Organization of auditory cortex in the owl monkey (Aotus Trivirgatus). J. Comp. Neurol. 171:111–128.

Kelly, J. P. 1991. Hearing. In Kandel, E. R., Schwartz, J. H., and Jessell, T. M. (eds.), Principles of Neural Science, 3rd ed. New York: Elsevier, pp. 481–499.

Kelly, J. P. 1991. The sense of balance. In Kandel, E. R., Schwartz, J. H., and Jessell, T. M. (eds.), Principles of Neural Science, 3rd ed. New York: Elsevier, pp. 500–511.

Merzenich, M. M., and Brugge, J. F. 1973. Representation of the cochlear partition on the superior temporal plane of the macaque monkey. Brain Res. 50:275–296.

Moore, J. K., and Osen, K. K. 1979. The human cochlear nuclei. In Creutzfeldt, O., Scheich, H., and Schreiner, C. (eds.), Hearing Mechanisms and Speech. Berlin: Springer-Verlag, pp. 36–44.

Roth, G. L., Aitkin, L. M., Andersen, R. A., et al. 1978. Some features of the spatial organization of the central nucleus of the inferior colliculus of the cat. J. Comp. Neurol. 182:661–680.

Schwartz, I. R. 1992. The superior olivary complex and lateral lemniscal nuclei. In Webster, D. B., Popper, A. N., and Fay, R. R. (eds.), The Mammalian Auditory Pathway: Neuroanatomy. New York: Springer-Verlag, pp. 117-167.

Strominger, N. L., Nelson, L. R., and Dougherty, W. J. 1977. Second order auditory pathways in the chimpanzee. J. Comp. Neurol. 172:349–366.

Webster, D. B. 1992. An overview of mammalian auditory pathways with an emphasis on humans. In Webster, D. B., Popper, A. N., and Fay, R. R. (eds.), The Mammalian Auditory Pathway: Neuroanatomy. New York: Springer-Verlag, pp. 1–22.

8

The Gustatory, Visceral Afferent, and Olfactory Systems

TASTE AND SMELL ARE CHEMICAL SENSES. The neural systems that mediate these sensations, the gustatory and olfactory systems, are among the phylogenetically oldest systems of the brain. In perceiving chemicals in the oral and nasal cavities, the gustatory and olfactory systems work jointly. For example, even though the gustatory system is concerned with the four primary taste sensations—sweet, sour, salty, and bitter—the perception of richer and more complex flavors such as those present in wine is dependent on a properly functioning sense of smell. Damage to the olfactory system, as a result of head trauma, or even the common cold, which impairs conduction of air-borne molecules in the nasal passages, can dull our perception of flavor even though the basic taste sensations of sweet, sour, salty, and bitter are preserved.

When we eat our food, we perceive the sensory messages that the gustatory and olfactory systems provide. Yet when food and drinks are swallowed from the mouth into the esophagus and then the stomach, most chemical perceptions typically are lost. In fact, we are not consciously aware of most chemical and many other stimuli that are present within our body despite the fact that our internal organs are richly innervated by primary sensory neurons. Sensory messages from internal organs do, however, signal important ongoing events that are key to controlling essential body functions. These functions include maintaining blood glucose levels, regulating heart rate, and adjusting respiration in relation to the oxygen demands of the body. We become conscious of some of these events only under special circumstances, such as when we become nauseated after eating a certain food or when we feel "full" after eating a large meal. Some internal stimuli, however, are never perceived. A change in intra-arterial pressure, even a hypertensive episode, can proceed unnoticed. Most sensory information from the viscera does not reach consciousness.

Although taste and smell work jointly and share similarities in their neural substrates, the anatomical organization of these systems is different enough to be considered separately. The central projections of the primary sensory neurons that innervate the gut, the cardiovascular system, and the lungs—which mediate both regulation of body organs and visceral sensations—are similar to those for taste. For these reasons, we first examine the gustatory and visceral afferent systems together and then consider the olfactory system.

■ THE GUSTATORY AND VISCERAL AFFERENT SYSTEMS

Taste is mediated by the **facial** (seventh cranial), **glossopharyngeal** (ninth cranial), and **vagus** (tenth cranial) **nerves**. The glossopharyngeal and vagus nerves also mediate much of the afferent innervation of the gut, cardiovascular system, and lungs. This visceral afferent innervation provides the central nervous system with information about the internal state of the body, for example, blood oxygen content. As we saw in Chapter 2, both taste and visceral afferent information are **visceral afferent** modalities. Taste is distinguished as a special modality because it is mediated by specialized cranial receptor organs, the taste buds.

There Are Separate Gustatory and Visceral Afferent Ascending Pathways

Taste receptor cells are clustered in the **taste buds**, located on the tongue and at various intraoral sites (soft palate, pharynx, epiglottis, and larynx). Taste receptor cells are innervated by the distal branches of the primary afferent fibers in the facial, glossopharyngeal, and vagus nerves (Figure 8–1B). These afferent fibers have a pseudounipolar morphology, similar to that of the dorsal root ganglion neurons. In contrast to the nerves of the skin and mucous membranes, where generally the **terminal portion** of the pseudounipolar afferent fiber is sensitive to stimulus energy, gustatory receptor cells are separate from the primary afferent fibers. For taste, the role of the primary afferent fiber is simply to transmit sensory information to the central nervous system (Figures 8–1B and 8–2A). For touch, the role of the primary afferent fiber is both to transduce stimulus energy and transmit information to the central nervous system.

The central branches of the afferent fibers, after entering the brain stem, collect into the **solitary tract** of the dorsal medulla. This tract is surrounded by the **solitary nucleus**, in which the afferent fibers terminate. The solitary nucleus is divided into two functionally distinct parts (Figure 8–1A): a rostral **gustatory nucleus** and a caudal **cardiorespiratory nucleus**. The gustatory nucleus, the medullary origin of the path for taste perception, is where gustatory afferent fibers synapse. The axons of second-order neurons in this nucleus ascend **ipsilaterally** in the brain stem, in the **central tegmental tract**, and terminate in the most **medial portion of the ventral posterior medial nucleus**, in the **parvocellular** division (Figure 8–1A, B). From the thalamus, third-order neurons project to the **frontal operculum and the anterior portion of the insular cortex**, where the gustatory cortical areas are located. This pathway is thought to mediate the **discriminative aspects of taste**, which enable us to distinguish one quality from another.

The caudal solitary, or **cardiorespiratory, nucleus** is critically involved in regulating body functions in relation to afferent information from visceral receptors. It plays a role in transmitting information to the cortex for conscious sensory experiences arising from these receptors. Most important among its visceral regulatory tasks is controlling blood pressure and respiration rate. Visceral afferents from the gut also synapse in the caudal solitary nucleus for regulating gastrointestinal motility and secretions.

Neurons in the cardiorespiratory nucleus have three kinds of projections for controlling body functions (Figure 8–1C):

- **Local projections** in the medulla and pons participate in the reflex control of respiration, and basic cardiovascular function.

- **Descending projections** contact autonomic neurons in the thoracic, lumbar, and sacral spinal cord.

- **Ascending projections,** via the parabrachial nucleus of the pons, transmit afferent information from the viscera to the amygdala, hypothalamus, and other sites for regulating visceral functions and food intake.

What are the connections that mediate conscious visceral sensations? A candidate set of connections consists of the pathway from the parabrachial nucleus to the thalamus and then to the insular cortex. Studies in animals have shown that these thalamic and cortical areas receiving afferent information from the viscera are distinct from the gustatory areas.

Although taste and visceral afferent information are distinct, as are their central pathways, the two modalities do interact. In fact, linking information about the taste of a food and its effect on body functions upon ingestion is key to an individual's survival. One of the most robust forms of learning, called **conditioned taste aversion**, associates the taste of tainted food with the nausea that it causes when eaten. Another name for this learning is "bait shyness," referring to a method used by ranchers to discourage predators from attacking their livestock. In this technique, ranchers contaminate livestock meat with an emetic, such as lithium chloride, which causes nausea and vomiting after ingestion. Coyotes, after eating the bait, develop an aversion for the contaminated meat and will not attack the stock. Unfortunately, some of us also have experienced a phenomenon related to conditioned taste aversion; perhaps we became nauseated and vomited, for example, because of flu. Although the food we ate was not tainted or spoiled, we nevertheless may develop an intense aversion to it. Experimental studies in rats have shown that such interactions between the gustatory and viscerosensory systems, leading to conditioned taste aversion, may occur in the insular cortex.

In the next three sections, we consider in detail the regional anatomy of the gustatory and visceral afferent systems, beginning in the periphery.

■ REGIONAL ANATOMY

Branches of the Facial, Glossopharyngeal, and Vagus Nerves Innervate Different Parts of the Oral Cavity

Gustatory receptor cells are epithelial cells that transduce soluble chemical stimuli into neural signals. They are present in complex sensory organs, called **taste buds** (Figure 8–2A). In addition to the **receptor cells**, taste buds contain two additional types of cells: **basal cells**, which may differentiate to become receptor cells, and **support cells** (Figure 8–2A), which may provide structural or trophic support. Receptor cells have a synaptic contact with the distal processes of primary afferent fibers (Figure 8–2A).

A

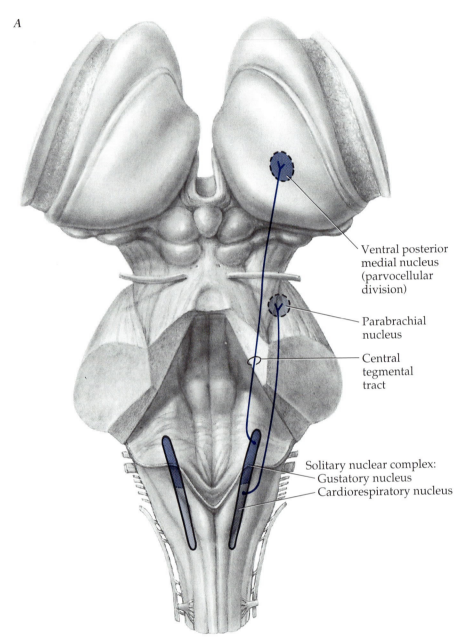

Figure 8–1. General organization of the gustatory and viscerosensory systems. *A.* Dorsal view of brain stem illustrating the location of the solitary nucleus and the differential projections of the rostral or gustatory and caudal or cardiorespiratory divisions. *B.* Ascending gustatory pathway. *C.* Ascending viscerosensory pathway. (*A,* Adapted from Beckstead, R. M., Morse, J. R., and Norgren, R. 1980. The nucleus of the solitary tract in the monkey: Projections to the thalamus and brain stem nuclei. J. Comp. Neurol. 190:259–282.)

Taste buds are present on the tongue, the soft palate, epiglottis, pharynx, and larynx. Taste buds on the tongue are clustered on papillae (Figure 8–2B), whereas those at the other sites are located in pseudostratified columnar epithelium or stratified squamous epithelium rather than distinct papillae. Taste receptor cells that are located on the **anterior two thirds of the tongue** are innervated by the **chorda tympani** nerve, a

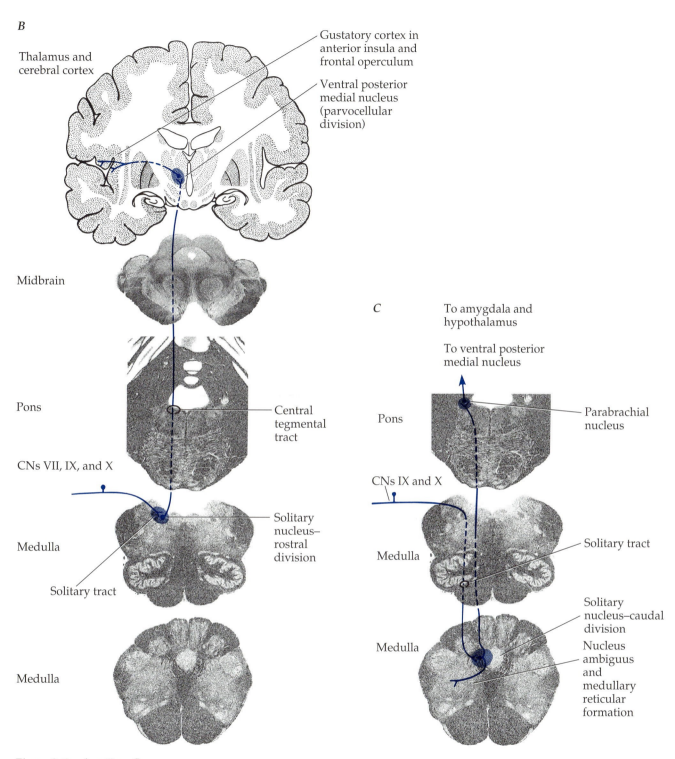

B

Thalamus and cerebral cortex

Gustatory cortex in anterior insula and frontal operculum

Ventral posterior medial nucleus (parvocellular division)

Midbrain

C

To amygdala and hypothalamus

To ventral posterior medial nucleus

Pons

Central tegmental tract

Pons

Parabrachial nucleus

CNs VII, IX, and X

CNs IX and X

Solitary nucleus–rostral division

Medulla

Solitary tract

Medulla

Solitary tract

Solitary nucleus–caudal division

Medulla

Medulla

Nucleus ambiguus and medullary reticular formation

Figure 8–1.   (continued)

branch of the facial nerve. (The facial nerve consists of two separate roots [Figure 8–3], a motor root commonly known as the **facial nerve** and a combined sensory and autonomic root called the **intermediate nerve**.) These anterior taste buds are clustered in the fungiform and foliate papillae (Figure 8–2B).

A

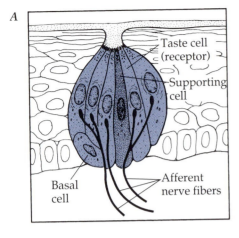

Taste cell
(receptor)

Supporting
cell

Basal
cell

Afferent
nerve fibers

B

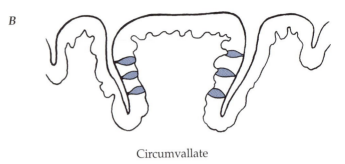

Circumvallate

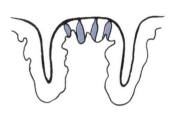

Foliate

Fungiform

Figure 8–2. Taste buds *(A)* consist of taste receptor cells, supporting cells, and basal cells (not shown). The three types of papillae are shown in *B*, circumvallate, foliate, and fungiform. Taste buds in papillae are shown in blue.

Taste buds on the **posterior third of the tongue** (Figure 8–3), which are located primarily in the circumvallate and foliate papillae, are supplied by the **glossopharyngeal (ninth cranial) nerve.** Taste buds are also located on the palate and are innervated by a branch of the seventh cranial nerve. Taste buds on the epiglottis and larynx are innervated by the vagus (tenth cranial) nerve, whereas those on the pharynx are innervated by the glossopharyngeal nerve.

The viscera are served by the glossopharyngeal and vagus nerves, which project to brain stem nuclei, as well as by branches of spinal nerves, which synapse on neurons in the dorsal horn. Here we focus on the cranial nerve innervation of the viscera. In addition to gustatory afferents, the glossopharyngeal and vagus nerves have other visceral afferent fibers that innervate arterial blood pressure receptors (baroreceptors) in the **carotid sinus** and **aortic arch.** The vagus nerve also innervates respiratory structures and the portion of the gut rostral to the splenic flexure (general visceral afferent innervation). Visceral afferent fibers are pseudounipolar neurons, similar to the primary afferent fibers that innervate the skin, muscle, and mucous membranes (see Figure 12–2).

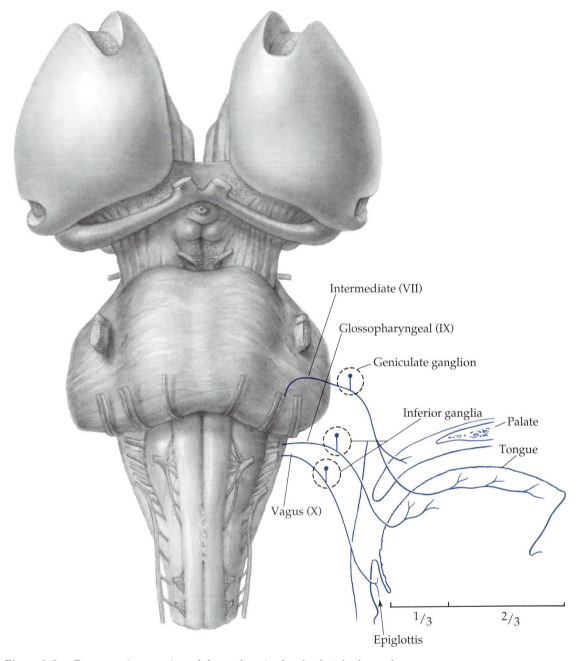

Intermediate (VII)

Glossopharyngeal (IX)

Geniculate ganglion

Inferior ganglia

Palate

Tongue

Vagus (X)

$^1/_3$ $^2/_3$

Epiglottis

Figure 8–3. Gustatory innervation of the oral cavity by the facial, glossopharyngeal, and vagus nerves. In the periphery, the chorda tympani nerve (CN VII) supplies taste buds on the anterior two-thirds of the tongue, lingual branches of the glossopharyngeal nerve (CN IX), taste buds on the posterior third, and the superior laryngeal nerve (CN X), taste buds on the epiglottis. The greater petrosal nerve (CN VII) supplies taste buds on the palate.

The cell bodies of the afferent fibers in the facial, glossopharyngeal, and vagus nerves are located in separate peripheral sensory ganglia. The cell bodies of afferent fibers in the intermediate branch of the facial nerve are found in the **geniculate ganglion**. Those of the vagus and glossopharyngeal nerves are located in their respective **inferior ganglia**. (We also call the inferior ganglion of the glossopharyngeal nerve the petrosal ganglion and the inferior ganglion to the vagus nerve, the nodose ganglion.) The glossopharyngeal and vagus nerves also contain afferent fibers that innervate **cranial skin and mucous membranes**; we find the cell bodies of these afferent fibers in ganglia separate from those innervating the viscera. This modality will be discussed in Chapter 12, along with the trigeminal nerve.

The afferent fibers of the intermediate branch of the facial nerve enter the brain stem at the **pontomedullary junction**, immediately lateral to the root that contains somatic motor axons (Figure 8–3). The gustatory and visceral afferent fibers of the glossopharyngeal and vagus nerves enter the brain stem in the rostral medulla.

The Solitary Nucleus Is the First Central Nervous System Relay For Taste and Visceral Afferent Information

Gustatory fibers innervating the taste buds enter the brain stem and collect in the **solitary tract**, located in the dorsal medulla. The axons of the facial nerve enter the tract rostral to those of the glossopharyngeal and vagus nerves. After entering, however, the fibers send branches that ascend and descend within the tract, similar to the terminals of afferent fibers in Lissauer's tract of the spinal cord. The axon terminals leave the tract and synapse on neurons in the surrounding **solitary nucleus**. Second-order neurons in the gustatory nucleus (Figures 8–1A and 8–4) send their axons into the ipsilateral **central tegmental tract** (Figure 8–5) and ascend to the thalamus (see below). Note that the medial lemniscus, which carries the ascending somatic sensory projection from the dorsal column nuclei, is located ventral to the central tegmental tract at the levels shown in Figure 8–5.

The **cardiorespiratory nucleus** receives input from visceral receptors, both chemoreceptors, such as receptors sensitive to blood carbon dioxide, and mechanoreceptors, such as arterial pressure receptors. As we saw earlier, neurons in this nucleus have diverse projections which together mediate the reflex control of the cardiovascular, respiratory, and gastrointestinal systems. The descending spinal projections of the caudal solitary nucleus contact sympathetic preganglionic neurons in the **intermediolateral**

Figure 8–4. The gustatory component of the solitary nucleus is illustrated in this myelin-stained transverse section through the medulla. The inset shows the plane of section.

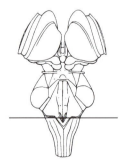

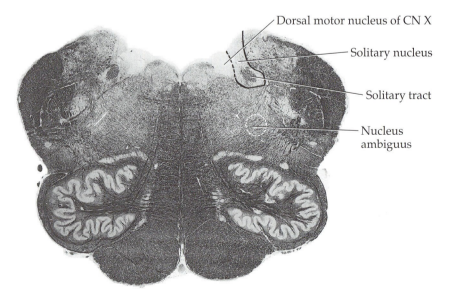

Dorsal motor nucleus of CN X

Solitary nucleus

Solitary tract

Nucleus ambiguus

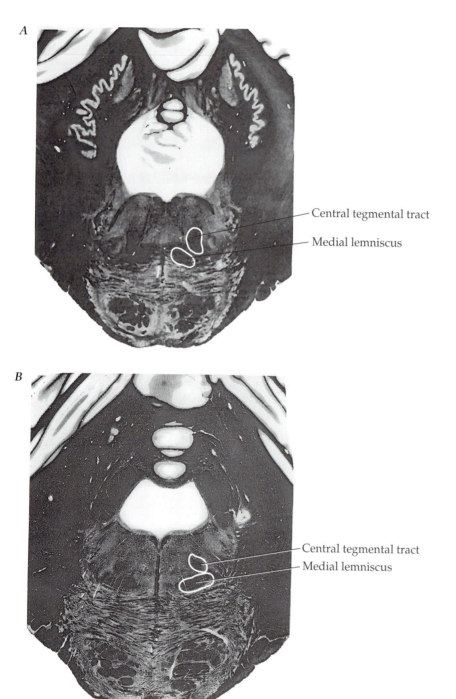

A

Central tegmental tract

Medial lemniscus

B

Central tegmental tract

Medial lemniscus

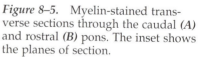

Figure 8–5. Myelin-stained transverse sections through the caudal *(A)* and rostral *(B)* pons. The inset shows the planes of section.

nucleus of the thoracic and lumbar spinal cord (see Chapter 14 and Figure 14–19). These projections mediate essential control of heart rate and blood pressure. The descending projections are either direct or via **adrenergic** neurons in the ventrolateral medulla. Projections of the neurons in the cardiorespiratory nucleus to the medullary preganglionic parasympathetic neurons are important in heart rate regulation and in controlling the motility and secretions of the gut. The caudal solitary nucleus also projects to parasympathetic preganglionic neurons and somatic motor neurons in the

nucleus ambiguus, which innervate pharyngeal and laryngeal muscles (see Chapter 13).

The ascending projections of the cardiorespiratory nucleus are focused on the **parabrachial nucleus** (Figure 8–1C; see AII–12). This nucleus is located in the pons adjacent to the principal output path of the cerebellum, the superior cerebellar peduncle (see Chapter 10). (Another name for the superior cerebellar peduncle is the brachium conjunctivum; hence the term parabrachial.) The parabrachial nucleus transmits visceral afferent information rostrally to the **hypothalamus** and the **amygdala** (see Figure 8–12B), two brain structures that are thought to participate in a variety of autonomic and endocrine functions, for example, feeding and reproductive behaviors (see Chapters 14 and 15). Thus, both the local connections of the caudal solitary nucleus as well as its ascending and descending projections are critically involved in integrating visceral afferent information and autonomic function.

The Parvocellular Portion of the Ventral Posterior Medial Nucleus Relays Gustatory Information to the Frontal Operculum and Anterior Insular Cortex

As with somatic sensation, vision, and hearing, there is a particular thalamic relay nucleus that receives gustatory information and projects this information to an area of the cerebral cortex. The ascending projection from the rostral solitary nucleus terminates in the **parvocellular division of the ventral posterior medial nucleus**. This nucleus has a characteristic pale appearance on myelin-stained sections (Figure 8–6). The axons of thalamocortical projection neurons in the thalamic gustatory nucleus project into the **posterior limb of the internal capsule** and ascend to the **frontal operculum and anterior insular cortex** (Figure 8–7).

Figure 8–6. A myelin-stained coronal section through the thalamic taste nucleus, the parvocellular portion of the ventral posterior medial nucleus. The medial dorsal nucleus is also shown on this section; a portion of this nucleus may play a role in olfactory perception. The inset shows the plane of section.

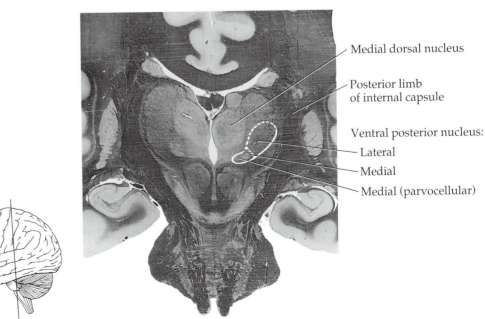

Medial dorsal nucleus

Posterior limb
of internal capsule

Ventral posterior nucleus:

Lateral

Medial

Medial (parvocellular)

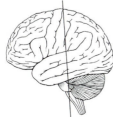

A

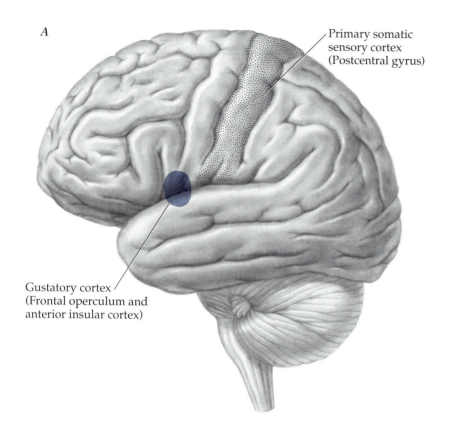

Primary somatic
sensory cortex
(Postcentral gyrus)

Gustatory cortex
(Frontal operculum and
anterior insular cortex)

B

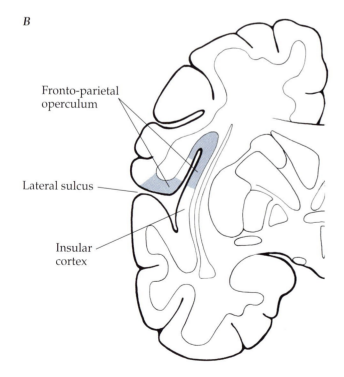

Fronto-parietal
operculum

Lateral sulcus

Insular
cortex

Figure 8–7. Cortical gustatory area.
A. Lateral view of human cerebral
hemisphere; the blue tinted field corresponds approximately to gustatory
areas. These areas, identified in the
rhesus monkey, are located entirely
beneath the cortical surface on the
frontal operculum and the anterior
insular cortex. The dotted area corresponds to primary somatic sensory
cortex. *B.* Schematic coronal section
through the anterior insular cortex
and frontoparietal operculum showing
the approximate locations of the gustatory areas.

A schematic coronal section through the cerebral hemisphere (Figure 8–7B), reveals the operculum of the frontal lobe overlying the insular cortex and the approximate locations of the cortical gustatory areas. Even though the sensory receptors mediating taste and touch on the tongue are intermingled, the cortical areas to which these sensory receptors project their information are distinct. The face areas of the primary and secondary somatic sensory cortical areas, where information from mechanoreceptors is relayed, is located on the cortical surface in the postcentral gyrus while the gustatory areas are located deep (Figure 8–7A). The presence of separate cortical areas for processing oral tactile and gustatory stimuli is a reflection of an important principle of cortical organization: **There is a separate cortical representation for each sensory modality.**

■ THE OLFACTORY SYSTEM

The sense of smell is a special visceral afferent modality mediated by the first cranial nerve, the **olfactory nerve**. There are two major differences between smell and the other sensory modalities. First, information about airborne chemicals impinging on the nasal mucosa is relayed to a part of the cerebral cortex without first relaying in the thalamus. The thalamic nucleus that processes olfactory information receives input from the cortical olfactory areas. Second, the cortical olfactory areas are phylogenetically older than the primary cortical regions that process other stimuli. The olfactory cortex is **allocortex**; the other sensory cortical areas are **isocortex** (see Chapter 3).

The Olfactory Projection to the Cerebral Cortex Does Not Relay in the Thalamus

We find primary olfactory neurons in the olfactory epithelium, a portion of the nasal cavity lining (Figure 8–8A). The primary olfactory neurons have a bipolar morphology (see Figure 12–2). The peripheral portion of the primary olfactory neuron is **chemosensitive**, and the central process is an **unmyelinated axon** that projects to the central nervous system. Recall that taste receptor cells, which transduce chemical stimuli on the tongue, and the primary taste fibers, which transmit information to the brain stem, are separate cells. The unmyelinated axons of the olfactory receptors collect into numerous small fascicles, which together form the **olfactory nerve**, the first cranial nerve. Olfactory nerve fascicles pass through foramina in a portion of the **ethmoid bone** termed the **cribriform plate** (Figure 8–8A) and synapse on second-order neurons in the **olfactory bulb** (Figures 8–8 and 8–10). Head trauma can shear off these delicate fascicles as they traverse the bone, resulting in **anosmia**, the inability to perceive odors.

The next link in the olfactory pathway is the projection of second-order neurons in the olfactory bulb through the **olfactory tract**, directly to numerous regions of the paleocortex on the ventral surface of the cerebral hemispheres. There are five separate areas of the cerebral hemisphere that receive a direct projection from the olfactory bulb (Figure 8–8B): (1) the **anterior olfactory nucleus**, which modulates information processing in the olfactory bulbs; (2) the **amygdala** and (3) the **olfactory tubercle**, which together are thought to be important in the emotional, endocrine, and visceral consequences of odors; (4) the adjacent **piriform and periamygdaloid cortex**, which may be important for olfactory perception; and (5)

A

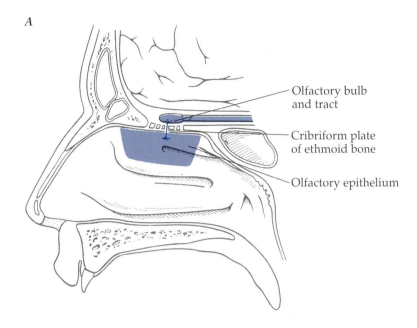

Olfactory bulb
and tract

Cribriform plate
of ethmoid bone

Olfactory epithelium

B

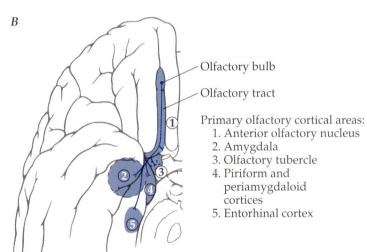

Olfactory bulb

Olfactory tract

Primary olfactory cortical areas:
1. Anterior olfactory nucleus
2. Amygdala
3. Olfactory tubercle
4. Piriform and
   periamygdaloid
   cortices
5. Entorhinal cortex

Figure 8–8. Olfactory pathway. *A.* Olfactory epithelium (blue) on the superior nasal concha. An olfactory receptor neuron is shown projecting from the olfactory epithelium to the olfactory bulb (blue). The nasal septum is not shown. *B.* Schematic of inferior surface of cerebral hemisphere illustrating the five main termination sites of olfactory tract fibers.

the **rostral entorhinal cortex**, which is thought to be important in olfactory memories.

The central projections of the olfactory bulb do not appear to have the precise topographic organization like that of other sensory systems. Recall, for example, the retinotopic organization of the visual system, present in both subcortical visual nuclei and in various visual cortical areas. In the following sections, we discuss first the peripheral components of the olfactory system and then the cortical olfactory areas.

■ REGIONAL ANATOMY

The Primary Olfactory Neurons Are Located in the Nasal Mucosa

Most of the lining of the nasal cavity is part of the respiratory epithelium, which warms and humidifies inspired air. The **olfactory mucosa** is a

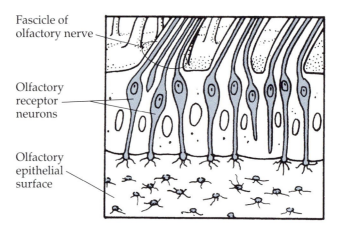

Fascicle of olfactory nerve

Olfactory receptor neurons

Olfactory epithelial surface

Figure 8–9. The primary olfactory neurons are shown in relation to the olfactory epithelium.

specialized portion of the nasal epithelial surface located on the superior nasal concha on each side as well as the midline septum and roof. There are approximately ten million olfactory receptor cells in the olfactory mucosa. Odorant molecules are carried into the olfactory mucosa with inhaled air.

These bipolar receptor neurons have an apical portion with hairlike structures (olfactory cilia) that contain the biochemical machinery for receiving chemical stimuli (Figure 8–9). In addition to the receptor cells, there are three other cell types in the olfactory mucosa: (1) **supporting cells**, which secrete mucus; (2) **microvillar cells**; and (3) **basal cells**, which are stem cells that differentiate into receptor cells.

The initial step in olfactory perception is the interaction of an odorant molecule with an **olfactory receptor,** a complex transmembrane protein located in the membrane of primary olfactory sensory neurons. Using molecular techniques, an important series of recent discoveries has shown that there are approximately 1000 different types of olfactory receptors, and that individual primary olfactory sensory neurons each contain **one olfactory receptor type or a small number of different receptor types.** It is thought that olfactory receptors and, as a consequence, primary olfactory neurons, recognize particular molecular characteristics of an odorant.

The Olfactory Bulb Is the First Central Nervous System Relay For Olfactory Input

The olfactory bulb (Figures 8–8, 8–10, and 8–11) is actually a part of the cerebral hemispheres. It develops as a small outpouching on the ventral surface of the telencephalon, rostral to the lamina terminalis (see Figure 2–15). The olfactory bulb is reduced in size in monkeys, apes, and humans. This is in contrast to many other components of the cerebral hemispheres, which reach their largest size in the brains of these species. Similar to most other components of the cerebral hemisphere, neurons in the olfactory bulb are organized into discrete laminae.

The central processes of olfactory receptor cells synapse on three types of neurons in the olfactory bulb (Figure 8–10A): on **mitral cells** and **tufted cells**, which are the two projection neurons of the olfactory bulb, and on interneurons called **periglomerular cells**. The terminals of the

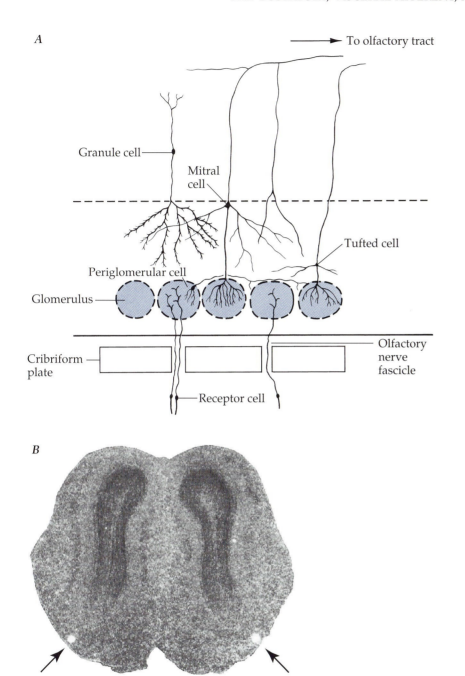

Figure 8–10. Projection of primary olfactory sensory neurons to the olfactory bulb. *A.* The axons of bipolar cells synapse on the projection neurons of the olfactory bulb, the mitral cells, and the tufted cells, as well as the periglomerular cells, a type of inhibitory interneuron. Also illustrated are the granule cells, another inhibitory interneuron. *B. In situ* hybridization of olfactory receptor mRNA in the axon terminals of primary olfactory sensory neurons in a single glomerulus in the olfactory bulb of the rat. The two bright spots on the ventral surface of the bulb (*arrows*) correspond to the two labelled glomeruli (*A.* Adapted from Shepard, G. M. 1972. Synaptic organization of the mammalian olfactory bulb. Physiol. Rev. 52:864–917. *B.* Vassar et al., 1994. Cell 79:981–991. Courtesy of Dr. Robert Vassar, Columbia University.)

olfactory receptor cells and the dendrites of mitral, tufted, and periglomerular cells form a morphological unit called the **glomerulus** (Figure 8–10), which may correspond to a functional unit (see Box 8–1). Within a glomerulus certain presynaptic and postsynaptic elements are ensheathed by **glial cells**. This sheath ensures specificity of action, limiting the spread of neurotransmitter released by the presynaptic terminal. While structures called glomeruli are located in other central nervous system locations, including the cerebellar cortex (see Chapter 10), those in the olfactory bulb are among the largest and most distinct.

Mitral and **tufted cells** are the projection neurons of the olfactory bulb. Their axons project from the olfactory bulb through the **olfactory tract** to the primary olfactory cortical areas (Figures 8–8B and 8–11).The periglomerular cell, which receives a direct input from the primary olfactory neurons, is an inhibitory interneuron. This neuron inhibits mitral cells in the same and adjacent glomeruli. Another inhibitory interneuron in the olfactory bulb is the granule cell (Figure 8–10A). This cell receives excitatory synaptic input from mitral cells to which it feeds back inhibition.

The Olfactory Bulb Projects to Structures on the Ventral Brain Surface Through the Olfactory Tract

The olfactory tract, together with the olfactory bulb, lies in the olfactory sulcus on the ventral surface of the frontal lobe (Figure 8–11). The gyrus rectus (or straight gyrus) is located medial to the olfactory bulb and tract (Figure 8–11). As the olfactory tract approaches the region where it fuses with the cerebral hemispheres, it bifurcates into a prominent lateral olfactory stria (Figures 8–11 and 8–12A) and a small medial olfactory stria (Figure 8–11). The lateral olfactory stria contains the axons from the olfactory bulb, whereas the medial olfactory stria contains axons from other brain regions that are projecting to the olfactory bulb.

Box 8–1. Molecular Analysis of the Projection of Primary Olfactory Sensory Neurons to the Olfactory Bulb

Recent experiments have used molecular techniques for analyzing the organization of the mammalian olfactory system. These studies have examined the locations of primary olfactory neurons that express the genes for olfactory receptors in the olfactory epithelium and their projections into the olfactory bulb. These molecular studies have revealed that the olfactory epithelium has a zonal organization. In rodents, the mammals that have been examined so far, there are four zones in the olfactory epithelium. Primary sensory neurons that contain a particular receptor type (i.e., express a particular receptor gene) appear to be distributed randomly within one of the zones. This suggests that different odorant molecules are initially processed by sensory neurons that are distributed widely throughout the olfactory epithelium.

Even though primary olfactory neurons that contain a particular type of olfactory receptor are widely distributed throughout part of the olfactory epithelium, they project to *one or a small number of glomeruli* in the olfactory bulb. The autoradiograph in Figure 8–10B shows the location of one glomerulus in each olfactory bulb of the rat that receives projections from primary olfactory neurons that express a particular receptor gene and thus contain olfactory receptors of a particular type. In addition to the labeled glomeruli on this histological section, there were a small number of additional labeled glomeruli elsewhere in the olfactory bulb.

Researchers have suggested that, because there are about 1000 different receptor genes and about 1000 to 3000 glomeruli, each glomerulus may receive projections from olfactory sensory neurons that have a particular type of receptor. This finding suggests that the neuronal processes within the glomerulus, the dendrites of mitral, tufted, and periglomerular cells, comprise a functional unit.

Other experiments examining more directly the function of glomeruli are entirely consistent with this view. These studies have used anatomical techniques that allow us to visualize the locations of neurons whose activity has been changed by a particular event, such as exposure of the organism to a particular odorant. Using these approaches, it is thought that different molecular characteristics of odorants are represented at different places in the olfactory bulb. This may be similar to the functional organization of other sensory systems, for example, how different characteristics of a visual stimulus (such as form, color, and motion) are represented in different parts of the thalamus and cortex.

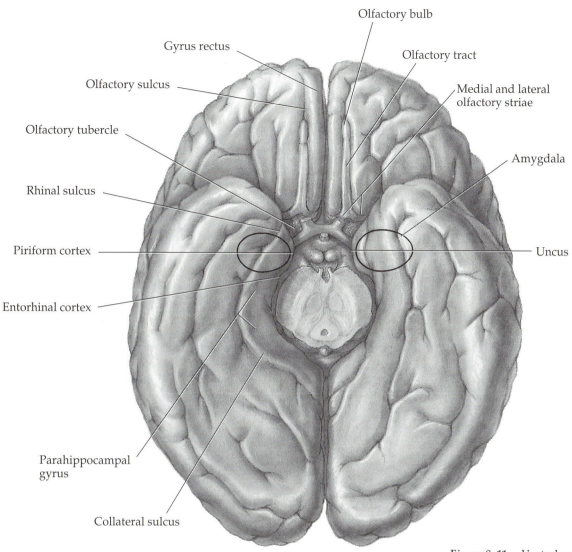

Gyrus rectus

Olfactory sulcus

Olfactory tubercle

Rhinal sulcus

Piriform cortex

Entorhinal cortex

Parahippocampal gyrus

Collateral sulcus

Olfactory bulb

Olfactory tract

Medial and lateral olfactory striae

Amygdala

Uncus

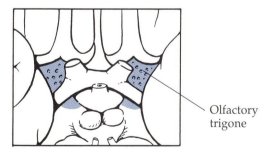

Olfactory trigone

Figure 8–11. Ventral surface of the cerebral hemisphere. The parahippocampal gyrus contains numerous anatomical and functional divisions, two of which are the entorhinal cortex and piriform cortex. Allocortex is located medial to the collateral sulcus and rhinal fissure. The approximate location of the amygdala is indicated. The inset shows the location of the olfactory tubercle within the region of the anterior perforated substance *(blue)*.

A triangular-shaped region on the ventral brain surface, called the **olfactory trigone**, is formed by the olfactory striae (Figure 8–11, inset). Caudal to the olfactory trigone is the **anterior perforated substance**. Tiny branches of the anterior cerebral artery perforate the ventral brain surface in this region. These branches provide the arterial supply for parts of the basal ganglia and internal capsule. The anterior perforated substance is gray matter (see below), whereas the olfactory striae are pathways on the

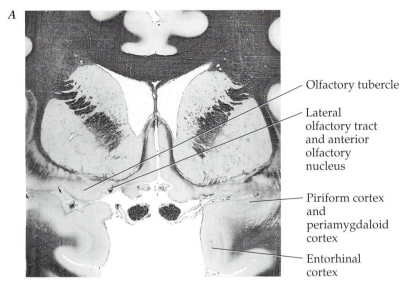

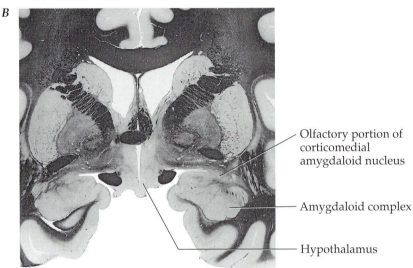

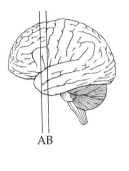

Figure 8–12. Myelin-stained coronal section through the region of the anterior perforated substance *(A)* and amygdala *(B)*. The inset shows the planes of section.

brain surface. The **olfactory tubercle**, one of the gray matter regions to which the olfactory bulb projects, is located in the anterior perforated substance (Figures 8–11, inset, and 8–12A). This tubercle and other parts of the anterior perforated substance are part of the **basal forebrain**. One nucleus of the basal forebrain is the basal nucleus of Meynert, which is comprised of neurons containing acetylcholine that project diffusely throughout the cortex and regulate cortical excitability (see Chapter 3; Figure 3–17A).

The Primary Olfactory Cortex Receives a Direct Input From the Olfactory Bulb

The olfactory bulb projects directly to the cerebral hemispheres; these areas are termed the **primary olfactory cortex**. However, there are three important distinctions between the primary olfactory cortex and the other primary cortical sensory areas. First, the primary olfactory cortex is not a single area but rather five structurally disparate regions on the ventral and medial surfaces of the cerebral hemisphere. Recall that these areas are: (1)

anterior olfactory nucleus, (2) amygdala, (3) olfactory tubercle, (4) piriform and periamygdaloid cortex, and (5) rostral entorhinal cortex. Second, some of the olfactory cortical areas are allocortex, and thus are distinct from the neocortical areas for the other sensory modalities. Third, as already mentioned, the olfactory input from the epithelium is relayed directly to the primary olfactory cortex.

Some of the primary olfactory areas on the ventral and medial surfaces of the cerebral hemispheres (Figure 8–8B) have a cytoarchitecture that is characteristically different from the nonolfactory cortical regions located lateral to it. Most of the cerebral cortex has six cell layers. Recall that this morphological type of cortex is termed isocortex; it is also termed neocortex because it dominates the brains of phylogenetically more recent animals. Somatic sensory, visual, auditory, and gustatory cortical areas are all part of the neocortex. In contrast, the olfactory cortex has fewer than six layers. Cortex with fewer than six layers is termed **allocortex**; there are two major kinds of allocortex: (1) archicortex, and (2) paleocortex (Figure 8–13). **Archicortex** is located primarily in the hippocampal formation (see Chapter 15). (See Figure 3–15, which compares the morphology of neocortex and allocortex.) **Paleocortex** is located on the basal surface of the cerebral hemispheres, in part of the insular cortex, and caudally along the parahippocampal gyrus and retrosplenial cortex (the area of cortex located caudal to the splenium of the corpus callosum; see AI–4). In addition to archicortex and paleocortex, there are various forms of transitional cortex with characteristics of both isocortex and allocortex. On the ventral brain surface, allocortex remains medial to the **rhinal sulcus** and its caudal extension, the **collateral sulcus** (Figures 8–11 and 8–13). The paleocortical olfactory areas each have three morphologically distinct layers. Axons of the olfactory tract course in the most superficial layer before synapsing on neurons in the deeper layers.

Neurons in the Anterior Olfactory Nucleus Modulate Information Transmission in the Olfactory Bulbs Bilaterally

The anterior olfactory nucleus is located caudal to the olfactory bulb on either side of the olfactory tract, where it fuses with the cerebral hemispheres (Figure 8–12A). Neurons of the anterior olfactory nucleus are also scattered along the olfactory tract (Figure 8–8B). Neurons in this olfactory nucleus project their axons back to the olfactory bulbs, both ipsilaterally and contralaterally. In Alzheimer's disease, a progressive neurological degenerative disease in which individuals become severely demented, the anterior olfactory nucleus undergoes characteristic structural changes. By contrast, other parts of the olfactory system, in particular the olfactory bulb and the piriform cortex, are relatively unchanged. Damage of the anterior olfactory nucleus may underlie the impaired sense of smell in Alzheimer's patients.

Projections of the Olfactory Bulb to the Amygdala and Olfactory Tubercle Play a Role in Olfactory Regulation of Behavior

A major projection of the olfactory bulb is to the **amygdala** (Figures 8–11 and 8–12B), a heterogeneous structure with numerous component nuclei, located in the anterior temporal lobe. The amygdala has three major nuclear divisions: the corticomedial nuclear group, the basolateral nuclear group, and the central nucleus. The olfactory bulb projects to a portion of the **corticomedial** nuclear group (Figure 8–12B). It is thought that this projection is important in the olfactory regulation of various

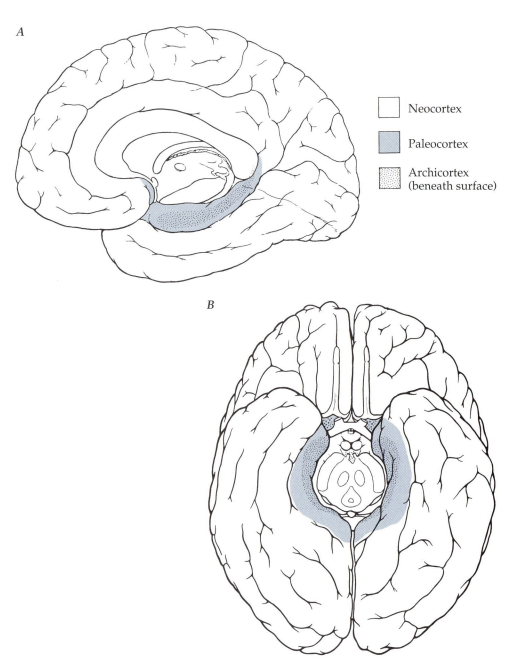

Figure 8–13.   Allocortex (archicortex, paleocortex, and other transitional regions) and isocortex (neocortex) on views of medial *(A)* and lateral *(B)* cerebral hemispheres.

behaviors rather than in perception of odors. For example, neurons in the corticomedial nuclear group are part of a circuit transmitting olfactory information to the hypothalamus (Figure 8–12B), for the regulation of food intake. Also, in certain animals it has been shown that the corticomedial nuclear group plays an essential role in the olfactory regulation of **reproductive behaviors**. The organization of the amygdala will be considered in detail in Chapter 15.

The **olfactory tubercle** is a part of the basal forebrain located medial to the olfactory tract (Figure 8–12 A). Compared with the amygdala, which receives a major olfactory projection in most animal species, the olfactory projections to the olfactory tubercle are fewer in number in primates. Neurons in the olfactory tubercle receive input from and project their axons to brain regions that play a role in **emotions** (Chapter 15).

The Olfactory Areas of the Frontal and Temporal Lobes May Be Important in Olfactory Perceptions and Discriminations

The olfactory bulb also projects directly to the caudolateral frontal lobe and the rostromedial temporal lobe. These areas consist of the rostral entorhinal cortex, the piriform cortex, as well as the periamygdaloid cortex, overlying the amygdala (Figures 8–12 and 8–14). The **rostral entorhinal cortex** is located on the parahippocampal gyrus. This area is thought to be important in allowing a particular smell to evoke far-distant memories of a place or event; this cortex projects to the hippocampal formation, which has been shown to be essential for consolidation of short-term memories into long-term memories (see Chapter 15).

The piriform cortex, named for its appearance in certain mammals (for example, the cat), where the rostral temporal lobe is shaped like a **pear** (Latin: *pirum*, pear), may be important in the initial processing of odors leading to perception. We deduce this because the piriform cortex projects to neocortical areas of the orbital frontal cortex that are implicated in olfactory perception (Figure 8–14). Lesions of the orbital frontal olfactory area in monkeys impair **olfactory discrimination**. This portion of the orbitofrontal cortex also receives a projection from the part of the **medial dorsal nucleus** (Figure 8–6) of the thalamus that receives an olfactory projection from the

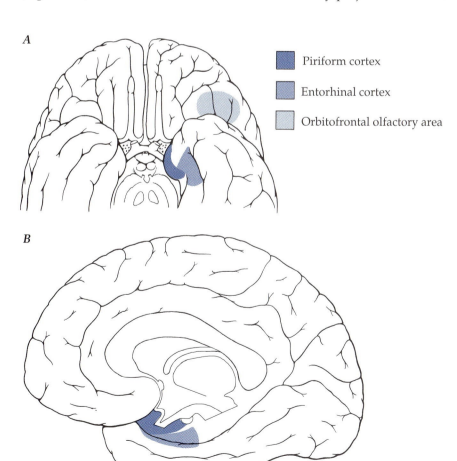

A

Piriform cortex

Entorhinal cortex

Orbitofrontal olfactory area

B

Figure 8–14. Olfactory cortical areas that may play a role in perception. Primary olfactory regions of the temporal lobe and the medial orbital surfaces of the frontal lobe *(blue)*. The orbitofrontal cortex receives a projection from the primary olfactory areas (as well as the medial dorsal nucleus of the thalamus).

piriform cortex. The indirect path for odorant information to the orbital frontal cortex, transmitted from the piriform cortex through the medial dorsal nucleus, may be functionally similar to the thalamocortical projections of the visual, somatic sensory, gustatory, and auditory systems.

Summary

■ GUSTATORY SYSTEM

Sensory Receptors and Peripheral Nerves

Gustatory receptors are clustered in **taste buds** (Figure 8–2), which are located on the tongue, palate, pharynx, larynx, and epiglottis (Figure 8–3). The **facial (seventh cranial) nerve** innervates taste buds on the **anterior two thirds of the tongue** and the **palate**; the **glossopharyngeal (ninth cranial) nerve**, innervates taste buds on the **posterior one third of the tongue and pharynx**; and the **vagus (tenth cranial) nerve**, on the epiglottis and larynx (Figure 8–3).

Brain Stem, Thalamus, and Cerebral Cortex

Afferent fibers of the three cranial nerves serving taste enter the solitary tract and terminate principally in the **rostral** portion of the **solitary nucleus**, also termed the **gustatory nucleus** (Figures 8–1 and 8–4). Projection neurons from the solitary nucleus ascend ipsilaterally, in the **central tegmental tract** (Figure 8–5), to the **parvocellular portion of the ventral posterior medial nucleus** (Figure 8–6). The cortical areas to which the thalamic neurons project are located on the **frontal operculum** and **anterior insular cortex** (Figure 8–7). These areas are separate from the representation of tactile sensation on the tongue.

The **caudal solitary nucleus** (Figure 8–1) receives visceral afferent input from cardiovascular, respiratory, and gastrointestinal structures. This portion is also termed the **cardiorespiratory nucleus**. The axons of ascending projection neurons synapse in the **parabrachial nucleus** (Figures 8–1A, C), which, in turn, projects to the hypothalamus and the amygdala. Other neurons in the caudal solitary nucleus project to **cranial nerve motor nuclei**, the **spinal cord**, and the reticular formation to mediate reflex functions (e.g., blood pressure regulation).

■ OLFACTORY SYSTEM

Receptors and Olfactory Nerve

Primary olfactory neurons, located in the **olfactory epithelium**, are **bipolar neurons** (Figures 8–8 and 8–9). The distal process is sensitive to chemical stimuli and the central process projects to the olfactory bulb (Figure 8–10) as the **olfactory (first cranial) nerve**. The olfactory nerve is formed by multiple small fascicles of axons of primary olfactory neurons that pass through foramina in a portion of the **ethmoid bone** termed the **cribriform plate** (Figures 8–9 and 8–10).

Telencephalon

Olfactory nerve fibers synapse on **mitral** and **tufted cells**, the projection neurons of the **olfactory bulb** (Figure 8–10). The axons of mitral and tufted cells project via the **olfactory tract** to five regions of the cerebral hemisphere (Figure 8–8B): (1) **anterior olfactory nucleus** (Figure 8–12A), (2) **olfactory tubercle** (a portion of the **anterior perforated substance**) (Figures 8–11 and 8–12), (3) **amygdala** (Figures 8–11 and 8–12), (4) **piriform cortex** and **periamygdaloid cortex** (Figure 8–12A), and (5) **rostral entorhinal cortex** (Figures 8–11 and 8–14). The piriform cortex is **allocortex** (Figure 8–13) and has fewer than six layers, similar to archicortex of the hippocampus, which has three layers. In contrast, isocortex has six layers. The path from piriform cortex to the **medial dorsal nucleus** and then to the **orbitofrontal cortex** may be important in olfactory discrimination. ■

KEY STRUCTURES AND TERMS

Gustatory and Visceral Afferent Systems
facial (seventh cranial) nerve
   intermediate nerve
   chorda tympani
glossopharyngeal (ninth cranial) nerve
vagus (tenth cranial) nerve
taste buds
   taste receptor cells
   basal cells
   support cells
fungiform and foliate papillae
circumvallate papillae
geniculate ganglion
inferior ganglia
solitary tract
solitary nucleus
   gustatory nucleus
   cardiorespiratory nucleus
central tegmental tract

parabrachial nucleus
ventral posterior medial nucleus–
      parvocellular division
internal capsule–posterior limb
frontal operculum and anterior
     insular cortex
amygdala
hypothalamus

Olfactory System
olfactory receptors
olfactory nerve
olfactory mucosa
   primary olfactory neurons
   supporting cells
   microvillar cells
   basal cells
cribriform plate
olfactory bulb
   glomerulus
   mitral cells

   tufted cells
   periglomerular cells
   granule cell
   glial cells
olfactory tract
olfactory sulcus
gyrus rectus
lateral olfactory stria
olfactory trigone
anterior perforated substance
basal forebrain
olfactory cortex
   anterior olfactory nucleus
   amygdala (corticomedial
     nucleus)
   olfactory tubercle
   piriform and periamygdaloid
     cortex
   rostral entorhinal cortex
medial dorsal nucleus
orbitofrontal cortex

Selected Readings

Dodd, J., and Castellucci, V. 1991. Smell and taste: The chemical senses. In Kandel, E. R., Schwartz, J. H., and Jessell, T. M. (eds.), Principles of Neural Science, 3rd ed. New York: Elsevier, pp. 512–529.

Finger, T. E. 1987. Gustatory nuclei and pathways in the central nervous system. In Finger, T. E., and Silver, W. L. (eds.), Neurobiology of Taste and Smell. New York: John Wiley and Sons, pp. 331–353.

Haberly, L.B. 1990. Olfactory Cortex. In Shepherd, G. M. (ed.), The Synaptic Organization of the Brain. New York: Oxford University Press, pp. 317–345.

Norgren, R. 1990. Gustatory system. In Paxinos, G. (ed.), The Human Nervous System. San Diego: Academic Press, pp. 845–860.

Price, J. L. 1990. Olfactory system. In Paxinos, G. (ed.), The Human Nervous System. San Diego: Academic Press, pp. 979–998.

Shepard, G. M. 1972. Synaptic organization of the mammalian olfactory bulb. Physiol. Rev. 52:864–917.

References

Beckstead, R. M., Morse, J. R., and Norgren, R. 1980. The nucleus of the solitary tract in the monkey: Projections to the thalamus and brain stem nuclei. J. Comp. Neurol. 190:259–282.

Braak, H. 1980. Architectonics of the Human Telencephalic Cortex. Berlin: Springer-Verlag, pp. 147.

Buck, L. B., and Axel, R. 1991. A novel multigene family may encode odorant receptors: A molecular basis for odor recognition. Cell 65:175–187.

Cechetto, D. F., and Saper, C. B. 1987. Evidence for a viscerotopic sensory representation in the cortex and thalamus in the rat. J. Comp. Neurol. 262:27–45.

Nauta, W. J. H., and Haymaker, W. 1969. Hypothalamic nuclei and fiber connections. In Haymaker, W., Anderson, E., Nauta, W. J. H. (eds.), The Hypothalamus. Springfield, Ill.: Charles C Thomas, pp. 136–209.

Potter, H., and Nauta, W. J. H. 1979. A note on the problem of olfactory associations of the orbitofrontal cortex in the monkey. Neurosci. 4:361–367.

Pritchard, T. C., Hamilton, R. B., Morse, J. R., et al. 1986. Projections of thalamic gustatory and lingual areas in the monkey, Macaca fascicularis. J. Comp. Neurol. 244:213–228.

Reis, D. J., Ruggiero, D. A., and Granata, A. 1986. Central nervous system control of the heart: Brainstem mechanisms governing the tonic and reflex control of the circulation. In Stober, T., Schimrigk, K., Ganten, D., and Sherman, D. G. (eds.), Central Nervous System Control of the Heart. Boston: Martinus Nijhoff Publishing, pp. 19–36.

Ressler, K. J., Sullivan, S. L., and Buck, L. B. 1993. A zonal organization of odorant receptor gene expression in the olfactory epithelium. Cell 73:597–609.

Ressler, K. J., Sullivan, S. L., and Buck, L. B. 1994. Information coding in the olfactory system: Evidence for a stereotyped and highly organized epitope map in the olfactory bulb. Cell 79:1245–1255.

Ressler, K. J., Sullivan, S. L., and Buck, L. B. 1994. A molecular dissection of spatial patterning in the olfactory system. Curr. Opin. Neurobiol. 4:588–596.

Shepherd, G. M., and Greer, C. A. 1990. Olfactory Bulb. In Shepherd, G. M. (ed.), The Synaptic Organization of the Brain. New York: Oxford University Press, pp. 133–169.

Steward, W. B., Kauer, J. S., and Shepherd, G. M. 1979. Functional organization of rat olfactory bulb, analyzed by the 2-deoxyglucose method. J. Comp. Neurol. 185:715–734.

Vassar, R., Chao, S. K., Sticheran, R., Nuñez, J. M., Vosshall, L. B., and Axel, R. 1994. Topographic organization of sensory projections to the olfactory bulb. Cell 79:981–991.

Vassar, R., Ngai, J., and Axel, R. 1993. Spatial organization of odorant receptor expression in the mammalian olfactory epithelium. Cell 74:309–318.

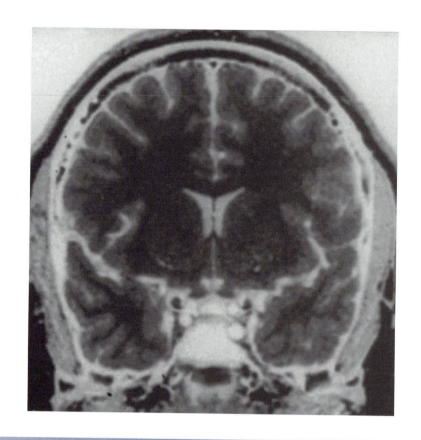

III

Motor Systems

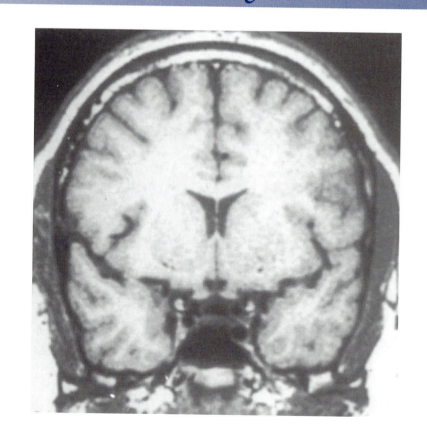

9

Descending Projection Systems and the Motor Function of the Spinal Cord

THE MOTOR SYSTEMS OF THE BRAIN AND SPINAL CORD work together to control skeletal muscle. The task of these systems is diverse because the functions of the various skeletal muscles differ remarkably. Contrast, for instance, the fine control required of the muscles of the hand as it grasps a china cup with the gross strength required of the muscles of the back and legs in lifting a box full of books. In fact, so complex and varied are these jobs, that the motor systems utilize virtually all of the major divisions of the central nervous system in producing even simple motor behaviors. We will see that different brain regions comprise separate components of the motor systems, each with distinct roles in controlling movement.

In this chapter, we first examine the general features of the functional anatomy of the motor systems. Next, we survey the key features of the functional organization of the descending motor pathways and the spinal cord motor nuclei to which they project. Finally, we explore the regional anatomy of the motor system at its different levels, beginning with the cerebral cortex and ending with the spinal cord. In this chapter we primarily focus on the pathways controlling skeletal muscles of the limbs and trunk. We save the pathways that control skeletal muscles of the head and the cranial nerve motor nuclei for Chapter 13.

FUNCTIONAL ANATOMY OF THE MOTOR SYSTEMS AND THE DESCENDING PATHWAYS

Diverse Central Nervous System Structures Comprise the Motor Systems

Four separate components of the central nervous system comprise the motor systems (Figure 9–1A): (1) descending projection pathways, (2) motor neurons and interneurons, (3) basal ganglia, and (4) cerebellum. These regions drive movements of the limbs and trunk by regulating skeletal muscle.

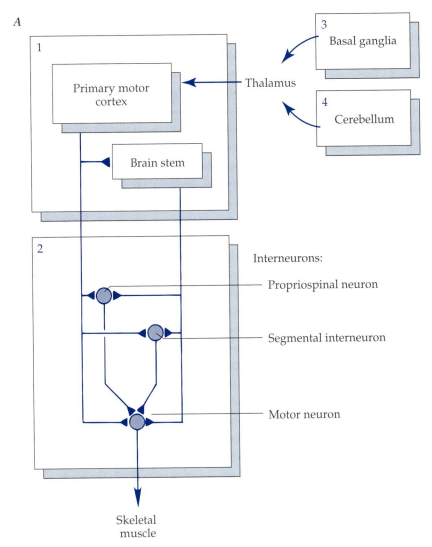

Figure 9–1. *A.* General organization of the motor systems. There are four major components to the motor systems (each enclosed by shaded box): descending pathways, motor neurons and interneurons, basal ganglia, and cerebellum. This figure also illustrates the parallel and hierarchical organization of the motor systems. In this example there are two parallel pathways one from the motor cortex and the other from the brain stem to motor neurons. There are three hierarchical pathways originating in the motor cortex but contacting three different sets of neurons in the brain stem, propriospinal neurons, and segmental interneurons. *B.* Key cortical regions for controlling movement. The limbic and prefrontal association areas are involved in the initial decision to move, in relation to motivational and emotional factors. In reaching to grasp an object, the visual areas process the information about the location and shape of the object. This information is transmitted, via the posterior parietal lobe, to the premotor areas, which are important in movement planning. From there, information is transmitted to the primary motor cortex, from which descending control signals are sent to the motor neurons.

The first component, regions of the cerebral cortex and brain stem that contribute to the **descending projection pathways**, is organized much like the sensory pathways. But rather than beginning in the periphery and ascending to the brain, the descending pathways have the reverse organization. Descending projection neurons in the cerebral cor-

B

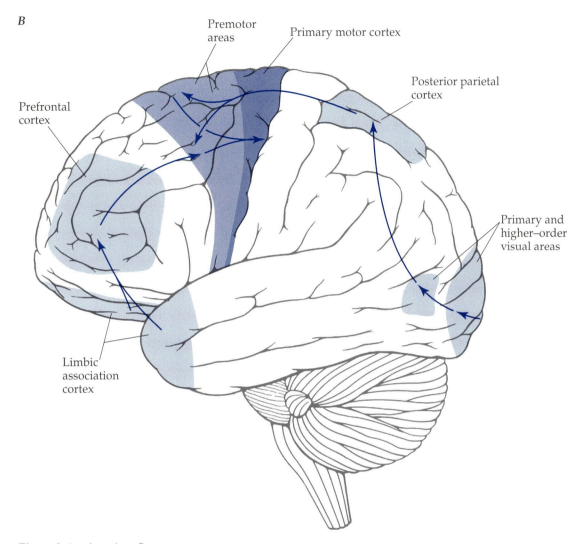

Figure 9–1. (continued)

tex and brain stem either synapse directly on motor neurons or synapse on interneurons that, in turn, synapse on motor neurons.

These motor neurons and interneurons comprise the second component of the motor systems. For muscles of the limbs and trunk, motor neurons and most interneurons are found in the **ventral horn and intermediate zone of the spinal cord**. For the head, these neurons are located in the **cranial nerve motor nuclei and the reticular formation**. There is an analogy between components of the motor systems of the spinal cord and brain stem: The cranial nerve motor nuclei are analogous to the ventral horn motor nuclei, and the reticular formation, to the intermediate zone.

The third and fourth components of the motor system, the **basal ganglia** and the **cerebellum** (see Chapters 10 and 11), do not contain neurons that project directly to motor neurons (Figure 9–1A). Nevertheless, these structures have a powerful regulatory influence over motor behavior. The cerebellum and basal ganglia act indirectly in motor behavior through their effects on the descending pathways. While only the path through the thalamus to the cortex is shown in Figure 9–1A, both the basal ganglia and cerebellum also project directly to the brain stem.

Other areas of the brain provide the different motor system components with information essential for accurate movement control (Figure 9–1B). For example, if we examine a visually guided behavior—reaching to grasp the cup introduced earlier—it becomes clear that even this common task engages the coordinated actions of the entire brain. The process of translating our thoughts and sensations into action begins with the initial decision to move, which is dependent on such brain structures as the **limbic and prefrontal association areas** (Figure 9–1B), which are involved in emotions, motivation, and cognition (see Chapters 14 and 15).

The **visual system**, especially the magnocellular system, processes sensory information for visually guiding our movements. We saw in Chapter 6 that the magnocellular system projects to the **posterior portion of the parietal lobe**, a cortical area important for identifying salient objects in the environment and in attention (Figure 9–1B). Visual information, consisting of the location and shape of the cup, is distributed next to **premotor** areas of the frontal lobe, where the **plan of action** to reach to the cup is formulated. Planning a movement is a process that involves specifying the particular motor act that will be executed to achieve the goal. Whereas the decision to move and where to move are conscious experiences, much of the planning of a movement is subconscious.

The next step in translating our decision to reach into action (Figure 9–1B) is directing the muscles to contract. This is accomplished by the **primary motor cortex**, which receives inputs from all of the premotor areas, and, in turn, projects to the spinal cord. This projection, termed the **corticospinal tract**, is thought to be the most important descending projection pathway in humans for controlling voluntary movements. This pathway transmits control signals directly to motor neurons, or indirectly, to interneurons.

What are the specific contributions of the cerebellum and basal ganglia to movement control? Surprisingly, the answer remains elusive. We do know that the cerebellum receives convergent inputs from the various sensory systems and from the descending projection pathways themselves. In this way, the cerebellum is thought to compare the intended action, derived from control signals from the various descending pathways, with the action that took place, monitored by using sensory information arising as a consequence of the movement itself (feedback). When the cerebellum detects a disparity between the intended and actual movement, it may generate an error-correcting control signal. This signal is transmitted to the premotor and motor cortex via the thalamus (Figure 9–1A), as well as to the brain stem. From there, descending pathways transmit these error-correcting signals to the motor neurons. The cerebellum is also important in coordinating movements by specifying the precise timing of control signals to different muscles.

Our understanding of basal ganglia function is even less informed than our understanding of the cerebellum. The basal ganglia have a unique anatomical property: they receive projections from the entire cerebral cortex—including the sensory, motor, and association cortical areas, as well as from the limbic system—but their output is focused on the frontal lobe. Like most subcortical structures, the basal ganglia project to the cortex via the thalamus. Certainly, the basal ganglia are important in the planning and execution of movements since the premotor and motor areas are located in the frontal lobe and receive basal ganglia input.

Moreover, movements become disordered in patients with Parkinson's disease, a neurodegenerative disease that primarily affects the basal ganglia. However, the specific contribution of the basal ganglia to formulating a plan of motor action or executing movement is not yet known.

The basal ganglia also play a key role in cognition and in emotions. Much of the output of the basal ganglia is directed to the prefrontal cortex and limbic association cortex, which are important in the highest levels of organizing our thoughts and behavior.

We have seen that the cortical motor areas—the primary and premotor cortices—receive input from both the cerebellum and basal ganglia via relays in the thalamus. The brain stem motor nuclei contributing to descending pathways (Figure 9–1A) also receive input from the cerebellum and basal ganglia. The brain stem descending pathways, together with the cerebellum and basal ganglia, are thought to mediate relatively automatic control of movements and posture as well as rapid correction of misdirected movements.

There Are Three Functional Classes of Descending Pathways

Descending pathways can be classified as: (1) motor control pathways, (2) pathways that regulate somatic sensory processing, and (3) pathways that regulate the functions of the autonomic nervous system. **Motor control pathways** mediate the voluntary and involuntary (or automatic) control of movement. As we have seen, they originate in the cerebral cortex and brain stem and synapse, directly or indirectly, on motor neurons that innervate skeletal muscle. The pathways that are involved in the control of limb and axial muscles synapse on motor neurons in the motor nuclei in the **ventral horn** of the spinal cord. The motor control pathways also terminate on interneurons that, in turn, synapse on motor neurons. These interneurons are dispersed throughout the spinal cord gray matter, but are primarily located in the intermediate zone and ventral horn. As we saw earlier, the pathways for controlling cranial muscles have an analogous organization: They terminate in cranial nerve motor nuclei, which contain the motor neurons, and in the reticular formation, which contains the interneurons that synapse on the motor neurons.

The descending pathways that regulate **somatic sensory processing** also originate in the cerebral cortex and brain stem, similar to the motor control pathways, but terminate primarily on **dorsal horn neurons** and in brain stem **somatic sensory relay nuclei.** These pathways are important for controlling the flow of somatic sensory information into the central nervous system, which has an important effect on perception. For example, the raphespinal path mediates pain suppression (see Chapter 5).

Somatic sensory information is also important for the control of movement. Sensory information triggers motor reflexes, such as the knee-jerk reflex (Figure 3–2), and is used in the guidance of limb movements and in posture. The importance of such control can be seen in patients with sensory neuropathies, such as damage to large-diameter fibers conveying mechanical information, which can occur in certain toxicity syndromes. These patients are incapable of performing such routine motor tasks such as buttoning a shirt or reaching accurately for a glass of water.

Many of the movement disorders produced by brain damage, such as **spasticity**, are believed to be due, in part, to changes in the regulation of flow of somatic sensory information into the central nervous system. Because there is overlap in the functions of the motor control and sensory regulatory pathways, it is not surprising that there is also overlap in their connections.

The descending pathways that regulate the **autonomic nervous system** originate in diverse brain structures, including the cerebral cortex, amygdala, hypothalamus, and brain stem. The neurons comprising these pathways synapse on preganglionic autonomic neurons in the brain stem and spinal cord. In this chapter, we consider only the anatomical organization of the descending spinal projection systems that are important in the control of limb and trunk musculature and in the sensory regulation of movement. The autonomic pathways, together with the autonomic nervous system itself, are considered along with the hypothalamus (see Chapter 14).

Seven major descending motor pathways originate in the cerebral cortex and in various nuclei in the brain stem (Table 9–1). Three originate in the cortex, primarily in the frontal lobe: (1) **lateral corticospinal tract**,

Table 9–1. Descending pathways for controlling movement.

Tract	Site of origin	Decussation	Spinal cord column	Site of termination	Function
Cerebral Cortex					
Corticospinal					
Lateral	Areas 6, 4, 1, 2, 3, 5, 7	Crossed—Pyramidal decussation	Lateral	Dorsal horn, lateral intermediate zone, ventral horn	Sensory control, voluntary movement (limb muscles)
Ventral	Areas 6, 4	Uncrossed[1]	Ventral	Medial intermediate zone, ventral horn	Voluntary movement (axial muscles)
Corticobulbar	Areas 6, 4, 1, 2, 3, 5, 7	Crossed and uncrossed[2]	Brain stem only	Cranial nerve sensory and motor nuclei, reticular formation	Sensory control, voluntary movement (cranial muscles)
Brain Stem					
Rubrospinal	Red nucleus (magnocellular)	Ventral tegmentum	Lateral	Lateral intermediate zone and ventral horn	Voluntary movement, limb muscles
Vestibulospinal					
Lateral	Dieters' nucleus (lateral vestibular nucleus)	Ipsilateral[1]	Ventral	Medial intermediate zone and ventral horn	Balance
Medial	Medial vestibular nucleus	Bilateral	Ventral	Medial intermediate zone and ventral horn	Head position/neck muscles
Reticulospinal					
Pontine	Pontine reticular formation	Ipsilateral[1]	Ventral	Medial intermediate horn and ventral horn	Automatic movement, axial and limb muscles
Medullary	Medullary reticular formation	Ipsilateral[1]	Ventrolateral	Medial intermediate zone and ventral horn	Automatic movement, axial and limb muscle
Tectospinal	Deep superior colliculus	Dorsal tegmentum	Ventral	Medial intermediate zone and ventral horn	Coordinates neck with eye movements

[1]Whereas these tracts descend ipsilaterally, they terminate on interneurons whose axons decussate in the ventral commissure and thus influence axial musculature bilaterally.

[2]Most of the projections to the cranial nerve motor nuclei are bilateral; those to the part of the facial nucleus that innervates upper facial muscles are bilateral and those to the lower facial muscles are contralateral (see Chapter 13).

(2) **ventral (or anterior) corticospinal tract**, and (3) **corticobulbar tract**. The corticobulbar tract terminates primarily in cranial motor nuclei in the pons and medulla and is the cranial equivalent of the corticospinal tracts. It will be considered in detail in Chapter 13. The remaining four pathways originate from brain stem nuclei: (4) **rubrospinal tract**, (5) **reticulospinal tracts**, (6) **vestibulospinal tracts**, and (7) **tectospinal tract**. In addition to these seven descending motor pathways, neurotransmitter-specific systems—including the raphe nuclei, locus ceruleus, and midbrain dopaminergic neurons—have diffuse projections to the spinal cord intermediate zone and ventral horn. Other than pain regulation, the functions of these descending pathways are not understood (see Chapter 3).

Descending Pathways Synapse on Segmental Interneurons and Propriospinal Neurons in Addition to Motor Neurons

Each of the descending pathways influences skeletal muscle via **monosynaptic, disynaptic, and polysynaptic connections** between descending projection neurons and **motor neurons** (Figure 9–1A). Typically, the axon of a descending projection neuron makes all types of connections with motor neurons. Whether disynaptic or polysynaptic, the connections are mediated by two kinds of spinal cord interneurons: segmental interneurons and propriospinal neurons. The **segmental interneuron** (sometimes termed **intrasegmental neuron**) has a short axon that distributes branches within a single spinal cord segment to synapse on motor neurons. In addition to receiving input from the descending systems, segmental interneurons receive convergent input from different classes of somatic sensory receptors for the reflex control of movement. For example, particular interneurons receive input from nociceptors and mediate limb withdrawal reflexes in response to a painful stimulus, such as when we jerk our hand away from a hot stove. Segmental interneurons are located primarily in the intermediate zone and the ventral horn.

The **propriospinal neuron** has an axon that projects for multiple spinal segments before synapsing on motor neurons (Figure 9–1A). Another name for the propriospinal neuron is **intersegmental neuron**. Propriospinal neurons comprise two major systems with distinct axonal terminations. One system connects widely separate spinal segments, such as the cervical and lumbar segments. These **long propriospinal neurons** play a role in posture through connections with axial and girdle motor neurons. These long propriospinal neurons may participate in coordinating motions of the upper and lower extremities. The other kind of propriospinal neuron connects neighboring segments, for example, within the cervical enlargement. These **short propriospinal neurons** are important in transmitting control signals from the descending pathways to limb motor neurons.

The Descending Pathways Have a Parallel and Hierarchical Organization

The descending projection systems, similar to the ascending systems (see Chapter 5), have a parallel and hierarchical organization (Figure 9–1A). The **parallel organization** of the motor systems is revealed in their multiple descending pathways that transmit control signals from the brain to the spinal cord. We have already briefly considered that seven separate pathways project directly from distinct cortical and brain stem sites to the spinal cord to influence the excitability of motor circuitry. We are also beginning to learn that different parts of the cerebellum and basal ganglia are part of functionally distinct parallel paths, because they may primarily influence different descending pathways.

Descending projection neurons contact motor neurons directly through monosynaptic connections; they also contact motor neurons indirectly by synapsing on propriospinal and segmental interneurons. Moreover, pathways originating in the cortex also synapse on descending projection neurons in the brain stem. This is the **hierarchical organization** of the descending systems (Figure 9–1A). For example, the cerebral cortex controls motor neurons through direct connections with the spinal cord (the corticospinal tracts) and indirect connections to brain stem nuclei that, in turn, give rise to descending pathways to the spinal cord (e.g., the reticulospinal tracts). In this indirect path, projection neurons of the cerebral cortex constitute the higher level in the sequence (or hierarchy). The intermediate levels are formed by brain stem nuclei as well as spinal cord segmental interneurons and propriospinal neurons. The lowest level of the hierarchy consists of the motor neurons.

The Functional Organization of the Descending Pathways Parallels the Somatotopic Organization of the Motor Nuclei in the Ventral Horn

The motor neurons innervating **limb muscles**, and the interneurons from which they receive input, are located in the **lateral ventral horn and intermediate zone** (Figure 9–2A). In contrast, motor neurons innervating **axial and girdle muscles**, and their associated interneurons, are located in the **medial ventral horn and intermediate zone**. The locations of the motor neurons and interneurons correspond to the locations of the various descending motor pathways in the spinal cord white matter that innervate them. The **lateral** motor nuclei and interneurons, which control limb muscles, receive projections from pathways that primarily descend in the lateral portion of the spinal cord white matter. In contrast, the **medial** motor nuclei and interneurons, for controlling **axial** and **girdle muscles** (i.e., neck and shoulder), receive projections from pathways that primarily descend in the **medial** portion of the white matter.

In addition to the mediolateral organization there is a dorsoventral organization: motor neurons that innervate flexor muscles are located dorsal to extensor motor neurons (Figure 9–2A). The mediolateral somatotopic organization and dorsoventral flexor–extensor organization of the intermediate zone and ventral horn are easy to remember because they mimic the form of the body (Figure 9–2B). Not surprisingly, in the snake, which has only axial muscles, there are only medial motor nuclei.

The Laterally Descending Pathways Control Limb Muscles and Regulate Voluntary Movement

There are two laterally descending pathways: lateral corticospinal tract, which originates in the cerebral cortex, and rubrospinal tract, which descends from the midbrain (see Table 9–1). The neurons that give rise to both of these pathways are **somatotopically** organized. Moreover, the lateral corticospinal and rubrospinal tracts control muscles on the **contralateral** side of the body. The **lateral corticospinal tract** is the principal motor control pathway in humans. A lesion of this pathway anywhere along its path to the motor neuron has a devastating and persistent effect on limb

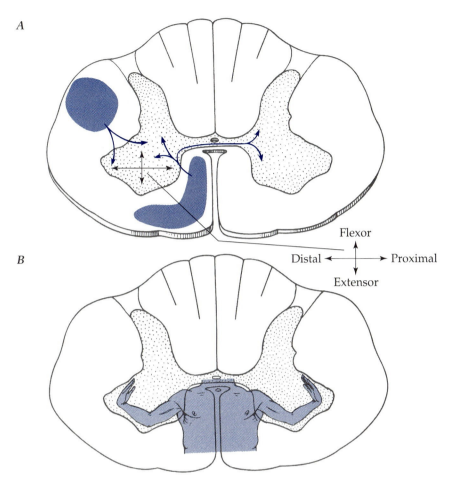

Flexor

Distal ←————————→ Proximal

Extensor

Figure 9–2. The somatotopic organization of the ventral horn. *A.* Schematic diagram of the spinal cord, indicating the general locations of motor neurons innervating limb and axial muscles and flexor and extensor muscles. *B.* A partial "homunculus" is superimposed on the ventral horns. (*B,* Adapted from Crosby, E. C., Humphrey, T., and Lauer, E. W. 1962. Correlative Anatomy of the Nervous System. New York: Macmillan.)

use. One motor deficit produced by a lateral corticospinal tract lesion is the loss of the ability to **fractionate movements**, to move one finger independently from the others. Manual dexterity depends on fractionation, without which movements of our hands are clumsy and imprecise.

The major site of origin of the lateral corticospinal tract is the primary motor cortex (Figure 9–3A); axons also originate from the premotor cortical regions and the somatic sensory cortical areas. Descending axons in the tract course within the cerebral hemisphere in the **posterior limb of the internal capsule** and, in the midbrain, on its ventral surface in the **basis pedunculi** (Figure 9–3A). Next on its caudal course, the tract disappears beneath the ventral surface of the pons only to reappear on the ventral surface of the medulla as the **pyramid**. At the junction of the spinal cord and medulla, the axons **decussate** and descend in the dorsolateral portion of the **lateral** column of the spinal cord white matter. Hence the name lateral corticospinal tract (see Figure 9–5). This pathway terminates primarily in the lateral portions of the intermediate zone and ventral horn of the cervical and lumbosacral cord, the locations of neurons that control distal limb muscles of the hand and foot.

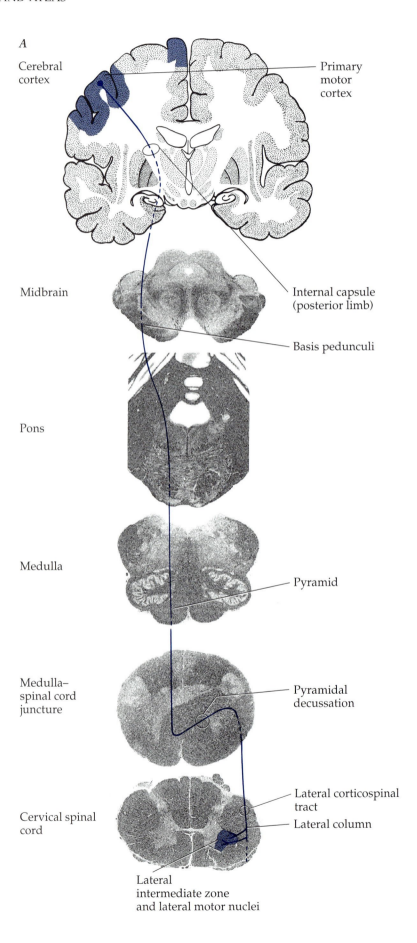

Figure 9–3. Laterally descending pathways. *A.* Lateral corticospinal tract. *B.* Rubrospinal tract. Note that the lateral corticospinal tract also originates from neurons located in area 6 and the parietal lobe.

B

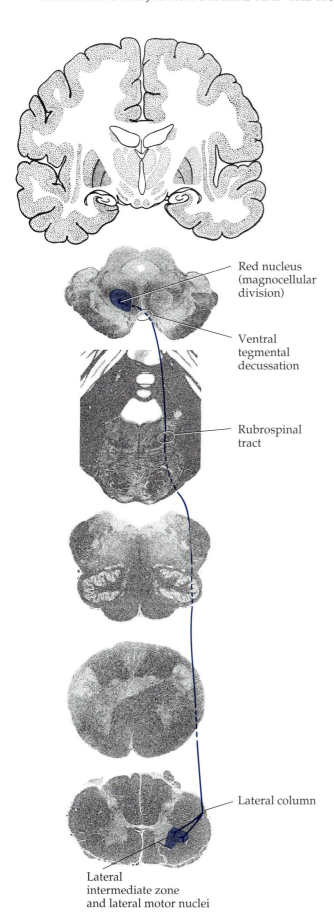

Red nucleus
(magnocellular
division)

Ventral
tegmental
decussation

Rubrospinal
tract

Lateral column

Lateral
intermediate zone
and lateral motor nuclei

Figure 9–3. *(continued)*

The **rubrospinal tract** (Figure 9–3B) has fewer axons than the corticospinal tract. The rubrospinal tract originates from neurons in the caudal portion of the **red nucleus**, a portion termed **magnocellular** because rubrospinal tract neurons are characteristically large. The rubrospinal tract decussates in the midbrain and descends in the dorsolateral portion of the brain stem. Similar to the lateral corticospinal tract, the rubrospinal tract is found in the dorsal portion of the lateral column (see Figure 9–5) and terminates primarily in the **lateral portions of the intermediate zone and ventral horn** of the cervical cord.

Despite its small size, the rubrospinal tract may be clinically important because it is thought to subserve some residual motor function after damage of the lateral corticospinal tract. The red nucleus is one of the largest midbrain nuclei (see Figure 9–10), yet in humans the magnocellular division is much smaller than the other component of the red nucleus, the **parvocellular** (or small-celled) division. Neurons of the parvocellular division are part of a multisynaptic pathway from the cerebral cortex to the cerebellum (see Chapter 10).

The Medially Descending Pathways Control Axial and Girdle Muscles and Regulate Posture

Axial and girdle muscles are controlled primarily by the four medially descending pathways: ventral corticospinal tract, reticulospinal tracts, vestibulospinal tracts, and tectospinal tract (Table 9–1). Even though individual pathways may project unilaterally (either ipsilateral or contralateral) they synapse on interneurons whose axons decussate in the ventral spinal commissure. Thus, overall, the medial descending pathways have bilateral projections to spinal cord neurons and thus exert **bilateral control** over axial and girdle muscles. An important clinical consequence of this organization is that **unilateral** brain stem or cerebral cortical lesions that interrupt descending motor pathways do not produce profound deficits of axial and girdle muscle control. Such protection results from a sustaining contralateral projection of the medially descending systems. Bilateral control of axial and girdle muscles contrasts with crossed unilateral control of distal limb muscles by the lateral corticospinal and rubrospinal tracts.

Many of the medially descending pathways only project to the cervical spinal cord, a pattern that is consistent with a preferential role in the control of neck, upper trunk, and shoulder musculature as opposed to lower trunk and leg muscles. Animal experiments, however, have shown that propriospinal neurons located in the upper cervical spinal cord can transmit control signals from the medial pathways to more caudal levels (see below). Thus, pathways terminating in the cervical cord may also influence trunk and lower limb muscles.

The **ventral corticospinal tract** (Figure 9–4A) originates predominantly from the **primary motor cortex** and the **supplementary motor area**. Similar to the lateral corticospinal tract, the ventral corticospinal tract descends through the internal capsule, the basis pedunculi, the ventral pons, and the medullary pyramid. At the junction of the spinal cord and the medulla, where the lateral corticospinal tract decussates, the ventral corticospinal tract does not cross over but descends in the **ipsilateral ventral column** of the spinal cord (Figure 9–5). The ventral corticospinal tract terminates in the medial gray matter. This pathway synapses on motor neurons in the **medial** ventral horn and segmental interneurons and propriospinal neurons in the **medial** intermediate zone.

Many ventral corticospinal tract axons have branches that decussate in the spinal cord. As a consequence, the ventral corticospinal tract on one side influences axial and girdle muscles bilaterally. The ventral corticospinal tract projects to the cervical and upper thoracic spinal cord and thus may be preferentially involved in the control of the neck, shoulder, and upper trunk muscles.

The two separate reticulospinal tracts (Figure 9–4B) originate from different regions of the **reticular formation**: the **pontine reticulospinal tract** and the **medullary reticulospinal tract** (Figure 9–5). (Few neurons from the midbrain reticular formation project to the spinal cord.) The pontine reticulospinal tract descends in the ventral column of the spinal cord, whereas the medullary reticulospinal tract descends in the ventrolateral quadrant of the lateral column. The reticulospinal tracts descend predominantly in the ipsilateral spinal cord and are thought to help control more automatic movements, such as maintaining posture or walking over even terrain.

As its name implies, the **tectospinal tract** (Figure 9–4B) originates primarily from neurons in the **tectum**, the portion of midbrain located dorsal to the cerebral aqueduct (see Figure 3–8). Most of these neurons are located in the deeper layers of the **superior colliculus**. The tectospinal tract also has a limited rostrocaudal distribution, projecting only to the cervical spinal segments. It therefore is believed to participate primarily in the control of neck, shoulder, and upper trunk muscles. Because the superior colliculus also plays a key role in controlling eye movements (see Chapter 6), it is likely that the tectospinal tract is important for **coordinating head movements with eye movements**.

The two **vestibulospinal tracts** (Figure 9–4C) originate primarily from different vestibular nuclei. The **lateral vestibulospinal tract**, which begins at the **lateral vestibular nucleus** (also termed **Deiters' nucleus**), descends ipsilaterally in the white matter to all spinal levels. This pathway is crucial in maintaining balance. Despite its name, the lateral vestibulospinal tract is one of the medial descending pathways. The **medial vestibulospinal tract**, which starts at the **medial vestibular nucleus**, descends bilaterally in the white matter, but only to the cervical and upper thoracic spinal cord. The medial vestibulospinal tract plays a role in controlling head position.

The various descending pathways in the spinal cord are illustrated on the right side of Figure 9–5; the ascending somatic sensory pathways (see Chapter 5) are illustrated on the left side. The two spinocerebellar pathways, which transmit sensory information to the cerebellum for controlling movement (see Chapter 10) also are illustrated.

■ REGIONAL ANATOMY

In the rest of this chapter, we examine the brain and spinal cord with the aim of understanding the anatomy of the descending projection pathways and their spinal terminations. In the chapter on the somatic sensory system (Chapter 5), we examined key levels through the brain and spinal cord from caudal to rostral, following the natural flow of sensory information. In this chapter, we begin with the cerebral cortex—the highest level of movement control—and proceed caudally to the spinal cord.

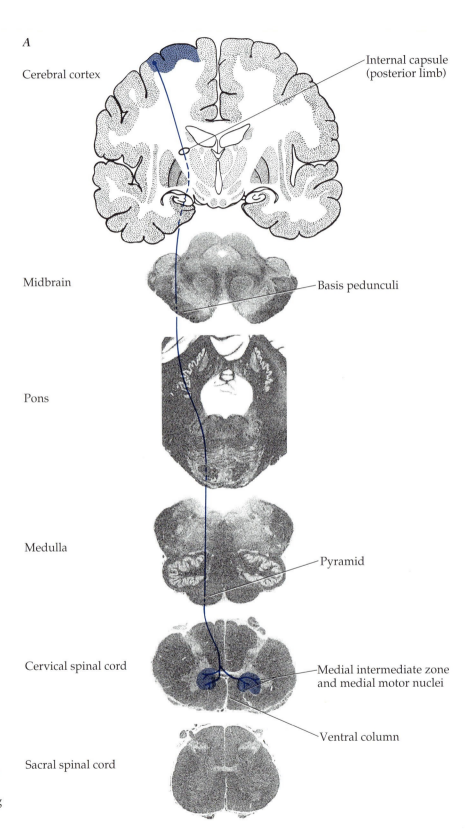

A

Cerebral cortex

Internal capsule
(posterior limb)

Midbrain

Basis pedunculi

Pons

Medulla

Pyramid

Cervical spinal cord

Medial intermediate zone
and medial motor nuclei

Ventral column

Sacral spinal cord

Figure 9–4. Medially descending pathways. *A.* Ventral corticospinal tract. *B.* Tectospinal tract, pontine, and medullary reticulospinal tracts. *C.* Lateral and medial vestibulospinal tracts. Another name for the medial vestibulospinal tract is the descending medial longitudinal fasciculus.

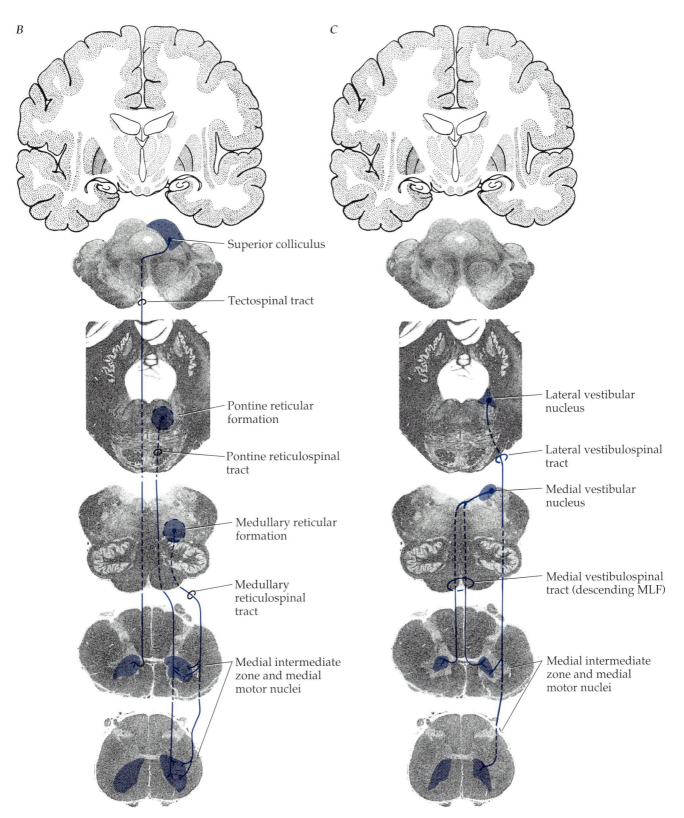

B

Superior colliculus

Tectospinal tract

Pontine reticular formation

Pontine reticulospinal tract

Medullary reticular formation

Medullary reticulospinal tract

Medial intermediate zone and medial motor nuclei

C

Lateral vestibular nucleus

Lateral vestibulospinal tract

Medial vestibular nucleus

Medial vestibulospinal tract (descending MLF)

Medial intermediate zone and medial motor nuclei

Figure 9–4. *(continued)*

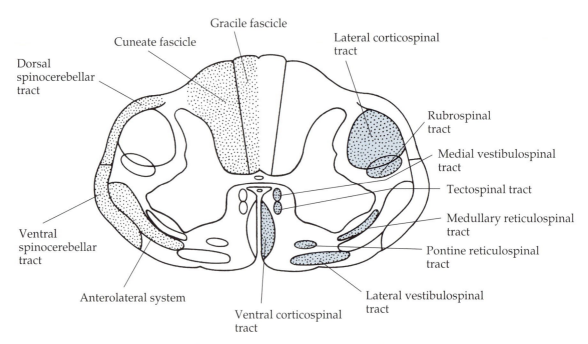

Figure 9–5. Schematic diagram of the spinal cord indicating the locations of the ascending *(left)* and descending *(right)* pathways.

Motor Regions of the Cerebral Cortex Are Located in the Frontal Lobe

In Chapters 5 through 8, we learned that each sensory modality is represented at multiple cortical sites. Motor systems are similarly organized, with multiple regions of the frontal lobe serving motor control functions (Figure 9–6A). Four separate motor areas have been identified: the primary motor cortex, the supplementary motor area (SMA), premotor cortex, and cingulate motor area (Figure 9–6). In the monkey, these areas have been carefully studied and many of them have been shown to consist of distinct subregions.

The **primary motor cortex** (Figure 9–6) gives rise to most of the fibers in the corticospinal tracts and has a complete and somatotopically organized body representation (see below). It plays a key role in the execution of skilled movement. We find the primary motor cortex in the caudal part of the **precentral gyrus**, extending from the lateral sulcus to the medial surface of the cerebral hemisphere, in cytoarchitectonic **area 4**. The **premotor cortical regions** are located rostral to the primary motor cortex. These areas, which include the **supplementary motor area**, the **premotor cortex**, and the **cingulate motor area** (Figure 9–6), are believed to help us plan our movements.

The traditional view of the anatomical organization of the various frontal motor areas stresses the spinal projections of the primary motor cortex. However, we now know from research conducted in monkeys, which have motor systems similar to those of humans, that many of the premotor cortical areas have dense spinal projections. In fact, the density of corticospinal neurons in parts of these premotor regions may be as great as that of corticospinal neurons in the primary motor cortex! An important challenge is to determine the respective roles of the projections of the different frontal motor areas to the spinal cord.

Insights into the function of the motor regions of the frontal lobe have come from examining the motor capacity of patients who have sustained damage to these areas from stroke and other trauma. Damage to the primary motor cortex produces profound weakness of the body part represented at the site of the stroke. Such lesions also produce changes in muscle tone (see below). This suggests that the primary motor cortex is important in the direct production of movements. Lesions of the premotor cortical regions produce complex movement disorders. When weakness occurs, it is never as severe as with primary motor cortical damage.

The Premotor Cortical Regions Integrate Information From Diverse Sources

The **supplementary motor area** is located primarily on the **medial surface** of the cerebral hemisphere, in area 6 (Figure 9–6). Its major subcortical input arises from the **ventral anterior nucleus** of the thalamus, through which a major portion of the basal ganglia projects. One key cortical input is from the prefrontal cortex, which we saw earlier is important in the highest level of planning motor behavior. A supplementary motor area lesion, such as might occur after infarction of a branch of the anterior cerebral artery (see Chapter 4, Figure 4–8B), impairs the combined use of both hands for purposeful movements, suggesting an important role in **bimanual coordination**.

The **premotor cortex** is located **laterally** in area 6 (Figure 9–6A). There are at least two distinct motor fields within the premotor cortex (Figure 9–6A): the dorsal and ventral premotor cortices. In contrast to the supplementary motor area, which gets its input from the basal ganglia, the premotor cortex receives its major input from the **cerebellum**, relayed by the **ventral lateral nucleus** of the thalamus. Parts of the premotor cortex have a major descending projection to the **reticular formation**. This path may be important for controlling the actions of girdle muscles by a projection to neurons that give rise to the **reticulospinal tracts**. Dorsal premotor cortex lesions, for example by infarction of cortical branches of the middle cerebral artery, alter the normal sequence of muscle activation during movement, producing defective rhythmical movements, such as the action of pedaling a bicycle. This suggests a role in **interjoint coordination**. Based on examining motor defects after lesion, we have no insight into the function of the ventral premotor cortex. This is because a lesion here also involves the motor cortex.

We find the **cingulate motor area** on the **medial surface** of the cerebral hemisphere, in cytoarchitectonic areas 6, 23, and 24 deep within the cingulate sulcus (Figure 9–6B). Curiously, this motor area, which in the monkey comprises three separate subfields, is located in a cortical gyrus that we consider part of the system for emotions (limbic system). It is not known if this motor area plays a preferential role in regulating motor behaviors triggered, for example, by emotions, motivation, and drives.

The Primary Motor Cortex Gives Rise to Most of the Fibers of the Corticospinal Tract

The primary motor cortex receives input from three major sources: the premotor cortical regions, the somatic sensory areas, and the thalamus. These input pathways transmit neural control signals that motor cortical neurons integrate to produce accurately directed voluntary movements.

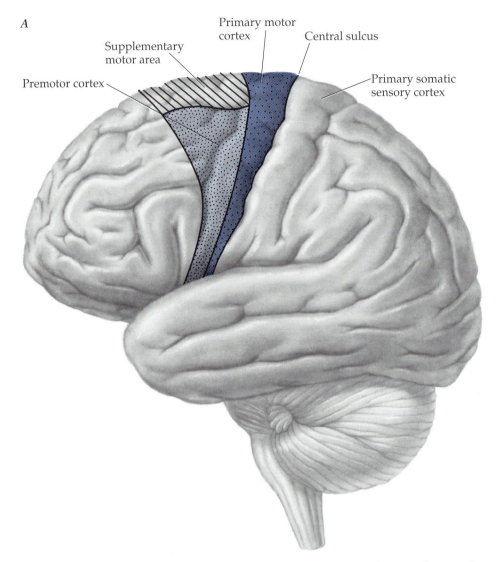

Figure 9–6. Lateral *(A)* and medial *(B)* views of the human brain, indicating the locations of the primary motor cortex, premotor cortex, supplementary motor area, and the cingulate motor area. The primary somatic sensory cortex is also shown.

As we saw earlier, premotor cortical regions receive input from diverse cortical and subcortical sources and project both subcortically and to the primary motor cortex. The somatic sensory cortical areas (primary, secondary, and higher-order areas) have privileged access to the primary motor cortex. Other sensory cortical areas do not. This may be because somatic sensory information is essential to coordinate and guide movements. Thalamic input to the primary motor cortex comes primarily from the **ventral lateral nucleus** (see Figure 9–10A), the principal thalamic relay nucleus for the **cerebellum**. The motor cortex also receives input from the basal ganglia, relayed by the **ventral anterior nucleus**. Thus, the cerebellum and basal ganglia can influence the motor cortex by two separate routes: through direct thalamic projections to motor cortex and through corticocortical projections from the premotor cortex and the supplementary motor areas, respectively.

B

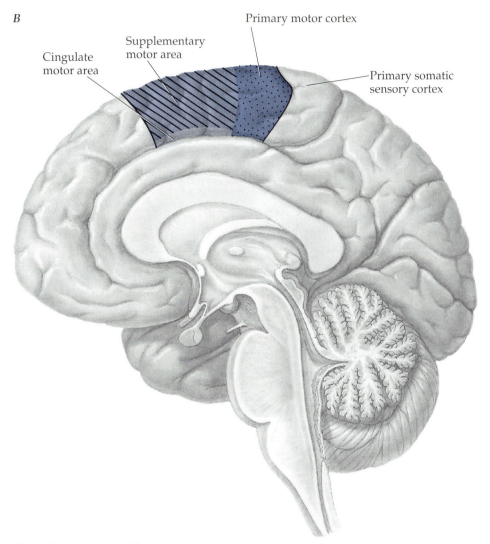

Cingulate
motor area

Supplementary
motor area

Primary motor cortex

Primary somatic
sensory cortex

Figure 9–6.   (continued)

The cytoarchitecture of the primary motor cortex is different from that of sensory areas in the parietal, temporal, and occipital lobes (see Figure 3–16). Whereas the sensory areas have a thick layer 4 and a thin layer 5, the motor cortex has a **thin layer 4** and **thick layer 5**. Recall that layer 4 is the principal input layer of the cerebral cortex, where most of the axons from the thalamic relay nuclei terminate, and that layer 5 is the layer from which descending projections originate. In the motor areas, thalamic terminations have a wider laminar distribution than sensory areas.

The cytoarchitecture of the primary motor cortex is further distinguished from that of other motor areas by **Betz cells**, which are large pyramidal cells in layer 5. Betz cells are the largest neurons in the mammalian central nervous system. They were once thought to be the only cortical neuron to project to the spinal cord. However, there are only about 30,000 to 40,000 Betz cells in the precentral gyrus on one side of the brain, whereas there are about one million axons in one medullary pyramid. This difference suggests that other cortical neurons contribute axons to the corticospinal tracts.

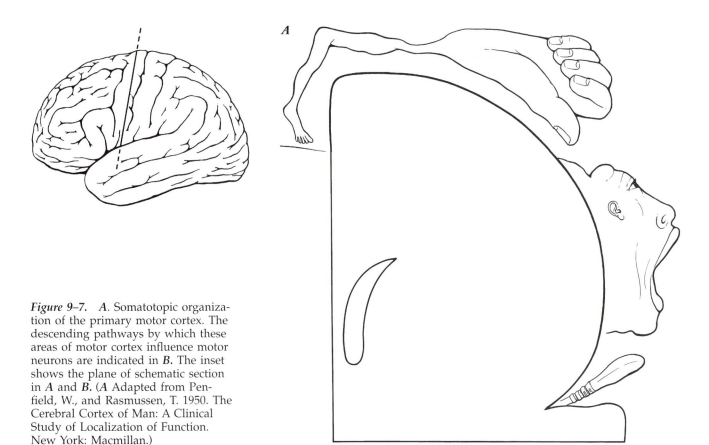

Figure 9–7. *A.* Somatotopic organization of the primary motor cortex. The descending pathways by which these areas of motor cortex influence motor neurons are indicated in *B.* The inset shows the plane of schematic section in *A* and *B.* (*A* Adapted from Penfield, W., and Rasmussen, T. 1950. The Cerebral Cortex of Man: A Clinical Study of Localization of Function. New York: Macmillan.)

We can answer the question of which motor cortex neurons project to the spinal cord by using a retrograde tracer, for example, horseradish peroxidase (see Chapter 1). Tracer injected into the spinal cord gray matter is taken up by the axon terminals of cortical neurons that project into the injected region of the cord. The substance is then retrogradely transported back to the cell bodies. This experimental approach has shown that in addition to the larger Betz cells, smaller pyramidal cells in layer 5 project to the spinal cord. These tracer studies have also shown that primary motor cortex, premotor cortical regions, and somatic sensory areas in the parietal lobe project to the spinal cord.

The primary motor cortex, like the somatic sensory cortex (see Chapter 5) is somatotopically organized (Figure 9–7A). In motor cortex, somatotopy is revealed by electrical stimulation of the cortical surface, a procedure often used during neurosurgery. Stimulation evokes contraction of individual and groups of muscles. This approach has shown that regions controlling facial muscles (through projections to the cranial nerve motor nuclei) are located in the lateral portion of the precentral gyrus, close to the lateral sulcus. Regions controlling other body parts are, from lateral to medial: neck, arm, and trunk areas. We find the leg and foot areas on the medial surface of the brain. The motor representation in the precentral gyrus forms the **motor homunculus;** it is distorted in a similar way as the **sensory homunculus** of the postcentral gyrus (see Figure 5–19).

Magnetic resonance imaging (MRI), typically used to probe brain structure, can also be used as a noninvasive tool to image brain function. This technique, termed **functional MRI,** has recently been used to eluci-

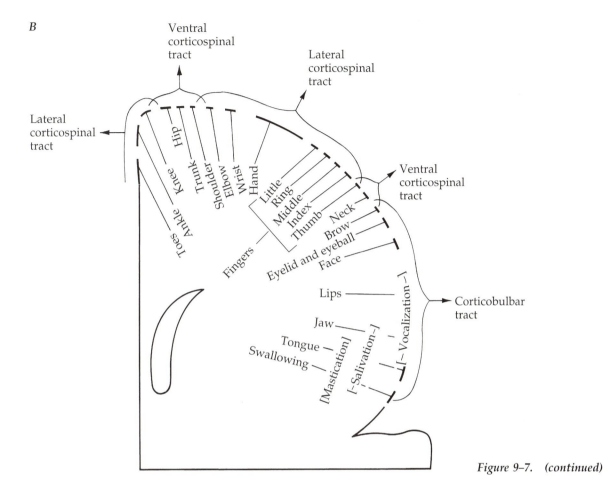

Figure 9–7. (continued)

date the somatotopic organization of the human motor cortex. Functional MRI can detect minute changes in **deoxyhemoglobin** concentration that result from changes in neural activity. Neural activation results in an increase in local blood flow and a decrease in capillary and venous deoxyhemogloblin concentrations. Functional MRI thereby provides a map of the distribution of brain regions that are active while the image is obtained. Figure 9–8 shows an example of two functional MR images of the motor cortex while the person made simple movements. In part A, the person alternated between making hand and foot movements. As predicted from the homunculus obtained by electrical stimulation, a horizontal functional MRI slice through the cortex shows that hand movements produced an active area in the lateral precentral gyrus, and foot movements, in the medial precentral gyrus, within the interhemispheric fissure. In part B, the person made repetitive oppositional movement of the thumb and each of the remaining four fingers. This resulted in activation only on the lateral convexity of the precentral gyrus. These simple examples illustrate how noninvasive imaging tools can be used to probe basic brain functions. Functional imaging tools, like MRI or PET, are also being used to examine more complex aspects of cortical motor functions, such as what kinds of movements produce changes in the different premotor and motor regions.

Within the representations of the individual major body parts in motor cortex—face, arm, trunk, and leg—the somatotopic organization does not seem to be as precise as that in the primary somatic sensory cor-

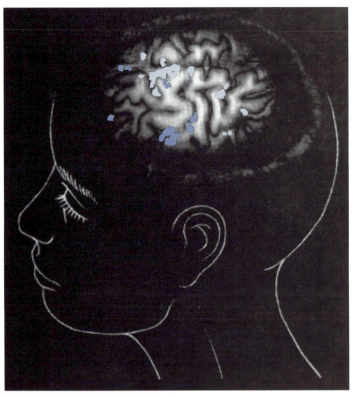

A

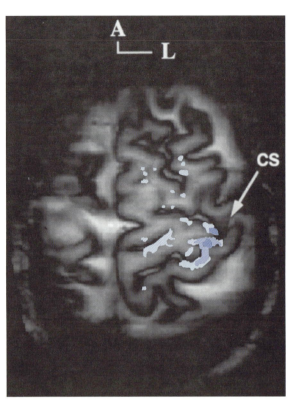

B

Figure 9–8. Functional imaging of human motor cortex. **A.** Horizontal slice through the cerebral hemispheres while the person made alternating hand and foot movements. Increased neural activity, as monitored by changes in deoxyhemogloblin detected by the MRI scan, occurred laterally (dark blue)—corresponding to the hand area—and medially, within the interhemispheric fissure (light blue)—corresponding to the foot area. **B.** Horizontal slice obtained while the person made oppositional movements of thumb with the remaining digits. This task activated only the lateral motor cortex. The strength of activation is indicated by the depth of blue: light blue, weak activation; dark blue, strong activation. (Abbreviations: A, anterior; L, lateral; cs, central sulcus.) (**A.** Courtesy of Drs. S. G. Kim, J. Ashe, A.P. Georgopoulos, and K. Ugurbil; **B.** Courtesy of Drs. S. G. Kim, J. Ashe, A.P Georgopoulos and colleagues. 1993. J. Neurophysiol 69:297–302.)

tex. Studies in monkeys and other species suggest that the primary motor cortex may have an organization that is more complex than a somatotopic one. For example, muscles of a body part that act together to produce a particular motor behavior, such as reaching, may be represented together in a local cortical area.

Somatotopic organization means that different mediolateral regions of the primary motor cortex contribute differently to the three descending corticospinal paths (Figure 9–7B). As described above, limb muscles are preferentially controlled by the **lateral corticospinal tract**, and girdle and axial muscles by the **ventral corticospinal tract**. It follows that arm and leg areas contribute preferentially to the lateral corticospinal tract, and neck, shoulder, and trunk regions, to the ventral corticospinal tract. The face area of the motor cortex projects to the cranial nerve motor nuclei and thus contributes axons to the **corticobulbar projection** (see Chapter 13). In addition, the limb and trunk areas project to the reticular formation of the pons and medulla and dorsal column nuclei. This projection is sometimes considered part of the corticobulbar tract.

The Projection From Cortical Motor Regions Passes Through the Internal Capsule En Route to the Brain Stem and Spinal Cord

Descending axons from the various motor areas, but all originating from pyramidal neurons in layer 5, course in the **internal capsule**. The internal capsule, which is shaped like a curved fan (Figure 9–9), has three main parts: (1) the rostral component, termed the **anterior limb**; (2) the caudal component, termed the **posterior limb**; and (3) the **genu** (Latin, knee), which joins the two limbs. These three components can be seen in Figure 9–10A, which is a horizontal section through the diencephalon and cerebral hemispheres.

The anterior limb separates the caudate nucleus and the putamen, the two principal components of the striatum. The posterior limb separates the caudate nucleus and thalamus from the putamen. Ascending thalamocortical projections, termed **thalamic radiations**, are located in the internal capsule (Figure 9–10A). The projections from the ventral anterior and ventral lateral nuclei of the thalamus (Figure 9–10A) also course here. The ascending thalamocortical projections, together with descending corticopontine projections, form the bulk of the axons in the

Figure 9–9. Three-dimensional view of fibers in the white matter of the cerebral cortex. The regions corresponding to the internal capsule, basis pedunculi, and pyramid are indicated. The dashed line indicates the approximate plane of section in Figure 9–13A. (Adapted from Carpenter, M. B., and Sutin, J. 1983. Human Neuroanatomy. Baltimore: Williams & Wilkins.)

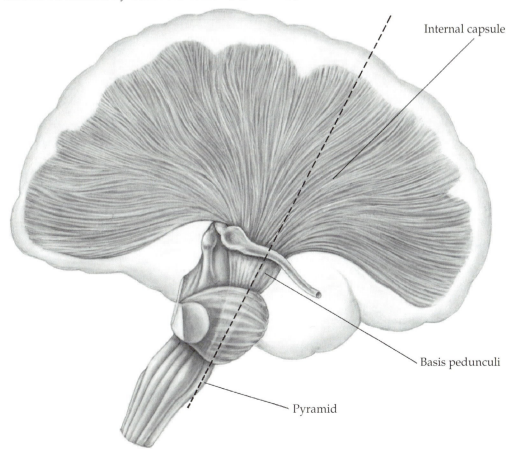

Internal capsule

Basis pedunculi

Pyramid

various parts of the internal capsule. The descending motor projection to the spinal cord courses in the posterior limb (labeled A, T, and L for projections controlling muscles of the arm, trunk, and leg in Figure 9–10A), whereas the projection to the caudal brain stem—via the corticobulbar tract—descends in the genu (labeled F for face in Figure 9–10A). The entire internal capsule appears to condense to form the **basis pedunculi** of the midbrain (Figure 9–10B). Because the internal capsule contains both ascending thalamocortical fibers and descending cortical fibers, it is larger than the basis pedunculi, which contains only descending fibers.

The Corticospinal Tract Courses in the Base of the Midbrain

Each division of the brain stem contains three regions from its dorsal to ventral surfaces: **tectum**, **tegmentum**, and **base** (see Chapter 3).

Figure 9–10. *A.* Myelin-stained horizontal section through the internal capsule. Note how the thalamus extends rostrally as far as the genu. The head of the caudate nucleus and the putamen are separated by the anterior limb of the internal capsule. The fiber constituents and somatotopic organization of the internal capsule are indicated. The *arrow* indicates the plane of section shown in Figure 9–13A. *B.* Myelin-stained transverse section through the rostral midbrain. The composition of axons in the basis pedunculi and the somatotopic organization of the corticospinal fibers are shown on right. (Abbreviations: F, face; A, arm; T, trunk; L, leg.) The inset shows the planes of section.

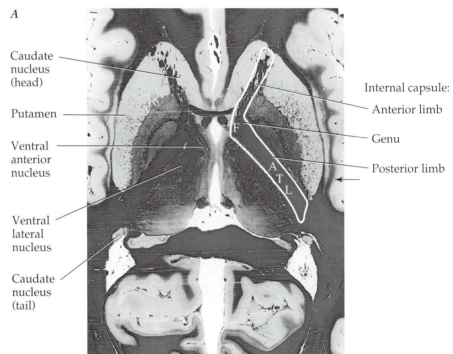

A

Caudate nucleus (head)

Putamen

Ventral anterior nucleus

Ventral lateral nucleus

Caudate nucleus (tail)

Internal capsule:

Anterior limb

Genu

Posterior limb

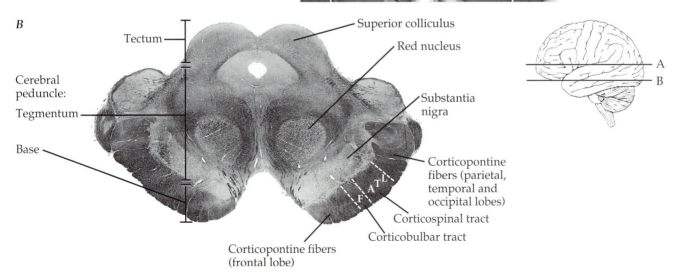

B

Tectum

Cerebral peduncle:

Tegmentum

Base

Superior colliculus

Red nucleus

Substantia nigra

Corticopontine fibers (parietal, temporal and occipital lobes)

Corticospinal tract

Corticobulbar tract

Corticopontine fibers (frontal lobe)

A

B

The tectum is well developed only in the midbrain and, in the rostral midbrain (Figure 9–10B), the tectum consists of the **superior colliculus**. The midbrain base is termed the **basis pedunculi** (or crus cerebri). Together, the tegmentum and basis pedunculi constitute the **cerebral peduncle**.

Corticospinal tract axons course within the basis pedunculi where they are somatotopically organized (Figure 9–10B). Coursing within the middle of the basis pedunculi, the corticospinal fibers are flanked medially and laterally by corticopontine axons (see Chapter 10). Figure 9–11 shows that although some repositioning occurs between the descending fibers in the internal capsule and in the basis pedunculi, the fibers maintain the same spatial interrelations and mediolateral relations.

The rostral midbrain is a key level in the motor system because three nuclei that subserve motor function are located in the midbrain tegmentum: the superior colliculus, the red nucleus, and the substantia

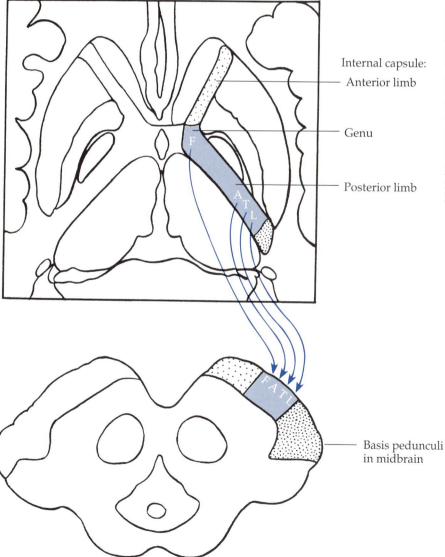

Internal capsule:

— Anterior limb

— Genu

— Posterior limb

— Basis pedunculi
   in midbrain

Figure 9–11. The relationship between descending fibers in the internal capsule *(top)* and the basis pedunculi *(bottom)*. The anterior limb of the internal capsule contains fronto-pontine fibers and fibers projecting to the brain stem. The caudal part of the posterior limb contains parieto-, temporo-, and occipitopontine fibers as well as a brain stem projection. These schematic drawings correspond to the sections shown in Figure 9–10. Note that the bottom section is inverted dorso-ventrally relative to Figure 9–10B.

nigra. Neurons from the deeper layers of the **superior colliculus** (Figure 9–10; see Figure 6–7) give rise to the **tectospinal tract**, one of the medial descending pathways. The **red nucleus** (Figures 9–10B, 9–13A) is the origin of the **rubrospinal tract**, a lateral descending pathway that begins at the **magnocellular portion** of this nucleus. The tectospinal and rubrospinal tracts cross over in the midbrain near the level of their origins, in the dorsal tegmental and ventral tegmental decussations, respectively. The **substantia nigra** is a part of the basal ganglia (see Chapter 11). Neurons in this nucleus that contain the neurotransmitter dopamine degenerate in Parkinson's disease.

Descending Cortical Fibers Separate Into Small Fascicles in the Ventral Pons

Sections through the pons reveal that the descending cortical fibers no longer occupy the ventral brain stem surface, but rather are located deep within the base of the pons. The characteristic appearance of these fibers in the midbrain, as a discrete tract that is clearly separated from nuclei of the tegmentum, is no longer present in the rostral pons (Figure 9–12). The compact group of descending cortical fibers divides into many small fascicles, each separated from the other by the pontine nuclei and the efferent axons of these nuclei, the pontocerebellar fibers.

The pontine nuclei receive their principal input from the cerebral cortex via fibers that descend in the anterior and posterior limbs of the internal capsule and through the basis pedunculi (Figures 9–10B and 9–11). The corticopontine projection is an important path by which information from all cerebral cortex lobes influences the cerebellum (see Chapter 10). In the caudal pons, fewer separate fascicles are apparent because the corticopontine axons have terminated in the pontine nuclei (see Figure 9–14B1). Box 9–1 shows the course of the descending cortical axons in the internal capsule, basis pedunculi, and pons in the human.

Figure 9–12. Myelin-stained transverse section through the rostral pons. The inset shows the plane of section.

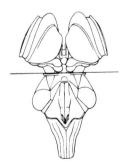

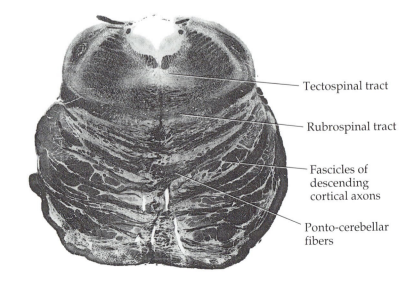

Tectospinal tract

Rubrospinal tract

Fascicles of descending cortical axons

Ponto-cerebellar fibers

The Vestibular Nuclei Are Located in the Dorsal Pons and Medulla

The four vestibular nuclei are the first central nervous system relays for the vestibular labyrinth, the group of cranial sensory structures that contain receptors sensitive to head position and movement (see Chapter 7). Together, these four nuclei (Figure 9–14A) play an essential role in maintaining balance and head position by controlling axial and girdle muscles via the vestibulospinal tracts. The **lateral vestibulospinal tract**, an ipsilateral descending pathway that projects to all levels of the spinal cord, originates from neurons in the **lateral vestibular nucleus** (also termed **Deiters' nucleus**). This pathway is important in maintaining balance.

The **medial vestibulospinal tract**, a bilateral tract that descends only as far as the cervical segments, originates primarily from neurons in the **medial vestibular nucleus**, with a lesser contribution from the **superior** and **inferior vestibular nuclei**. The tract is important in neck muscle control. As the caudal extension of the **medial longitudinal fasciculus** (MLF), the medial vestibulospinal tract is also known as the descending medial longitudinal fasciculus. The medial longitudinal fasciculus, which is located close to the midline (Figures 9–14B and 9–15), is a brain stem pathway that contains axons from numerous sources that are crucial for controlling eye movements (see Chapter 13). Lesions of this pathway (or the nuclear regions contributing axons to it) produce characteristic deficits in eye movements. All four vestibular nuclei also contribute ascending axons to the medial longitudinal fasciculus. Note that the tectospinal tract, which coordinates head movements with eye movements, is located ventral to the medial longitudinal fasciculus (Figure 9–14B1). Like the medial vestibulospinal tract, the tectospinal tract descends only as far as the cervical spinal cord.

Neurons in the pontine and medullary reticular formation (Figure 9–14A) give rise to the **pontine** and **medullary reticulospinal tracts**. Whereas some fibers of the reticulospinal tracts originate from discrete nuclei, most fibers arise from neurons scattered in the medial tegmentum of the pons and medulla. We think the reticulospinal tracts control relatively automatic motor responses, such as stepping when we walk and postural adjustments. When these automatic responses must occur during voluntary movements, such as maintaining an upright posture when we reach to lift something heavy, we think that the corticoreticulospinal path is engaged.

The reticular formation and the intermediate zone of the spinal cord share two features. First, their locations are similar, forming the central region of the brain stem and spinal cord gray matter. Second, both the reticular formation and the intermediate zone contain neurons that have a widespread projection pattern that often includes an axon with both an ascending and a descending branch.

What is the significance of this morphological pattern? Individual neurons can distribute information both to lower levels of the motor systems that are directly involved in executing movements, and to higher levels that are thought to be involved in the adaptation and correction of ongoing movements. In the intermediate zone, neurons with this morphology can transmit information to motor neurons, for commanding muscles to contract, and to brain stem nuclei, that are important for integrating sensory and motor information. In the reticular formation, neurons can transmit information both to the spinal motor nuclei and to rostral brain stem and diencephalic integrative centers. Because of these similarities, we consider the reticular formation to be the rostral extension of the intermediate zone.

Box 9–1. Magnetic Resonance Imaging of Degeneration in the Descending Cortical Projection

The major descending projections from the cerebral cortex include the corticospinal, corticobulbar, and corticopontine tracts. The path that these fibers take in their descent through the cerebral hemisphere and brain stem is revealed on magnetic resonance imaging (MRI) scans from a patient who suffered from a lesion of the internal capsule.

For orientation, the myelin-stained section in Figure 9–13A is approximately in the same plane as the MRI scan in Figure 9–13B1. This myelin-stained section is through the **posterior limb** of the internal capsule. (The approximate level of this section is indicated by the arrow in Figure 9–10A.) The descending cortical pathway can be followed from rostral to

caudal: posterior limb of the internal capsule, basis pedunculi, and medullary pyramids.

In the MRI scan, we see a discrete lesion in the posterior limb of the internal capsule, just lateral to the ventricle. The lesion produces a bright spot (i.e., hyperintense signal) on the image. This scan also shows axons that are undergoing Wallerian degeneration (see Chap-

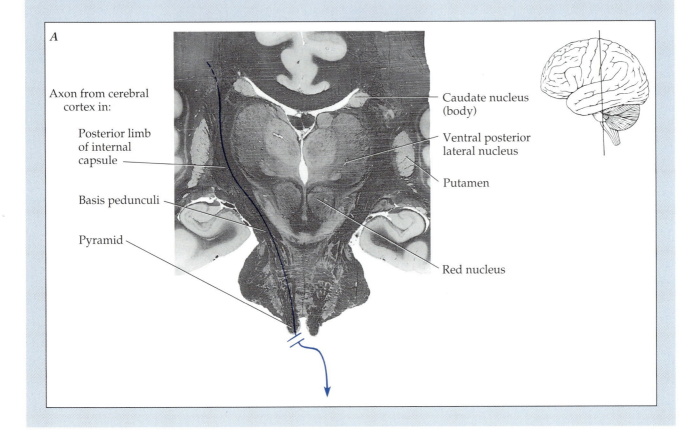

A

Axon from cerebral cortex in:

Posterior limb of internal capsule

Basis pedunculi

Pyramid

Caudate nucleus (body)

Ventral posterior lateral nucleus

Putamen

Red nucleus

The Lateral Corticospinal Tract Decussates in the Caudal Medulla

The path of the descending cortical fibers into the medulla can be followed in the sagittal section shown in Figure 9–15. The numerous fascicles of the caudal pons collect on the ventral surface of the medulla to form the **pyramids** (Figures 9–15 and 9–16). The axons of the lateral and ventral corticospinal tracts, which originated from the **ipsilateral frontal**

Box 9–1 (continued)

ter 1). Streaming caudally from the lesion, farther down the posterior limb of the internal capsule, are **degenerating axons**, which also produce a hyperintense signal on the MRI. Although a bit more subtle,

these degenerating axons can be followed through the midbrain and into the pons. Compare the configurations of the MRI slices through these two brain stem levels with their myelin-stained counterparts

(Figures 9–13B2 and 9–13B3). In the last section of this chapter, we consider the common causes of damage to the descending cortical projection and the neurological signs that the damage produces.

Figure 9–13. Descending cortical projection paths. *A.* Myelin-stained coronal section through the posterior limb of the internal capsule. Note that the component of the internal capsule is identified as the posterior limb in this section because the thalamus is located medial to the internal capsule. *B1.*

Magnetic resonance imaging (MRI) scan from a patient with an internal capsule lesion. Coronal slice through the posterior limb of the internal capsule showing bright vertically oriented band extending from the lesion caudally into the pons. This band corresponds to degenerated axons in the internal

capsule, basis pedunculi, and pons. *B2.* Transverse slice through the midbrain (horizontal slice through cerebral hemispheres) showing site of degeneration. *B3.* Same as *B2* but through the pons and cerebellum. (Courtesy of Dr. Jesús Pujol; from Pujol et al. 1990. Stroke 21:404–409.)

B1

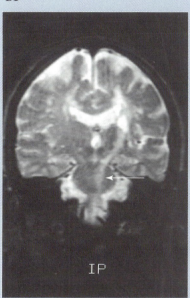

B2

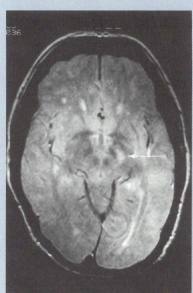

B3

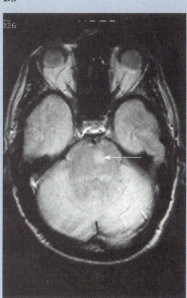

lobe, are located in each pyramid. This is why the terms **corticospinal tract** and **pyramidal tract** are often—and inaccurately—used interchangeably. These terms are *not* synonymous because the pyramids also contain **corticobulbar fibers** that terminate in the medulla.

The pyramidal decussation (i.e., decussation of the lateral corticospinal tract) is seen in Figure 9–16B. Note that the decussation of internal arcuate fibers (see Chapter 5) occurs rostral (Figure 9–16A) to that of

A

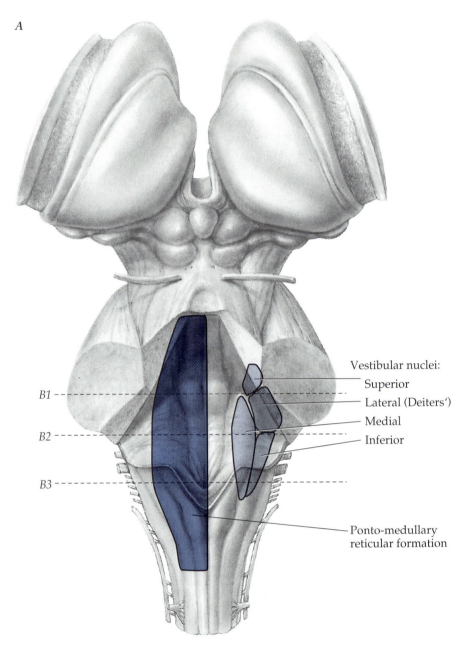

Vestibular nuclei:

Superior

Lateral (Deiters')

Medial

Inferior

Ponto-medullary reticular formation

B1

B2

B3

Figure 9–14. **A.** Locations of the vestibular nuclei *(right)* and pontomedullary reticular formation *(left)* are shown in this dorsal view of the brain stem with the cerebellum removed. **B.** Three myelin-stained transverse sections through the pons and medulla *(B1–B3)*. Note that the medial longitudinal fasciculus and central tegmental tract are only labeled in part *B1* but are present in parts *B2–B4.*

the lateral corticospinal tract. The positions of the other descending pathways are also indicated in Figure 9–16. The rubrospinal tract, which is located **dorsolaterally** in the brain stem, joins the lateral corticospinal tract at the medulla–spinal cord junction and descends in the lateral column (Figure 9–5). In contrast, the vestibulospinal tracts, the reticulospinal tracts, and the tectospinal tract remain medial and assume a more ventral position as they descend in the spinal cord.

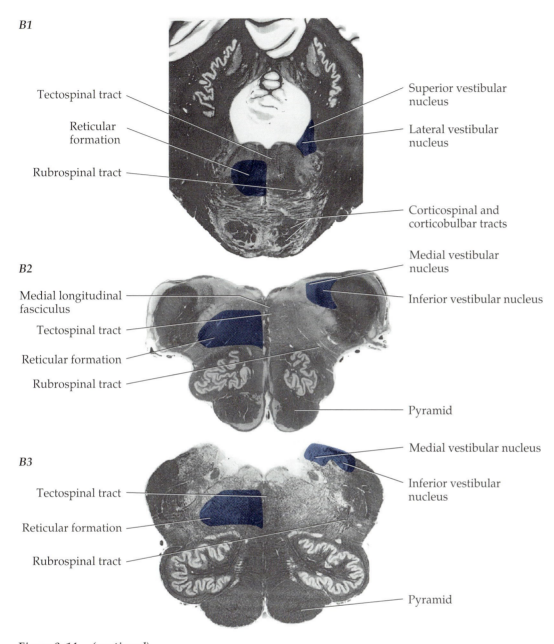

B1

Tectospinal tract

Reticular formation

Rubrospinal tract

Superior vestibular nucleus

Lateral vestibular nucleus

Corticospinal and corticobulbar tracts

Medial vestibular nucleus

B2

Medial longitudinal fasciculus

Tectospinal tract

Reticular formation

Rubrospinal tract

Inferior vestibular nucleus

Pyramid

B3

Tectospinal tract

Reticular formation

Rubrospinal tract

Medial vestibular nucleus

Inferior vestibular nucleus

Pyramid

Figure 9–14.   (continued)

The Intermediate Zone and Ventral Horn of the Spinal Cord Receive Input From the Descending Pathways

The motor pathways descend in the ventral and lateral columns of the spinal cord (Figure 9–5). The lateral corticospinal tract is located in the lateral column. The section in Figure 9–17 was taken at autopsy from the lumbosacral enlargement of an individual who had a lesion of the internal capsule at some time prior to death. The lateral corticospinal tract corresponds to the lightly stained region, showing degeneration. (Note that the ventral corticospinal tract descends only as far as the cervical spinal cord. Thus, there are no degenerating fibers in the ventral column.) Part A shows a section from a normal individual for comparison.

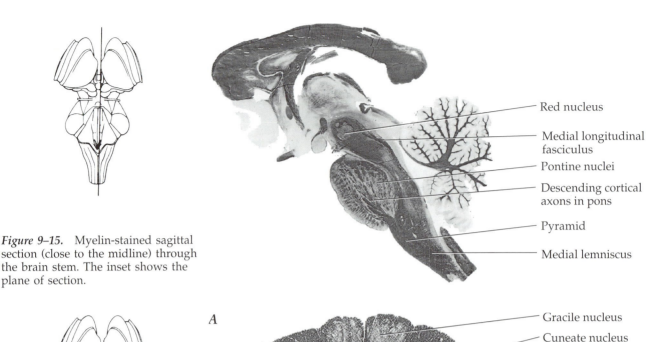

Figure 9–15. Myelin-stained section (close to the midline) through the brain stem. The inset shows the plane of section.

Red nucleus

Medial longitudinal fasciculus

Pontine nuclei

Descending cortical axons in pons

Pyramid

Medial lemniscus

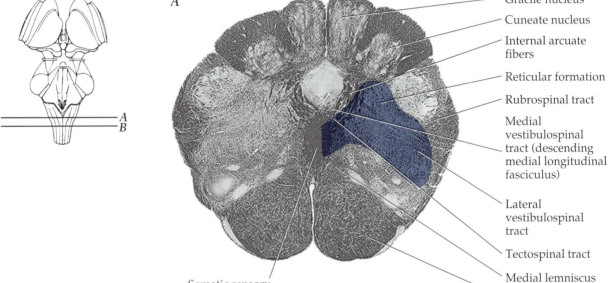

A

Gracile nucleus

Cuneate nucleus

Internal arcuate fibers

Reticular formation

Rubrospinal tract

Medial vestibulospinal tract (descending medial longitudinal fasciculus)

Lateral vestibulospinal tract

Tectospinal tract

Medial lemniscus

Pyramid

Somatic sensory decussation

B

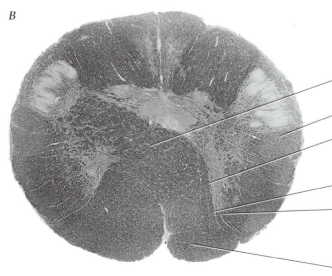

Pyramidal decussation

Rubrospinal tract

Medial vestibulospinal tract

Tectospinal tract

Lateral vestibulospinal tract and reticulospinal tract

Pyramid

Figure 9–16. Myelin-stained transverse sections through the decussation of the internal arcuate fibers, or "somatic sensory decussation" *(A)*, and the pyramidal or "motor" decussation *(B)*. The reticular formation is highlighted in part *A.* The inset shows the planes of sections.

A

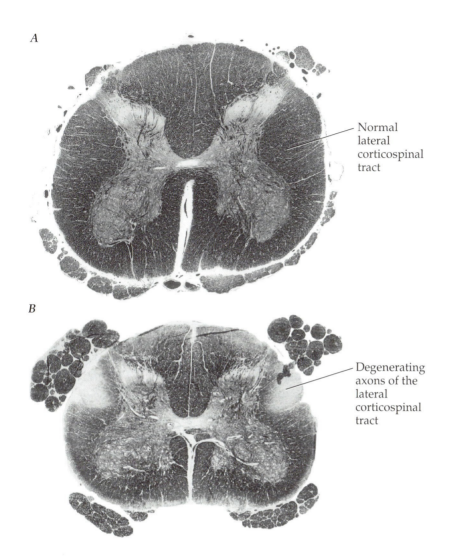

Normal
lateral
corticospinal
tract

B

Degenerating
axons of the
lateral
corticospinal
tract

Figure 9–17. Myelin-stained section through the lumbar spinal cord from a normal individual (*A*) and from an individual who suffered from an internal capsule lesion before death (*B*). Region showing degeneration in the lateral column (lightly stained) corresponds to the location of the lateral corticospinal tract.

The motor pathways, including the corticospinal tracts, synapse on motor neurons in the ventral horn and on segmental interneurons and propriospinal neurons in the intermediate zone (Figure 9–18). As we saw in Chapter 5 (see Table 5–1), the dorsal horn corresponds to Rexed's laminae 1 through 6, the intermediate zone to lamina 7, and the ventral horn to laminae 8 and 9. Lamina 10 surrounds the spinal cord central canal. While both the primary motor cortex and the primary somatic sensory cortex project to the spinal cord, their target laminae differ. The somatic sensory cortex projects dorsally in the gray matter—preferentially to the dorsal horn—and could regulate sensory processing. The motor cortex, on the other hand, projects ventrally to the intermediate zone and ventral horn to regulate directly motor neuron excitability.

Earlier we saw that the pathways that descend in the medial portion of the spinal cord white matter terminate in the medial portions of the intermediate zone and ventral horn. These regions of the spinal cord gray matter contain the neuronal machinery for controlling **girdle and axial muscles**. Propriospinal neurons in the medial intermediate zone have long axons that project to many spinal cord segments, up to the entire length of the spinal cord. Many of these neurons (as well as some segmental interneurons) have an axon branch that decussates in the ven-

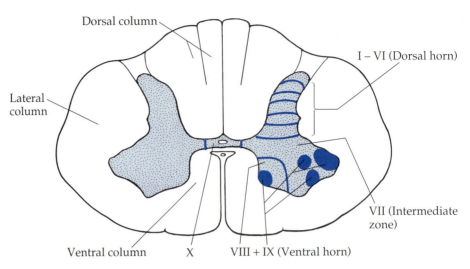

Figure 9–18. Schematic drawing of the general organization of the spinal cord gray matter and white matter.

tral commissure of the spinal cord. This pattern of connectivity is thought to provide the anatomical linkages for the **coordinated contraction of axial and girdle muscles during postural adjustments.** In contrast, the lateral descending pathways terminate in the lateral parts of the intermediate zone and ventral horn, where neurons controlling **distal limb muscles** are located. Propriospinal neurons located laterally have short axons that course only a few segments.

Motor neurons, propriospinal neurons, and segmental interneurons, in addition to receiving input from the descending pathways, receive sensory input from the various functional categories of primary afferent fibers. Reflexes are mediated by this afferent input. Motor neurons receive monosynaptic input from only one functional afferent fiber category, group 1a (or A-α) fibers (see Table 5–1), which carry action potentials from the **primary muscle spindle receptors** to the spinal cord. This monosynaptic input is the basis of the knee-jerk reflex (see Chapter 3; Figure 3–2).

Segmental interneurons and propriospinal neurons receive monosynaptic input from virtually all afferent fiber classes: mechanoreceptors, thermoreceptors, and nociceptors. This difference in the patterns of afferent input onto motor neurons, interneurons, and propriospinal neurons is significant. Information from the primary muscle spindle receptors has privileged access to the motor neurons. In contrast, other sensory input to motor neurons can be regulated by the brain by adjusting the excitability of interneurons that transmit this information to the motor neurons.

The Lateral and Medial Motor Nuclei Have Different Rostrocaudal Distributions

Motor neurons in the cervical enlargement (which corresponds to C5–T1 in the human spinal cord) and in the lumbosacral enlargement (L1–S2) innervate distal limb muscles (lateral motor nuclei) as well as girdle and axial muscles (medial motor nuclei) (Figure 9–19). Between approximately T2 and T12 (Figure 9–19B), and at the extreme rostral and caudal poles of the spinal cord, we find only medial motor nuclei. There is a simple way of understanding the rostrocaudal organization of the

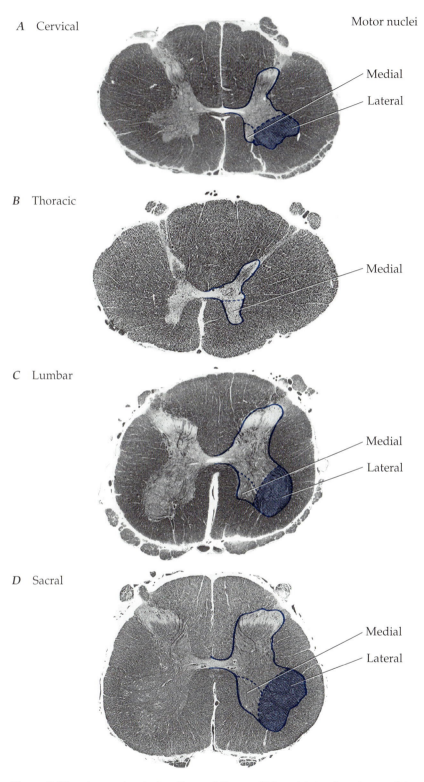

A Cervical

Motor nuclei

Medial

Lateral

B Thoracic

Medial

C Lumbar

Medial

Lateral

D Sacral

Medial

Lateral

Figure 9–19. Approximate locations of the medial and lateral motor nuclei are shown at four spinal cord levels: cervical *(A)*, thoracic *(B)*, lumbar *(C)*, and sacral *(D)*.

motor nuclei. Both the medial and lateral motor nuclei form separate columns consisting of adjacent motor nuclei extending rostrocaudally in the spinal cord. The column formed by the medial motor nuclei is **continuous**, running from the upper cervical to the lower sacral segments. In contrast, the column formed by the lateral motor nuclei is **interrupted**, present only in the cervical and lumbosacral enlargements.

In the spinal cord, autonomic preganglionic motor neurons are also arranged in a column (see Chapter 14) and, together with the motor nuclei, have a three-dimensional organization that is similar to that of the brain stem cranial nerve nuclei columns (see Chapters 2 and 12). The longitudinal organization of the somatic and autonomic motor nuclei and the cranial nerve nuclei underscores the common architecture of the spinal cord and brain stem (see Chapter 2, section on spinal cord and brain stem development).

Lesions of the Descending Cortical Pathway in the Brain and Spinal Cord Produce Flaccid Paralysis Followed by Spasticity

Lesions involving the posterior limb of the internal capsule, ventral brain stem, and spinal cord release motor neurons from their normal voluntary control, producing a common set of motor signs. Initially these signs include **flaccid paralysis** and **reduced myotatic reflexes** (e.g., the knee-jerk reflex). Clinical examination reveals **decreased muscle tone**, signaled by the marked reduction in resistance felt by the examiner to passive movement of the limb. Even though the corticoreticular and corticopontine fibers are damaged, these signs are attributable largely to interruption of the corticospinal fibers.

A few weeks after the occurrence of the lesion, a similar examination reveals **increased muscle tone** and **exaggerated myotatic reflexes.** The increased muscle tone is due to increased reflex activity when the limb is in motion. This is termed **spasticity**. Spasticity is thought to result from damage of pathways other than the corticospinal tract, for example, the corticoreticular tract. This is because in animal experiments selective damage of the pyramid in the caudal medulla produces decreased, not increased, muscle tone.

In addition to producing spasticity, lesions of the descending cortical projection pathway result in the emergence of abnormal reflexes, the most notable of which is the **Babinski sign**. This sign involves dorsiflexion of the big toe in response to scratching the lateral margin and ball of the foot. The Babinski sign is thought to be a withdrawal reflex. Normally such withdrawal of the big toe is produced by scratching its ventral surface. After damage to the descending cortical fibers, the reflex can be evoked from a much larger area than normal. In addition to extension of the big toe, scratching the lateral margin of the foot also produces fanning of the other toes. Hoffman's sign, which is thumb adduction in response to flexion of the distal phalanx of the third digit, is an example of an abnormal upper limb reflex caused by damage to the descending cortical fibers.

Occlusion of Deep Branches of the Middle Cerebral Artery Damages the Internal Capsule

Whereas damage to different portions of the descending motor pathways can produce similar effects on muscle tone, vascular lesions of the **internal capsule** are more common than lesions of the ventral brain

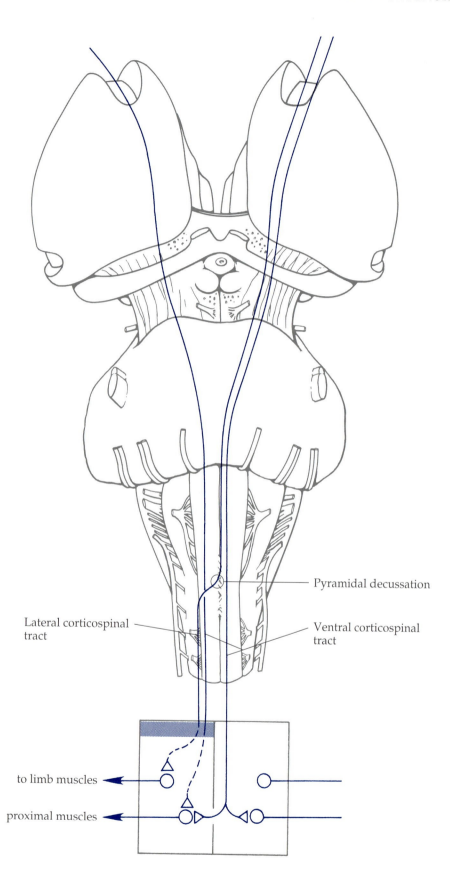

Lateral corticospinal
tract

Ventral corticospinal
tract

Pyramidal decussation

to limb muscles

proximal muscles

Figure 9–20. Brown–Séquard syndrome. Spinal cord hemisection produces motor and somatic sensory signs. This figure shows the cortical pathways producing motor signs; see Figure 5–9 for the effect of such a lesion on touch, position sense, vibration sense, pain, and temperature senses. The lateral descending pathways, which target distal limb muscle motor neurons, decussate in the medulla. In contrast, the medial descending pathways, which target proximal limb motor neurons, typically descend ipsilateraly and terminate bilaterally in the spinal cord. As a consequence of this pattern, spinal cord hemisection affects distal muscles on the ipsilateral limb and, to a much lesser extent, proximal and axial musculature.

stem and spinal cord. The arterial supply of the internal capsule is provided mainly by deep branches of the **middle cerebral artery** and, for the most inferior portions of the internal capsule, by the **anterior choroidal artery** (a large branch of the internal carotid artery) (see Figure 4–1). Small branches of these arteries commonly occlude and produce focal (laccunar) infarctions. Following even a small capsular infarction, it is rare for only the arm or leg to be affected. This is because the axons that descend from the arm and leg areas of the primary motor cortex, even though their cells of origin are widely separated in the cortex, converge within a small space in the posterior limb of the internal capsule (Figure 9–10A.)

Spinal Cord Hemisection Produces Ipsilateral Limb Motor Signs

In Chapter 5, we saw that spinal cord hemisection produces characteristic sensory deficits below the level of the lesion: a loss of **tactile sense**, **vibration sense**, and **limb position sense** on the **ipsilateral side** and loss of **pain and temperature sense** on the **contralateral side** (see Figure 5–9). These are the somatic sensory signs of the **Brown–Séquard syndrome**. Motor deficits are also a key feature of spinal cord hemisection (Figure 9–20). Initially, **flaccid paralysis** and **reduced myotatic (stretch) reflexes** occur in the limb innervated by motor neurons located caudal to the lesion. As with a capsular lesion, after a variable period of a few weeks **spastic paralysis** develops, the **Babinski sign** emerges, and **myotatic reflexes become exaggerated**. These effects are all expressed on the ipsilateral side because the lateral descending motor pathways decussate in the brain stem (Figure 9–20). Because the medial descending pathways terminate bilaterally, axial motor function is usually not seriously affected with unilateral spinal cord lesions.

Summary

Descending Pathways

There are six descending motor pathways that course in the white matter of the spinal cord (Figures 9–3 and 9–5; Table 9–1): **lateral corticospinal tract**, **rubrospinal tract**, **ventral corticospinal tract**, **reticulospinal tract** (which is further subdivided into separate medullary and pontine components), **vestibulospinal tract** (which is subdivided into separate medial and lateral components), and **tectospinal tract**. These pathways project directly on spinal motor neurons, through monosynaptic connections, and indirectly by synapsing first on segmental interneurons and propriospinal neurons.

Lateral Descending Systems

The locations of the descending axons in the spinal cord provide insight into their functions (Figures 9–2, 9–3, and 9–4). Those that control **limb muscles** descend in the **lateral column** of the spinal cord and terminate in the **lateral intermediate zone** and **lateral ventral horn** (Figures 9–2, 9–3, and 9–5). The **lateral corticospinal tract** and the **rubrospinal tract** are the two laterally descending pathways. In humans, the lateral corticospinal tract has more axons than the rubrospinal tract. The **primary motor cortex** (area 4), located on the precentral gyrus, contributes most of the fibers of the lateral corticospinal tract (Figures 9–6 and 9–7). (The other major contributors to the lateral corticospinal tract are the higher-order motor cortical regions located rostral to the primary motor

cortex, mainly in cytoarchitectonic **area 6** and the parietal lobe.) The descending projection neurons of the cortex are located in **layer 5** and their axons course through the **posterior limb of the internal capsule** (Figure 9–10A), then along the ventral brain stem surface (Figures 9–10B through 9–12 and 9–14). The lateral corticospinal tract decussates in the ventral medulla in the **pyramidal decussation**, at the junction of the medulla and the spinal cord (Figure 9–16B). In the spinal cord, the lateral corticospinal tract courses in the dorsal portion of the **lateral column** (Figures 9–5 and 9–17) and terminates in cervical and lumbosacral segments. The other laterally descending pathway, the **rubrospinal tract**, originates from the **magnocellular portion of the red nucleus** (Figure 9–10). The axons decussate in the midbrain, descend in the **dorsolateral portion of the brain stem and spinal cord** (Figures 9–3B and 9–5), and terminate in the cervical cord. The other division of the red nucleus, the **parvocellular** component, is part of a circuit that involves the cerebellum.

Medial Descending Pathways

The remaining four pathways course in the medial portion of the spinal cord white matter, the **ventral column**, and influence axial and girdle muscles. These medially descending pathways (Figure 9–5) terminate in the medial ventral horn—where axial and girdle motor neurons are located—and the medial intermediate zone (Figure 9–4). These pathways influence motor neurons bilaterally: after descending into the cord, the axon of the projection neuron either decussates in the ventral commissure or its terminals synapse on interneurons and propriospinal neurons whose axons decussate. The **ventral corticospinal tract**, which originates mostly in the primary motor cortex and area 6, descends in the brain stem along with the lateral corticospinal tract, but does not decussate in the medulla and courses in the ventral column of the spinal cord (Figures 9–3A and 9–4A). The **reticulospinal tracts** (pontine and medullary) originate in the **reticular formation** (Figure 9–14) and descend ipsilaterally for the entire length of the spinal cord and function in posture and automatic responses, like locomotion. There are two vestibulospinal tracts. The **medial vestibulospinal tract** (also termed the **descending medial longitudinal fasciculus**) originates primarily from the **medial vestibular nucleus** (Figure 9–14) and descends bilaterally in the white matter only as far as the cervical cord. This pathway is important in control of head position. The **lateral vestibulospinal tract**, important in maintaining balance, originates from the **lateral vestibular nucleus (Deiters' nucleus)** (Figure 9–14) and descends in the ipsilateral white matter to all levels of the spinal cord. The **tectospinal tract** originates from the deeper layers of the **superior colliculus** (Figure 9–10B), decussates in the midbrain, and descends medially in the caudal brain stem and spinal cord. This path only descends to the cervical spinal cord and plays a role in coordination of head and eye movements. ■

KEY STRUCTURES AND TERMS

medial and lateral descending
    systems
  lateral corticospinal tract
  ventral (or anterior) corticospinal
      tract
  corticobulbar tract
  rubrospinal tract
  reticulospinal tracts
      pontine reticulospinal tract
      medullary reticulospinal tract
  vestibulospinal tracts
      medial
      lateral
  tectospinal tract
cerebellum
basal ganglia
cortical motor areas
  primary motor cortex (area 4)

premotor cortex (lateral area 6)
supplementary motor area (medial
    area 6)
cingulate motor area
internal capsule
  anterior limb
  posterior limb
  genu
ventral lateral nucleus
ventral anterior nucleus
superior colliculus
red nucleus
  magnocellular
  parvocellular
substantia nigra
basis pedunculi
medial longitudinal fasciculus
cranial nerve motor nuclei

reticular formation
vestibular nuclei
  medial
  superior
  inferior
  lateral
pyramid (pyramidal tract)
ventral horn
  motor neurons
intermediate zone
  segmental interneuron
  propriospinal neuron
motor signs
  flaccid paralysis and reduced
      myotatic reflexes
  spasticity
  Babinski sign

Selected Readings

Davidoff, R. A. 1990. The pyramidal tract. Neurology 40:332–339.

Dum, R. P., and Strick, P. L. 1992. Medial wall motor areas and skeletomotor control. Curr. Opin. Neurobiol. 2:836–839.

Freund, H.-J. 1991. What is the evidence for multiple motor areas in the human brain? In Humphrey, D. R. (ed.), Motor Control: Concepts and Issues. New York: John Wiley, pp. 399–411.

Ghez, C. 1991. The control of movement. In Kandel, E. R., Schwartz, J. H., and Jessell, T. M. (eds.), Principles of Neural Science, 3rd ed. New York: Elsevier, pp. 533–547.

Ghez, C. 1991. Voluntary movement. In Kandel, E. R., Schwartz, J. H., and Jessell, T. M. (eds.), Principles of Neural Science, 3rd ed. New York: Elsevier, pp. 609–625.

Jankowska, E., and Lundberg, A. 1981. Interneurons in the spinal cord. Trends in Neurosci. 4:230–233.

Kalaska, J. F., and Crammond, D. J. 1992. Cerebral control of reaching movements. Science 255:1517–1523.

Lance, J. W., and McLeod, J. G. 1981. A Physiological Approach to Clinical Neurology. London: Butterworths.

Schieber, M. H., Hibbard, L. S. 1993. How somatotopic is the motor cortex hand area? Science 261:489–492.

Wise, S. P. 1985. The primate premotor cortex: Past, present, and preparatory. Ann. Rev. Neurosci. 8:1–19.

References

Asanuma, H. 1981. The pyramidal tract. In Brooks, V. B. (ed.), Handbook of Physiology, Section I: The Nervous System, Vol. II, Motor Control. Bethesda, Md.: American Physiological Society, pp. 703–733.

Betz, V. 1874. Anatomischer Nachweis zweier Gehirncentra. Centralbl. Med. Wiss. 12:578–580, 595–599.

Crosby, E. C., Humphrey, T., and Lauer, E. W. 1962. Correlative Anatomy of the Nervous System. New York: Macmillan.

Dum, R. P., and Strick, P. L. 1991. The origin of corticospinal projections from the premotor areas in the frontal lobe. J. Neurosci. 11:667–689.

Freund, H.-J., and Hummelsheim, H. 1984. Premotor cortex in man: Evidence for innervation of proximal limb muscles. Exp. Brain Res. 53:479–482.

Kim, S. G., Ashe, J., Georgopoulos, A. P., Merkle, H., Ellermann, J. M., Menon, R. S., Ogawa, S., and Ugurbil, K. 1993. Functional imaging of human motor cortex at high magnetic field. J. Neurophysiol. 69:297–302.

Kuypers, H. G. J. M. 1981. Anatomy of the descending pathways. In Brooks, V. B. (ed.), Handbook of Physiology, Section I: The Nervous System, Vol. II, Motor Control. Bethesda, Md.: American Physiological Society, pp. 597–666.

Kuypers, H. G. J. M., and Brinkman, J. 1970. Precentral projections to different parts of the spinal intermediate zone in the rhesus monkey. Brain Res. 24:151–188.

Lu, M.-T., Present, J. B., and Strick, P. L. 1994. Interconnections between the prefrontal cortex and the premotor areas in the frontal lobe. J. Comp. Neurol. 341:375–392.

Molenaar, I., and Kuypers, H. G. J. M. 1978. Cells of origin of propriospinal fibers and of fibers ascending to supraspinal levels. An HRP study in cat and rhesus monkey. Brain Res. 152:429–450.

Muakkassa, K. F., and Strick, P. L. 1979. Frontal lobe inputs to primate motor cortex: Evidence for four somatotopically organized 'premotor' areas. Brain Res. 177:176–182.

Murray, E. A., and Coulter, J. D. 1981. Organization of corticospinal neurons in the monkey. J. Comp. Neurol. 195:339–365.

Nathan, P. W., and Smith, M. C. 1982. The rubrospinal and central tegmental tracts in man. Brain 105:223–269.

Penfield, W., and Rasmussen, T. 1950. The Cerebral Cortex of Man: A Clinical Study of Localization of Function. New York: Macmillan.

Pujol J., Martí-Vilalta, J. L., Junqué, C., Vendrell, P., Fernández, J., and Capdevila, A. 1990. Wallerian degeneration of the pyramidal tract in capsular infarction studied by magnetic resonance imaging. Stroke 21:404–409.

Schell, G. R., and Strick, P. L. 1984. The origin of thalamic inputs to the arcuate premotor and supplementary motor areas. J. Neurosci. 4:539–560.

Sterling, P., and Kuypers, H. G. J. M. 1967. Anatomical organization of the brachial spinal cord of the cat. III. The propriospinal connections. Brain Res. 4:419–443.

Wiesendanger, M. 1981. Organization of secondary motor areas of cerebral cortex. In Brooks, V. B. (ed.), Handbook of Physiology, Section I: The Nervous System, Vol. II, Motor Control. Bethesda, Md.: American Physiological Society, pp. 1121–1147.

10

The Cerebellum

T HE CEREBELLUM PLAYS A KEY ROLE IN MOVEMENT by regulating the functions of the descending motor pathways. When this major brain structure is damaged, movements that were smooth and steered accurately become uncoordinated and erratic. Important insights into the general role of the cerebellum in motor control can be gained by considering its connections with other brain regions. Unique among the components of the central nervous system, the cerebellum receives input from virtually all brain regions, as well as the spinal cord.

Its output is focused on the descending projection pathways (Figure 10–1). The cerebellum provides the major input to the red nucleus and is one of the major sources of input (via the thalamus) to the primary motor cortex (area 4) and premotor cortex (lateral portion of area 6). Thus, the cerebellum controls movement not by affecting the excitability of motor neurons directly, but indirectly, through its actions on the descending motor pathways.

◾ GROSS ANATOMY OF THE CEREBELLUM

Because the three-dimensional organization of the cerebellum is so complex, rivaling that of the cerebral cortex, we consider the gross anatomy first and then its functional organization. Next, we discuss the cytoarchitecture of the cerebellar cortex. Finally, sections through the spinal cord, brain stem, diencephalon, and cerebral hemisphere are examined to identify the locations of key components of the cerebellum and its associated afferent connections and efferent projections.

The Convoluted Surface of the Cerebellar Cortex Is Organized Into Three Lobes

Located in the **posterior cranial fossa**, dorsal to the pons and medulla (Figure 10–2), the cerebellum is separated from the overlying cerebral cortex (Figure 10–3) by a tough flap in the dura, the **cerebellar**

291

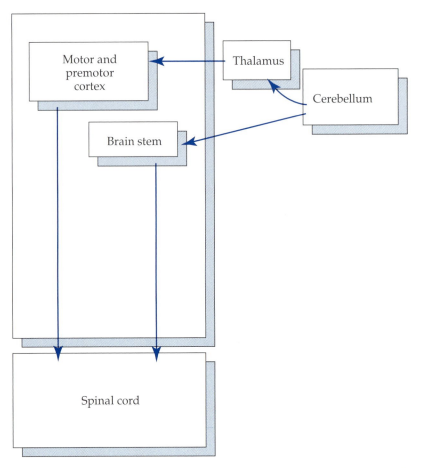

Figure 10–1. The relationship between the cerebellum and the descending spinal projection systems.

tentorium (see Chapter 4, Figure 4–14). The superior surface of the cerebellum is somewhat flattened. Inferiorly, it is incompletely divided into symmetrical halves by the **posterior cerebellar incisure**, which contains a small dural flap, the **falx cerebelli.** The cerebellum is attached to the brain stem by three **peduncles** (Figures 10–2B and C). Afferent axons, projecting to and from the cerebellum, and efferent axons, exiting from the cerebellum, course through the peduncles: the **superior cerebellar peduncle** contains mostly **efferent axons**, the **middle cerebellar peduncle** contains only **afferent axons**, and the **inferior cerebellar peduncle** contains both **afferent and efferent axons**. The cerebellar peduncles have an alternate nomenclature that is often used in the clinical and scientific literature. The superior cerebellar peduncle is also called the brachium conjunctivum; the middle cerebellar peduncle, the brachium pontis; and the inferior cerebellar peduncle, the restiform body. The various peduncles are distinguished in Figures 10–2B and C because each one has been given a different cut surface in the dissection. Three distinct peduncles would not be apparent had a single cut been made.

The cerebellum is covered by an outer cortex (or gray matter) containing neuronal cell bodies overlying a region that contains predominantly myelinated axons (or white matter). The cerebellar cortex contains an extraordinary number of neurons, rivaling that of the rest of the brain! The large number of neurons in the cerebellar cortex reflects the difficult

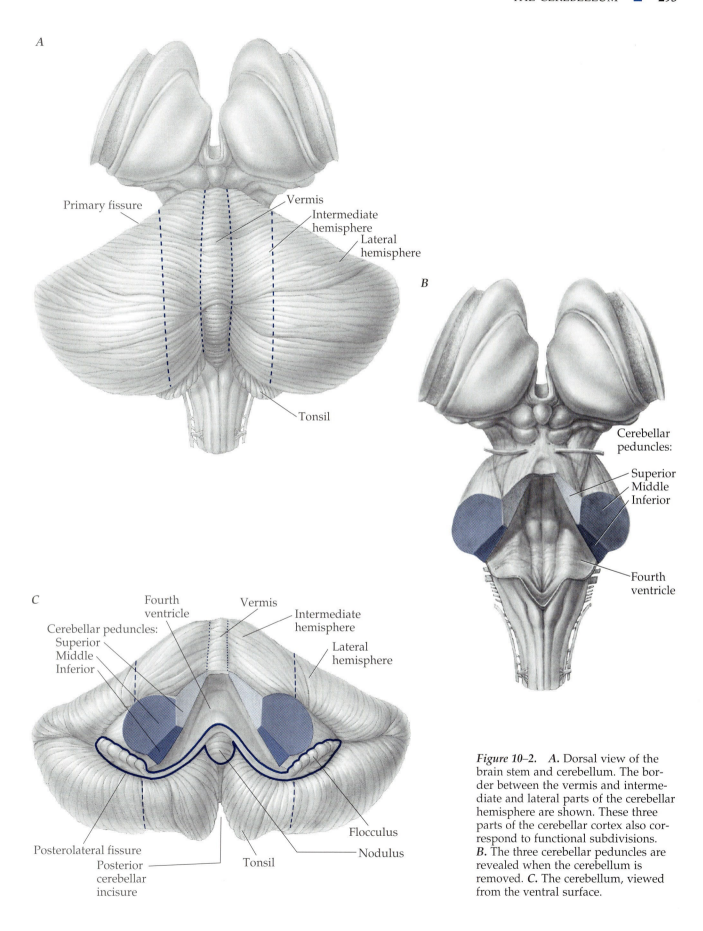

A

Primary fissure

Vermis

Intermediate hemisphere

Lateral hemisphere

Tonsil

B

Cerebellar peduncles:

Superior
Middle
Inferior

Fourth ventricle

C

Fourth ventricle

Vermis

Intermediate hemisphere

Cerebellar peduncles:
Superior
Middle
Inferior

Lateral hemisphere

Flocculus

Nodulus

Posterolateral fissure

Posterior cerebellar incisure

Tonsil

Figure 10–2. **A.** Dorsal view of the brain stem and cerebellum. The border between the vermis and intermediate and lateral parts of the cerebellar hemisphere are shown. These three parts of the cerebellar cortex also correspond to functional subdivisions. **B.** The three cerebellar peduncles are revealed when the cerebellum is removed. **C.** The cerebellum, viewed from the ventral surface.

A

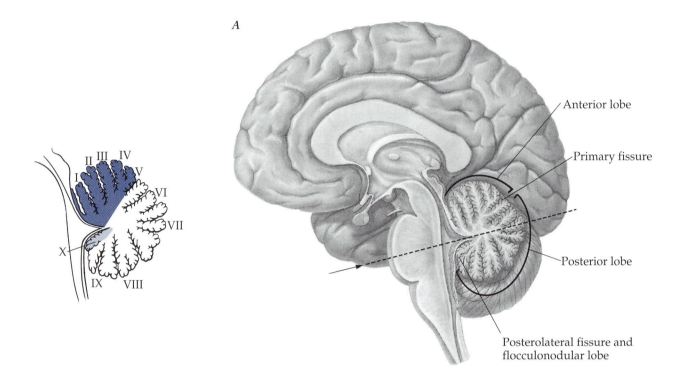

Anterior lobe

Primary fissure

Posterior lobe

Posterolateral fissure and flocculonodular lobe

B

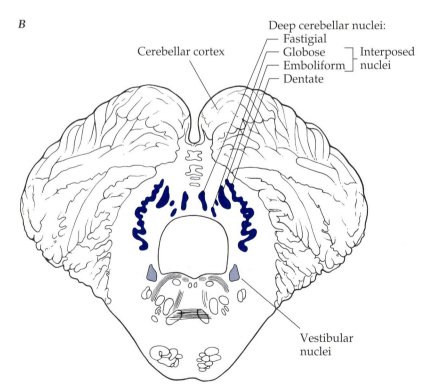

Deep cerebellar nuclei:
— Fastigial
— Globose ⎤ Interposed
— Emboliform ⎦ nuclei
— Dentate

Cerebellar cortex

Vestibular nuclei

Figure 10–3. *A.* Midsagittal cut through the brain revealing the cerebellar vermis. Inset shows the 10 cerebellar lobules. Lobules I through V comprise the anterior lobe, VI through IX, the posterior lobe, and X, the flocculonodular lobe. *B.* Schematic transverse section through the pons and cerebellum illustrating the location of the deep cerebellar nuclei. The plane of *B* is shown as the dashed line in *A*.

task of controlling the skeletal muscles of the body. In addition to the large numbers of neurons, there also is a rich array of neuron types (see below). Two prominent neurons are the projection neurons of the cerebellum, the **Purkinje cells**, and a class of cerebellar interneurons, **granule cells**. Most cerebellar neurons belong to this interneuron class.

Two shallow grooves running from rostral to caudal divide the cerebellar cortex into the **vermis**, located along the midline, and **two hemispheres** (Figures 10–2A and C). This anatomical distinction marks the specific functional divisions of the cerebellar cortex. Like the cerebral cortex, the cerebellar cortex is highly convoluted. These characteristic folds, termed **folia**, are equivalent to the gyri of the cerebral cortex. They vastly increase the amount of cerebellar cortex that can be packed into the posterior cranial fossa.

The cerebellar cortex is organized into groups of folia, termed **lobules**, that are separated from one another by fissures. In a section through the vermis, the lobules appear to radiate from the apex of the roof of the fourth ventricle (Figure 10–3A, inset). Anatomists recognize ten lobules, whose nomenclature is used largely by specialists studying the cerebellum. Two fissures are particularly deep and divide the various lobules into **three lobes** (Figures 10–2 and 10–3A). The **primary fissure** separates the **anterior lobe** from the **posterior lobe**. Together the anterior and posterior lobes are important in the planning, execution, and control of **movements of the limbs and trunk**. The **flocculonodular lobe** is separated from the posterior lobe by the **posterolateral fissure**. This lobe consists of the **nodulus**, located on the midline (i.e., the vermis), and the **flocculus**, on either side. The flocculonodular lobe plays a key role in **maintaining balance and eye movement control**.

Beneath the cerebellar cortex is the **white matter**, which contains axons coursing to and from the cortex (Figure 10–3). The branching pattern of the white matter of the cerebellum inspired early anatomists to refer to it as the **arbor vitae** ("tree of life"); hence the name folia (leaves) rather than gyri is used to describe the cortical convolutions. Embedded within the white matter of the cerebellum are four bilaterally paired nuclei, the **deep cerebellar nuclei**, shown in the schematic transverse section through the pons and cerebellum (Figure 10–3B): **fastigial nucleus**, **globose nucleus**, **emboliform nucleus**, and **dentate nucleus**. The globose and emboliform nuclei are collectively termed the **interposed nuclei**. The deep cerebellar nuclei are key elements in the neural circuit of the cerebellum (see below).

■ FUNCTIONAL ANATOMY OF THE CEREBELLUM

All Three Functional Divisions of the Cerebellum Display a Similar Input–Output Organization

The cerebellum has three functional divisions, each consisting of a portion of the cerebellar cortex and one or more deep nuclei (Figures 10–2 and 10–4):

- The **spinocerebellum**—which receives highly organized somatic sensory inputs from the spinal cord—is important in controlling the **posture and movement** of the trunk and limbs. While this division is named for its major source of input, the spinocerebellum also receives information from structures other than the spinal cord. This

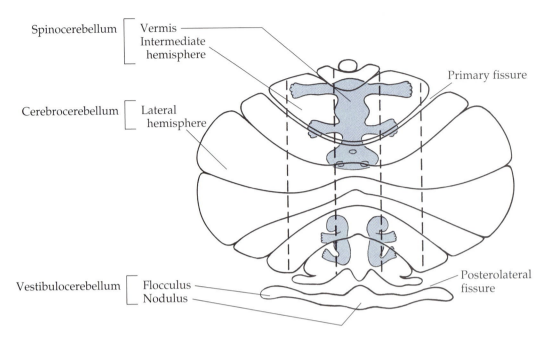

Spinocerebellum
— Vermis
— Intermediate hemisphere

Cerebrocerebellum
— Lateral hemisphere

Vestibulocerebellum
— Flocculus
— Nodulus

Primary fissure

Posterolateral fissure

Figure 10–4. The three functional divisions are shown in schematic view of the cerebellum. The topographic organization of somatic sensory inputs to the spino-cerebellum is also shown. These inputs are somatotopically organized. Visual, auditory, and vestibular inputs are directed predominantly to the "head" areas.

division is comprised of the **vermis** and the paravermal cerebellar cortex, termed the **intermediate hemisphere**, of both the anterior and posterior lobes. These cortical areas project to the fastigial and interposed nuclei, respectively (see below).

- The **cerebrocerebellum**—which receives input from the **cerebral cortex** (via a relay in the pontine nuclei)—participates in the **planning of movement**. Located lateral to the spinocerebellum in both the anterior and posterior lobes, the cerebrocerebellum consists of those cortical regions collectively termed the **lateral hemisphere**. There is, however, no gross anatomical boundary between the intermediate hemisphere of the spinocerebellum and the lateral hemisphere of the cerebrocerebellum (Figure 10–4). The cortex of the cerebrocerebellum projects to the dentate nucleus.

- The **vestibulocerebellum**—which receives input from the **vestibular labyrinth**—helps us to **maintain balance** and **control head and eye movements**. This cerebellar division corresponds to the **flocculonodular lobe**. The output of the vestibulocerebellar cortex is not to the deep nuclei, but rather to the vestibular nuclei. The vestibular nuclei are thus analogous to the deep nuclei (see below).

Each functional division of the cerebellar cortex has a similar generalized pattern of afferent and efferent connections (Figure 10–5). However, each division differs from the other with respect to the specific input sources and the specific structures to which it projects (Figure 10–6). Figure 10–5 shows the basic organizational plan of the cerebellar functional divisions. There are two major sets of inputs to the cerebellum, and with some exceptions, both sets of inputs are directed to neurons in the deep nuclei as well as cortical neurons (Figure 10–5). We consider the intrinsic organization of the cerebellar cortex in detail in a later section.

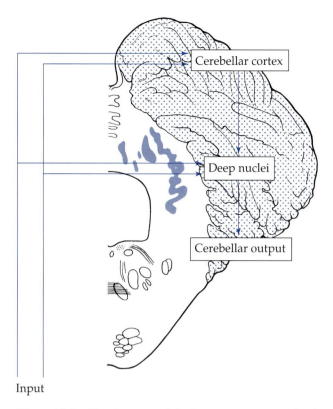

Input

Figure 10–5. Key features of the input–output organization of the cerebellum.

Figure 10–6. Key features of the functional organization of the spinocerebellum *(A)*, cerebrocerebellum *(B)*, and vestibulocerebellum *(C)*.

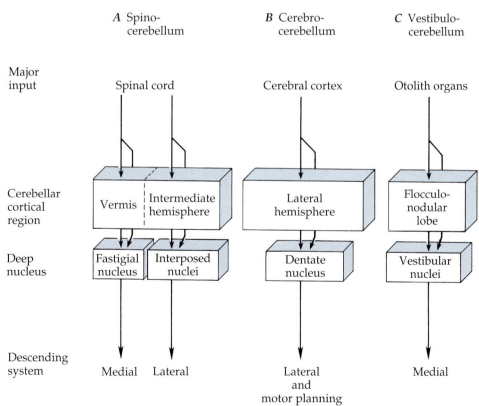

*The Vermis and the Intermediate Hemisphere Are the
Anatomical Components of the Spinocerebellum*

The **spinocerebellum** (Figures 10–6A, 10–7, and 10–8) is important in
the control of body musculature. It is somatotopically organized: the vermis and the intermediate hemisphere control axial muscles and limb muscles, respectively (Figure 10–4). This mediolateral somatotopic arrange-

Figure 10–7. ***A.*** Spinocerebellar pathways relaying sensory feedback (dorsal
spinocerebellar and cuneocerebellar tracts). ***B.*** Spinocerebellar pathway relaying
information about the amount of activity in descending pathways (ventral spinocerebellar tract).

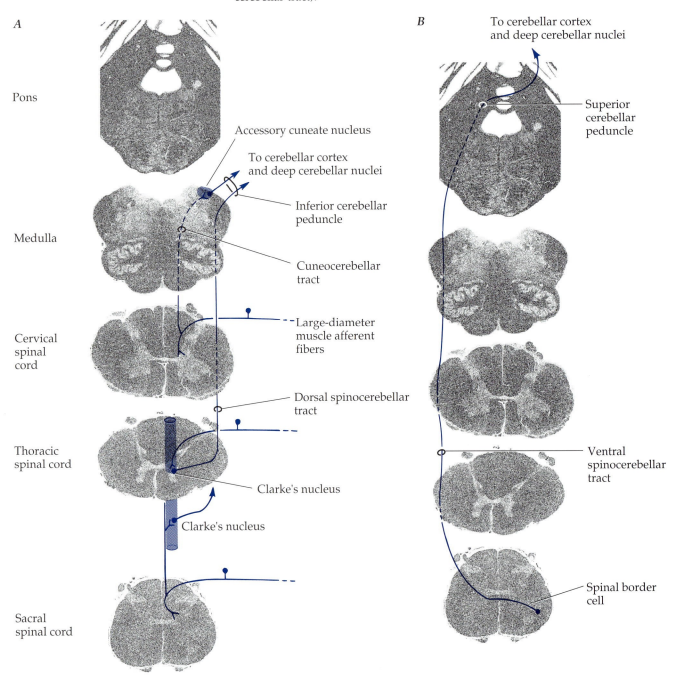

ment recalls the somatotopic organization of the ventral horn, where medial motor neurons innervate **axial** and **proximal limb muscles** (such as neck and shoulder muscles), and those located laterally innervate more **distal muscles** (such as those of the wrist and hand) (see Chapter 9).

The **spinocerebellar tracts** transmit somatic sensory information from the limbs and trunk to the spinocerebellum, whereas the trigeminocerebellar tract transmits information from the head. Somatic sensory information is projected to the spinocerebellum in a somatotopic fashion. Distinct zones can be distinguished that process information from the head, neck, arms, trunk, and legs. The vermis receives somatic sensory information primarily from the head, neck, and trunk; the intermediate hemisphere processes signals from the limbs. Within each of these zones, the representation of sensory information has a more complex organization. Information from a particular part is represented at multiple sites, and conversely, a single site in the cortex of the spinocerebellum may represent different parts of a body region. Termed **fractured somatotopy**, this organization is thought to be important in bringing together information from different parts of the limbs, trunk, or head for coordinating complex movements. In addition, the vermis receives a direct projection from primary sensory neurons of the **vestibular labyrinth**, as well as **visual** and **auditory** input relayed by brain stem nuclei. Here we focus on the spinocerebellar pathways, the major input to this part of the cerebellum. In Chapter 12, the cerebellar projections of the spinal trigeminal nucleus will be considered.

There are four spinocerebellar tracts, termed: dorsal spinocerebellar, cuneocerebellar, ventral spinocerebellar, and rostral spinocerebellar (Table 10–1). The **dorsal spinocerebellar and cuneocerebellar tracts** (Figure 10–7) transmit somatic sensory information from the leg, trunk, and arm. The dorsal spinocerebellar tract originates in **Clarke's nucleus**, which is located in the intermediate zone. This nucleus has a columnar shape and has a restricted rostrocaudal location (see below). (Clarke's nucleus is sometime called Clarke's column.) Clarke's nucleus receives input directly from large-diameter primary afferent fibers, such as those that innervate muscle spindles (see Table 5–1), from the **lower limb and lower trunk**. Neurons giving rise to the dorsal spinocerebellar tract send their axons into the **ipsilateral lateral column**.

The cuneocerebellar tract originates from neurons in the **accessory cuneate nucleus**, which is located in the caudal medulla (Figure 10–7A). Like Clarke's nucleus, the accessory cuneate nucleus receives inputs from large-diameter afferent fibers, but only from the **upper trunk** and **upper limb**. It is thus analogous to Clarke's nucleus, but for the upper extremity. Both the dorsal spinocerebellar tract and the cuneocerebellar tract enter the cerebellum via the **ipsilateral inferior cerebellar peduncle**. Their axons synapse on neurons of the fastigial and interposed nuclei as well as on cortical neurons in the vermis and intermediate hemisphere. The pattern of cortical termination is somatotopic, forming the separate **homunculi** rostrally in the anterior lobe and caudally in the posterior lobe (Figure 10–4).

The **ventral** and **rostral spinocerebellar tracts**, rather than transmitting **sensory information** from the periphery, are believed to relay **internal feedback signals** to the cerebellum that reflect the amount of neural activity in descending motor pathways. The ventral spinocerebellar pathway, similar to the dorsal pathway, transmits information about the lower limb and lower trunk, whereas the **rostral spinocerebellar tract** transmits information about the upper trunk and upper limb. The ventral spinocerebellar tract (Figure 10–7B) originates from neurons that are spread throughout

A

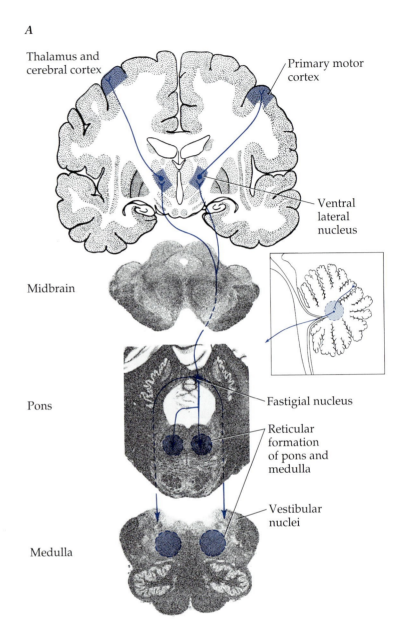

Figure 10–8. Efferent pathways from the vermis of the spinocerebellum *(A)* and the intermediate hemisphere *(B)*. Note that the ascending projection of the fastigial nucleus to the thalamus is much smaller than the descending projection to the pons and medulla. Insets show projection from cerebellar cortex to the fastigial nucleus *(A)* and interposed nuclei *(B)*.

the intermediate zone and ventral horn of the sacral, lumbar, and lower thoracic cord. Many of these neurons are located along the gray matter border; these neurons are called the **spinal border cells**. The axons of the ventral spinocerebellar path decussate in the spinal cord and ascend in the ventral portion of the lateral column (Figure 10–7B). In the pons, the axons enter the cerebellum via the **superior cerebellar peduncle**. Once in the cerebellum, some axons decussate again and terminate in the ipsilateral cerebellum. This "doubly crossed" contingent is smaller than the crossed group. Very little is known about the rostral spinocerebellar tract. It is an ipsilateral pathway and enters the cerebellum via both the inferior and the superior cerebellar peduncles.

As their names reveal, these are direct pathways from the spinal cord to the cerebellum: the axon of a neuron in the spinal cord terminates in the cerebellum. In addition, there exist indirect routes from the spinal cord. These pathways synapse in the reticular formation and the inferior olivary

B

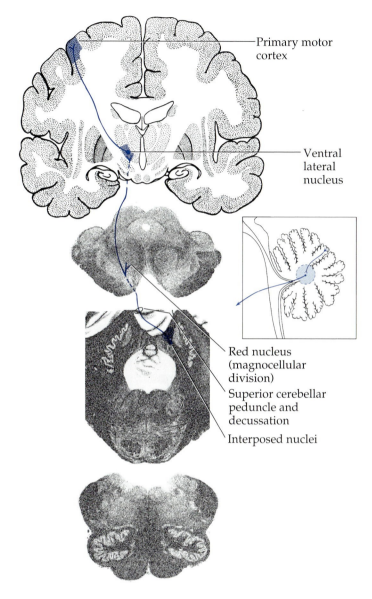

Primary motor cortex

Ventral lateral nucleus

Red nucleus (magnocellular division)

Superior cerebellar peduncle and decussation

Interposed nuclei

Figure 10–8.   (continued)

nuclear complex, adding at least one additional synapse. Information transmitted by these indirect paths is also subject to more extensive processing and may play more complex roles in movement than information transmitted by the direct paths.

Some spinal neurons that give rise to indirect cerebellar paths also serve other functions. One such neuron that has been studied extensively is also a propriospinal neuron located in the rostral cervical spinal cord important for transmitting descending control signals to motor neurons. These particular propriospinal neurons have a descending axon branch, which contacts motor neurons, and an ascending branch, which is thought to transmit information to the cerebellum for correcting movement inaccuracy.

The two cortical components of the spinocerebellum project to two deep cerebellar nuclei: the **vermis** projects to the **fastigial nucleus** and the **intermediate hemisphere** projects to the **interposed nuclei** (Figure 10–6).

Table 10–1. Spinocerebellar pathways.

Pathway	Origin	Decussation	Cerebellar peduncle	Body parts
Dorsal spinocerebellar	Clarke's nucleus	Uncrossed	Inferior	Lower limb, lower trunk
Cuneocerebellar	Accessory cuneate nucleus	Uncrossed	Inferior	Upper trunk, upper limb, neck
Ventral spinocerebellar	Spinal border cells	Crossed, doubly crossed	Superior	Lower limb
Rostral spinocerebellar	Spinal cord neurons	Uncrossed	Inferior	Upper limb

These deep nuclei, in turn, influence motor neurons primarily through their projections onto the descending systems (Figure 10–6). The fastigial nucleus projects most of its axons through the **inferior cerebellar peduncle** to brain stem nuclei, giving rise to **medial descending pathways**, the reticulospinal and vestibulospinal tracts (Figure 10–8A). The fastigial nucleus also has a small ascending projection, via a thalamic relay in the ventral lateral nucleus, to the cells of origin of the ventral corticospinal tract. This efferent projection exits through the superior cerebellar peduncle. The interposed nuclei project through the **superior cerebellar peduncle** to the magnocellular component of the red nucleus and, via the thalamus, to portions of the motor areas of the frontal lobe (Figure 10–8B). These components of the motor systems give rise to the **lateral descending systems**: the rubrospinal and lateral corticospinal tracts.

The Lateral Hemisphere and Dentate Nucleus Correspond to the Cerebrocerebellum

The **cerebrocerebellum** (Figures 10–4 and 10–6) is primarily involved in the planning of movement and is interconnected with the **cerebral cortex**. This is in contrast to the spinocerebellum, which is interconnected with the spinal cord. The afferent and efferent connections of the cerebrocerebellum are illustrated in Figure 10–9. The major input to the cerebrocerebellum is from the **contralateral cerebral cortex**. This projection is not direct, but rather is relayed by neurons in the **pontine nuclei**. The pontine nuclei, in turn, project to the contralateral cerebellar cortex through the **middle cerebellar peduncle**. The efferent projection from the cortex of the cerebrocerebellum is to the **dentate nucleus**, the largest and most lateral of the deep nuclei. The dentate nucleus, in turn, projects its axons to two main sites. The first is the ventral lateral nucleus, the motor relay nucleus of the thalamus. The second site is the **red nucleus**; however, it projects to the **parvocellular** portion of the red nucleus, not the magnocellular portion. Whereas the magnocellular portion of the red nucleus gives rise to the rubrospinal tract (see Chapter 9), the parvocellular division projects to the ipsilateral **inferior olivary nucleus**, a major source of input to the cerebellum (see below).

Recent studies in humans, including functional imaging, suggest that the most ventrolateral portion of the dentate nucleus participates in cognitive and linguistic functions. There may be a distinctive anatomical correlate for the dentate's role in higher brain functions. In the monkey, where anatomical tracer studies can be done, there is a portion of the dentate

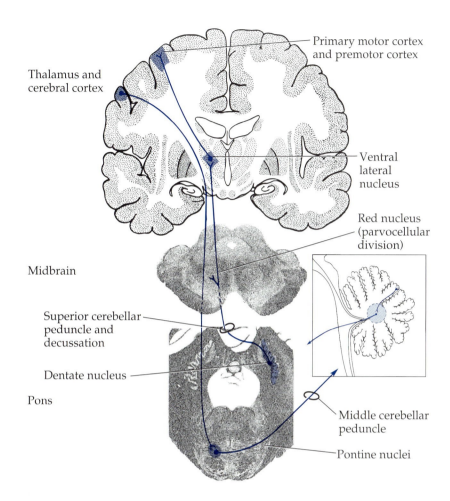

Primary motor cortex
and premotor cortex

Thalamus and
cerebral cortex

Ventral
lateral
nucleus

Red nucleus
(parvocellular
division)

Midbrain

Superior cerebellar
peduncle and
decussation

Dentate nucleus

Pons

Middle cerebellar
peduncle

Pontine nuclei

Figure 10–9. Afferent and efferent connections of the cerebrocerebellum. Note that the major input to the pontine nuclei is from the entire cerebral cortex, although input from only a single site is shown.

nucleus analogous to the ventrolateral dentate in the human. This portion in the monkey projects via the thalamus, to the **prefrontal association cortex**. This region of the frontal lobe is involved in spatial memory, such as remembering where objects are in the environment, and other cognitive functions.

The Flocculonodular Lobe Corresponds to the Vestibulocerebellum

The **vestibulocerebellum** (Figures 10–4 and 10–6) is crucial for maintaining balance and controlling eye movements. This particular division of the cerebellum corresponds to the flocculonodular lobe. The vestibulocerebellum receives afferent input from **primary vestibular afferents** and secondary vestibular neurons in the **vestibular nuclei**. In fact, the vestibular afferents are the only primary sensory neurons that project directly to the cerebellum. The cortical component of the vestibulocerebellum projects to the **vestibular nuclei**—the medial, inferior, and superior vestibular nuclei (Figure 10–10). These vestibular nuclei give rise to the **medial vestibulospinal tract** as well as to fibers in the **medial longitudinal fasciculus**. From the perspective of the projections of the cerebellum, the vestibular nuclei are anatomically similar to the deep cerebellar nuclei (see below). The cortex of the vestibulocerebellum also has a small projection to the fastigial nucleus (not shown in Figure 10–10).

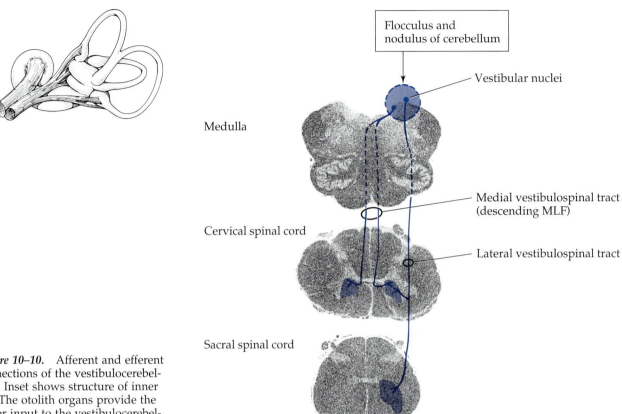

Flocculus and
nodulus of cerebellum

Vestibular nuclei

Medulla

Medial vestibulospinal tract
(descending MLF)

Cervical spinal cord

Lateral vestibulospinal tract

Sacral spinal cord

Figure 10–10. Afferent and efferent connections of the vestibulocerebellum. Inset shows structure of inner ear. The otolith organs provide the major input to the vestibulocerebellum.

■ REGIONAL ANATOMY

In the remaining sections of Chapter 10, we examine the regional anatomy of the cerebellum and associated nuclei and tracts. First, we explore the histology of the cerebellar cortex. The cellular constituents and synaptic connections of the cerebellum are among the best understood of the central nervous system. Then we view sections through key levels illustrating locations of the cerebellar peduncles, afferent and efferent pathways, and the deep cerebellar nuclei.

The Intrinsic Circuitry of the Cerebellar Cortex Is Similar For the Different Functional Divisions

The cerebellar cortex consists of three cell layers (Figure 10–11), progressing from its external surface inward: the **molecular layer**, the **Purkinje layer**, and the **granular layer**, which is adjacent to the white matter. There are five types of neurons in the cerebellar cortex, and they have a different laminar distribution (Table 10–2): (1) Purkinje cell, (2) granule cell, (3) basket cell, (4) stellate cell, and (5) Golgi cell. The cellular organization of the cerebellar cortex is considered in a stepwise fashion in Figures 10–12A through C, beginning with the two major classes of excitatory inputs.

A

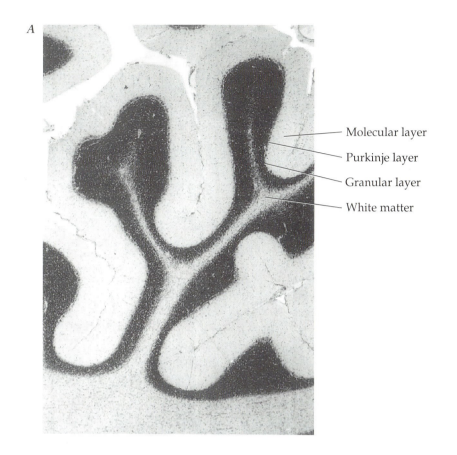

Molecular layer

Purkinje layer

Granular layer

White matter

Figure 10–11. Nissl-stained section through the cerebellar cortex. *A.* Low-power view. *B.* High-power view.

B

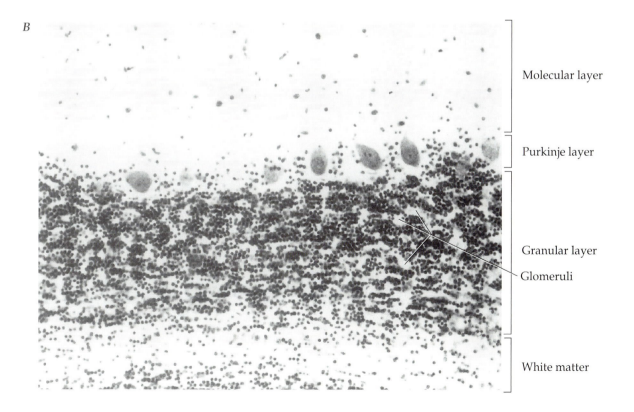

Molecular layer

Purkinje layer

Granular layer

Glomeruli

White matter

Table 10–2. Neurons and neurotransmitters of the cerebellar cortex.

Cell type	Neuro-transmitter	Laminar distribution	Postsynaptic action	Postsynaptic target
Projection Neuron				
Purkinje	GABA	Purkinje	Inhibitory	Deep nuclei, vestibular nuclei
Interneurons				
Granule	Glu/A	Granular	Excitatory	Purkinje, stellate, basket, and Golgi cells
Basket	GABA	Molecular	Inhibitory	Purkinje cells
Stellate	Taurine	Molecular	Inhibitory	Purkinje cells
Golgi	GABA	Granular	Inhibitory	Purkinje cells

GABA = γ-aminobutyric acid
Glu/A = glutamate/aspartate

Climbing and Mossy Fibers Are the Two Major Excitatory Inputs to the Cerebellar Cortex

Climbing fibers originate entirely from the **inferior olivary nuclear complex** (see Figure 10–16). **Mossy fibers** provide the other major input to the cerebellum. The cell bodies of mossy fibers are located primarily in the spinal cord (see Figure 10–15) and in two brain stem nuclear groups, pontine nuclei (see Figure 10–17), and nuclei of the reticular formation (see Figure 10–16).

Ultimately, the target of the mossy and climbing fibers is the **Purkinje cell**, the only type of neuron whose axon projects from the cerebellar cortex. The Purkinje layer contains Purkinje cells. Climbing fibers contact Purkinje cells directly (Figure 10–12A). There is a remarkable degree of specificity of the connections of climbing fibers and Purkinje cells: **each Purkinje cell receives input from a single climbing fiber.** Individual climbing fibers make contact with no more than ten Purkinje cells. Climbing fibers make multiple synapses with one Purkinje cell, forming one of the strongest excitatory connection in the central nervous system.

In contrast to climbing fibers, mossy fibers first synapse on **granule cells**—the only excitatory interneurons in the cerebellum. Located in the granular layer (Figure 10–11), granule cells have an axon that ascends through the Purkinje layer into the molecular layer. Here the axon bifurcates to form the **parallel fibers**, which synapse on Purkinje cells (Figure 10–12A) and other cerebellar interneurons. One parallel fiber will synapse with thousands of Purkinje cells, and each Purkinje cell receives synapses from thousands of parallel fibers. Unlike the climbing fiber, which makes multiple synaptic contacts with the Purkinje cell, the parallel fiber makes only a few synapses with each Purkinje cell.

The paucity of parallel fiber synaptic contacts on the Purkinje cell reflects the orientation of Purkinje cell dendrites to the parallel fibers. Briefly, the Purkinje cell dendritic tree (Figures 10–12 and 10–13) is planar and oriented orthogonal to the long axis of the folium in which it is located (much like coins stacked on top of one another). The parallel fiber courses at a right angle to the dendritic plane of the Purkinje cell (i.e., parallel to the long axis of the folium). The fiber makes only a few contacts with a single Purkinje cell as the axon passes through the dendritic tree. As

A

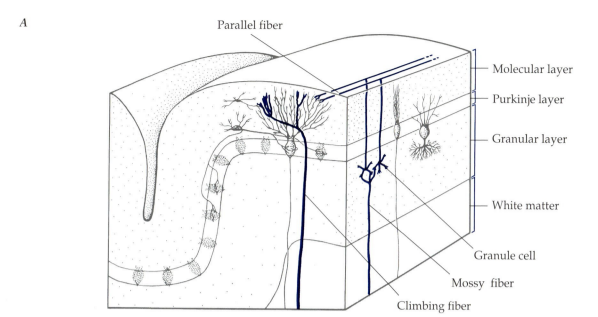

Parallel fiber

Molecular layer

Purkinje layer

Granular layer

White matter

Granule cell

Mossy fiber

Climbing fiber

B

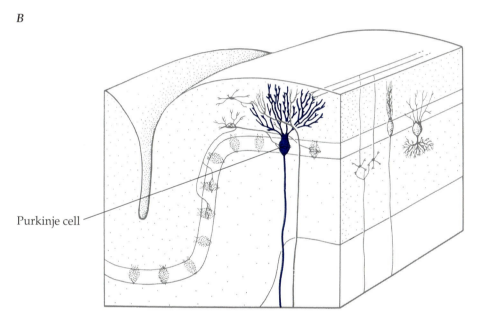

Purkinje cell

Figure 10–12. The circuitry of the cerebellar cortex is illustrated in a stepwise fashion. *A.* There are two major excitatory inputs to the cerebellum, climbing fibers and mossy fibers. Whereas the climbing fibers synapse directly on Purkinje cells, the mossy fibers first synapse on granule cells, which in turn give rise to the parallel fibers, which synapse on Purkinje cells. *B*. Purkinje cells are the output neurons of the cerebellum. *C.* There are three types of inhibitory interneurons: Golgi cells, basket cells, and stellate cells.

C

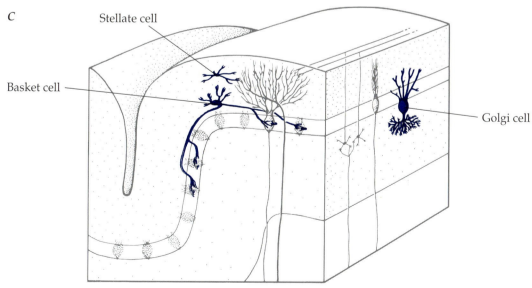

Stellate cell

Basket cell

Golgi cell

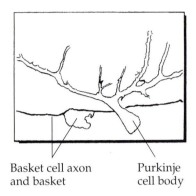

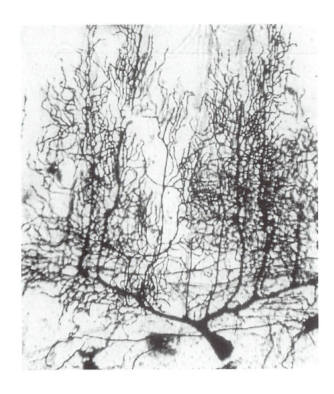

Basket cell axon
and basket

Purkinje
cell body

Figure 10–13. Golgi-stained section of the human cerebellar cortex showing a Purkinje cell and basket axons. The inset shows a schematic of the Purkinje cell body, proximal dendrites, basket cell axon, and basket synapse on an adjacent (unstained) Purkinje cell.

a consequence of the difference in the number of synaptic contacts, the strength of parallel fiber input to a Purkinje cell is much less than that of climbing fiber input. It has been suggested that the efficacy of parallel fiber input onto a given Purkinje cell is increased immediately after Purkinje cell activation by a climbing fiber.

Purkinje Cell Axons Synapse on Neurons of the Deep Cerebellar Nuclei and Vestibular Nuclei

Purkinje cells project their axons through the cerebellar white matter to synapse on neurons in the deep cerebellar nuclei (Figure 10–12B). To reach the vestibular nuclei, Purkinje axons travel through the inferior cerebellar peduncle after coursing in the cerebellar white matter. The Purkinje cell is an inhibitory projection neuron: when it discharges it hyperpolarizes the neurons in the deep cerebellar nuclei or vestibular nuclei with which it synapses. How then can neurons in the deep cerebellar nuclei and vestibular nuclei fire action potentials when they are inhibited by Purkinje cells? For the deep cerebellar nuclei, recall that the climbing fibers as well as many mossy fibers (from the spinal cord and reticular formation) have a direct excitatory synaptic connection (Figure 10–5). (Anatomical data suggest that most mossy fibers from the pontine nuclei bypass the deep nuclei, synapsing only in the cortex.) It is thought that these direct inputs to the deep nuclear cells increase their excitability and help to maintain their background neuronal activity at a high level. There are also intrinsic cell membrane properties, such as high resting ionic currents, that help to maintain high levels of activity. The high levels of neural activity in the deep nuclear cells is then reduced, or "sculpted," by the inhibitory actions of the Purkinje cells. Neurons in the vestibular nuclei receive major excitatory inputs from vestibular afferents—equivalent to mossy fiber input—as well as from climbing fibers. These inputs are major determinants of neuronal excitability in the vestibular nuclei.

Cerebellar Cortical Interneurons Inhibit Purkinje and Granule Cells

The Purkinje cell, in turn, is inhibited by two groups of interneurons (Figure 10–12C): **stellate cells**, located in the outer portion of the molecular layer, and **basket cells**, located close to the border between the molecular and Purkinje layers. Both of these neurons receive their predominant input from the parallel fibers.

The locations of the synaptic terminals of the basket and stellate cells on the Purkinje cells are different, which is important functionally in determining the strength of inhibition. The basket cell synapse is located on the Purkinje cell body, forming a dense meshwork, or "basket," of inhibitory synaptic contacts (Figure 10–13). The basket cell synapse is one of the strongest central nervous system inhibitory synapses. This is because of its close proximity to the spike initiation zone, at the axon hillock of the Purkinje cell, as well as the high density of synaptic contacts. The basket cell axon is oriented at a right angle to the folium (Figure 10–12); therefore, only Purkinje cells located in a band on either side of the basket cell are contacted. In contrast, the stellate cell synapse is located on the distal dendrites, far from the axon hillock, and hence the degree of inhibition it produces on Purkinje cells is much less than that of the basket cell. Whereas the inhibitory actions of basket cells can turn off the firing of the Purkinje cell, stellate cell inhibition only affects the integration of synaptic actions locally, in the region of its terminals on the distal dendrites of Purkinje cells.

The **Golgi** (Figure 10–12C) interneuron inhibits the granule cell. This inhibitory synapse is made in the granular layer, in a complex structure termed the **cerebellar glomerulus** (Figure 10–14). The cerebellar glomerulus consists of two presynaptic elements, the **mossy fiber terminal** and the **Golgi cell axon**, and one main postsynaptic element, the **granule cell dendrite**. The mossy fiber terminal is also termed the mossy fiber rosette because of the configuration of its enlarged terminal. Synaptic glomeruli ensure specificity of connections because this entire synaptic complex is contained within a **glial capsule**. The mossy fiber terminals are located in the clear zones seen under high power in the Nissl-stained section of the cerebellar cortex (Figure 10–11B). If we now take an inventory of the synaptic action of the interneurons of the cerebellar cortex (Table 10–2) we see that all but the granule cell are inhibitory. Even the projection neuron of the cerebellar cortex, the Purkinje cell, is inhibitory.

In the rest of this chapter, we follow the input and output pathways of the cerebellum as we examine sections through the spinal cord, brain stem, thalamus, and cerebral hemispheres.

Spinal Cord and Medullary Sections Reveal Nuclei and Paths Transmitting Somatic Sensory Information to the Cerebellum

Clarke's nucleus and the accessory cuneate nucleus are the principal nuclei that relay somatic sensory information to the spinocerebellum. We find **Clarke's nucleus** (Figure 10–15) in the medial portion of the intermediate zone of the spinal cord gray matter (lamina 7). This nucleus forms a column with a limited rostrocaudal distribution. In the human, Clarke's nucleus spans the **eighth cervical segment** (C8) to approximately the **second lumbar segment** (L2) and relays somatic sensory information from the lower limb and upper trunk. Most of the large-diameter afferent fibers that synapse in Clarke's nucleus course medially around the cap of the

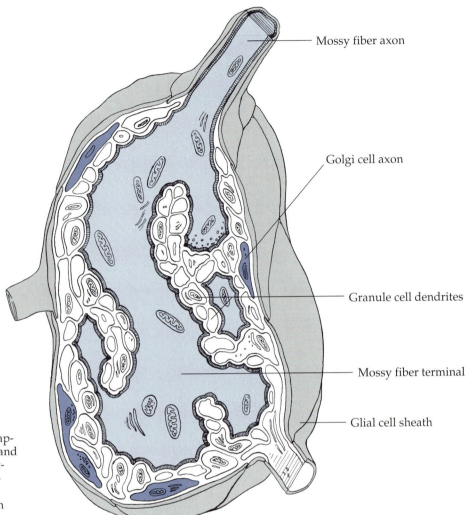

Mossy fiber axon

Golgi cell axon

Granule cell dendrites

Mossy fiber terminal

Glial cell sheath

Figure 10–14. The cerebellar glomerulus consists of two presynaptic elements, mossy fiber terminal and Golgi cell axon, and one main postsynaptic element, granule cell dendrite. These neural elements are ensheathed by glial cells. (Based on Eccles et al., 1967.)

dorsal horn and through the ipsilateral dorsal column en route to their termination site. In Figure 10–15A some of the axons can be seen following this trajectory. Afferent fibers arriving over dorsal roots caudal to the second lumbar segment first ascend in the **gracile fascicle**. Then they leave the white matter to terminate in Clarke's nucleus. Clarke's nucleus gives rise to the **dorsal spinocerebellar tract**, which ascends in the outermost portion of the lateral column (Figure 10–15B). The other pathway from the lower limb, the **ventral spinocerebellar tract**, is also shown in Figure 10–15B in relation to the ascending fibers of the anterolateral system. Many of the fibers of the ventral spinocerebellar tract are the axons of the spinal border cells.

In the cervical spinal cord and caudal medulla, the spatial relationship is maintained between the dorsal spinocerebellar and the ventral spinocerebellar tracts. More rostrally in the medulla, the dorsal spinocerebellar tract enters the cerebellum via the **inferior cerebellar peduncle** (Figure 10–16). The ventral spinocerebellar tract continues to ascend within the brain stem and enters the cerebellum via the **superior cerebellar peduncle** (see Figure 10–18).

In the caudal medulla we can identify the **accessory cuneate nucleus** (Figure 10–16A), which is located rostral to the cuneate nucleus. (The

A

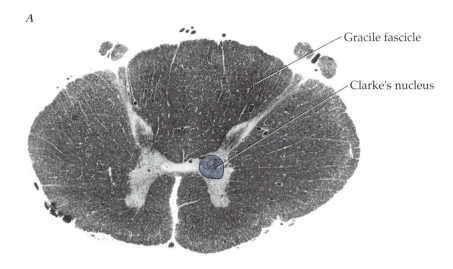

Gracile fascicle

Clarke's nucleus

B

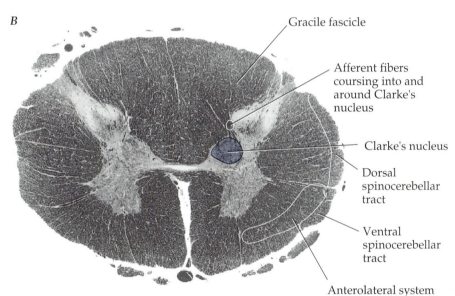

Gracile fascicle

Afferent fibers coursing into and around Clarke's nucleus

Clarke's nucleus

Dorsal spinocerebellar tract

Ventral spinocerebellar tract

Anterolateral system

Figure 10–15. Myelin-stained transverse sections through the thoracic *(A)* and lumbar *(B)* spinal cord. Clarke's nucleus is tinted blue.

accessory cuneate nucleus is also termed the lateral cuneate nucleus and the external cuneate nucleus.) The accessory cuneate nucleus relays somatic sensory information from the upper trunk and upper limb to the cerebellum, not for perception, but rather, for controlling movements. Recall that the cuneate nucleus is important in transmitting somatic sensory information to the thalamus for perception (see Chapter 5). To reach the accessory cuneate nucleus, afferent fibers from the upper trunk and arm first course rostrally within the cervical spinal cord in the **cuneate fascicle** of the dorsal column. Similar to the dorsal spinocerebellar tract, the cuneocerebellar projection courses in the **inferior cerebellar peduncle**.

The Vestibulocerebellum Receives Input From Primary and Secondary Vestibular Neurons

In addition to the accessory cuneate nucleus, there are three major groups of brain stem nuclei that project to the cerebellum: the **inferior oli-**

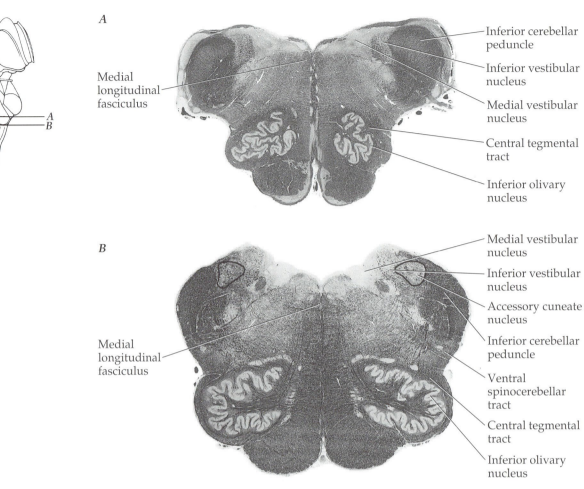

A

Medial longitudinal fasciculus

Inferior cerebellar peduncle

Inferior vestibular nucleus

Medial vestibular nucleus

Central tegmental tract

Inferior olivary nucleus

B

Medial longitudinal fasciculus

Medial vestibular nucleus

Inferior vestibular nucleus

Accessory cuneate nucleus

Inferior cerebellar peduncle

Ventral spinocerebellar tract

Central tegmental tract

Inferior olivary nucleus

Figure 10–16. Myelin-stained transverse sections through the medulla at the level of the accessory cuneate nucleus *(B)* and more rostrally *(A)*.

vary nucleus, the **vestibular nuclei**, and the **pontine nuclei**. Note the first two of these nuclei in the transverse sections through the medulla (Figure 10–16). The inferior olivary nucleus (or nuclear complex) is a collection of three nuclei: (1) the principal olivary nucleus, (2) the dorsal accessory olivary nucleus, and (3) the medial accessory olivary nucleus. The inferior olivary nucleus, from which all of the **climbing fibers** originate, is large, and forms an elevation on the ventral surface of the medulla termed the **olive**. The inferior olivary nucleus consists of a convoluted sheet of neurons surrounded by the axons of the central tegmental tract, which originated from the parvocellular component of the red nucleus (see below). Neurons in the inferior olivary nucleus are electrically coupled, resulting in a synchrony of action among local groups of olivary neurons.

The vestibular nuclei are located in the rostral medulla and caudal pons (Figures 10–16 and 10–17). Purkinje cells of the flocculonodular lobe send their axons primarily to these nuclei, rather than to the deep cerebellar nuclei, as do Purkinje cells in other regions of the cerebellum. (Exceptions exist and some Purkinje cells of the flocculonodular lobe project their axons to the fastigial nucleus. Similarly, some Purkinje cells of a small portion of the vermis of the posterior lobe project to the vestibular nuclei.)

The vestibular nuclei may serve as the anatomical equivalent of the deep cerebellar nuclei of the vestibulocerebellum. The vestibular nuclei

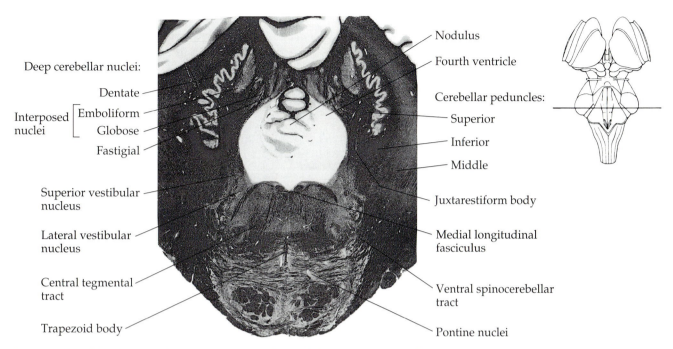

Deep cerebellar nuclei:

Dentate

Interposed nuclei { Emboliform
Globose

Fastigial

Superior vestibular nucleus

Lateral vestibular nucleus

Central tegmental tract

Trapezoid body

Nodulus

Fourth ventricle

Cerebellar peduncles:

Superior

Inferior

Middle

Juxtarestiform body

Medial longitudinal fasciculus

Ventral spinocerebellar tract

Pontine nuclei

Figure 10–17. Myelin-stained transverse section through the caudal pons and deep cerebellar nuclei.

and deep cerebellar nuclei share two similarities in the sources of afferent input. First, both groups of nuclei receive a projection from the inferior olivary nucleus. Other than the vestibular nuclei, deep cerebellar nuclei, and cerebellar cortex, no other structure receives a projection from the inferior olivary nucleus. Second, neurons in both the vestibular nuclei and the deep cerebellar nuclei are monosynaptically inhibited by Purkinje cells. The vestibular nuclei (Figure 10–16) give rise to major spinal pathways, the vestibulospinal tracts (see Chapter 9), and also contribute to the **medial longitudinal fasciculus** (Figures 10–16 through 10–18), which plays a key role in eye muscle control (see Chapter 13). Thus, the vestibulocerebellum has direct control of head and eye position via its influence on the vestibular nuclei.

The Pontine Nuclei Provide the Major Input to the Cerebrocerebellum

The pontine nuclei (Figures 10–17 and 10–18) relay input from the cerebral cortex to the cerebrocerebellum. Whereas virtually the entire cerebral cortex projects to the pontine nuclei, the densest projections arise from four major regions: (1) the **premotor areas (area 6)** (including the premotor cortex and supplementary motor area), (2) **primary motor cortex (area 4)**, (3) **primary somatic sensory cortex (areas 1, 2, and 3)**, and (4) **higher-order somatic sensory cortex (area 5)**. Corticopontine neurons originate in layer 5 of the cerebral cortex, the same layer that gives rise to the corticospinal and corticobulbar neurons. The descending axons course within the internal capsule and basis pedunculi to synapse in the pontine nuclei (see below). The axons of neurons of the pontine nuclei decussate in the pons and enter the cerebellum via the **middle cerebellar peduncle** (Figures 10–17 and 10–18). (The trapezoid body, which is the pontine auditory

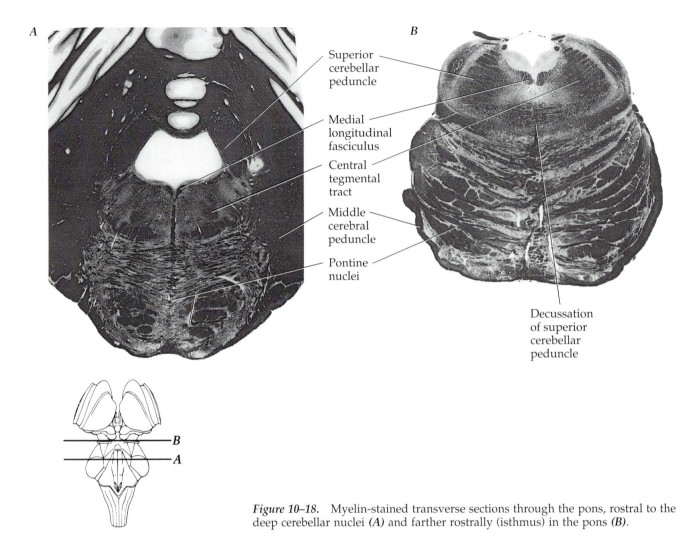

A

B

Superior cerebellar peduncle

Medial longitudinal fasciculus

Central tegmental tract

Middle cerebral peduncle

Pontine nuclei

Decussation of superior cerebellar peduncle

B

A

Figure 10–18. Myelin-stained transverse sections through the pons, rostral to the deep cerebellar nuclei *(A)* and farther rostrally (isthmus) in the pons *(B)*.

decussation, is located dorsal to the decussating pontine nucleus axons [Figure 10–17].)

The Deep Cerebellar Nuclei Are Located Within the White Matter

The deep cerebellar nuclei can be identified in the transverse section through the pons and cerebellum shown in Figure 10–17, from medial to lateral: fastigial, globose, emboliform, and dentate nuclei. Recall that the globose and emboliform nuclei collectively are termed the interposed nuclei. The efferent projections of the deep nuclei course through the inferior and superior cerebellar peduncles. The middle cerebellar peduncle carries afferent information to the cerebellum.

The fastigial, interposed, and dentate nuclei have differential projections that reflect their functions in maintaining balance, controlling limb movement, and movement planning, respectively. The major target of the output of the fastigial nucleus are nuclei in the pons and medulla. These fastigial efferent axons course in a particular portion of the inferior cerebellar peduncle termed the **juxtarestiform body** (Figure 10–17). This descending fastigial projection terminates in the vestibular nuclei and the reticular formation, two components of the medial descending systems that control balance and posture. The ascending projections from all of the deep nuclei course in the **superior cerebellar peduncle** (Figure 10–18). In Figure 10–18A, the superior cerebellar peduncle is dorsal to the pons and, farther rostrally (Figure 10–18B), it is located within the pontine **tegmentum**. The targets of the ascending projections are discussed below.

The Superior Cerebellar Peduncle Decussates in the Caudal Midbrain

The **decussation** of the superior cerebellar peduncle begins at the junction of the pons and midbrain and continues until the caudal midbrain, at the level of the inferior colliculus (Figure 10–19A). At the level shown in Figure 10–18A, the axons are located ipsilateral to the cells of origin in the deep cerebellar nuclei. Figure 10–18B shows a small contingent of axons crossing the midline; Figure 10–19A cuts through the middle of the decussation.

The ascending axons of the interposed nuclei synapse in the **magnocellular** portion of the red nucleus. The rubrospinal tract originates from

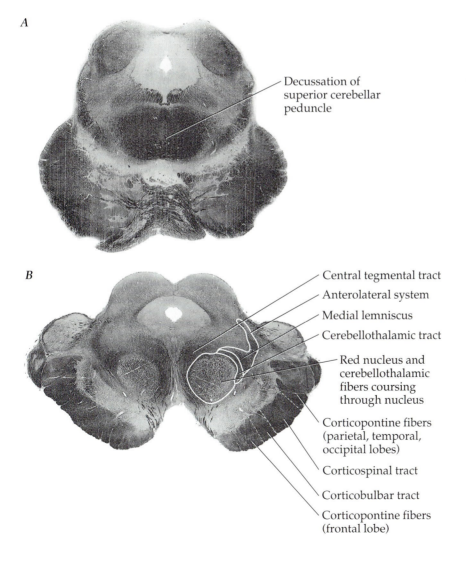

A

Decussation of superior cerebellar peduncle

B

Central tegmental tract
Anterolateral system
Medial lemniscus
Cerebellothalamic tract
Red nucleus and cerebellothalamic fibers coursing through nucleus
Corticopontine fibers (parietal, temporal, occipital lobes)
Corticospinal tract
Corticobulbar tract
Corticopontine fibers (frontal lobe)

Figure 10–19. Myelin-stained transverse sections through the caudal *(A)* and the rostral *(B)* midbrain. The organization of the fibers in the basis pedunculi is shown in *B*.

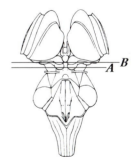

this division of the red nucleus. Neurons of the dentate nucleus synapse in the parvocellular portion of the red nucleus (Figure 10–19B). In humans the parvocellular division is much larger than the magnocellular division. The parvocellular division neurons send their axons to the ipsilateral inferior olivary nucleus via the **central tegmental tract** (Figures 10–16 and 10–17). The ascending projection from the dentate nucleus can be followed in the section shown in Figure 10–20. This section was cut obliquely, along the long axis of the superior cerebellar peduncle. The path taken by the axons of dentate nucleus neurons to the red nucleus as well as the thalamus (see below) is schematically illustrated.

The ventral surface of the midbrain is the basis pedunculi, where the descending corticopontine projection courses. The corticopontine projection (Figure 10–19B) from the frontal lobe is located in the medial basis pedunculi, whereas the projection from the parietal, temporal, and occipital lobes descends laterally. The corticospinal and corticobulbar fibers (see Chapter 9) are flanked between these two contingents of corticopontine fibers.

The Ventral Lateral Nucleus Relays Cerebellar Output to the Premotor and Primary Motor Cortices

Each of the deep cerebellar nuclei has an ascending projection that synapses in the ventral lateral nucleus of the thalamus. However, the projection from the dentate nucleus is much denser than that of the interposed nuclei, and that from the fastigial is the lightest. Collectively, the projection from all of the deep cerebellar nuclei is termed the cerebellothalamic tract. It courses directly through the red nucleus (Figure 10–20) as well as surrounding the nucleus, forming a dense ring of myelinated fibers (Figure 10–19B). The ventral lateral nucleus (Figure 10–21) is difficult to identify. One clue that makes identification a bit easier is the pres-

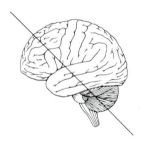

Internal capsule:

Anterior limb
Posterior limb

To primary motor cortex

Ventral lateral nucleus

Red nucleus

Decussation of superior cerebellar peduncle

Superior cerebellar peduncle

Dentate nucleus

Figure 10–20. Myelin-stained oblique section through the cerebellum, brain stem, and cerebral hemispheres. The path of the cerebellothalamic tract from the dentate nucleus to the ventral lateral nucleus and the path to the parvocellular red nucleus are shown.

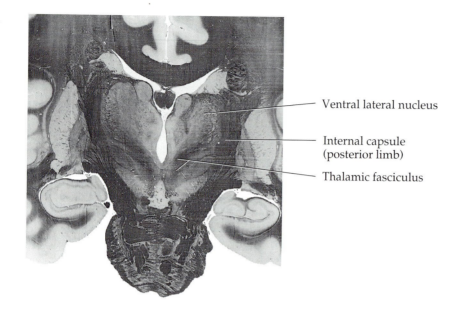

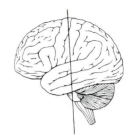

Ventral lateral nucleus

Internal capsule (posterior limb)

Thalamic fasciculus

Figure 10–21. Myelin-stained coronal section through the ventral lateral nucleus.

ence of the **thalamic fasciculus**. This band of myelinated fibers contains axons of the cerebellothalamic tract as well as axons of the basal ganglia projection to the thalamus (see Chapter 11).

The ventral lateral nucleus is one of the relay nuclei of the lateral thalamus (Figure 10–20). It is located rostral to the ventral posterior nucleus, which is the somatic sensory relay nucleus. In the rhesus monkey, on which much of the research on the motor functions of the thalamus has been conducted, an alternate nomenclature is used for this part of the thalamus. The most rostral portion of the ventral posterior lateral nucleus (the oral part, VPLo) projects to the motor cortex. This portion of the nucleus is located rostral to the sensory part of the ventral posterior nucleus, which projects to the primary somatic sensory cortex (the caudal part, VPLc). Although also likely to be complex in the human brain, the portion of the motor thalamus that transmits cerebellar input to the motor areas of the frontal lobe is described by the shorthand term, ventral lateral nucleus. The ventral lateral nucleus receives inputs from each of the deep cerebellar nuclei. Although inputs from the different nuclei are intermingled, they are largely not overlapping. In turn, the ventral lateral nucleus relays to the **primary motor cortex (area 4)** and the **premotor cortex (lateral area 6)**. The ventral lateral nucleus, like the ventral posterior nucleus, is somatotopically organized.

Damage to the Cerebellum Produces Neurological Signs on the Same Side as the Lesion

Now that we have examined the input and output paths of the cerebellum and the relationship between cerebellar projections and the descending pathways, we are in a position to consider neurological signs following cerebellar damage. There are three classic signs of cerebellar damage: ataxia, nystagmus, and tremor. **Ataxia** is inaccuracy in the speed, force, and distance of movement. In reaching for an object, the arm of a patient with cerebellar damage overshoots or undershoots the target. Ataxia of gait produces staggering and lurching. **Nystagmus** is a rhythmic

involuntary oscillation of the eyes. **Tremor** is involuntary oscillation of the limbs or trunk.

Cerebellar tremor is characteristically present when the patient is trying to perform an accurate reaching movement, such as touching the examiner's finger or bringing a forkful of food to the mouth. Ataxia and nystagmus typically occur after damage to cerebellar inputs, such as the spinocerebellar tracts or the inferior cerebellar peduncle (see below). In contrast, tremor is more often a consequence of damage to the cerebellar output pathways, such as the superior cerebellar peduncle. However, combinations of signs typically occur with damage to the cerebellum depending on the site and size of the lesion.

Knowledge of the anatomy of the descending projection systems is crucial for understanding why cerebellar damage typically produces **ipsilateral motor signs**. This is because both the cerebellar efferent projections are crossed as well as the descending pathways, which are the targets of cerebellar action. The combined decussations result in a system of connections that is "doubly crossed" (Figure 10–22). Damage to cerebellar input

Figure 10–22. The "doubly crossed" arrangement of the efferent projections of the cerebellum. Note that the cerebellar projection to the magnocellular division of the red nucleus is from the interposed nuclei (globose and emboliform nuclei) and the projection to the parvocellular division originates in the dentate nucleus. (Adapted from Carpenter, M. B., and Sutin, J. 1983. Human Neuroanatomy. Baltimore: Williams & Wilkins.)

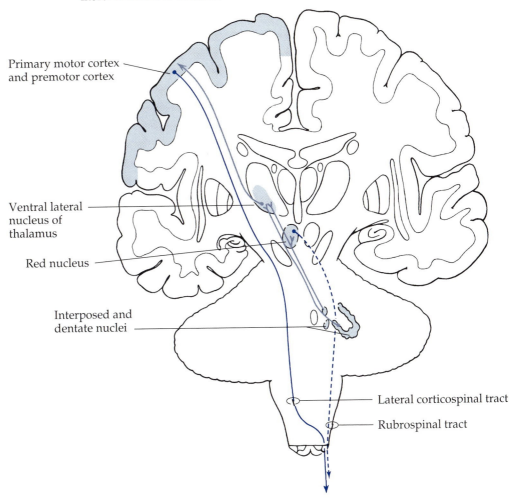

Primary motor cortex and premotor cortex

Ventral lateral nucleus of thalamus

Red nucleus

Interposed and dentate nuclei

Lateral corticospinal tract

Rubrospinal tract

from the spinal cord also produces ipsilateral signs because the principal spinocerebellar pathways, the dorsal spinocerebellars and cuneocerebellar tracts, ascend ipsilaterally. Thus, whether damage occurs to either cerebellar inputs or outputs, or to the cerebellum itself, neurological signs are present on the ipsilateral side.

Occlusion of the **posterior inferior cerebellar artery**, which produces infarction of the **inferior cerebellar peduncle**, also results in ipsilateral signs. Two key signs related to this infarction are nystagmus (also a consequence of damage to the vestibular nuclei) and ataxia. These are the cerebellar signs associated with the **lateral medullary**, or **Wallenberg's**, syndrome. Somatic sensory deficits are also present with posterior inferior cerebellar artery occlusion because infarction of the dorsolateral medulla interrupts ascending fibers of the anterolateral system (see Chapter 5) as well as the trigeminal spinal tract and nucleus (see Chapter 12). Damage to the decussation of the superior cerebellar peduncle produces bilateral signs.

Cerebellar Gross Anatomy

Summary

The cerebellum (Figure 10–1) participates in the control of movement through projections to the lateral and medial descending pathways. The cerebellar cortex overlies the white matter (Figure 10–3). The cerebellar cortex contains numerous **folia**, which are grouped into three **lobes** (Figures 10–2 and 10–3): **anterior lobe**, **posterior lobe**, and **flocculonodular lobe** (Figure 10–3). Embedded within the white matter of the cerebellum are four bilaterally paired deep nuclei, from medial to lateral (Figure 10–3B): **fastigial nucleus**, **globose nucleus**, **emboliform nucleus**, and **dentate nucleus**. The globose and emboliform nuclei are collectively termed the **interposed nuclei**.

Cerebellar Cortex

The cerebellar cortex consists of three cell layers, from the cerebellar surface to the white matter (Figure 10–11): **molecular**, **Purkinje**, and **granular** layers. Five neuron classes are found in the cerebellar cortex (Table 10–1, Figures 10–11 and 10–12): (1) **Purkinje cell** (Figure 10–13A), the **projection neuron** of the cerebellum—which is **inhibitory**, (2) **granule cell**, the only **excitatory interneuron** in the cerebellum, and the (3) **basket**, (4) **stellate**, and (5) **Golgi cells**—the **three inhibitory interneurons** (Figures 10–13 and 10–14).

Cerebellar Afferents

Two principal classes of afferent fibers reach the cerebellum: **climbing fibers** (Figures 10–5 and 10–12), which are the axons of neurons of the **inferior olivary nuclei** (Figure 10–16), and **mossy fibers**, which originate from numerous sources, including the **pontine nuclei** (Figure 10–17), **reticular formation nuclei**, **vestibular nuclei** (Figures 10–16 and 10–17), and **spinal cord** (Figure 10–15). Climbing and mossy fiber inputs are directed to both the deep cerebellar nuclei and the cerebellar cortex (Figure 10–5); but some mossy fiber sources do not project to the deep nuclei. The **climbing fibers make monosynaptic connections with the Purkinje cells**; the **mossy fibers synapse on granule cells**, which in turn synapse on Purkinje cells via their **parallel fibers**. The Purkinje cells project from the

cerebellar cortex to the deep nuclei (Figure 10–17) and the vestibular nuclei (Figures 10–16).

Cerebellar Functional Divisions

The cerebellum is divided into three functional regions (Figures 10–4 and 10–6). The **vestibulocerebellum** (1) (Figures 10–6C and 10–10) is important in balance and eye movement control; the cortical component corresponds anatomically to the **flocculonodular lobe**. It receives input from the **vestibular nuclei** and **primary vestibular afferents** and projects back to the **vestibular nuclei** via the **inferior cerebellar peduncle** (Figure 10–16).

The **spinocerebellum** (2) (Figures 10–6A, 10–7, and 10–8), which is important in posture and limb movement, is subdivided into two cortical regions that also have functional counterparts: the medial **vermis** subserves control of axial and girdle muscles, and the **intermediate hemisphere** controls **limb muscles**. The principal inputs to the spinocerebellum originate from the spinal cord. The **dorsal spinocerebellar tract** (Figure 10–7A) and the **ventral spinocerebellar tract** (Figure 10–7B) are the **lower limb pathways** and the **cuneocerebellar tract** (Figure 10–7A) and the **rostral spinocerebellar tract** (Figure 10–7B) are the **upper limb** homologues, respectively. Purkinje cells of the vermis project to the **fastigial nucleus** (Figure 10–17) which influences **medial descending pathways**: the reticulospinal, vestibulospinal, and ventral corticospinal tracts. The projection to the lower brain stem is via the **inferior cerebellar peduncle** (Figure 10–16), and the thalamic projection is via the **superior cerebellar peduncle** (Figures 10–18 and 10–19). The **intermediate hemisphere** projects to the interposed nuclei, which in turn influence the **lateral descending pathways**: the rubrospinal and lateral corticospinal tracts. All projections from the spinocerebellum course through the superior cerebellar peduncle.

The **cerebrocerebellum** (3) (Figure 10–6B) plays a role in planning movements; its cortical component is the **lateral hemisphere**. The cerebral cortex projects to the **pontine nuclei** (Figures 10–17 and 10–18), which provide the main input to the cerebrocerebellum. Purkinje cells of this functional division project to the **dentate nucleus** (Figure 10–17). From there, dentate neurons project to the contralateral **parvocellular red nucleus** (Figure 10–19B) and the **ventral lateral nucleus** of the thalamus (Figures 10–20 and 10–21), both via the **superior cerebellar peduncle**. The principal projections of the ventral lateral nucleus are to the **primary motor cortex** (area 4) and the **premotor cortex** (lateral area 6). ■

KEY STRUCTURES AND TERMS

posterior cranial fossa
cerebellar tentorium
folia
lobules
posterior cerebellar incisure
anterior lobe
posterior lobe
primary fissure
posterolateral fissure
peduncles
   superior cerebellar peduncle
   middle cerebellar peduncle
   inferior cerebellar peduncle
vermis
hemispheres
flocculonodular lobe
   nodulus
   flocculus
cerebellar cortex
   molecular layer
      basket cell
      stellate cell

Purkinje layer
   Purkinje cells
granular layer
   granule cells
   Golgi cell
   cerebellar glomerulus
climbing fibers
mossy fibers
deep cerebellar nuclei
   fastigial nucleus
   interposed nuclei (globose and
      emboliform nuclei)
   dentate nucleus
vestibular nuclei
spinocerebellum
cerebrocerebellum
vestibulocerebellum
dorsal spinocerebellar tract
   Clarke's nucleus
cuneocerebellar tract
   accessory cuneate nucleus

ventral and rostral spinocerebellar
   tracts
premotor areas (area 6)
primary motor cortex (area 4)
primary somatic sensory cortex
   (areas 1, 2, and 3)
higher-order somatic sensory cortex
   (area 5)
ventral lateral nucleus
pontine nuclei
medial longitudinal fasciculus
central tegmental tract
red nucleus
   parvocellular
   magnocellular
inferior olivary nucleus
ataxia
nystagmus
tremor
ipsilateral motor signs
posterior inferior cerebellar artery

Selected Readings

Brodal, A. 1981. Neurological Anatomy. New York: Oxford University Press.

Brooks, V. B. 1986. The Neural Basis of Motor Control. New York: Oxford University Press.

Brooks, V. B., and Thatch, W. T. 1981. Cerebellar control of posture and movement. In Brooks, V. B. (ed.), Handbook of Physiology, Section I: The Nervous System, Vol. II, Motor Control. Bethesda, Md.: American Physiological Society, pp. 877–946.

Eccles, J. C., Ito, M., and Szentágothai, J. 1967. The Cerebellum as a Neuronal Machine. New York: Springer-Verlag.

Ghez, C. 1991. The cerebellum. In Kandel, E. R., Schwartz, J. H., and Jessell, T. M. (eds.), Principles of Neural Science, 3rd ed. New York: Elsevier, pp. 626–646.

Glickstein M., and Yeo, C. 1990. The cerebellum and motor learning. J. Cog. Neurosci. 2:69–80.

Ito, M. 1984. The Cerebellum and Neural Control. New York: Raven Press.

Leiner, H. C., Leiner, A. L., and Dow, R. S. 1993. Cognitive and language functions of the human cerebellum. Trends Neurosci. 16:444–447.

Thach, W. T., Goodkin, H. P., and Keating, J. G. 1992. The cerebellum and the adaptive coordination of movement. Annu. Rev. Neurosci. 15:403–442.

References

Angevine, J. B., Jr., Mancall, E. L., and Yakovlev, P. I. 1961. The Human Cerebellum: An Atlas of Gross Topography in Serial Sections. Boston: Little, Brown.

Carpenter, M. B., and Sutin, J. 1983. Human Neuroanatomy. Baltimore: Williams & Wilkins.

Dietrichs, E., and Walberg, F. 1987. Cerebellar nuclear afferents—where do they originate? Anat. Embryol. 177:165–172.

Heimer, L. 1983. The Human Brain and Spinal Cord. New York: Springer-Verlag.

Kim, SS. -G., Ugurbil, K., and Strick, P. L. 1994. Activation of cerebellar output nucleus during cognitive processing. Science 265:949–951.

Massion, J. 1988. Red nucleus: Past and future. Behav. Brain Res. 28:1–8.

Middleton, F. A., and Strick, P. L. 1994. Anatomical evidence for cerebellar and basal ganglia involvement in higher cognitive function. Science 266:458–461.

Schell, G. R., and Strick, P. L. 1984. The origin of thalamic inputs to the arcuate premotor and supplementary motor areas. J. Neurosci. 4:539–560.

11

The Basal Ganglia

T*HE BASAL GANGLIA ARE A COLLECTION OF SUBCORTICAL NUCLEI* that have captured the fascination of clinicians for well over a century because of the remarkable range of behavioral dysfunction that is associated with basal ganglia disease. Movement control deficits are among the key signs, ranging from the tremor and rigidity of Parkinson's disease and the graceful writhing movements of Huntington's disease to the bizarre tics of Tourette's syndrome. These clinical findings suggest that one important set of basal ganglia functions is the control of our motor actions. How do the basal ganglia fit into an overall view of the organization of the motor systems? Unlike the motor cortex, which has direct connections with motor neurons, the basal ganglia influence movements of our eyes, limbs, and trunk indirectly by acting on the descending pathways. In this way the basal ganglia are more like the cerebellum than the structures that give rise to the descending motor pathways.

In addition to producing movement control deficits, basal ganglia disease can also impair intellectual capacity, suggesting an important role in cognition. Dementia is an early disabling consequence of Huntington's disease and is present in patients with advanced stages of Parkinson's disease. Recently, the basal ganglia have also been linked with emotional function, playing a role in aspects of drug addiction and psychiatric disease.

Although the basal ganglia are still among the least understood of all brain structures, their mysteries are now yielding to modern neurobiological techniques for elucidating neurochemistry and connections. For example, we now know that the basal ganglia contain virtually all of the major neuroactive agents that have been discovered in the various divisions of the central nervous system. While the reason for this biochemical diversity remains elusive, we can apply this knowledge to effectively treat some forms of basal ganglia disease. Indeed, the discovery that the brains of patients with Parkinson's disease are deficient in the neuroactive agent dopamine quickly led to the development of drug replacement therapy. Our knowledge about connections of the basal ganglia with the rest of the brain have led to a major revision of the traditional views of basal ganglia organization and function. Discoveries about basal ganglia circuitry and pathways have even led to therapeutic neurosurgical procedures.

In this chapter, we first consider the constituents of the basal ganglia and their three-dimensional shapes. Next, their functional organization is surveyed, emphasizing the role of the basal ganglia in movement control. This emphasis is chosen because we have more complete information on the motor functions of basal ganglia than their role in cognition and emotions. Finally, we examine the regional anatomy of the basal ganglia in a series of slices through the cerebral hemisphere and brain stem. In Chapter 15, we will consider basal ganglia anatomy in relation to emotions.

■ FUNCTIONAL ANATOMY OF THE BASAL GANGLIA

Separate Components of Basal Ganglia Process Incoming Information and Mediate the Output

To understand the organization of the basal ganglia we must first take an inventory of the various components. The nomenclature of the basal ganglia is more complex than that of other regions of the brain. On the basis of their connections, the various components of the basal ganglia can be divided into three categories: input nuclei, output nuclei, and intrinsic nuclei. The **input nuclei** receive afferent connections from brain regions other than the basal ganglia, and in turn, project to the intrinsic and output nuclei. The **output nuclei** project to regions of the diencephalon and brain stem that are not part of the basal ganglia. The connections of the **intrinsic nuclei** are largely restricted to the basal ganglia.

The general organization of the basal ganglia from input to output is shown in Figure 11–1. The key to understanding the anatomy of this brain region is that the four lobes of the cerebral cortex are the major source of input to the basal ganglia, but only the **frontal lobe receives their output**. The **striatum** is the **input** side of the basal ganglia, receiving afferent projections from the cerebral cortex. Three nuclei comprise the striatum: **caudate nucleus**, **putamen**, and **nucleus accumbens**. It should be recalled (see Chapter 2) that the striatum has a complex shape (Figure 11–2). The caudate nucleus has a C-shape, which is a consequence of the extensive development of the cerebral cortex (see Chapter 2). Although it is one continuous structure, three separate names are given to portions of the caudate nucleus: head, body, and tail (Figure 11–2). The putamen, when viewed from its lateral surface, is shaped like a disk. The caudate nucleus and putamen are connected by **cell bridges**, which resemble spokes on a wheel. The nucleus accumbens (Figure 11–2) is located ventromedial to the caudate nucleus and putamen. The three components of the striatum are joined rostrally.

There are three nuclei on the **output** side of the basal ganglia (Figure 11–1): **internal segment of the globus pallidus**, **ventral pallidum**, and **substantia nigra pars reticulata**. The output nuclei send their axons primarily to thalamic nuclei which, in turn, project to different areas of the frontal lobe. These thalamic nuclei include the **ventral lateral nucleus** (to a part distinct from the one receiving cerebellar input), the **ventral anterior nucleus**, and the **medial dorsal nucleus**. Thalamic nuclei also have a major projection back to the striatum that may serve an important behavioral regulatory function (see below).

There are four intrinsic nuclei of the basal ganglia and their connections are closely related to the input and output nuclei: **external segment of the globus pallidus**, **subthalamic nucleus**, **substantia nigra pars compacta**, and **ventral tegmental area**. The external segment of the globus pal-

B

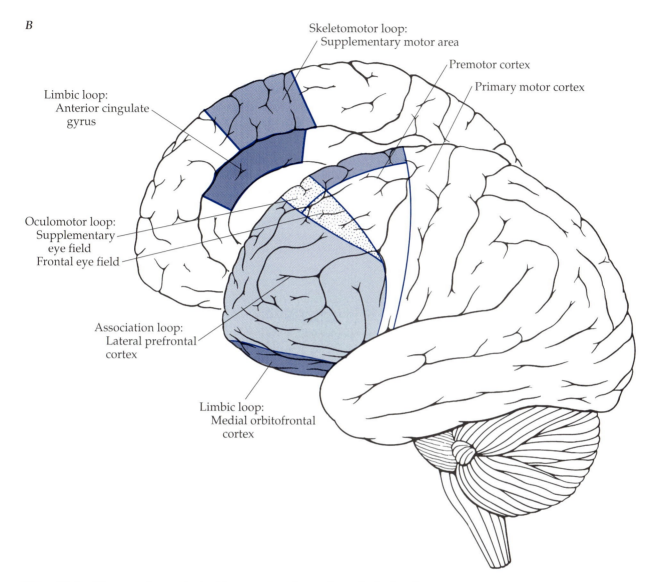

Skeletomotor loop:
Supplementary motor area

Premotor cortex

Primary motor cortex

Limbic loop:
Anterior cingulate
gyrus

Oculomotor loop:
Supplementary
eye field
Frontal eye field

Association loop:
Lateral prefrontal
cortex

Limbic loop:
Medial orbitofrontal
cortex

Figure 11–3. There are four principal input–output loops through the basal ganglia. *A.* Block diagrams illustrating the general organization of the loops. (1) Skeletomotor loop, (2) oculomotor loop, (3) association loop, and (4) limbic loop. (Abbreviations: GPi, globus pallidus internal segment; SNr, substantia nigra pars reticulata.) *B.* Lateral and medial views of cerebral cortex, illustrating the approximate location of the "target" regions in the frontal lobe. Note that the medial orbitofrontal cortex is located ventral to the lateral prefrontal cortex and is tinted dark blue.

motor fields. Even the prefrontal association cortex, important in organizing goal-directed behaviors and complex thought and reasoning, has relatively direct connections with premotor areas that, in turn, have motor cortical and even spinal projections.

Even though there are numerous parallel basal ganglia circuits, integration across circuits must take place. For example, how can the limbic loop influence motor behavior, such as reaching for a cup of coffee, if its connections always remain distinct from those of the motor loop? Basal ganglia research is beginning to point to a second organization whereby interactions occur between circuits. Using our example of limbic system–motor interactions, we know that both the ventral and dorsal parts of the striatum—which serve limbic and motor functions, respectively—project to the substantia nigra. The terminals of axons comprising these two loops may converge on nigral neurons and thus be sites for integration. Researchers are beginning to uncover other examples where integration between the parallel loops can take place. For example, the dendrites of striatal neurons may extend beyond their own loop into adjacent loops.

Knowledge of the Connections and Neurotransmitters of the Basal Ganglia Provides Insight Into Their Function in Health and Disease

Although each loop through the basal ganglia helps to shape our thoughts, emotions, and motor behaviors, the particular roles played by these loops and the operations performed by their component nuclei remain elusive. We do not know, for example, how neural information is transformed as it passes from the input nuclei to the output nuclei and then through the thalamus back to the cerebral cortex. We can, however, gain important insights for developing an understanding of the function of the basal ganglia by examining the kinds of neuroactive compounds present in the various basal ganglia nuclei and the patterns of neuronal connections.

Basal Ganglia Contain Diverse Neurotransmitters and Neuromodulators

Many of the classic neurotransmitters, which have rapid postsynaptic actions, are present in the various basal ganglia nuclei (Figure 11–4), including γ-aminobutyric acid (GABA) and glutamate (acting on non-N-methyl-D-aspartate [NMDA] receptors). In addition, many **neuromodulatory** substances, which have slow synaptic actions, such as dopamine, acetylcholine, and glutamate (acting on NMDA receptors), are also present.

Figure 11–4. The neurotransmitters of the basal ganglia (boldface labels) are shown in relation to the organization of basal ganglia circuits. (Abbreviations: GABA, γ-aminobutryic acid; GPi, globus pallidus, internal segment; GPe, globus pallidus, external segment; SNr, substantia nigra pars reticulata; SNc, substantia nigra pars compacta; STN, subthalamic nucleus; VTA, ventral tegmental area.) (Adapted from Haber, S. N. 1986. Neurotransmitters in the human and nonhuman primate basal ganglia. Human Neurobiol. 5:159–168.)

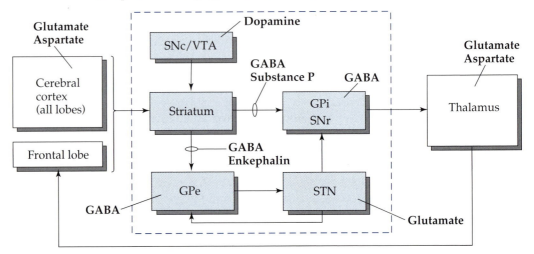

In this section, we briefly survey the neurotransmitters and neuro-modulatory agents that are present in the various components of the basal ganglia. Later, we will use examples of histochemical staining to reveal the distribution of these compounds in the input and output nuclei.

The excitatory neurotransmitter **glutamate** is present in the terminals of the corticostriatal neurons (the major input to the basal ganglia), thalamic neuron terminals in the striatum, and the projection neurons of the subthalamic nucleus. The major neurotransmitter of the basal ganglia is **GABA**, which is **inhibitory**. In the striatum, GABA is located in the projection neurons, the **medium spiny neurons**. These neurons, which have abundant dendritic spines (see Figure 1–1), project their axons to the two segments of the globus pallidus and the substantia nigra pars reticulata. In addition to GABA, medium spiny neurons also contain neuropeptides, with two distinct neuron classes containing either **enkephalin** or, on the other hand, **substance P** and **dynorphin**. Projection neurons of the internal and external segments of the globus pallidus and the substantia nigra pars reticulata also contain GABA. Thus, the output of the basal ganglia, similar to that of the cerebellar cortex, is **inhibitory**. The significance of this common synaptic organization is not yet apparent.

Neurons in the pars compacta of the substantia nigra and the ventral tegmental area contain **dopamine**. The term substantia nigra, which means black substance, derives from the presence of the black pigment **neuromelanin**, a polymer of the catecholamine precursor dihydroxy-phenylalanine (or Dopa), which is contained in the neurons in the pars compacta. In the movement disorder **Parkinson's disease**, the midbrain dopaminergic neurons are destroyed and striatal dopamine is profoundly reduced (see below). Replacement therapy using a precursor to dopamine, **L-dopa**, leads to a dramatic improvement in the neurological signs of this disease. Not surprisingly, neuromelanin is not present in the substantia nigra pars compacta of Parkinson's patients. Dopaminergic neurons in other parts of the central nervous system also become destroyed. Dopamine loss in the basal ganglia, however, apparently produces the most debilitating neurological signs.

Acetylcholine is also a common neurotransmitter in the basal ganglia. It is present in striatal interneurons, where it is an important neurotransmitter in the function of **local neuronal circuits**.

Parkinson's Disease Is a Hypokinetic Movement Disorder
Whereas Hemiballism Is a Hyperkinetic Disorder

In Parkinson's disease, with its loss of striatal dopamine, there is a major impairment in initiating movements, termed **akinesia**, and a reduction in the extent and speed of movements, called **bradykinesia**. These are called **hypokinetic** signs because movements become impoverished. In addition, patients exhibit a resting **tremor,** and when their limbs are moved by an examiner, a characteristic stiffness or **rigidity** can be noted.

Recently, researchers have fortuitously acquired an important tool in the study of Parkinson's disease. They discovered that a certain kind of synthetic heroin produces a permanent clinical syndrome in humans that is remarkably similar to Parkinson's disease. This substance contains the neurotoxin MPTP (1-methyl-4-phenyl-1,2,3,6-tetrahydropyridine), which kills the dopaminergic neurons of the substantia nigra pars compacta (as well as other dopaminergic neurons in the central nervous system). When monkeys are administered MPTP, they too develop parkinsonian signs, including akinesia, bradykinesia, rigidity, and tremor.

Box 11–1. *Knowledge of the Intrinsic Circuitry of the Basal Ganglia Helps to Explain Hypokinetic and Hyperkinetic Signs*

Recently, scientists have begun to study disordered movement control during basal ganglia disease in terms of two sets of connections in the skeletomotor loop (see Figure 11–3A1), termed the **direct** and **indirect** striatal output pathways (Figure 11–5A). These paths are thought to have antagonistic effects on the thalamus, with the **direct path exciting thalamic target neurons** and **the indirect path, inhibiting**.

Projection neurons of the putamen in the direct path synapse on internal pallidal neurons, which in turn, project to the ventral lateral and ventral anterior nuclei of the thalamus. This circuit contains two inhibitory neurons, in the putamen and globus pallidus. Thus, cortical excitation of the putamen is first transformed into an inhibitory message to the internal segment of the globus pallidus. However, the output of the internal pallidum is also

inhibitory. So inhibition from the putamen **reduces the amount of inhibition of the thalamus from the internal pallidal segment**. Inhibition of an inhibitory signal is termed **disinhibition**; functionally, this "double negative" is equivalent to excitation. For example, in a motor behavior such as reaching for a cup of coffee, neurons in premotor areas, as well as corticospinal tract neurons in primary motor cortex, may be excited by the actions of the direct path.

The indirect path has the opposite effect on the thalamus and cerebral cortex as the direct path. The key to understanding the indirect path is that the subthalamic nucleus is excitatory. Putamen neurons of the indirect path, which are inhibitory, project to the **external pallidal segment**, the output of which is also inhibitory. Because the external globus pallidus projects to the subthalamic nucleus, the putamen disinhibits the subthal-

amic nucleus. This disinhibition will excite the output of the subthalamic nucleus, the internal globus pallidus and substantia nigra reticulata and thereby increase the strength of the inhibitory output signal that is directed to the thalamus.

Currently, this model is helping us understand the mechanisms of some hypokinetic and hyperkinetic signs seen in basal ganglia disease. Dopamine is deficient in Parkinson's disease, which produces hypokinetic signs. Dopamine is thought to excite striatal neurons of the direct path and inhibit striatal neurons of the indirect path (Figure 11–5B). Reduced striatal dopamine in Parkinson's disease would be expected to diminish the excitatory effects of the direct path on cortical motor areas and enhance the inhibitory effects of the indirect path. Together the reduced excitatory drive of the direct path and increased inhibitory drive

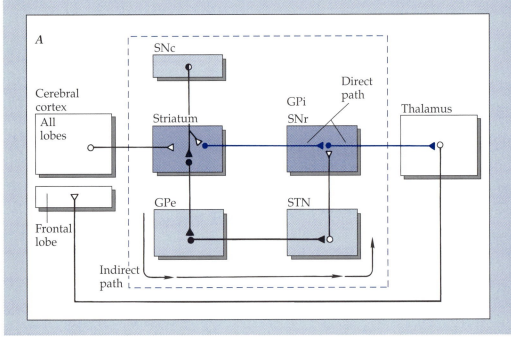

Box 11–1. *(continued)*

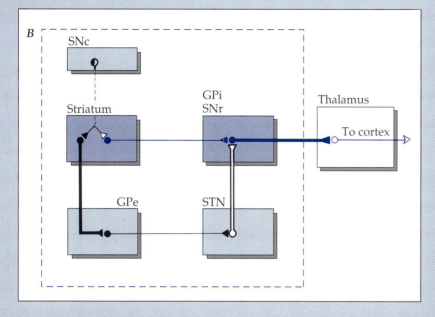

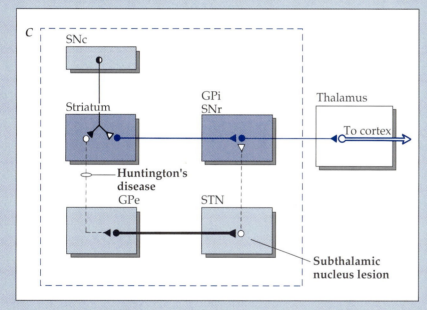

of the indirect path would drastically reduce the thalamic signals to the cortex. For the premotor and motor cortex, this would reduce cortical outflow along the corticospinal tract and favor reduced production of motor behaviors (i.e., hypokinesia).

In hyperkinetic disorders (Figure 11–5C), the opposite changes take place: there are enhanced excitatory effects of the indirect path on the cortex. For example, hemiballism is produced by subthalamic nucleus lesions and this nucleus normally exerts an excitatory action on the internal segment of the globus pallidus. When the subthalamic nucleus becomes lesioned, the internal globus pallidus would be expected to inhibit the thalamus less, thereby increasing outflow to the cerebral cortex. In Huntington's disease, another hyperkinetic disorder, recent studies suggest that there is a loss of striatal enkephalin, a neuroactive substance localized to neurons of the indirect path. Like hemiballism, Huntington's disease would also result in greater thalamic outflow to the cortex, but by a decreasing striatal inhibition of the external globus pallidus.

Figure 11–5. Functional basal ganglia circuits. *A.* Summary of the direct and indirect paths of the basal ganglia. *B* and *C.* Model for changes in the direct and indirect path that could account for hypokinetic *(B)* and hyperkinetic *(C)* signs of basal ganglia disease. Filled neurons indicate inhibitory actions and open, excitatory. (See Figure 11–4 for basal ganglia neurotransmitters.) Neurons of the direct path are colored blue, whereas neurons of the indirect path are black. Dashed lines indicate degenerating neurons. (Abbreviations: SNc, substantia nigra pars compacta; SNr, substantia nigra pars reticulata; GPe, globus pallidus, external segment; GPi, globus pallidus, internal segment; STN, subthalamic nucleus.)

In contrast to Parkinson's disease, which is a hypokinetic disorder because movements are slowed, **Huntington's disease** is a hyperkinetic disorder, inherited as an autosomal dominant. The Huntington's gene is located on the short arm of chromosome 4. In most patients, Huntington's disease presents during midlife. One hyperkinetic sign of this disorder is **chorea**, which is characterized by involuntary rapid and random movements of the limbs and trunk. Patients with Huntington's disease also have dementia. Another hyperkinetic disorder is **hemiballism**. This remarkable clinical disturbance occurs after vascular lesion of the **subthalamic nucleus**. As its name suggests, the stricken patient makes uncontrollable, rapid **ballistic** (or flinging) movements of the contralateral limbs. These movements are produced by motion at proximal limb joints, such as the shoulder and elbow. There also may be involuntary distal limb movements, such as writhing of the hand (athetosis). Box 11–1 presents a recently developed model for understanding some of the general signs of hypokinetic and hyperkinetic movement disorders in terms of the circuitry and biochemistry of the basal ganglia.

■ REGIONAL ANATOMY

Having considered the functional organization of the basal ganglia, we next examine the regional anatomy of the parts of the brain that contain the components and associated nuclei of the basal ganglia. We begin with a horizontal slice through the cerebral hemispheres and diencephalon because it permits visualization of the various components of the internal capsule, which form major subcortical landmarks, and then move to coronal slices. In addition to learning the regional anatomy of the basal ganglia, we also begin to synthesize an overall view of the deep structures of the cerebral hemisphere.

The Anterior Limb of the Internal Capsule Separates the Head of the Caudate Nucleus From the Putamen

The dominant structure of the horizontal section (Figure 11–6) is the **internal capsule**, which contains ascending thalamocortical fibers and descending cortical fibers. The three main segments of the internal capsule include (see Chapter 3): the **anterior limb**, the **posterior limb**, and the **genu**, which connects the two limbs (Figure 11–6). A three-dimensional view of the internal capsule is shown in Figure 11–7. Complementing these three main segments are the retrolenticular and sublenticular portions of the internal capsule (Figure 11–7), named for their locations with respect to the **lenticular nucleus**, which comprises the putamen and globus pallidus. The striatum is shown in relation to the internal capsule in Figure 11–7. While the putamen and nucleus accumbens are located lateral to the internal capsule, the caudate nucleus is located medial.

In horizontal section, the internal capsule is shaped like an arrowhead pointed toward the midline (Figure 11–6). The anterior limb separates the **head of the caudate nucleus from the putamen** (Figure 11–6). This limb contains axons projecting to and from the frontal association cortex, including the **prefrontal cortex**. The posterior limb separates the **putamen** and **globus pallidus** (lenticular nucleus) from the **thalamus** and **body and tail of the caudate nucleus** (Figure 11–6). The posterior limb

6. **Lateral medullary lamina.** Axons that separate the putamen from the external segment of the globus pallidus.

7. **External segment of the globus pallidus.** Projects to the subthalamic nucleus.

8. **Medial medullary lamina.** Separates the external and internal segments of the globus pallidus.

9. **Internal segment of the globus pallidus.** Projects to the thalamus.

10. **Posterior limb of the internal capsule.** Contains descending corticospinal axons as well as other descending fibers and ascending thalamocortical fibers.

11. **Thalamus.** Contains the principal sensory and motor relay nuclei for the cerebral cortex.

12. **Thalamic adhesion** (or massa intermedia). A small portion of the thalamus that physically adheres to its counterpart on the contralateral side, spanning the third ventricle.

An important feature of the complex three-dimensional structure of the caudate nucleus can be identified in Figure 11–6. Because the caudate nucleus has a C-shape, it can be seen in two locations in this section. The head of the caudate nucleus is located rostromedially and the tail of the caudate nucleus, caudolaterally. (The body of the caudate nucleus is located dorsal to the plane of section.) Later we will discover that in certain coronal sections, the caudate nucleus is also seen in two locations (dorsomedially and ventrolaterally).

Cell Bridges Link the Caudate Nucleus and the Putamen

A coronal slice through the anterior limb of the internal capsule (Figure 11–8) reveals the three components of the striatum: (1) **caudate nucleus** (at this level, the head of the caudate nucleus), (2) **putamen**, and (3) **nucleus accumbens**. Although the internal capsule courses between the caudate nucleus and the putamen, **striatal cell bridges** link the two structures. These cell bridges are a reminder that, in the developing brain

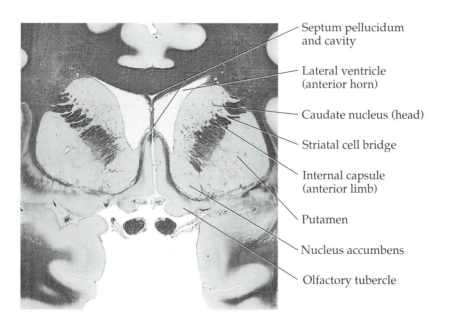

- Septum pellucidum and cavity
- Lateral ventricle (anterior horn)
- Caudate nucleus (head)
- Striatal cell bridge
- Internal capsule (anterior limb)
- Putamen
- Nucleus accumbens
- Olfactory tubercle

Figure 11–8. Myelin-stained coronal section through the head of the caudate nucleus.

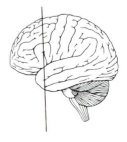

(see Chapter 2), axons coursing to and from the cortex incompletely divide the group of neuroblasts in the floor of the lateral ventricle that give rise to the striatum.

The nucleus accumbens, together with the ventromedial portions of the caudate and putamen (Figure 11–8), comprise the **ventral striatum**, the striatal component of the limbic loop (Figure 11–3A4). (The olfactory tubercle is sometimes included within the ventral striatrum; it is located on the basal surface of the forebrain. A portion of the tubercle receives olfactory inputs. The boundary between the olfactory portion of the tubercle and the part that is contained within the limbic loop is not clearly understood.)

The **septum pellucidum** (Figure 11–8) is a thin connective tissue membrane that forms the medial walls of the anterior horn and body of the lateral ventricles. Between the two septa is a cavity in which fluid may accumulate. The cavity is large in the fetus, and it can be imaged noninvasively using ultrasound. There is normal variation in the size of the cavity in mature brains. However, the size of the cavity is consistently large in certain pathological conditions, for example, in the brains of boxers suffering from dementia pugilistica, a degenerative condition similar to Parkinson's disease, characterized by loss of cognitive functions and disordered movements.

Figure 11–9. Histochemical localization of acetylcholinesterase *(A)* and enkephalin *(B)* in the human striatum. (Courtesy of Dr. Suzanne Haber, University of Rochester School of Medicine.)

A

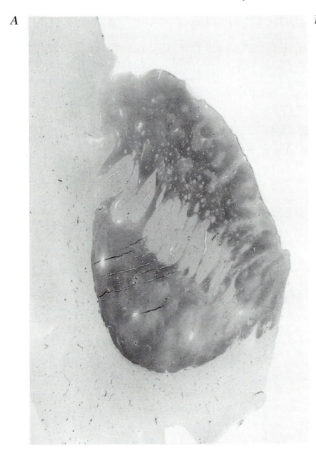

B

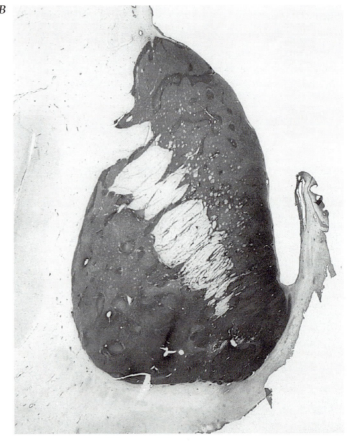

The Striatum Has a Compartmental Organization

In myelin-stained sections, the three striatal components appear identical and homogeneous, as they also do in Nissl-stained sections. Histochemical staining of the striatum also demonstrates similarities. For example, each striatal component stains positive for the enzyme **acetylcholinesterase**, a marker for the neurotransmitter **acetylcholine** (Figure 11–9A), or **enkephalin** (Figure 11–9B).

Histochemical staining, however, also reveals a striking lack of homogeneity in which there is a nonuniform distribution of neurotransmitters and neuromodulators within local regions of the components of the striatum. For acetylcholinesterase, "patches" of low concentration are surrounded by a "matrix" of tissue containing a higher concentration (Figure 11–9A). Enkephalin (Figure 11–9B), as well as numerous other neuroactive substances that are present in the striatum, also has a patchy distribution. The functional significance of striatal compartmentalization has remained elusive and, among the many unresolved questions concerning basal ganglia organization, is one of the most important. Recent experimental findings have shown that neurons in the patch and matrix have different connections. These studies point to an important functional role for the patch–matrix organization in integrating information.

The projections of cortical neurons also have a nonuniform distribution to local striatal regions. This is shown in Figure 11–10 for projections from the prefrontal association cortex of the rhesus monkey to the head of

Figure 11–10. Autoradiograph of the cerebral hemispheres showing the patchy distribution of labeled corticostriatal axon terminals in the head of the caudate nucleus of the rhesus monkey. In the center of the figure is the corpus callosum, with the cingulate gyri above and the anterior horns of the lateral ventricles below. As in the human, the head of the caudate nucleus also bulges into the anterior horn of the lateral ventricle. Radioactive tracer, consisting of a mixture of ^{3}H proline and ^{3}H leucine, was injected into the prefrontal cortex. Tracer was incorporated into cortical neurons and transported anterogradely to their axons and terminals. This resulted in an intricate pattern of labeling in the caudate nucleus. Also note that axons were labeled in the white matter, including in the corpus callosum. This is because the tracer labels callosal neurons as well as a variety of descending projection neurons. (Courtesy of Dr. Patricia Goldman-Rakic; Goldman-Rakic, P. S. 1978. Science 202:768–770)

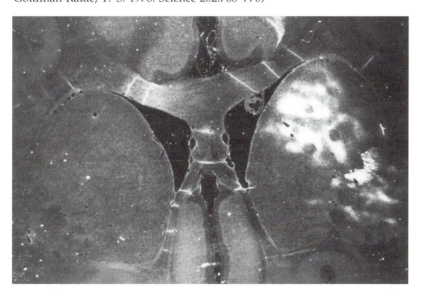

the caudate nucleus. Other studies have shown that the unlabeled regions receive projections from other cortical association areas, such as the posterior parietal cortex.

The Head of the Caudate Nucleus Is a Radiological Landmark

The head of the caudate nucleus bulges into the anterior horn of the lateral ventricle (Figure 11–8). This can be seen on a magnetic resonance imaging (MRI) scan of a normal individual (Figure 11–11). Gross changes in the structure of the caudate nucleus in a Huntington's disease patient also can be seen (Figure 11–11). In patients with Huntington's disease, there is a loss of **medium spiny neurons**. This cell loss begins in the caudate nucleus and dorsal putamen. Because these neurons constitute more than three quarters of striatal neurons, in Huntington's patients the characteristic bulge of the head of the caudate nucleus into the lateral ventricle is absent.

Figure 11–11. Magnetic resonance imaging (MRI) scans of brain slices through the head of the caudate nucleus of a patient with Huntington's disease. Note that the head of the caudate nucleus is smaller in the patient with Huntington's disease compared with normal. The imaging planes and locations of the MRI scans in *A* and *B* are similar to the planes of section and locations of the myelin-stained sections in Figures 11–8 and 11–6, respectively. (Courtesy of Dr. Susan Folstein.)

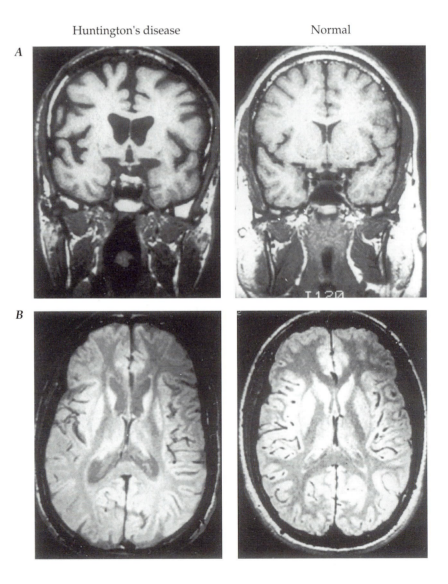

Huntington's disease   Normal

The External Segment of the Globus Pallidus and the Ventral Pallidum Are Separated by the Anterior Commissure

The external segment of the globus pallidus, as we saw earlier, is an intrinsic basal ganglia nucleus that sends its axons to the subthalamic nucleus. The ventral pallidum is the output nucleus for the limbic loop. The external segment of the globus pallidus and the ventral pallidum are separated by the **anterior commissure** (Figure 11–12). This commissure, like the corpus callosum, interconnects regions of the cerebral cortex of either hemisphere. Unlike the corpus callosum, which connects wide regions of the frontal, parietal, occipital, and posterior temporal lobes, the anterior commissure interconnects very restricted regions, parts of the **anterior temporal lobes** (see Chapter 15), **amygdaloid nuclear complex**, and **olfactory structures** (see Chapter 8). A parasagittal section through the internal segment of the globus pallidus is presented in Figure 11–13, in which it can be seen that the ventral pallidum extends to the ventral brain surface.

The Internal Segment of the Globus Pallidus Projects to the Thalamus Via the Ansa Lenticularis and the Lenticular Fasciculus

Two major laminae separate components of the basal ganglia (Figure 11–14A). The (1) **lateral medullary lamina** separates the external segment of the globus pallidus from the putamen; (2) the **medial medullary lamina** separates the internal and external segments of the globus pallidus. The internal segment of the globus pallidus is a major output of the basal ganglia. Neurosurgeons have been able to produce a lesion (by electrocoagulation) in the internal globus pallidus in patients with Parkinson's disease. In this surgical procedure, termed **pallidotomy**, by eliminating the abnormal output of the basal ganglia, the remaining portions of the motor systems appear to function better. Neurons of the internal segment of the globus pallidus project their axons to the thalamus. These axons course in two anatomically separate pathways: the **lenticular fasciculus** and the **ansa lenticularis**. The axons of the lenticular fasciculus course directly

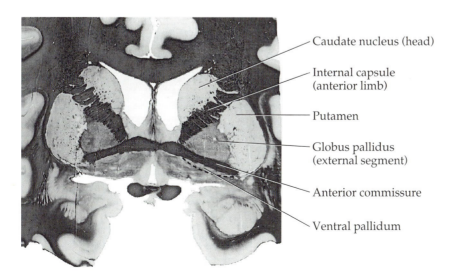

Caudate nucleus (head)

Internal capsule (anterior limb)

Putamen

Globus pallidus (external segment)

Anterior commissure

Ventral pallidum

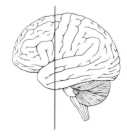

Figure 11–12. Myelin-stained coronal section through the external segment of the globus pallidus and ventral pallidum.

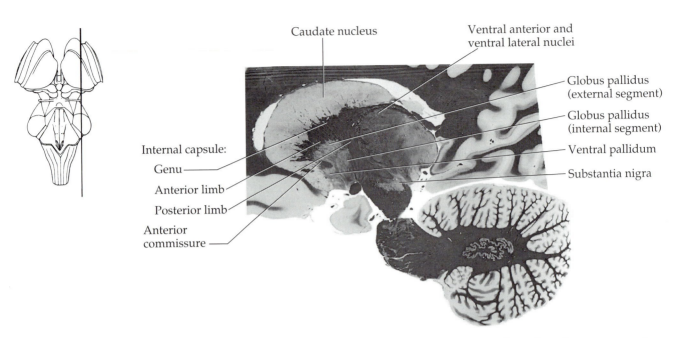

Figure 11–13. Myelin-stained parasagittal section through various components of the basal ganglia.

through the internal capsule, but these axons are not clearly visualized until they collect medial to the internal capsule (Figure 11–14B).

The internal capsule appears to be a barrier for fibers of the ansa lenticularis; these fibers course around it to reach the thalamus (Figures 11–14A and B). The ansa lenticularis and lenticular fasciculus converge beneath the thalamus and join fibers of the cerebellothalamic tract to form the **thalamic fasciculus** (Figure 11–14B). There is an alternate nomenclature for lenticular and thalamic fasciculi that is sometimes used. The lenticular fasciculus is also termed **Forel's field H2** and the thalamic fasciculus, **Forel's field H1**. A third Forel's field, termed **H**, is the region ventromedial to field H1 and is continuous with the tegmentum of the midbrain.

The three major thalamic targets of the output nuclei of the basal ganglia (see Figure 11–3A) can be identified in Figures 11–13 through 11–15: the **medial dorsal**, **ventral lateral**, and **ventral anterior nuclei**. Most of the fibers of the deep cerebellar nuclei also terminate in the **ventral lateral nucleus**, but in a separate portion as axons from the basal ganglia. Two intralaminar thalamic nuclei (see Chapter 3), **centromedian** and **parafascicular nuclei**, are anatomically closely related to the basal ganglia because they provide a major direct input to the striatum. In addition, these thalamic nuclei also project to the frontal lobe, the cortical target of the basal ganglia. Whereas the centromedian nucleus (Figure 11–14B) is part of the basal ganglia circuitry for motor control, the parafascicular nucleus is thought to be part of the circuitry for emotions and cognitive functions. Because the intralaminar nuclei have widespread cortical projections, they are diffuse-projecting thalamic nuclei and not relay nuclei.

While GABA is present in both structures, the neuropeptide content of the internal segment of the globus pallidus is different from that of the external segment (Figure 11–16). **Substance P** is in greater abundance in the **internal segment** of the globus pallidus, whereas **enkephalin** is restricted largely to the **external segment** of the globus pallidus.

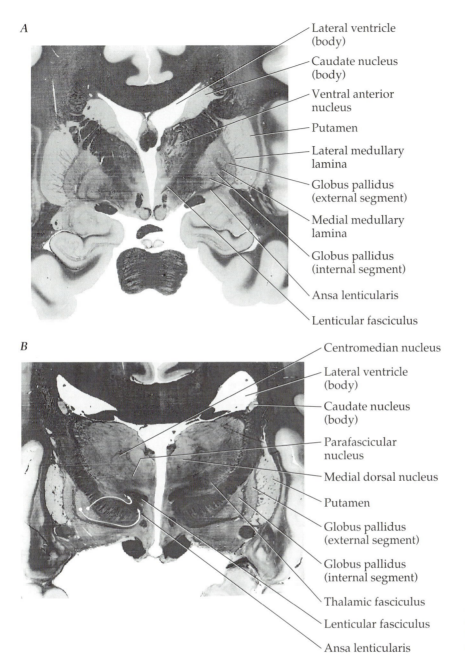

A

Lateral ventricle (body)

Caudate nucleus (body)

Ventral anterior nucleus

Putamen

Lateral medullary lamina

Globus pallidus (external segment)

Medial medullary lamina

Globus pallidus (internal segment)

Ansa lenticularis

Lenticular fasciculus

B

Centromedian nucleus

Lateral ventricle (body)

Caudate nucleus (body)

Parafascicular nucleus

Medial dorsal nucleus

Putamen

Globus pallidus (external segment)

Globus pallidus (internal segment)

Thalamic fasciculus

Lenticular fasciculus

Ansa lenticularis

Figure 11–14. Myelin-stained coronal *(A)* and oblique *(B)* sections through the internal and external segments of the globus pallidus.

Lesion of the Subthalamic Region Produces a Movement Disorder

Ventral to the thalamus is the subthalamic region, which consists of a disparate collection of nuclei. Two major nuclei in this poorly understood brain region are the **subthalamic nucleus** and **zona incerta** (Figure 11–15). A lesion of the subthalamic nucleus produces **hemiballism**, characterized by ballistic movements of the contralateral limbs. By examining patients with small vascular accidents in this area, we know that the subthalamic nucleus is somatotopically organized. Damage to one portion may involve the upper limb; damage to the other area, the lower limb. The connections of the subthalamic nucleus are complex. Receiving input from the external

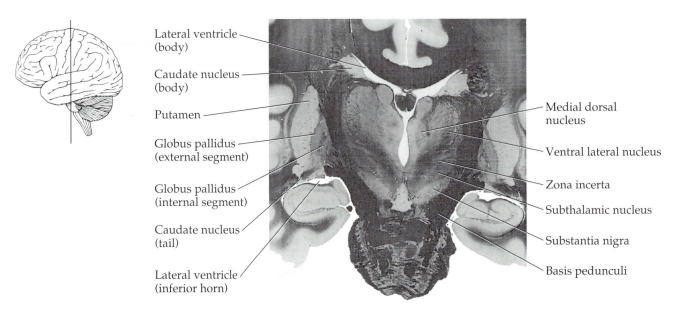

Lateral ventricle (body)

Caudate nucleus (body)

Putamen

Globus pallidus (external segment)

Globus pallidus (internal segment)

Caudate nucleus (tail)

Lateral ventricle (inferior horn)

Medial dorsal nucleus

Ventral lateral nucleus

Zona incerta

Subthalamic nucleus

Substantia nigra

Basis pedunculi

Figure 11–15. Myelin-stained coronal section through the thalamus and subthalamic region.

pallidal segment as well as from the motor cortex, the subthalamic nucleus projects back to both the **external and internal pallidal segments.** The subthalamic nucleus is also reciprocally connected with the ventral pallidum.

Very little is known of the function of the zona incerta, a nuclear region that is interposed between the subthalamic nucleus and the thalamus. The zona incerta receives projections from a variety of sources, including the spinal cord and cerebellum. Many of the neurons in the zona incerta contain GABA and, in turn, have diffuse cortical projections.

The Substantia Nigra Contains Two Anatomical Divisions

The posterior limb of the internal capsule separates the internal segment of the globus pallidus from the substantia nigra, a separation that can be seen both in coronal (Figure 11–15) and parasagittal section (Figure 11–13). The **substantia nigra pars reticulata,** which is located adjacent to the basis pedunculi, contains GABA (Figure 11–4). The substantia nigra pars reticulata also projects to the superior colliculus (Figure 11–17A). In rhesus monkeys, this projection has been shown to play a role in controlling **saccadic eye movements** to remembered visual targets.

The other division of the substantia nigra is the **substantia nigra pars compacta,** which consists of neurons containing dopamine. The projection of these neurons to the striatum forms the **nigrostriatal tract.** While the neurons of the compact part of the nigra play such a pivotal role in movement control, it is surprising that we have little specific information on their particular motor control functions. In fact, the results of physiological experiments in monkeys suggest that the activity of many of the compacta neurons is related to salient stimuli for the animal rather than particular features of the movement the animals perform. This may not be surprising since the compact part of the substantia nigra receives a projection from the **amygdala,** which is involved in motivation and emotions, and from the **reticular formation,** which is involved in arousal.

A

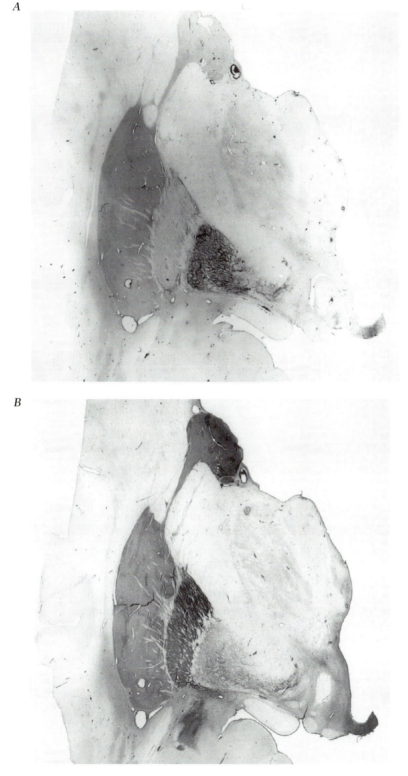

B

Figure 11–16. Histochemical localization of substance P-like immunoreactivity *(A)* and enkephalin-like immunoreactivity *(B)* in the human globus pallidus. (Courtesy of Dr. Suzanne Haber, University of Rochester School of Medicine.)

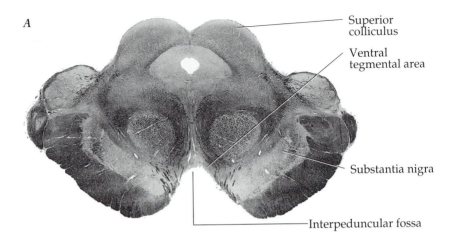

A

Superior
colliculus

Ventral
tegmental area

Substantia nigra

Interpeduncular fossa

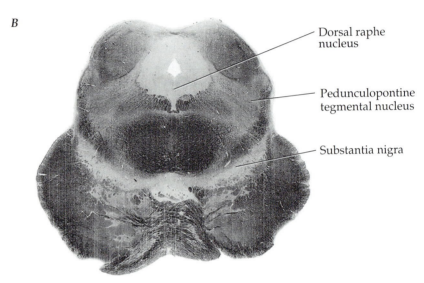

B

Dorsal raphe
nucleus

Pedunculopontine
tegmental nucleus

Substantia nigra

Figure 11–17. Myelin-stained transverse sections through the superior colliculus (*A*) and the inferior colliculus (*B*).

The compact part is not the only midbrain region that contains dopamine. The **ventral tegmental area** is located dorsomedial to the substantia nigra, beneath the floor of the interpeduncular fossa (Figure 11–17A). Dopaminergic neurons in the ventral tegmental area send their axons to the striatum via the **medial forebrain bundle** (see Chapters 14 and 15) as well as to the frontal lobe (see Figure 3–17B). The dendrites of dopaminergic neurons extend into the substantia nigra pars reticulata. This is thought to be functionally important for integrating information between the various parallel loops. For example, the dopaminergic neurons can receive inputs to their distal and proximal dendrites from diverse sources and, in turn, influence wide areas of the striatum via their diffuse projections.

In the coronal section through its rostral portion, we see that the substantia nigra (Figure 11–15) is interposed between the subthalamic nucleus and the basis pedunculi. The transverse sections through the rostral and caudal midbrain (Figure 11–17) reveal the substantia nigra dorsal to the base of the midbrain in both sections. The substantia nigra is the largest nuclear structure in the midbrain. As a consequence of its large size, vascular injury rarely disrupts substantia nigra function and parkinsonian signs are typically absent.

Two other brain stem nuclei are closely associated with the basal ganglia, the **dorsal raphe nucleus**, located in the caudal midbrain, and the **pedunculopontine tegmental nucleus**, found at the junction of the pons and midbrain (Figure 11–17B). The dorsal raphe nucleus gives rise to a **serotonergic** projection to the striatum. In addition to projecting to the striatum, the dorsal raphe nucleus has extensive projections to most of the cerebral cortex and to other forebrain nuclei. The basal ganglia also have "descending" projections to the brain stem that can play an important behavioral role. The globus pallidus internal segment projects to the **reticular formation** in the region of pedunculopontine tegmental nucleus. Many of the neurons in this region are cholinergic. This brain stem region has diverse functions, including regulating arousal—through diffuse ascending projections to the thalamus and cortex—and movement control—through reticulospinal projections.

The Vascular Supply of the Basal Ganglia Is Provided by the Middle Cerebral Artery

As described in Chapter 4, the vascular supply to the deep structures of the cerebral hemisphere—**thalamus**, **basal ganglia**, and **internal capsule**—is provided by branches of the internal carotid artery and the three cerebral arteries. Most of the striatum is supplied by perforating branches of the middle cerebral artery; however, regions located rostromedially are supplied by perforating branches of the anterior cerebral artery (see Figures 4–6 and 4–7). Collectively, these penetrating branches of the anterior and middle cerebral arteries are termed the **lenticulostriate arteries**. Most of the globus pallidus is supplied by the **anterior choroidal artery**, which is a branch of the internal carotid artery.

Basal Ganglia Nuclei

Summary

The basal ganglia contain numerous component nuclei (Figures 11–1 and 11–2) that can be divided into three groups based on their connections (Figure 11–1). The **input nuclei** (1) include the **caudate nucleus**, the **putamen**, and the **nucleus accumbens** (Figures 11–2, 11–8, and 11–12) and collectively are termed the **striatum**. The ventromedial portions of the caudate nucleus and putamen, together with the nucleus accumbens, comprise the **ventral striatum**. The **output nuclei** (2) include the **internal segment** of the **globus pallidus** (Figures 11–13 and 11–14), the **ventral pallidum** (Figures 11–12 and 11–13), and the **substantia nigra pars reticulata** (Figure 11–17). The **intrinsic nuclei** (3) include the **external segment** of the **globus pallidus** (Figures 11–12 and 11–13), the **subthalamic nucleus** (Figure 11–15), the **substantia nigra pars compacta** (Figure 11–17), and the **ventral tegmental area** (Figure 11–17A).

Basal Ganglia Functional Loops

The basic input–output pathway through the basal ganglia links wide regions of the cerebral cortex with, in sequence, the input nuclei of the basal ganglia (striatum), the output nuclei, the thalamus, and a portion of the frontal lobe (Figures 11–1 and 11–3). Four functional "loops" through the basal ganglia have been studied (Figure 11–3). The **skeleto-motor** (1) and **oculomotor** (2) loops play important roles in the control of body musculature and extraocular muscles; the **association** (3) loop may subserve such functions as cognition, spatial memory, and evaluation of the effectiveness of behavior; and the **limbic** (4) loop may subserve emotions and their visceral consequences. The **skeletomotor, oculomotor, and association** loops begin in the **somatic sensory, motor,** and **association areas** of the cerebral cortex and pass through the **caudate nucleus** and **putamen** (Figures 11–2, 11–6, and 11–8). The output nuclei of these loops are the **internal segment of the globus pallidus** (Figures 11–6, 11–13, and 11–14) and the **substantia nigra pars reticulata** (Figures 11–15 and 11–17). They, in turn, synapse in the **ventral lateral, ventral anterior,** and **medial dorsal nuclei** of the thalamus (Figures 11–6A and 11–13). There are two pathways by which the internal segment of the globus pallidus projects to the thalamus: the **ansa lenticularis** and the **lenticular fasciculus** (Figure 11–14B). However, components of the various loops synapse on neurons that are located in different nuclei or different portions of the same nuclei.

The **limbic** loop begins in **association cortical** areas. The **ventral striatum** is the principal input nucleus of the limbic loop; the output and thalamic nuclei of the limbic loop are the **ventral pallidum** and the **medial dorsal nucleus**. The cortical targets of the four loops are (Figure 11–3B) **supplementary motor areas, premotor cortex, and primary motor cortex** for the skeletomotor loop, **frontal and supplementary eye fields** for the oculomotor loop, **prefrontal association cortex** for the association loop, and **anterior cingulate gyrus** (and **orbitofrontal gyri**) for the limbic loop.

Intrinsic Basal Ganglia Connections

The intrinsic nuclei have interconnections with the input and output nuclei. Dopaminergic neurons of the **substantia nigra pars compacta** (Figure 11–15) and **ventral tegmental area** project to the **striatum;** dopaminergic neurons of the **ventral tegmental area** also project directly to parts of the **frontal lobe** (Figure 11–8). The **external segment of the globus pallidus** projects to the **subthalamic nucleus** which, in turn, projects to both the **internal and external segments of the globus pallidus,** the **substantia nigra pars reticulata,** and the **ventral pallidum.** ■

KEY STRUCTURES AND TERMS

input–output loops
    skeletomotor
    oculomotor
    association
    limbic
striatum
    caudate nucleus
    putamen
    nucleus accumbens
globus pallidus
    internal segment
    external segment
    ventral pallidum
substantia nigra
    pars compacta
    pars reticulata
ventral tegmental area
subthalamic nucleus
lenticular nucleus
dorsal raphe nucleus
pedunculopontine tegmental
    nucleus
thalamic nuclei
    medial dorsal
    ventral lateral

ventral anterior
centromedian
parafascicular
frontal lobe
    prefrontal cortex
    orbitofrontal cortex
    supplementary motor area
    premotor cortex
    primary motor cortex
    cingulate gyrus
nigrostriatal tract
lenticular fasciculus
ansa lenticularis
thalamic fasciculus
Forel's fields
neurotransmitters and
      neuromodulators
    γ-aminobutyric acid (GABA)
    glutamate
    dopamine
    acetylcholine
    enkephalin
    substance P
    dynorphin
    serotonin

neuromelanin
L-dopa
medium spiny neurons
Parkinson's disease
Huntington's disease
dyskinesias
    bradykinesia
    akinesia
    rigidity
    chorea
    hemiballism
    athetosis
hypokinetic and hyperkinetic signs
direct and indirect striatal output
      pathways
extreme capsule
claustrum
external capsule
thalamic adhesion
striatal cell bridges
septum pellucidum
zona incerta
lenticulostriate arteries
anterior choroidal artery

Selected Readings

Alexander, G. E., and Crutcher, M. D. 1990. Functional architecture of basal ganglia circuits: Neural substrates of parallel processing. Trends Neurosci. 13:266–271.

Alexander, G. E., DeLong, M. R., and Strick, P. L. 1986. Parallel organization of functionally segregated circuits linking basal ganglia and cortex. Ann. Rev. Neurosci. 9:357–381.

Carpenter, M. 1981. Anatomy of the corpus striatum and brain stem integrating systems. In Brooks, V. B. (ed.), Handbook of Physiology, Section I: The Nervous System, Vol. II, Motor Control. Bethesda, Md.: American Physiological Society, pp. 947–995.

Case record of the Massachusetts General Hospital (#2–1992). New Engl. J. Med. 326:117–125.

Côté, L., and Crutcher, M. D. 1991. The basal ganglia. In Kandel, E. R., Schwartz, J. H., and Jessell, T. M. (eds.), Principles of Neural Science, 3rd ed. New York: Elsevier, pp. 646–659.

DeLong, M. R. 1990. Primate modes of movement disorders of basal ganglia origin. Trends Neurosci. 13:281–285.

DeLong, M. R., and Georgopoulos, A. P. 1981. Motor function of the basal ganglia. In Brooks, V. B. (ed.), Handbook of Physiology, Section I: The Nervous System, Vol. II, Motor Control. Bethesda, Md.: American Physiological Society, pp. 1017–1061.

Gerfen, C. R. 1992. The neostriatal matrix: Multiple levels of compartmental organization. Trends Neurosci. 15:133–139.

Goldman-Rakic, P. S. 1984. Modular organization of prefrontal cortex. Trends Neurosci. 7:419–429.

Graybiel, A. M. 1990. Neurotransmitters and neuromodulators in the basal ganglia. Trends Neurosci. 13:244–254.

Gunilla, R., Öberg, E., and Divac, I. 1981. Commentary: The basal ganglia and the control of movement. Levels of motor planning, cognition and the control of movement. Trends Neurosci. 4:122–125.

Haber, S. N. 1986. Neurotransmitters in the human and nonhuman primate basal ganglia. Human Neurobiol. 5:159–168.

Heimer, L., Switzer, R. D., and Van Hoesen, G. W. 1982. Ventral striatum and ventral pallidum. Trends Neurosci. 5:83–87.

Parent, A. 1990. Extrinsic connections of the basal ganglia. Trends Neurosci. 13:254–258.

Special issue on the basal ganglia. 1990. Trends Neurosci. 13:241–308.

References

Alheld, G. F., Heimer, L., Switzer, R. C. III. 1990. Basal ganglia. In Paxinos, G. (ed.), The Human Nervous System. San Diego: Academic Press, pp. 483–582.

Goldman-Rakic, P. S. 1978. Neuronal plasticity in primate telencephalon: Anomalous projections induced by prenatal removal of frontal cortex. Science 202:768–770.

Gusella, J. F., Wexler, N. S., Conneally, P. M., et al. 1983. A polymorphic DNA marker genetically linked to Huntington's disease. Nature 306:234–238.

Haber, S. N., Groenewegen, H. J., Grove, E. A., et al. 1985. Efferent connections of the ventral pallidum: Evidence of a dual striato-pallidofugal pathway. J. Comp. Neurol. 235:322–335.

Haber, S. N., and Watson, S. J. 1985. The comparative distribution of enkephalin, dynorphin and substance P in the human globus pallidus and basal forebrain. Neuroscience 4:1011–1024.

Hoover, J. E., and Strick, P. L. 1993. Multiple output channels in basal ganglia. Science 259:819–821.

Jones, E. G., and Leavitt, R. Y. 1974. Retrograde axonal transport and the demonstration of non-specific projections to the cerebral cortex and striatum from thalamic intralaminar nuclei in the rat, cat and monkey. J. Comp. Neurol. 154:349–378.

Poirier, L. J., Giguère, M., and Marchand, R. 1983. Comparative morphology of the substantia nigra and ventral tegmental area in the monkey, cat and rat. Brain Res. Bull. 11:371–397.

Reiner, A., Albin, R. L., Anderson, K. D., D'Amato, C. J., Penney, J. B., and Young, A. B. 1988. Differential loss of striatal projection neurons in Huntington disease. Proc. Natl. Acad. Sci. USA 85:5733–5737.

Schell, G. R., and Strick, P. L. 1984. The origin of thalamic inputs to the arcuate premotor and supplementary motor areas. J. Neurosci. 4:539–560.

Schutz, W., Romo, R. 1990. Dopamine neurons of the monkey midbrain: Contingencies of response to stimuli eliciting immediate behavioral reactions. J. Neurophysiol. 63:607–624.

Selemon, L. D., and Goldman-Rakic, P. S. 1985. Longitudinal topography and interdigitation of corticostriatal projections in the rhesus monkey. J. Neurosci. 5:776–794.

Yeterian, E. H., and Van Hoesen, G. W. 1978. Cortico-striate projections in the rhesus monkey: The organization of certain cortico-caudate connections. Brain Res. 139:43–63.

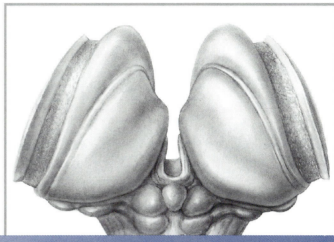

IV

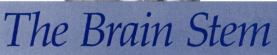

The Brain Stem

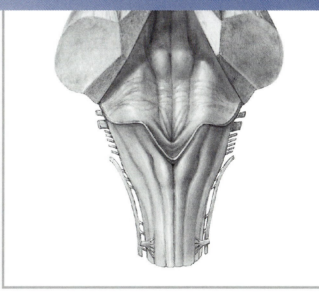

12

General Organization of the Cranial Nerve Nuclei and the Trigeminal System

IN NEUROANATOMY, THE STUDY OF SENSATION and motor control of cranial structures has traditionally been separate from that of the limbs and trunk. This is because the head is innervated by the cranial nerves, and the limbs and trunk by the spinal nerves. We can see similarities, however, in the functional organization of the cranial and spinal nerves, and of the parts of the central nervous system with which they directly connect. Sensory axons in cranial nerves synapse in sensory cranial nerve nuclei. This is similar to sensory axons in spinal nerves, which synapse on neurons of the dorsal horn of the spinal cord and the dorsal column nuclei. The motor cranial nerve nuclei, like the motor nuclei of the ventral horn, contain the motor neurons whose axons project to the periphery. Extending this parallel further, the autonomic cranial nerve nuclei which contain autonomic preganglionic neurons are analogous to autonomic nuclei of the intermediate zone of the spinal cord.

In this chapter, we examine the general organization of the cranial nerves and the columnar organization of the cranial nerve nuclei, topics introduced in Chapter 2. The columnar organization helps us to understand how the sensory and motor functions of the cranial nerves and nuclei are organized. In earlier chapters, certain cranial nerve sensory functions were considered when we examined the anatomical substrates of perception. We now complete this discussion by examining the trigeminal system, which mediates somatic sensation from the face and head. This system is analogous to the dorsal column–medial lemniscal and anterolateral systems of the spinal cord (see Chapter 5). In the next chapter, the motor functions of the cranial nerves will be examined.

■ CRANIAL NERVES AND NUCLEI

In contrast to the spinal nerves, which number approximately 31 pairs, there are only 12 pairs of cranial nerves (Figure 12–1; Table 12–1). The first two cranial nerves—olfactory (I) and optic (II)—are purely sensory. The olfactory nerve directly enters the **telencephalon** and the optic nerve, the **diencephalon**. Recall that the optic nerve contains the axons of

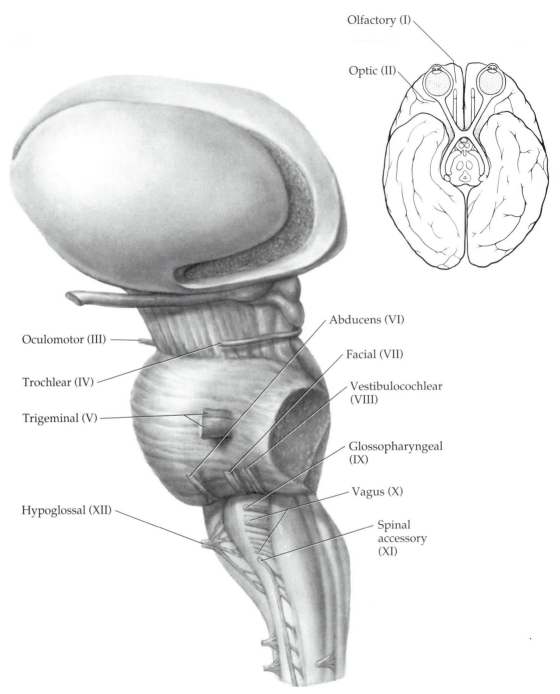

Figure 12–1. A lateral view of the brain stem, showing the locations of the cranial nerves that enter and exit the brain stem and diencephalon. The inset indicates that the olfactory nerve (I) enters the olfactory bulb, part of the telencephalon, and the optic nerve (II) enters the diencephalon via the optic tract.

retinal ganglion cells (see Chapter 6). Because the retina develops from the diencephalon, the optic nerve is actually a displaced central nervous system pathway and not a peripheral nerve.

The other 10 cranial nerves enter and leave the **brain stem**. The oculomotor (III) and trochlear (IV) nerves, which are motor nerves, exit from the midbrain. The trochlear nerve is further distinguished as the only cranial nerve found on the dorsal brain stem surface. The oculomotor and trochlear nerves serve visuomotor functions.

There are four cranial nerves of the pons. The trigeminal (V) nerve is located at the middle of the pons. It is termed a **mixed nerve** because it subserves both sensory and motor functions. The trigeminal nerve consists of separate sensory and motor roots, a separation reminiscent of the segregation of function in the dorsal and ventral spinal roots. The sensory root provides the somatic sensory innervation both of the facial skin and mucous membranes of oral and nasal cavities. The motor root contains axons that innervate jaw muscles.

We find the remaining pontine nerves at the pontomedullary junction. The abducens (VI) nerve is a motor nerve and its functions are coordinated with those of the oculomotor and trochlear nerves. The facial (VII) nerve is a mixed nerve, and like the trigeminal nerve, has separate sensory and motor roots. The motor root innervates the muscles of facial expression, while the sensory root innervates taste buds and mediates taste (see Chapter 8). Another name for the facial sensory root is the intermediate nerve. (In Chapter 13 we will see that the intermediate nerve also contains axons that innervate various cranial autonomic ganglia.) The vestibulocochlear (VIII) nerve is a sensory nerve and also contains two separate roots. The vestibular component of the nerve innervates the semicircular canals, saccule, and utricle, whereas the cochlear component innervates the organ of Corti (see Chapter 7).

The medulla has four cranial nerves and each contain numerous roots that leave from different rostrocaudal locations. Although the glossopharyngeal (IX) nerve is a mixed nerve, its major function is to provide the sensory innervation of the pharynx and to innervate taste buds of the posterior one third of the tongue. The motor function of the glossopharyngeal nerve is that of innervating a single pharyngeal muscle and peripheral autonomic ganglion (Table 12–1). The vagus (X), a mixed nerve, has myriad sensory and motor tasks that include somatic and visceral sensation, innervation of pharyngeal muscles, and much of the visceral autonomic innervation. The spinal accessory (XI) and the hypoglossal (XII) nerves subserve motor function, innervating neck and tongue muscles, respectively (Table 12–1).

In the medulla, the roots of a single cranial nerve enter and exit from different rostrocaudal levels. We do not yet understand whether this organization is related to the differential projections of sensory and motor axons in the different roots or reflects the segmental organization of the developing hindbrain (see Chapter 2 and Figure 2–5).

There Are Important Differences Between the Sensory and Motor Innervation of Cranial Structures and That of the Limbs and Trunk

In general, the peripheral organization of sensory (afferent) fibers in cranial nerves is similar to that of spinal nerves. In fact, the organization of the primary afferent neurons that innervate the **skin and mucous membranes of the head**—mediating tactile, thermal, and pain senses—is virtually identical to that of the limbs and trunk (Figure 12–2). In both cases, the distal portion of the axon of **pseudounipolar** primary sensory neurons is sensitive to stimulus energy and the cell bodies of these primary sensory neurons are located in **peripheral ganglia**. The proximal portion of the axon projects into the central nervous system to synapse on neurons in the

Table 12–1. The cranial nerves.

Cranial nerve and root	Function	Cranial formaina	Peripheral sensory ganglia
I Olfactory	SVA	Cribriform plate	
II Optic	SSA	Optic	
III Oculomotor	GSM	Superior orbital fissure	
	GVM		
IV Trochlear	GSM	Superior orbital fissure	
V Trigeminal	GSA	Superior orbital fissure (Ophthalmic) Rotundum (Maxillary)	Semilunar
	SVM	Ovale (Mandibular)	
VI Abducens	GSM	Superior orbital fissure	
VII Intermediate	SVA GSA GVM	Internal auditory meatus	Geniculate Geniculate
Facial	SVM	Internal auditory meatus	
VIII Vestibulocochlear	SSA SSA	Internal auditory meatus	Spiral Vestibular
IX Glossopharyngeal	GSA GVA	Jugular	Superior Petrosal (inferior)
	SVA GVM SVM		Petrosal
X Vagus	GSA GVA SVA GVM	Jugular	Jugular (superior) Nodose (inferior) Nodose (inferior)
	SVM		
XI Spinal accessory	SVM	Jugular	
	Unclassified[1]	Jugular	
XII Hypoglossal	GSM	Hypoglossal	

CNS nucleus	Peripheral autonomic ganglia	Peripheral structure innervated
Olfactory bulb		Olfactory receptors of olfactory epithelium
Lateral geniculate nucleus		Retina (ganglion cells)
Oculomotor		Medial, superior, inferior, rectus, inferior oblique, and levator palpebrae muscles
Edinger–Westphal	Ciliary	Constrictor muscles of iris, ciliary muscle
Trochlear		Superior oblique muscle
Spinal nucleus, main sensory nucleus, mesencephalio nucleus of CN V		Skin and mucous membranes of the head, muscle receptors, meninges
Motor nucleus of CN V		Jaw muscles, tensor tympani, tensor palati, and digastric (anterior belly)
Abducens		Lateral rectus muscle
Solitary nucleus		Taste (anterior two thirds of tongue), palate
Spinal nucleus of CN V		Skin of external ear
Superior salivatory	Pterygopalatine submandibular	Lacrimal glands, glands of nasal mucosa, salivary glands
Facial		Muscles of facial expression, digastric (posterior belly), and stapedius
Cochlear		Hair cells in organ of Corti
Vestibular		Hair cells in vestibular labyrinth
Spinal nucleus of CN V		Skin of external ear
Solitary nucleus (caudal)		Mucous membranes in pharyngeal region, middle ear, carotid body, and sinus
Solitary nucleus (rostral)		Taste (posterior one third of tongue)
Inferior salivatory nucleus	Otic	Parotid gland
Ambiguus (rostral)		Striated muscle of pharynx
Spinal nucleus of CN V		Skin of external ear, meninges
Solitary nucleus (caudal)		Larynx, trachea, gut, aortic arch receptors
Solitary nucleus (rostral)		Taste buds (posterior oral cavity, larynx)
Dorsal motor nucleus of CN X	Peripheral autonomic	Gut (to splenic flexure of colon), respiratory structures, heart
Ambiguus (middle region)		Striated muscles of palate, pharynx, and larynx
Ambiguus (caudal)		Striated muscles of larynx [Aberrant vague branches] sternocleidomastoid and portion of trapezius muscles
Accesory nucleus, pyramidal decussation to C3–C5		
Hypoglossal		Intrinsic muscles of tongue, hyoglossus, genioglossus, and styloglossus muscles

Abbreviation key: GSM, general somatic motor; SVM, special visceral motor; GVM, general visceral motor; GVA, general visceral afferent; SVA, special visceral afferent; SSA, special somatic afferent; GSA, general somatic afferent.

[1]The accessory nucleus is unclassified because some of the muscles (or compartments of muscles) innervated by this nucleus develop from the occipital somites.

medulla and pons. The peripheral sensory ganglia, in which the cell bodies of the primary sensory neurons of the different cranial nerves are located, are listed in Table 12–1.

Despite these similarities, three important differences are evident between the anatomical organization of primary sensory neurons in spinal and cranial nerves:

- First, for the senses of taste, vision, hearing, and balance, a separate **receptor cell** transduces stimulus energy (Figure 12–2). The primary sensory neuron transmits information, encoded in the form of action potentials, to the central nervous system. For cranial touch, jaw proprioception, pain, and thermal senses, the primary sensory neurons mediate both stimulus transduction and information transmission.
- Second, primary sensory neurons in cranial nerves have either a **pseudounipolar** or a **bipolar morphology** (Figure 12–2). (In vision, the ganglion cell is analogous to the primary sensory neurons because it transmits afferent information to the thalamus. This neuron, however, is a multipolar projection neuron of the central nervous system.)

Figure 12–2. Schematic illustration of morphology of primary sensory neurons, the location of cell bodies, and the approximate differences in actual sizes. Whereas primary afferent fibers in the spinal cord have a pseudounipolar morphology, in cranial nerves they have either a pseudounipolar or bipolar morphology. The primary sensory neuron for jaw proprioception is further distinguished because its cell body is located in the central nervous system. For hearing, balance, and taste, a separate receptor cell transduces stimulus information and primary afferent fiber transmits the resulting signals to the central nervous system. The sensory neurons for hearing, balance, and smell are bipolar. For touch, pain, temperature sense, jaw proprioception, and taste, the primary sensory neurons are pseudounipolar. For vision, the retina develops from the central nervous system and thus none of the neural elements are in the periphery.

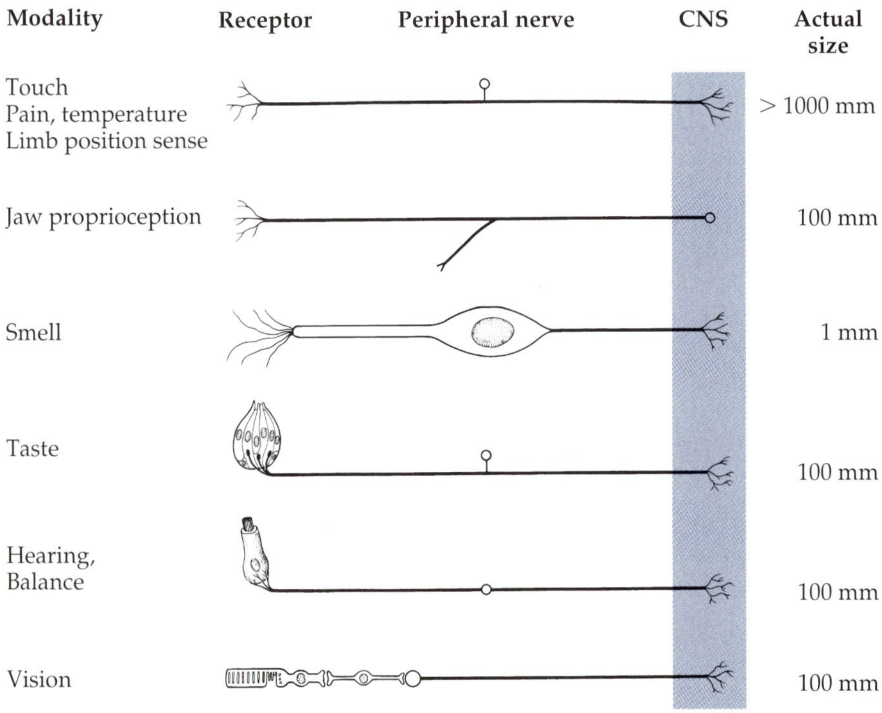

Modality	Receptor	Peripheral nerve	CNS	Actual size
Touch Pain, temperature Limb position sense				> 1000 mm
Jaw proprioception				100 mm
Smell				1 mm
Taste				100 mm
Hearing, Balance				100 mm
Vision				100 mm

- Third, stretch receptors in jaw muscles, which signal jaw muscle length and thus mediate **jaw proprioception**, are pseudounipolar primary sensory neurons, but their cell bodies are located within the central nervous system, not in peripheral ganglia. These neurons derive from neural crest cells (see Figure 2–1), that do not migrate from the central nervous system to the periphery.

The structures innervated by the motor fibers of cranial nerves, similar to motor fibers in spinal nerves, include striated muscle and autonomic postganglionic neurons. In contrast to striated muscle of the limbs and trunk, however, which develop from body somites, cranial striated muscle develops either from the cranial **somites** (somatic) or the **branchial arches** (visceral). The extraocular muscles and the tongue muscles are of somatic origin, whereas jaw, facial, laryngeal, palatal, and certain neck muscles are of visceral origin because they develop from the branchial arches.

Cranial Nerves Have a Complex Nomenclature

Seven functional categories of cranial nerve fibers are recognized on the basis of whether the individual axons provide the **afferent (sensory)** or **motor** innervation of the head and whether the innervated structures develop from the **somites** or the **viscera**. Four of these categories are shared by the cranial nerves and the spinal nerves:

1. **General somatic afferents** subserve somatic sensations, including touch, vibration sense, pain and temperature senses, and jaw (and limb) proprioception.
2. **General visceral afferents** mediate visceral sensations and chemoreception from body organs.
3. **General somatic motor** fibers are the axons of motor neurons that innervate striated muscle that develops from the somites.
4. **General visceral motor** fibers are the axons of autonomic preganglionic neurons.

Because cranial nerves are more complex than spinal nerves, there are three additional categories:

5. **Special somatic afferents** subserve vision (see Chapter 6), hearing, and balance (see Chapter 7).
6. **Special visceral afferents** mediate taste and smell (see Chapter 8).
7. **Special visceral motor** fibers are the axons of motor neurons that innervate striated muscle that develops from the branchial arches.

Cranial Nerve Nuclei Are Organized Into Rostrocaudal Columns

The primary sensory neurons in cranial nerves that enter the brain stem synapse in **sensory cranial nerve nuclei**; the cell bodies of motor axons in cranial nerves are located in **motor cranial nerve nuclei**. This is similar to the dorsal roots, which synapse in the dorsal horn and dorsal column nuclei, and the skeletal motor axons of the ventral roots, whose cell bodies are found in the spinal motor nuclei. Each cranial nerve nucleus subserves a single sensory or motor task. This is in contrast with many of the cranial nerves themselves, which contain a mixture of axons that have different functions (see Table 12–1).

As there are seven functional categories of cranial nerves, there are also seven categories of cranial nerve nuclei. Nuclei of each of these categories form discontinuous **columns that extend rostrocaudally through the brain stem** (Figures 12–3 and 12–4), reminiscent of the columnar organization of the spinal cord. This similar organization reflects their common developmental plan (Figure 2–7). Although there are seven functional categories of cranial nerves and nuclei, there are only six discrete columns. This is because two of the categories of afferent axons synapse on neurons in separate rostrocaudal locations in a single column (see following section).

Cranial Sensory Columns Are Located Lateral to the Motor Columns

There is a systematic relationship between the function subserved by each column and its location with respect to the midline (Figures 12–3 and 12–4). Knowing the approximate location of these nuclear columns greatly simplifies the study of the cranial nerve nuclei and the regional anatomy of the brain stem. The motor columns are located medial to the sensory columns. In the pons and medulla, nuclei on the ventricular floor are separated by the **sulcus limitans**. In the embryonic brain and spinal cord, the sulcus limitans separated the alar and basal plates (see Chapter 2).

Cell bodies of the three categories of motor axons in the cranial nerves are arranged in three separate columns of motor nuclei: general somatic motor column, special visceral motor column, and general visceral motor column. The **general somatic motor column** is found close to the midline in the medulla, pons, and midbrain. Nuclei in this column contain the cell bodies of motor neurons that innervate somatic striated muscle: the extraocular muscles and the tongue muscles. The **special visceral motor column** also contains motor neurons. Although located in the medulla and pons, it is displaced from the ventricular floor. The motor neurons in this column innervate visceral striated muscles that derive from the branchial arches. These muscles include: jaw, facial (i.e., for facial expressions), laryngeal, palatal, pharyngeal, and certain neck muscles. The **general visceral motor** column is located in the floor of the fourth ventricle in the medulla and pons and ventral to the cerebral aqueduct in the midbrain. This column contains parasympathetic preganglionic neurons. Motor nuclei are examined in Chapter 13.

The four categories of sensory, or afferent, axons in the cranial nerves synapse in three separate columns of nuclei: combined special and general visceral afferent column; special somatic afferent column; and general somatic afferent column. The single **visceral afferent** column has a special visceral component, located rostrally, subserving taste, and a general visceral component, located caudally, which subserves aspects of sensation from the visceral organs and processing of chemical stimuli. This column corresponds to a single nucleus, the **solitary nucleus** (see Chapter 8), and is located primarily in the medulla beneath the floor of the fourth ventricle. The **special somatic afferent** column is found in the pons and medulla and consists of the **vestibular** and **cochlear** nuclei (see Chapter 7). The **general somatic afferent** column stretches from the rostral spinal cord to the midbrain. This column consists of the three trigeminal sensory nuclei and mediates somatic sensation of cranial structures.

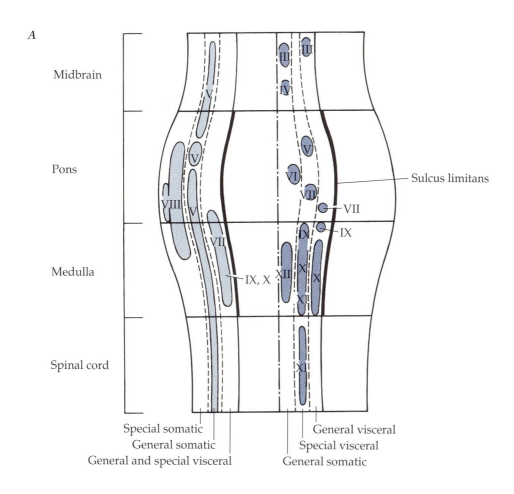

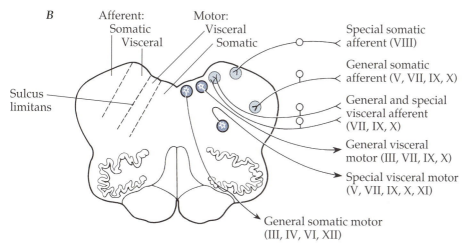

Figure 12–3. *A.* Schematic dorsal view of brain stem, showing that the cranial nerve nuclei are organized into discontinuous columns. The sulcus limitans separates the afferent and motor nuclei. *B.* Schematic cross section through the medulla, showing the locations of cranial nerve nuclear columns. (*A,* Adapted from Nieuwenhuys, R., Voogd, J., and van Huijzen, C. 1988. The Human Central Nervous System, A Synopsis and Atlas, 3rd ed. Berlin: Springer-Verlag.)

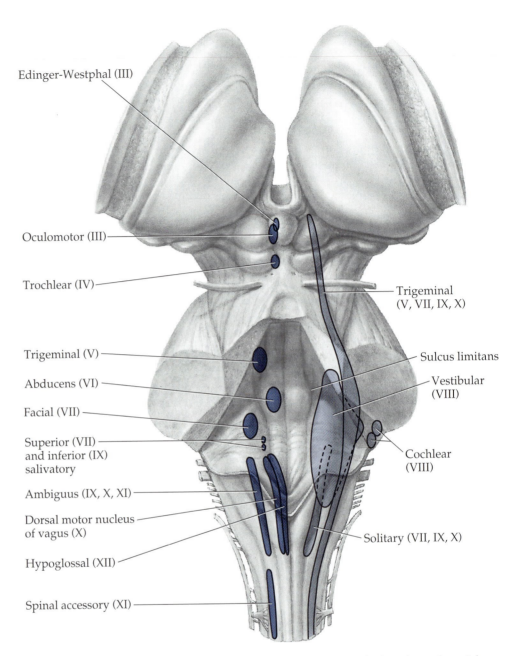

Figure 12–4. Dorsal view of the brain stem indicating the locations of cranial nerve nuclei.

The rest of this chapter examines the trigeminal system, which mediates touch, pain, and thermal sensations of the head as well as jaw proprioception. The functions of this system compare with those of the spinal nerves and the trigeminal pathways with the ascending spinal cord pathways (see Chapter 5).

■ FUNCTIONAL ANATOMY OF THE TRIGEMINAL SYSTEM

Somatic sensation of the head, including the oral cavity, is carried by general somatic afferent fibers in four cranial nerves. The **trigeminal nerve** (1) innervates most of the head and oral cavity and is the most important

of the four nerves. The **facial** (2), the **glossopharyngeal** (3), and the **vagus** (4) nerves innervate certain areas of the skin about the external ear, pharynx, larynx, nasal cavity and sinuses, and middle ear. The afferent fibers in these nerves that innervate surface skin project into central trigeminal nuclei (see below). On the other hand, the other afferent fibers that innervate visceral structures (e.g., laryngeal mucous membrane) project to the caudal portion of the solitary nucleus. It should be recalled that the facial, glossopharyngeal, and vagus nerves also contain visceral afferent fibers that mediate taste and chemoreception (see Chapter 8). Because of the modest overall contribution of facial, glossopharyngeal, and vagus nerves to cranial somatic sensation, we will focus primarily on the trigeminal nerve. This innervation is clinically significant, however, in signaling damage or infection to internal structures.

Three trigeminal sensory nuclei serve cranial somatic sensations from all of the cranial nerves (i.e., the general somatic afferent modalities). These afferent fibers terminate in two of the trigeminal sensory nuclei, the **main** (or **principal**) **trigeminal sensory nucleus** and the **spinal trigeminal nucleus**. The third trigeminal sensory nucleus, the **mesencephalic trigeminal nucleus**, is not a site of termination of primary afferent fibers. Rather, it is equivalent to a peripheral sensory ganglion because it contains the cell bodies of some of the trigeminal primary afferent fibers (see below).

Separate Trigeminal Pathways Mediate Touch and Pain and Temperature Senses

Just as in spinal nerves, functional differences distinguish individual afferent fibers in the trigeminal nerve. Mechanoreceptors mediate touch; their axons have large-diameter myelinated fibers. By contrast, nociceptors and thermoreceptors mediate pain and temperature senses and have small-diameter myelinated fibers and unmyelinated fibers. The cell bodies of the trigeminal primary afferent fibers are located in the **semilunar** (or **trigeminal**) **ganglion**.

These differences set the stage for two anatomically and functionally distinct trigeminal ascending systems (Figures 12–5 and 12–6). One system receives input primarily from mechanoreceptors, for cranial touch and dental mechanical senses, much as the dorsal column–medial lemniscal system is important for mechanoreceptions from the limbs and trunk. In the other system, which mediates cranial pain and temperature senses, nociceptors and thermoreceptors provide the principal inputs. Input from mechanoreceptors serves a less discriminative, or crude, form of touch (see Chapter 5). This system is analogous to the anterolateral system.

The Main Trigeminal Sensory Nucleus Mediates Facial Touch Sensation

Large-diameter axons of the trigeminal nerve that mediate tactile sense enter the ventral pons and course to the dorsal portion. Here, most afferent fibers emit a short ascending branch and a longer descending branch (Figure 12–5). The ascending branch terminates in the **main** (or **principal**) **trigeminal sensory nucleus**. The descending branch travels in the **spinal trigeminal tract** (see below). Most neurons in the main sensory nucleus give rise to axons that decussate in the pons and ascend dorsomedial to fibers from the dorsal column nuclei in the medial lemniscus. The ascending second-order trigeminal fibers—which are collectively termed the **trigeminal lemniscus**—synapse in the thalamus, in its **ventral posterior medial nucleus** (Figure 12–6A). From here, the axons of thalamic neu-

A

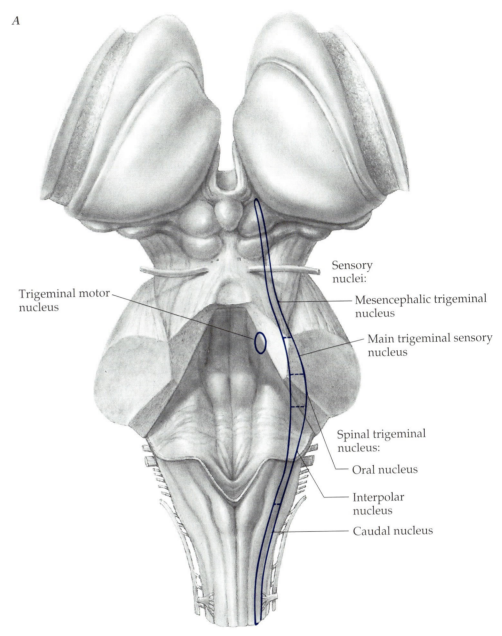

Trigeminal motor nucleus

Sensory nuclei:

Mesencephalic trigeminal nucleus

Main trigeminal sensory nucleus

Spinal trigeminal nucleus:

Oral nucleus

Interpolar nucleus

Caudal nucleus

Figure 12–5. *A.* Dorsal view of the brain stem without cerebellum indicates the locations of trigeminal nuclei. *B.* Neuronal and synaptic organization of the trigeminal nuclei. (Arrows indicate directions of information flow for jaw-jerk reflex. Sensory information from jaw proprioceptors is transmitted to trigeminal motor neurons in the trigeminal motor nucleus.) (*B,* Adapted from Cajal, S. Ramón y. 1909, 1911. Histologie du système nerveux de l'homme et des vertèbres. 2 vols. Paris: Maloine.)

rons project, via the posterior limb of the internal capsule, to the lateral part of the **primary somatic sensory cortex**, close to the lateral sulcus, in the **postcentral gyrus**. The **secondary somatic sensory cortex**, which is located in the parietal operculum and posterior insular cortex (see Chapter 5), receives its major input from the primary somatic sensory cortex.

This principal pathway for tactile perception on the face is analogous to the dorsal column–medial lemniscal system. The axons of the primary

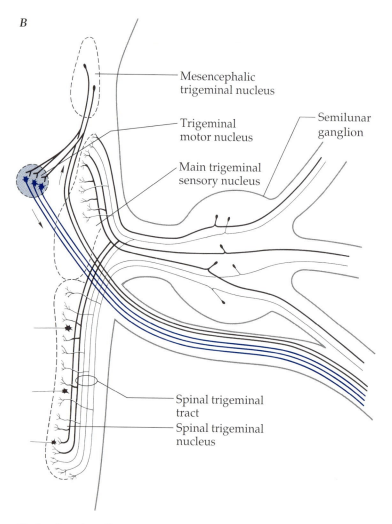

B

Mesencephalic
trigeminal nucleus

Trigeminal
motor nucleus

Semilunar
ganglion

Main trigeminal
sensory nucleus

Spinal trigeminal
tract

Spinal trigeminal
nucleus

Figure 12–5.   (continued)

sensory neurons that ascend in the spinal trigeminal tract are analogous to the dorsal column axons, and the main trigeminal sensory nucleus is anatomically and functionally similar to the dorsal column nuclei (gracile and cuneate nuclei).

A second, smaller ascending pathway originates from neurons in the dorsal portion of the main sensory nucleus (Figure 12–6A). This pathway ascends ipsilaterally through the dorsal tegmentum of the brain stem and, like the trigeminal lemniscus, terminates in the ventral posterior medial nucleus. This ipsilateral pathway processes mechanical stimuli from the teeth and soft tissues of the oral cavity.

The Spinal Trigeminal Nucleus Mediates Cranial Pain and Temperature Senses

Small-diameter myelinated and unmyelinated fibers enter the pons and descend in the spinal trigeminal tract (Figure 12–5B). These branches terminate in the **spinal trigeminal nucleus**. Few small-diameter axons ascend in the spinal trigeminal tract. Large-diameter fibers also descend in this tract to terminate in the spinal trigeminal nucleus. However, as we will discuss below, the large- and small-diameter afferent fibers have dif-

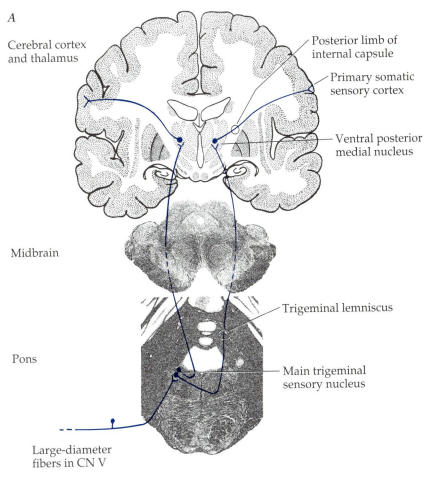

A

Cerebral cortex and thalamus

Posterior limb of internal capsule

Primary somatic sensory cortex

Ventral posterior medial nucleus

Midbrain

Trigeminal lemniscus

Pons

Main trigeminal sensory nucleus

Large-diameter fibers in CN V

Figure 12–6. General organization of the ascending trigeminal pathways for *(A)* touch and *(B)* pain and temperature senses.

ferent patterns of termination in the spinal nucleus. The spinal trigeminal nucleus and tract actually are located in the pons, medulla, and spinal cord and receive input from the facial, glossopharyngeal, and vagus nerves in addition to the trigeminal nerve.

The spinal trigeminal nucleus has a rostrocaudal anatomical and functional organization (Figures 12–5A and 12–6B) with three components: (1) **oral nucleus**, (2) **interpolar nucleus**, and (3) **caudal nucleus**. The functions of the spinal trigeminal nucleus are similar to those of the dorsal horn of the spinal cord, with which it is continuous, but the trigeminal nucleus mediates **facial** sensation. Similar to the dorsal horn, the spinal trigeminal nucleus plays an important role in **pain** and **temperature** senses, including dental pain, and a lesser role in tactile sensation. In addition, the interpolar and oral nuclei are also involved in trigeminal reflexes. For example, interneurons for the **jaw-opening reflex**, which opens the mouth in response to tactile stimulation of oral and perioral structures, are located in the interpolar and oral nuclei.

The ascending trigeminal pathway, important principally for facial and dental pain, starts at the spinal trigeminal nucleus, especially the caudal and interpolar nuclei, and terminates in the contralateral thalamus (Figure 12–6B). The organization of this path is similar to that of the **spinothalamic tract** (see Chapter 5). This ascending **trigeminothalamic**

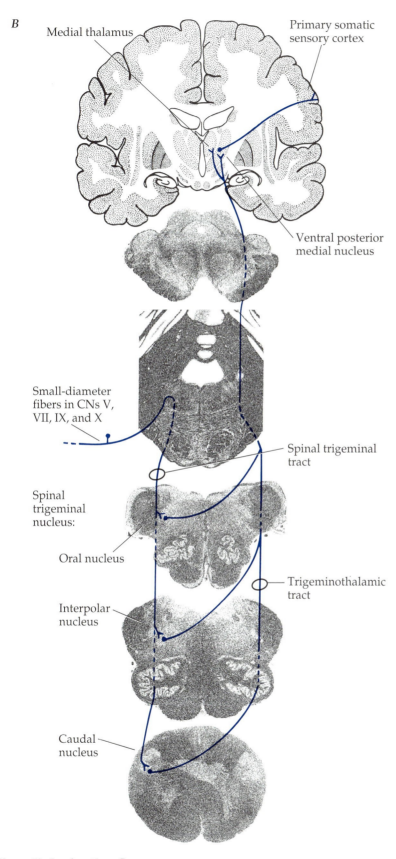

B

Medial thalamus

Primary somatic
sensory cortex

Ventral posterior
medial nucleus

Small-diameter
fibers in CNs V,
VII, IX, and X

Spinal trigeminal
tract

Spinal
trigeminal
nucleus:

Oral nucleus

Trigeminothalamic
tract

Interpolar
nucleus

Caudal
nucleus

Figure 12–6.   (continued)

tract is predominantly crossed and ascends with fibers of the **anterolateral system**. Subcomponents terminate in two locations in the thalamus: laterally, in the ventral posterior medial nucleus, and medially, in the intralaminar nuclei. As we saw in Chapter 5, projections to these two thalamic sites mediate different aspects of pain and temperature senses. The projection to the **ventral posterior medial nucleus** is thought to mediate discriminative aspects of facial pain and temperature senses, for example, stimulus localization. In contrast, the projection to the **intralaminar nuclei** is thought to participate in the affective and motivational aspects of facial pain and temperature senses. There is a further parallel between the trigeminal and spinal ascending systems: The ventral posterior medial nucleus projects to the facial representation of the primary somatic sensory cortex, in the lateral portion of the **postcentral gyrus**. The intralaminar nuclei have a more diffuse projection, which includes the anterior insular cortex, which plays a role in pain (see Box 5–1).

The spinal trigeminal nucleus, like the dorsal horn, also contains cells that project to other brain regions. For example, other contingents of ascending fibers arise from the spinal trigeminal nucleus to terminate in the reticular formation (trigeminoreticular tract), midbrain tectum (trigeminotectal tract), and the cerebellum (trigeminocerebellar pathways).

■ **REGIONAL ANATOMY**

Separate Sensory Roots Innervate Different Parts of the Face and Mucous Membranes of the Head

The trigeminal nerve consists of three sensory roots and one motor root. The sensory roots are analogous to dorsal spinal roots; the motor root, to a ventral spinal root. The analogy is functional only, because the two trigeminal roots are not located dorsal and ventral to one another. The motor root innervates the muscles of mastication and will be discussed in the next chapter. Each sensory root innervates the skin and mucous membranes of separate regions of the head: the **ophthalmic division**, the **maxillary division**, and the **mandibular division** (Figure 12–7A). The mandibular division also innervates the oral cavity, excluding the pharynx and posterior third of the tongue. Unlike dorsal roots of adjacent spinal cord segments, where the dermatomes overlap extensively, the trigeminal dermatomes (i.e., the area of skin innervated by a single trigeminal sensory nerve division) overlap very little. Thus, a peripheral anesthetic region is more likely to occur after damage to one trigeminal division than after damage to a single dorsal root.

In addition to the trigeminal nerve, the **intermediate** (a branch of the **facial nerve**), **glossopharyngeal**, and **vagus nerves** innervate portions of the skin and mucous membranes of the head. The skin of the ear and the external auditory meatus are innervated by the intermediate and vagus nerves (Figure 12–7A). The vagus nerve also innervates the mucous membranes of the larynx. The glossopharyngeal nerve innervates the posterior one third of the tongue, the pharynx, portions of the nasal cavity and sinuses, and the middle ear. The innervation of the pharynx and larynx by the glossopharyngeal and vagus nerves is essential for normal swallowing. In addition, normal vagal innervation of the larynx helps to maintain the airway clear of saliva and other liquids during swallowing. Both the trigeminal and vagus nerves innervate the dura.

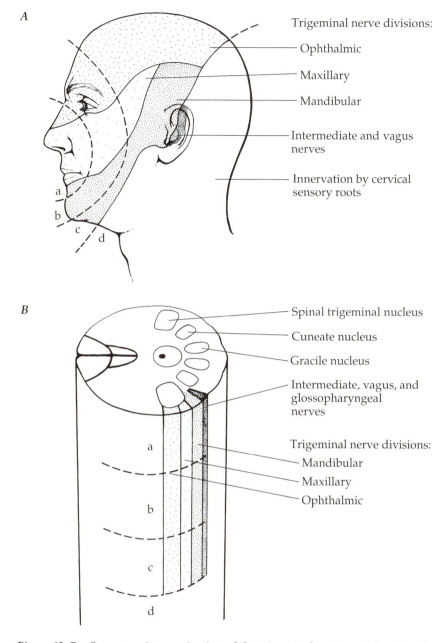

Figure 12–7. Somatotopic organization of the trigeminal system. *A.* Peripheral innervation territories of the three divisions of the trigeminal nerve and the intermediate and vagus nerves. *B.* The organization of the spinal trigeminal tract in relation to the three trigeminal nerve divisions and the intermediate, glossopharyngeal, and vagus nerves for the portion of the medulla that includes the caudal nucleus. The "onion skin" pattern of representation of trigeminal afferents in the caudal nucleus corresponds to **a**, **b**, and **c**; **d** corresponds to the rostral spinal cord representation. Regions marked **a** (located rostrally), **b**, and **c** (located caudally), correspond to the concentric zones on the face indicated in *A.* The intraoral representation is located rostral to region **a** in *B*; cervical representation is located caudally (i.e., region **d**). (Adapted from Brodal, A. 1981. Neurological Anatomy. New York: Oxford University Press.)

After entering the pons, the fibers of each nerve division occupy a discrete rostrocaudally oriented slice in the spinal trigeminal tract (Figure 12–7B). It is organized like an inverted face: the roots of the intermediate, glossopharyngeal, and vagus nerves as well as the mandibular division of the trigeminal nerve are located dorsal, the ophthalmic division of the trigeminal nerve is located ventral, and the maxillary division of the trigeminal nerve is in between. Axons in the spinal trigeminal tract, in turn, synapse on neurons in the spinal trigeminal nucleus (Figure 12–7B).

Cell Bodies of Primary Afferent Fibers Mediating Facial Somatic Sensations Are Located in the Peripheral Ganglia and in the Central Nervous System

The cell bodies of the primary afferent fibers that subserve cranial somatic sensation are located both in the periphery and in the central nervous system. For the afferent fibers mediating cranial touch, pain, and temperature senses, the cell bodies are found in peripheral sensory ganglia: the **semilunar ganglion** for the trigeminal nerve, the **superior ganglia** for the glossopharyngeal and vagus nerves, and the **geniculate ganglion** for the facial nerve. The cell bodies of vagal and glossopharyngeal afferent fibers that subserve visceral sensations (taste and chemoreception; sensations from mucous membranes) are located in the **inferior ganglia** of both nerves (see Chapter 8). This offers another example of the anatomical segregation of functionally dissimilar neurons.

The trigeminal nerve innervates stretch receptors found in jaw muscles, which mediate mastication. These receptors are unusual because their cell bodies are located in the central nervous system, in the **mesencephalic trigeminal nucleus** (Figure 12–5). The trigeminal nerve also innervates stretch receptors in the extraocular muscles, but these afferent fibers have their cell bodies located in the semilunar ganglion, and their axons course within the ophthalmic division of the trigeminal nerve.

The Key Components of the Trigeminal System Are Present at All Levels of the Brain Stem

The three trigeminal nuclei subserve distinct sensory functions. The **spinal trigeminal nucleus** (1) is important in facial pain and temperature senses and is located principally in the medulla and the caudal pons. Three nuclear subdivisions comprise the spinal trigeminal nucleus; from caudal to rostral: caudal nucleus; interpolar nucleus; and oral nucleus. The **main (principal) trigeminal sensory nucleus** (2) mediates facial tactile sense and oral mechanosensations and is located in the pons. The **mesencephalic trigeminal nucleus** (3) contains the cell bodies of stretch receptors that signal jaw muscle length, which is used by the brain for jaw proprioception and is located in the rostral pons and midbrain.

The Spinal Trigeminal Nucleus Is the Rostral Extension of the Spinal Cord Dorsal Horn

The dorsal horn extends rostrally into the medulla as the spinal trigeminal nucleus. To better understand this point, we should recall that the developing spinal cord and brain stem contain two zones of developing neurons, the **alar** and **basal plates**, that form rostrocaudally oriented columns of cells from the sacral spinal cord to the midbrain. In the spinal cord, these cells form the dorsal and ventral horns. As the central nervous system matures, the alar plate in the caudal medulla becomes further differentiated, forming the distinct **dorsal column nuclei**, located medially, and the **spinal trigeminal nucleus**, located laterally.

The most caudal portion of the spinal trigeminal nucleus, the **caudal nucleus**, and the dorsal horn of the spinal cord have three key similarities: (1) general morphology and lamination, (2) laminar distribution of afferent fiber terminals, and (3) laminar distribution of projection neurons. In fact, the caudal nucleus is sometimes called the **medullary dorsal horn** because its organization is similar to that of the spinal cord dorsal horn.

Comparing sections of the spinal cord and the caudal medulla reveals a similar morphology and lamination of the dorsal horn and caudal nucleus (Figure 12–8).

- **Lamina 1,** the outermost, is equivalent to the **marginal zone** of the dorsal horn.
- **Lamina 2** is equivalent to the **substantia gelatinosa**.

Figure 12–8. The spinal cord dorsal horn and the caudal nucleus have a similar organization. Myelin-stained transverse sections through the caudal nucleus—the level of pyramidal decussation *(A)*—and the cervical spinal cord *(B)*.

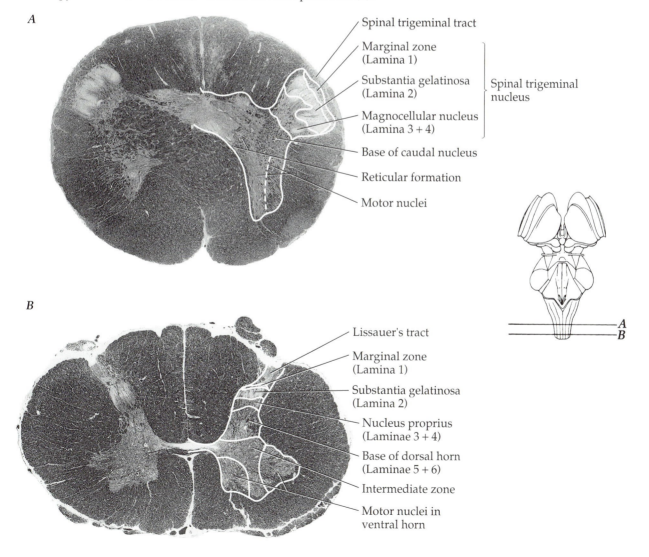

- **Laminae 3 and 4** are termed the **magnocellular nucleus** in the trigeminal system and are equivalent to the **nucleus proprius** of the spinal cord.
- **Laminae 5 and 6** (base of dorsal horn) of the spinal cord extend rostrally into the base of the spinal trigeminal nucleus.

As the nuclear components of the dorsal horn have counterparts in the trigeminal system, so too does the spinal sensory tract, Lissauer's tract, which extends into the medulla as the **spinal trigeminal tract**. Both Lissauer's tract and the spinal trigeminal tract are lightly stained (Figure 12–8) because they contain thinly myelinated and unmyelinated axons.

We also can draw an analogy between the organization of other portions of the spinal cord and that of the caudal medulla. The intermediate zone of the spinal cord is continuous with the portion of the medullary gray matter ventral to lamina 6. In the caudal medulla, this area is the **reticular formation**. Finally, the ventral horn extends rostrally into the medulla to form the cranial nerve motor nuclei.

Important insights into the functions of the spinal trigeminal nucleus and tract have been gained from a neurosurgical procedure to relieve intractable facial pain. This operation transects the spinal trigeminal tract and produces selective disruption of such pain and temperature senses with little effect on touch. (Spinal trigeminal tractotomy is rarely done today, however, because analgesic drugs have proved a more effective therapy.) If the tract is transected rostrally, near the border between the caudal and interpolar nuclei, facial pain and temperature senses over the entire face are disrupted. Transecting the tract between its rostral and caudal borders spares pain and temperature senses over the perioral region and nose.

This clinical finding shows that there is a rostrocaudal somatotopic organization in the spinal trigeminal tract in addition to a mediolateral organization (Figure 12–7B). Trigeminal fibers that innervate the portion of the head adjacent to the cervical spinal cord representation (Figure 12–7) project more caudally in the spinal trigeminal tract and terminate in more caudal regions of the caudal nucleus than those that innervate the oral cavity, perioral face, and nose.

Now we can understand the somatotopic organization of the rostral spinal cord and caudal medulla. Proceeding rostrally from the cervical spinal cord, neurons of the spinal dorsal horn process somatic sensory information (ie., pain and temperature senses) from the arm, neck, and occiput (i.e., region d in Figure 12–7B). Neurons of the caudal nucleus at the spinal cord–medulla border process somatic sensory information from the posterior face and ear (i.e., regions b and c in Figure 12–7B). Farther rostrally, the neurons process information from the perioral region and nose (i.e., region a in Figure 12–7B). Finally, neurons in the most rostral part of the caudal nucleus process pain and temperature information from the oral cavity, and in the adjacent interpolar nucleus (not shown in Figure 12–7B), from the **teeth.** This organization is termed "onion skin" because of the concentric ring configuration of the peripheral fields processed at a given level by the medullary dorsal horn.

A second similarity can be noted between the spinal dorsal horn and the caudal nucleus. As in the dorsal horn of the spinal cord (see Figure 5–6), afferent fibers of different diameters terminate in different laminae of the caudal nucleus. Whereas small-diameter trigeminal afferent fibers mediating pain and temperature senses terminate in laminae 1 and 2, large-diameter fibers mediating aspects of dental and other cranial mechanosensations terminate primarily in laminae 3 through 6.

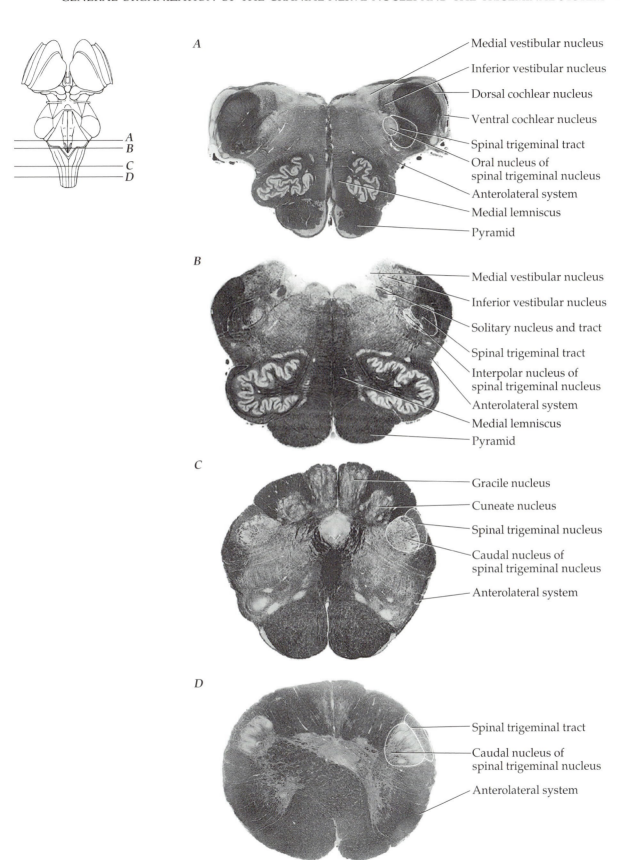

A

Medial vestibular nucleus

Inferior vestibular nucleus

Dorsal cochlear nucleus

Ventral cochlear nucleus

Spinal trigeminal tract

Oral nucleus of
spinal trigeminal nucleus

Anterolateral system

Medial lemniscus

Pyramid

B

Medial vestibular nucleus

Inferior vestibular nucleus

Solitary nucleus and tract

Spinal trigeminal tract

Interpolar nucleus of
spinal trigeminal nucleus

Anterolateral system

Medial lemniscus

Pyramid

C

Gracile nucleus

Cuneate nucleus

Spinal trigeminal nucleus

Caudal nucleus of
spinal trigeminal nucleus

Anterolateral system

D

Spinal trigeminal tract

Caudal nucleus of
spinal trigeminal nucleus

Anterolateral system

Figure 12–9. Myelin-stained transverse sections through the three divisions of
the spinal trigeminal nucleus: oral nucleus *(A)*; interpolar nucleus *(B)*; and caudal
nucleus *(C, D)*.

The third similarity between the spinal dorsal horn and the caudal nucleus is the laminar distribution of ascending projection neurons. The ascending pathway for facial pain is the trigeminothalamic tract and the ascending projection neurons are principally located in laminae 1 and 5. These neurons project primarily to the contralateral thalamus. Cells that project to other brain stem sites, such as the reticular formation, have a broader laminar distribution. The projection to the reticular formation also has a larger ipsilateral component.

The three subdivisions of the spinal trigeminal nucleus—caudal, interpolar, and oral nuclei—are shown in Figure 12–9. The section shown in Figure 12–8A is duplicated in Figure 12–9D to facilitate comparison of these subdivisions and continuity from the spinal cord to the brain stem. Although the boundaries between subdivisions are not precise, the different components of the trigeminal spinal nuclear complex can be identified with respect to brain stem landmarks (see Figure 12–5A). The **caudal nucleus** extends from approximately the first or second cervical segment of the spinal cord to the medullary level, at which the central canal "opens" to form the fourth ventricle. The **interpolar nucleus** extends from the rostral boundary of the caudal nucleus to the rostral medulla. Finally, the **oral nucleus** extends from the rostral boundary of the interpolar nucleus to the level at which the trigeminal nerve enters the pons. The other cranial nerve sensory (afferent) nuclei—solitary nucleus, vestibular nuclei, and cochlear nuclei—also are labeled in Figure 12–9.

Occlusion of the Posterior Inferior Cerebellar Artery Interrupts Pain and Temperature Senses on the Same Side of the Face But on the Opposite Side of the Body

As we saw in earlier chapters, the posterior inferior cerebellar artery (PICA) provides the arterial supply to the dorsolateral portion of the medulla (Figure 12–10) and caudal pons. The posterior inferior cerebellar artery is an **end-artery with little collateral flow** from other vessels into the territory it serves. As a consequence, the dorsolateral region of the medulla becomes infarcted when the artery is occluded (Figure 12–10). The major cause of posterior inferior cerebellar artery stroke is **vertebral artery** occlusion where the posterior inferior cerebellar artery branches off (Figure 12–10, inset). The medial region of the medulla is spared infarction with such an occlusion because of the collateral blood supply to this area from the contralateral vertebral artery and the anterior spinal artery.

Occlusion of the posterior inferior cerebellar artery produces a complex set of sensory and motor deficits (the **lateral medullary syndrome** or **Wallenberg's syndrome**). Signs include loss of pain and temperature senses on the contralateral side of the body (see Chapter 5). This is due to interruption of the ascending axons of the anterolateral system in the **lateral medulla**. Sensory loss is on the contralateral side because fibers of the anterolateral system decussate in the spinal cord.

Posterior inferior cerebellar artery occlusion also produces **deficits in pain and temperature senses of the face**. Such deficits reveal that the neurons that mediate these senses—the descending primary afferent fibers in the spinal trigeminal tract and the neurons in the spinal trigeminal nucleus—are also located within the territory supplied by the posterior inferior cerebellar artery in the lateral medulla. Sensory deficits are on the **side ipsilateral to the occlusion** because the primary afferent fibers are destroyed. Since the axons of ascending projection neurons decussate rostral to their cell bodies, similar to the anterolateral system of the spinal

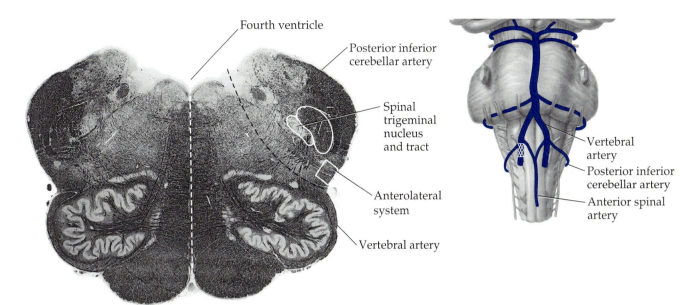

Figure 12–10. The arterial supply of the medulla. The inset shows the vasculature on a portion of the ventral brain stem. The shaded portion on the vertebral artery is the site of occlusion that prevents blood flow into the posterior inferior cerebellar artery. Collateral blood flow from the contralateral vertebral artery supplies the territory of the vertebral artery on the occluded side.

cord (see Figure 5–9), posterior inferior cerebellar artery occlusion rarely destroys the axons of decussated trigeminothalamic tract fibers.

Other sensory and motor deficits are also common neurological signs of the lateral medullary syndrome because the solitary nucleus, vestibular nuclei, and the inferior cerebellar peduncle are located in the dorsolateral medulla. These signs, introduced in Chapter 10, will be examined further in Chapter 13.

The Main Trigeminal Sensory Nucleus Is the Trigeminal Equivalent of the Dorsal Column Nuclei

Rostral to the spinal trigeminal nucleus is the **main trigeminal sensory nucleus** (Figure 12–11). This part of the trigeminal nuclear complex subserves tactile sensation of the face and head, including mechanosensation from the teeth. Neurons located primarily in the ventral two thirds of this nucleus give rise to axons that decussate and ascend to the **ventral posterior medial nucleus** of the thalamus. Their axons are located in the **trigeminal lemniscus**. The main trigeminal sensory nucleus may be the trigeminal equivalent of the dorsal column nuclei because: (1) both nuclei project to the contralateral ventral posterior nucleus (but to different subdivisions); and (2) both structures subserve tactile sensation (but from different body regions). The trigeminal lemniscus at brain stem levels caudal to the main sensory nucleus contains axons from neurons in the spinal trigeminal nucleus. This contingent, which may be analogous to the group of dorsal column axons that originate from dorsal horn neurons (see Chapter 5), joins with the ascending fibers from the main sensory nucleus in the rostral pons.

The dorsal one third of the main sensory nucleus receives mechanoreceptive signals from the soft tissues of the oral cavity and the teeth. Neurons from this portion of the main sensory nucleus give rise to

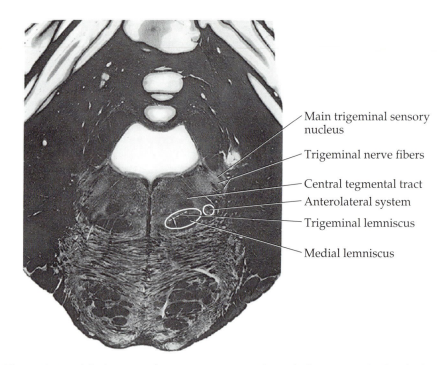

Main trigeminal sensory nucleus

Trigeminal nerve fibers

Central tegmental tract

Anterolateral system

Trigeminal lemniscus

Medial lemniscus

Figure 12–11. Myelin-stained transverse section through the pons at the level of the main sensory nucleus and the trigeminal motor nucleus.

an **ipsilateral pathway** that ascends dorsally in the pons and midbrain (Figure 12–11) and terminates in the ipsilateral ventral posterior medial nucleus of the thalamus. It follows that the ventral posterior medial nucleus receives bilateral inputs from intraoral structures: a contralateral projection from the **trigeminal lemniscus** and an ipsilateral projection from the **dorsal pathway.** This bilateral representation in the thalamus, and presumably also in the somatic sensory cortex, may reflect the function of oral structures on each side, which typically work together during such behaviors as chewing or talking. In contrast, the representation of the arms and legs is unilateral (i.e., crossed), an organization that may reflect how the limbs on either side can function independently.

The Mesencephalic Trigeminal Nucleus and Tract Course in Parallel With the Cerebral Aqueduct and Contain the Axons of Jaw Muscle Stretch Receptors

The mesencephalic trigeminal nucleus is found in the lateral portion of the periventricular and periaqueductal gray matter. The mesencephalic nucleus is equivalent to a peripheral sensory ganglion because cell bodies of primary afferent neurons are located there. Like those in the semilunar ganglion, the cells of the mesencephalic nucleus are also pseudounipolar neurons (Figure 12–2) with separate peripheral and central axonal branches. The peripheral branch, carrying afferent information to the central nervous system, ascends to the mesencephalic trigeminal nucleus in close association with the ventricular system, in the **mesencephalic trigeminal tract**. The central branch also projects through the mesencephalic trigeminal tracts, to terminate in various brain stem sites that are important for motor control and proprioception of the jaw. For example, the projection to the trigeminal motor nucleus mediates jaw reflexes, including the monosynaptic jaw closure—or **jaw-jerk**—reflex, which is analogous to the knee-jerk reflex (Figure 12–5).

The mesencephalic trigeminal tract, located lateral to the nucleus, can be identified by its myelinated axons (Figure 12–12). Although the mesencephalic nucleus and tract are present from the level of the main trigeminal sensory and motor nuclei in the pons to the superior colliculus in the midbrain, the tract can be more easily identified in the midbrain.

At the midbrain level shown in Figure 12–12, the medial lemniscus and trigeminal lemniscus have migrated laterally; however, the ascending trigeminal fibers are located dorsomedially. The trigeminal lemniscus terminates in the **medial** division of the ventral posterior nucleus.

The Ventral Posterior Nucleus Contains Separate Divisions That Mediate Somatic Sensation of the Face and Body

The ventral posterior nucleus contains two principal divisions that mediate somatic sensation (see Chapter 5). The **ventral posterior lateral** nucleus mediates somatic sensation from the limbs and trunk, and the **ventral posterior medial** nucleus (Figure 12–13) processes somatic sensation from the head. The ventral posterior medial nucleus is further subdivided into a lateral portion with medium size neurons and a medial **parvocellular** division. The division with medium-size neurons receives the projection from the trigeminal lemniscus. Although this portion is difficult to distinguish from the ventral posterior lateral nucleus, the **parvocellular** portion, which mediates taste (see Chapter 8), has a characteristic pale appearance in myelin-stained sections (Figure 12–13). Once the parvocellular portion is identified, the position of the magnocellular portion can be inferred.

The second major site receiving trigeminal input is the intralaminar nuclei. In contrast to the ventral posterior medial nucleus, which is a thalamic sensory relay nucleus that projects to a restricted portion of the postcentral gyrus (see below), the intralaminar nuclei project in a more diffuse projection pattern. The projection to the intralaminar nuclei is thought to be important in the emotional aspects of pain perception, whereas the projection to the ventral posterior medial nucleus is important in the discrim-

Figure 12–12. Myelin-stained transverse section through the rostral midbrain.

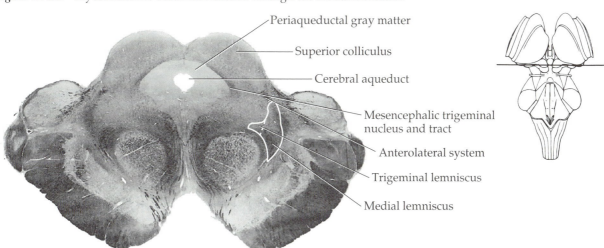

Periaqueductal gray matter

Superior colliculus

Cerebral aqueduct

Mesencephalic trigeminal nucleus and tract

Anterolateral system

Trigeminal lemniscus

Medial lemniscus

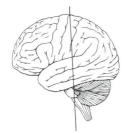

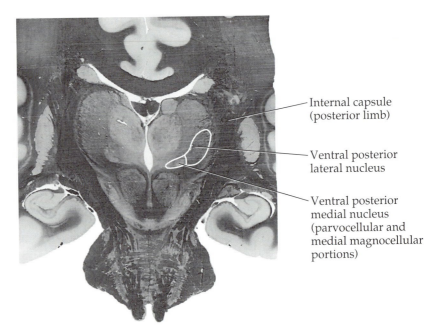

Internal capsule
(posterior limb)

Ventral posterior
lateral nucleus

Ventral posterior
medial nucleus
(parvocellular and
medial magnocellular
portions)

Figure 12–13. Myelin-stained coronal section through the ventral posterior nucleus of the thalamus. The magnocellular and parvocellular portions of the medial division (ventral posterior medial nucleus) are the trigeminal and taste relay nuclei, whereas the lateral division (ventral posterior lateral nucleus) is the relay nucleus for the medial lemniscus (i.e., spinal sensory input).

inative aspects of pain (see discussion of the roles of the medial and lateral thalamus in pain in Chapter 5).

The Ventral Posterior Medial Nucleus Projects to the Primary Somatic Sensory Cortex

The somatic sensory thalamic relay nucleus is the ventral posterior nucleus. Neurons in this nucleus project to the primary somatic sensory cortex, located in the postcentral gyrus (Figure 12–14) through the internal capsule (Figure 12–13). The lateral division of the nucleus, or the **ventral posterior lateral nucleus**, projects to the arm, trunk, and leg areas of the primary somatic sensory cortex (Figure 12–14A; see also Chapter 5). The medial division of the nucleus, or the **ventral posterior medial nucleus**, projects to the **face area** of the primary somatic sensory cortex.

The face area of the primary somatic sensory cortex is located on the lateral portion of the postcentral gyrus (Figure 12–14). The representation of the body surface takes the form of a map in which body parts extensively used are overrepresented (see Chapter 5). In humans, the representations of the fingers, tongue, and perioral region in the primary somatic sensory cortex are larger than the cortical representations of other body parts. In many species of rodents and carnivores, the face representation is more extensive than that of the fingers or tongue and perioral regions, because their large whiskers are their principal tactile discriminative organs. Two other cortical areas are important in processing somatic sensory information: (1) the **secondary somatic sensory cortex**, located largely on the parietal operculum; and (2) the **posterior parietal cortex**, located laterally in area 5 (see Figure 5–18).

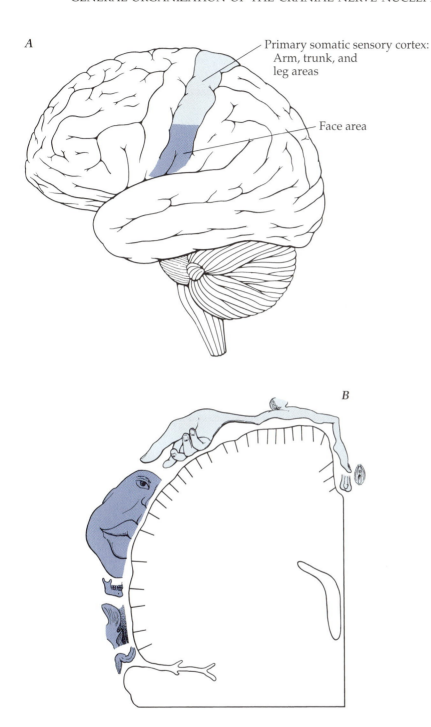

A

Primary somatic sensory cortex:
Arm, trunk, and
leg areas

Face area

B

Figure 12–14. *A.* Lateral view of cerebral hemisphere, with the representations of the limbs, trunk, and face indicated on the postcentral gyrus. *B.* Somatotopic organization of the postcentral gyrus. (*B,* Adapted from Penfield, W., and Rasmussen, T. 1950. The Cerebral Cortex of Man: A Clinical Study of Localization of Function. New York: Macmillan.)

The Cranial Nerves

Of the 12 cranial nerves (Table 12–1, Figure 12–1), the first two, the **olfactory** and the **optic** nerves, are sensory, and enter the telencephalon and diencephalon directly. The third through twelfth cranial nerves enter and exit from the brain stem directly. Two cranial nerves—both motor—are located in the midbrain, the **oculomotor** (III) and the **trochlear** (IV). The pons contains the **trigeminal** (V), a mixed nerve; the **abducens** (VI), a motor nerve; the **facial** (VII), a mixed nerve; and the **vestibulocochlear**

Summary

(VIII), a sensory nerve. The medulla also contains four cranial nerves: **glossopharyngeal** (IX) and **vagus** (X) are mixed nerves, whereas the **spinal accessory** (XI) and **hypoglossal** (XII) are motor nerves.

Cranial Nerve Nuclei Columns

Separate columns of cranial nerve nuclei course through the brain stem along its rostrocaudal axis (Figures 12–3 and 12–4). Each column subserves a separate sensory (afferent) or motor function, and the nomenclature conforms to that for the cranial nerves: (1) **general somatic motor**; (2) **special visceral motor**; (3) **general visceral motor**; (4) **general and special visceral afferent**; (5) **general somatic afferent**; (6) **special somatic afferent** (Table 12–1). Each column has its own mediolateral location (Figures 12–3 and 12–4). The **sulcus limitans** separates the sensory from the motor nuclear columns.

Trigeminal Sensory System

Somatic sensation of cranial structures is mediated predominantly by the trigeminal nerve, which has three sensory divisions (Figure 12–7A): the **ophthalmic**, the **maxillary**, and the **mandibular**. The cell bodies of the primary sensory neurons that innervate the skin and mucous membranes of the head are located in the **semilunar** (or **trigeminal**) **ganglion**. Three other cranial nerves also innervate portions of the head. The **intermediate nerve** (a branch of the **facial nerve**) (VII) innervates the skin of the **ear**, the **glossopharyngeal** (IX) nerve innervates the posterior tongue and portions of the oral cavity, nasal cavity, pharynx, and middle ear (Figure 12–7A). The **vagus** (X) nerve innervates the skin of the **ear** and mucous membranes of the **larynx.** The cell bodies of the primary afferent fibers in the facial nerve are located in the **geniculate ganglion**, and those of the glossopharyngeal and vagus nerves, in the **superior ganglion** of each nerve. Afferent fibers in these four cranial nerves enter the brain stem and ascend and descend in the **spinal trigeminal tract** (Figures 12–7 and 12–8). The fibers of the trigeminal nerve, whose cell bodies lie in the semilunar ganglion, terminate in two of the three major components of the trigeminal nuclear complex (Figure 12–5): the **main (principal) trigeminal sensory nucleus** (Figures 12–5 and 12–11) and the **spinal trigeminal nucleus** (Figures 12–1, 12–5, and 12–8), which has three subdivisions (Figures 12–5 and 12–11)— the **oral nucleus**, the **interpolar nucleus**, and the **caudal nucleus**. The afferent fibers of the facial, glossopharyngeal, and vagus nerves terminate in the spinal trigeminal nucleus.

Mechanoreceptive afferent fibers of the trigeminal nerve terminate predominantly in the **main trigeminal sensory nucleus**. The majority of the ascending projection neurons of this nucleus (Figure 12–6A) send their axons to the **contralateral ventral posterior medial nucleus** of the thalamus (Figure 12–13). From here, thalamic neurons project, via the posterior limb of the internal capsule, to the face representation of the **primary somatic sensory cortex**, which is located in the lateral portion of the **postcentral gyrus** (Figure 12–14). There is also a small component that ascends ipsilaterally to the thalamus and cortex.

Pain and **temperature** afferents from cranial structures enter and descend in the spinal trigeminal tract. The ascending pathway for pain and temperature sensations originates from the **spinal trigeminal nucleus,**

primarily from the **caudal and interpolar nuclei** (Figure 12–6B). The axons of projection neurons of this nucleus either remain on the ipsilateral side or decussate. The ascending fibers course with the anterolateral system in the lateral medulla and pons en route to the rostral brain stem and thalamus. The thalamic nuclei in which the fibers terminate are the **ventral posterior medial** nucleus and the **intralaminar nuclei**.

Afferent fibers carrying proprioceptive information from the jaw muscles form the **mesencephalic trigeminal tract** (Figure 12–12). Their cell bodies are located in the **mesencephalic trigeminal nucleus** and are unique because they are the only primary sensory neurons with their cell bodies located in the central nervous system (Figure 12–2). ■

KEY STRUCTURES AND TERMS

olfactory nerve (I)
optic nerve (II)
oculomotor nerve (III)
trochlear nerve (IV)
trigeminal nerve (V)
abducens nerve (VI)
facial nerve (VII)
vestibulocochlear nerve (VIII)
glossopharyngeal nerve (IX)
vagus nerve (X)
spinal accessory nerve (XI)
hypoglossal nerve (XII)
sulcus limitans
general somatic afferent
general visceral afferent
general somatic motor
general visceral motor
special somatic afferent
special visceral afferent

special visceral motor
trigeminal nerve
    ophthalmic division
    maxillary division
    mandibular division
intermediate nerve
pseudounipolar primary sensory
    neurons
bipolar sensory neurons
semilunar ganglion
superior ganglia
inferior ganglia
geniculate ganglion
spinal trigeminal nucleus
    oral nucleus
    interpolar nucleus
    caudal nucleus (medullary dorsal
        horn)
        marginal zone

substantia gelatinosa
magnocellular nucleus
main (or principal) trigeminal
    sensory nucleus
mesencephalic trigeminal nucleus
spinal trigeminal tract
trigeminal lemniscus
trigeminothalamic tract
ventral posterior medial nucleus
intralaminar nuclei
primary somatic sensory cortex
postcentral gyrus
secondary somatic sensory cortex
posterior inferior cerebellar artery
vertebral artery
lateral medullary syndrome
jaw-jerk reflex

Selected Readings

Brodal, A. 1957. The Cranial Nerves, Anatomical and Anatomicoclinical Correlations. Oxford: Blackwell Scientific Publications.

Brodal, A. 1981. Neurological Anatomy. New York: Oxford University Press.

Dodd, J., and Kelly, J. P. 1991. Trigeminal system. In Kandel, E. R., Schwartz, J. H., and Jessell, T. M. (eds.), Principles of Neural Science, 3rd ed. New York: Elsevier, pp. 701–710.

Dubner, R., and Bennett, G. J. 1983. Spinal and trigeminal mechanisms of nociception. Annu. Rev. Neurosci. 6:381–418.

Role, L., and Kelly, J. P. 1991. The brain stem: Cranial nerve nuclei and the monoaminergic systems. In Kandel, E. R., Schwartz, J. H., and Jessell, T. M. (eds.), Principles of Neural Science, 3rd ed. New York: Elsevier, pp. 684–699.

References

Arvidsson, J., and Gobel, S. 1981. An HRP study of the central projections of primary trigeminal neurons which innervate tooth pulp in the cat. Brain Res. 210:1–16.

Burton, H., and Craig, A. D. Jr. 1979. Distribution of trigeminothalamic projection cells in cat and monkey. Brain Res. 161:515–521.

Cajal, S. Ramón y. 1909, 1911. Histologie du système nerveux de l'homme et des vertèbres. 2 vols. Paris: Maloine.

Craig, A. D. Jr., and Burton, H. 1981. Spinal and medullary lamina 1 projection to nucleus submedius in medial thalamus: A possible pain center. J. Neurophysiol. 45:443–466.

Fukushima, T., and Kerr, F. W. L. 1979. Organization of trigeminothalamic tracts and other thalamic afferent systems of the brainstem in the rat: Presence of gelatinosa neurons with thalamic connections. J. Comp. Neurol. 183:169–184.

Gobel, S., Hockfield, S., and Ruda, M. A. 1981. Anatomical similarities between medullary and spinal dorsal horns. In Kawamura, Y., and Dubner, R. Oral–Facial Sensory and Motor Functions. Tokyo: Quintessence Publishing Co., pp. 211–223.

Hayashi, H., Sumino, R., and Sessle, B. J. 1984. Functional organization of trigeminal subnucleus interpolaris: Nociceptive and innocuous afferent inputs, projections to thalamus, cerebellum, and spinal cord, and descending modulation from periaqueductal gray. J. Neurophysiol. 51:890–905.

Hu, J. W., and Sessle, B. J. 1984. Comparison of responses of cutaneous nociceptive and nonnociceptive brain stem neurons in trigeminal subnucleus caudalis (medullary dorsal horn) and subnucleus oralis to natural and electrical stimulation of tooth pulp. J. Neurophysiol. 52:39–53.

Jones, E. G., Schwark, H. D., and Callahan, P. A. 1984. Extent of the ipsilateral representation in the ventral posterior medial nucleus of the monkey thalamus. Exp. Brain Res. 63:310–320.

Kruger, L. Functional subdivision of the brainstem sensory trigeminal nuclear complex. In Bonica, J. J., Liebeskind, J. C., and Albe-Fessard, D. G. (eds.), Advances in Pain Research and Therapy, Vol. 3. New York: Raven Press, pp. 197–209.

Martin, G. F., Holstege, G., and Mehler, W. R. 1990. Reticular formation of the pons and medulla. In Paxinos, G. (ed.), The Human Nervous System. San Diego: Academic Press, pp. 203–220.

Nieuwenhuys, R., Voogd, J., and Huijzen, C. 1988. The Human Central Nervous System: A Synopsis and Atlas, 3rd ed. Berlin: Springer-Verlag.

Paxinos, G., Törk, I., Halliday, G., and Mehler, W. R. 1990. Human homologs to brainstem nuclei identified in other animals as revealed by acetylcholinesterase activity. In Paxinos, G. (ed.), The Human Nervous System. San Diego: Academic Press, pp. 149–202.

Shigenaga, Y, Nishimura, M., Suemune, S., et al. 1989. Somatotopic organization of tooth pulp primary afferent neurons in the cat. Brain Res. 477:66–89.

Smith, R. L. 1975. Axonal projections and connections of the principal sensory trigeminal nucleus in the monkey. J. Comp. Neurol. 163:347–376.

13

The Somatic and Visceral Motor Functions of the Cranial Nerves

A S WE SAW IN CHAPTER 12, the functional and anatomical organization of the trigeminal system parallels that of the spinal cord ascending pathways. A similar comparison can be made between motor control of cranial structures and that of the limbs and body axis: Cranial muscles are innervated by motor neurons that are found in the cranial nerve motor nuclei, whereas limb and axial muscles are innervated by motor neurons in the motor nuclei of the ventral horn. Also similar to the spinal cord, the control of the pupil and glands and smooth muscle of the head is mediated by parasympathetic preganglionic neurons that are located in cranial nerve autonomic nuclei. Some of these autonomic neurons also function in the control of thoracic and abdominal organs.

In this chapter, the three functional categories of cranial nerve motor nuclei are considered. Together with the skeletal motor nuclei of the brain stem, we also examine the control of cranial skeletal motor function by the frontal lobe of the cerebral cortex, which is mediated by the corticobulbar system. Knowing the patterns of corticobulbar connections with the cranial motor nuclei has important diagnostic value. In completing our study of the cranial nerve nuclei, greater knowledge of brain stem regional anatomy will emerge. Such knowledge is essential for clinical problem solving: for example, in identifying the locus of central nervous system damage. Because each of the cranial nerve nuclei has a clearly identifiable sensory or motor function, the integrity of such functions can be thoroughly tested by the physician.

◼ FUNCTIONAL ANATOMY OF CRANIAL MOTOR NUCLEI

The Cranial Motor Nuclei Are Controlled by the Cerebral Cortex and Diencephalon

As we saw in the preceding chapter, 10 of 12 cranial nerves enter and exit the brain stem (Figure 13–1A). The ten brain stem cranial nerves are directly connected to the sensory and motor cranial nerve nuclei. The locations of the cranial nerve nuclei are shown in Figure 13–1B. Six columns of

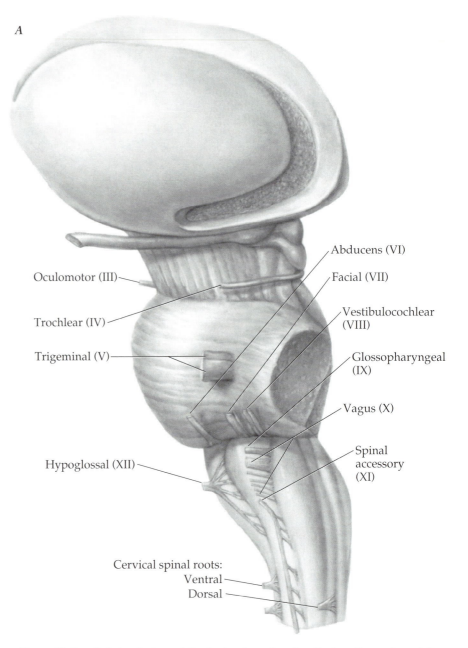

A

Oculomotor (III)

Trochlear (IV)

Trigeminal (V)

Hypoglossal (XII)

Abducens (VI)

Facial (VII)

Vestibulocochlear (VIII)

Glossopharyngeal (IX)

Vagus (X)

Spinal accessory (XI)

Cervical spinal roots:
Ventral
Dorsal

Figure 13–1. *A.* Lateral view of the brain stem showing the locations of cranial nerves. *B.* Dorsal view of brain stem (without cerebellum) showing the locations of cranial nerve nuclei.

cranial nerve nuclei course rostrocaudally in the brain stem (see Figure 12–3A). As we saw in Chapter 12, the columns containing nuclei that mediate cranial motor function are located medially, whereas the sensory columns are located laterally. On the floor of the fourth ventricle, the **sulcus limitans** serves as the boundary between the sensory and motor columns.

The three columns of cranial nerve motor nuclei (Figure 13–1B) include: (1) nuclei in the **general somatic motor** column, which contain motor neurons that innervate striated muscle of somatic origin (i.e., occipital somites); (2) nuclei of the **special visceral motor** column, which con-

B

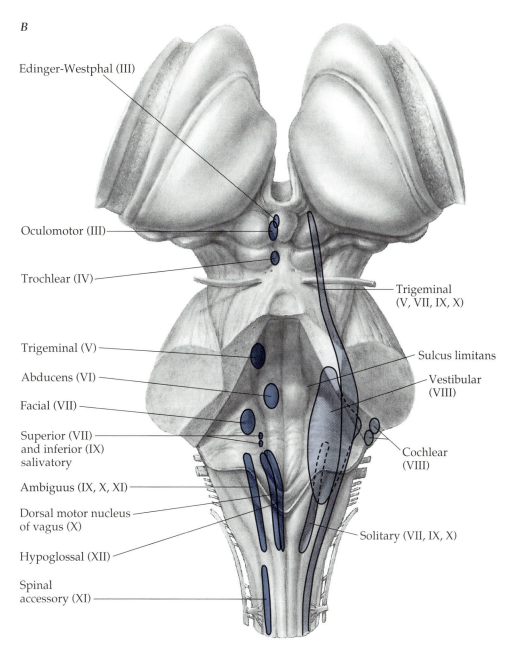

Edinger-Westphal (III)

Oculomotor (III)

Trochlear (IV)

Trigeminal (V, VII, IX, X)

Trigeminal (V)

Abducens (VI)

Facial (VII)

Superior (VII) and inferior (IX) salivatory

Ambiguus (IX, X, XI)

Dorsal motor nucleus of vagus (X)

Hypoglossal (XII)

Spinal accessory (XI)

Sulcus limitans

Vestibular (VIII)

Cochlear (VIII)

Solitary (VII, IX, X)

Figure 13–1.   (continued)

tain motor neurons innervating striated muscle of visceral (branchiomeric) origin; and (3) nuclei of the **general visceral motor** column, which contain the parasympathetic preganglionic neurons.

The nuclei that comprise the two columns that innervate cranial skeletal muscle, similar to the spinal motor nuclei in the ventral horn, receive projections from the cerebral cortex. Two key sets of descending cortical projections can be distinguished: (1) those controlling facial, jaw, laryngeal, pharyngeal, palatal, and neck muscles, which course in the **corticobulbar tract**; and (2) those controlling the extraocular muscles, which course along with other descending cortical fibers in the internal capsule and basis pedunculi. These systems mediate voluntary, and certain kinds of automatic, control of the cranial muscles.

The pattern of projections of the corticobulbar tract to cranial nerve nuclei innervating striated muscle is particularly important clinically. Corticobulbar axons terminate either contralaterally or bilaterally, depending on the particular nucleus (see below). Muscles innervated by motor nuclei that receive a **bilateral** projection from the corticobulbar tract do not become weak after a unilateral lesion of motor cortex (or some portion of its descending pathway). The intact projection is sufficient for normal (or near-normal) control of force production. This is not the case, however, for muscles receiving only contralateral motor cortical control. Here, weakness reveals unilateral damage. This relationship between the crossed and bilateral projections is similar to that of the corticospinal system. Recall that corticospinal projections to the limb motor neurons are mainly crossed (lateral corticospinal tract) and a unilateral lesion of these fibers produces unilateral weakness. In contrast, projections to axial motor neurons are mainly bilateral (ventral corticospinal tract) and a unilateral lesion typically does not produce weakness. Like skeletal motor neurons in the spinal motor nuclei, cranial motor neurons are also under involuntary and reflexive control by afferent fibers and brain stem motor circuits.

The nuclei that comprise the column that regulates cranial glands and body organs are also influenced by afferent fibers, brain stem motor circuits, and projections from higher levels of the nervous system. The principal structure regulating the autonomic nuclei is the **hypothalamus,** which receives inputs from diverse regions of the cerebral hemispheres, including the limbic association cortex. The autonomic nervous system is considered in detail with the hypothalamus (see Chapter 14).

Neurons in the General Somatic Motor Cell Column Innervate Striated Muscles That Develop From the Occipital Somites

Four nuclei comprise the motor column that contains motor neurons innervating striated muscles that derive from the **occipital somites**. Three of these nuclei contain motor neurons that innervate the extraocular muscles: (1) the **oculomotor nucleus** and (2) the **trochlear nucleus** are located in the rostral and caudal midbrain, respectively; whereas (3) the **abducens nucleus** is found in the pons. The fourth, the **hypoglossal nucleus,** is found in the medulla and innervates tongue muscles.

Three Extraocular Motor Nuclei Control Eye Movements

The oculomotor nucleus contributes most of the axons of the **oculomotor (III) nerve**, which exits the rostral midbrain from the medial aspect of the **cerebral peduncle**. The oculomotor nucleus (Figure 13–2) innervates four of the six extraocular muscles: **medial rectus, inferior rectus, superior rectus,** and **inferior oblique** (see Figure 13–14A). This nucleus also innervates the **levator palpebrae superioris muscle,** an elevator of the eyelid.

The other two extraocular motor nuclei are the trochlear and abducens nuclei (Figure 13–2). Motor neurons in the trochlear nucleus give rise to the fibers in the **trochlear (IV) nerve** (Figure 13–2B), which innervate the **superior oblique muscle** (see Figure 13–14A). This cranial nerve is the only one that exits from the **dorsal** brain stem surface. The trochlear nerve is further distinguished because all of its axons decussate within the central nervous system. The abducens nucleus contains the motor neurons that project their axons to the periphery through the **abducens (VI) nerve**.

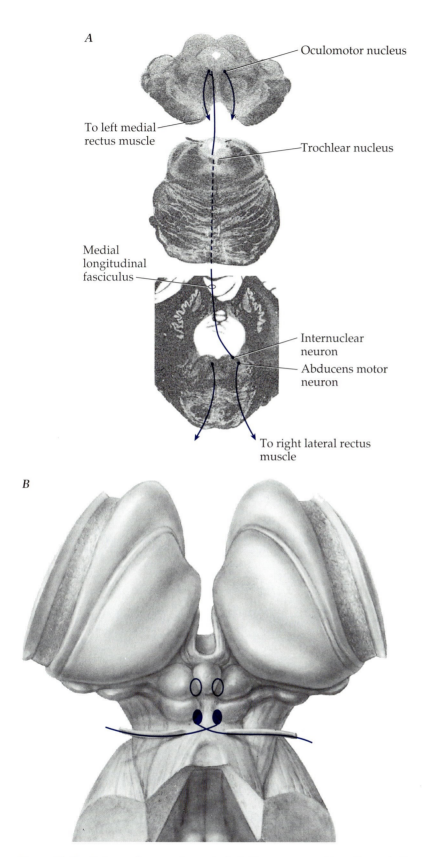

A

Oculomotor nucleus

To left medial rectus muscle

Trochlear nucleus

Medial longitudinal fasciculus

Internuclear neuron

Abducens motor neuron

To right lateral rectus muscle

B

Figure 13–2. Extraocular muscle control. *A.* Transverse sections through the oculomotor, trochlear, and abducens nuclei are shown. *B.* View of the dorsal brain stem showing the locations of the oculomotor nuclei (open ovals) and trochlear nuclei (filled ovals) and depicting the course of the trochlear nerve within the brain stem.

387

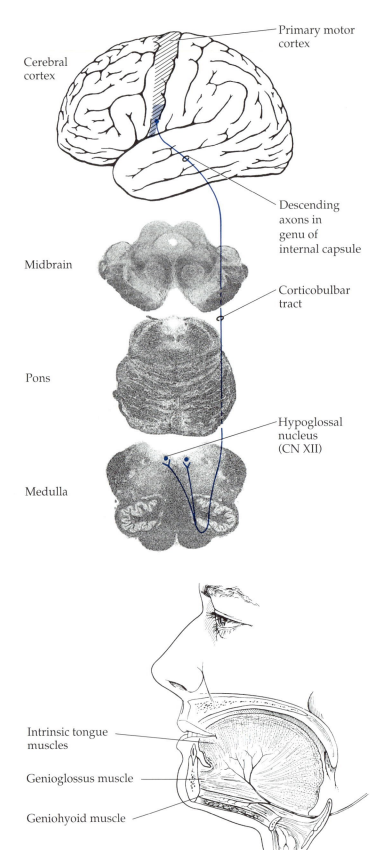

Figure 13–3. Cortical control of the hypoglossal nucleus. The descending cortical projection to the hypoglossal nucleus originates from the lateral motor cortex, which is the location of the cranial nerve motor representation. In most people the hypoglossal nucleus on one side is contacted by motor cortex neurons on both sides. A unilateral corticobulbar tract lesion typically does not produce unilateral weakness. Note that the geniohyoid muscle is innervated by cervical spinal cord motor neurons, whose axons course, for a portion, with the hypoglossal nerve.

This nerve exits the brain stem at the **pontomedullary junction**. Abducens motor neurons innervate the **lateral rectus** muscle (see Figure 13–14A). In contrast to the other cranial nuclei that innervate skeletal musculature, the primary motor cortex does not steer eye movements. Rather, distinct areas in the frontal lobe rostral to the primary motor cortex and in the parietal lobe play important roles in reflexive and voluntary eye movement control (see Box 13–1).

The Hypoglossal Nucleus Innervates Tongue Muscles

The **hypoglossal nucleus** is the fourth member of the general somatic motor column (Figure 13–3). The axons of motor neurons in the hypoglossal nucleus course in the hypoglossal (XII) nerve and innervate intrinsic tongue muscles, including: genioglossus, hypoglossus, and styloglossus. Similar to the control of limb muscles (and in contrast to the other three general somatic motor nuclei), the primary motor cortex does project to the hypoglossal nucleus. The axons descend in the **corticobulbar tract**, which courses through the genu of the internal capsule (as well as the rostral part of the posterior limb) and then in the basis pedunculi, medial to the spinal-projecting axons of the corticospinal tract (see Chapter 9). Neurons contributing axons to the corticobulbar tract, as well as all other cortical descending projection neurons, are located in layer 5. Cells of origin of the corticobulbar tract are located in the portion of the precentral gyrus close to the **lateral sulcus** (see Figure 9–7B).

This projection from the motor cortex to the hypoglossal nucleus is most commonly a **bilateral** one. Clinically, this is important in that a unilateral lesion of the descending path, for example in the genu of the internal capsule, typically does not produce weakness of tongue muscles. In some people, however, a unilateral infarction of the internal capsule produces contralateral tongue weakness. This suggests that in some individuals, the hypoglossal nucleus receives a crossed corticobulbar projection. By contrast, a lesion of the hypoglossal nucleus or nerve consistently produces a classical motor sign: When the patient is asked to protrude the tongue, it deviates to the side of the lesion. The hypoglossal nucleus and nerve can become lesioned with occlusion of the branches of the vertebral artery, which supplies the medial medulla (see Figure 4–3).

The Special Visceral Motor Cell Column Innervates Skeletal Muscles That Develop From the Branchial Arches

The special visceral motor cell column is located lateral to the general somatic motor column and is displaced ventrally from the ventricular floor (Figure 12–3B). The nuclei that comprise this column contain motor neurons that innervate striated muscles derived from the **branchial arches**. Three cranial nerve nuclei constitute this nuclear column: **trigeminal motor nucleus**, **facial motor nucleus**, and **nucleus ambiguus**. The special visceral motor nuclei in the brain stem each receive a projection from the primary motor cortex via the corticobulbar tract.

Trigeminal Motor Neurons Innervate Muscles of Mastication

The axons of motor neurons of the trigeminal motor nucleus course in the trigeminal (V) nerve and innervate principally the muscles of **mastication**: masseter, temporalis, and external and internal pterygoid muscles (see Table 12–1). Because the primary motor cortex projects **bilaterally** to the trigeminal motor nuclei (Figure 13–4A), unilateral cortical or

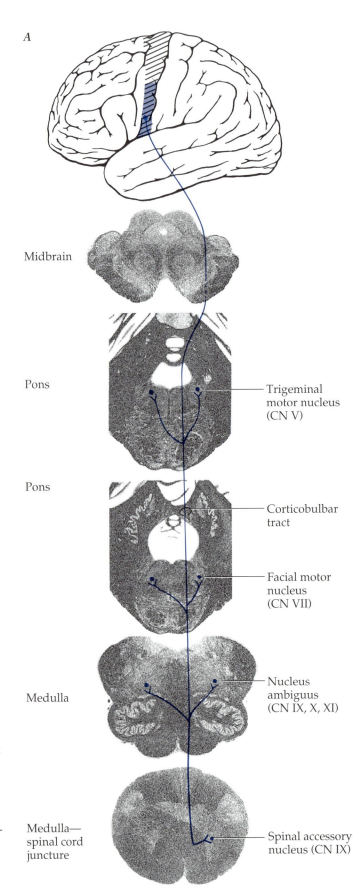

A

Midbrain

Pons

Pons

Medulla

Medulla—
spinal cord
juncture

Trigeminal
motor nucleus
(CN V)

Corticobulbar
tract

Facial motor
nucleus
(CN VII)

Nucleus
ambiguus
(CN IX, X, XI)

Spinal accessory
nucleus (CN IX)

Figure 13–4. *A.* Cortical control of nuclei of the special visceral motor cell column. Most of these nuclei receive a predominantly bilateral projection from the primary motor cortex so unilateral lesions have little or no effect. The spinal accessory nucleus is the exception. It receives a unilateral cortical projection. Lesion of this projection can produce unilateral weakness. *B.* Topography of cortical projections to the facial motor nucleus. *C.* Rostrocaudal organization of the nucleus ambiguus and spinal accessory nucleus.

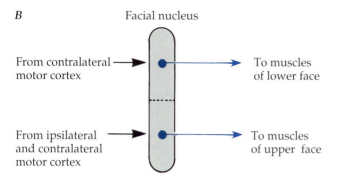

B

Facial nucleus

From contralateral motor cortex → To muscles of lower face

From ipsilateral and contralateral motor cortex → To muscles of upper face

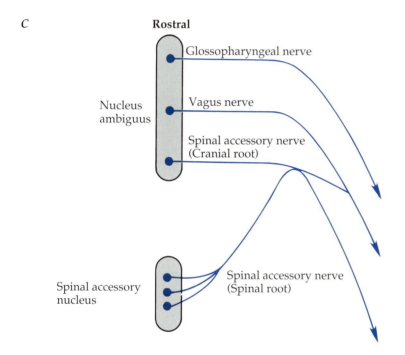

C

Rostral

Nucleus ambiguus

Glossopharyngeal nerve

Vagus nerve

Spinal accessory nerve (Cranial root)

Spinal accessory nucleus

Spinal accessory nerve (Spinal root)

Figure 13–4. (continued)

descending pathway lesions do not produce weakness of the muscles of mastication. Bilateral control by the primary motor cortex may reflect the fact that muscles of mastication on both sides of the mouth are typically activated in tandem during most motor acts, for example, chewing or talking. This is similar to the bilateral control of axial muscles, for maintaining posture, by the medial descending spinal cord pathways (see Chapter 9).

The Laterality of Cortical Projections to the Facial Motor Nucleus Is Complex

The facial (motor) nucleus contains the motor neurons that innervate the muscles of **facial expression** (Figure 13–4A). These axons course in the **facial (VII) nerve**. There is an interesting organization of descending control by the motor cortex to the facial nucleus (Figure 13–4B). Motor neurons that innervate muscles of the **upper face** receive a projection from the motor cortex in both hemispheres, whereas those innervating muscles of the lower face receive an input only from the **contralateral** motor cortex.

A unilateral lesion of the descending cortical fibers, for example in the genu of the internal capsule, will have differential effects on upper and lower facial muscles. After the lesion, upper facial muscles retain cortical control from the opposite side and, therefore, remain unaffected. In contrast, lower facial muscles, their cortical control interrupted, become weak on the side contralateral to the lesion, and facial expressions become asymmetrical. With a facial nerve or nucleus lesion, motor deficits occur on the **ipsilateral face** and muscles of **both the upper and lower face** are affected.

The Nucleus Ambiguus Receives a Bilateral Projection From the Primary Motor Cortex

The nucleus ambiguus contains motor neurons that innervate striated muscles of the **palate**, **pharynx**, and **larynx**. Most motor neurons in the nucleus send their axons through the **vagus (X) nerve**. Because the pharyngeal muscles are innervated by the vagus nerve, a lesion of the nucleus ambiguus produces difficulty in swallowing. The vagus nerve carries the fibers of the efferent limb of the **gag reflex**. In this reflex, mechanical stimulation of the pharynx, using a cotton swab for example, produces a reflex contraction of the pharyngeal muscles. The **glossopharyngeal nerve** contains the afferent fibers (i.e., general visceral afferent; see Chapter 12) that comprise the afferent limb of the gag reflex.

A minority of neurons in the nucleus ambiguus project through the glossopharyngeal (IX) and the spinal accessory (XI) nerves (Figure 13–4C). Motor neurons in the most rostral portion of the nucleus ambiguus (rostral to those projecting in the vagus nerve) course in the **glossopharyngeal (IX) nerve** (Figure 13–4C) and innervate one pharyngeal muscle, the stylopharyngeus. Because this muscle is located deep within the pharynx, its function cannot be tested noninvasively; thus, any dysfunction will remain unidentified on routine clinical examination.

The most caudal portion of the nucleus ambiguus contains laryngeal motor neurons whose axons course in a portion of the **spinal accessory (XI) nerve**. This cranial nerve consists of distinct **cranial and spinal roots** and only axons in the cranial root have their cell bodies in the **nucleus ambiguus**. These axons are actually **displaced vagal fibers** that join the vagus nerve as they exit from the cranium and innervate the same structure as the vagus. The motor cortex exerts a bilateral control of motor neurons located in the nucleus ambiguus (Figure 13–4A).

Axons in the spinal root of the spinal accessory nerve have their cell bodies located in the **spinal accessory nucleus** (see Figure 13–9); they innervate the **sternocleidomastoid muscle** and the upper part of the **trapezius muscle**. (The caudal portion of the trapezius is innervated by upper cervical ventral roots.) The spinal accessory nucleus is a part of the ventral horn of the upper cervical spinal cord. It begins at about the pyramidal decussation and extends as far caudally as the fourth or fifth cervical segments. Although located in line with the nucleus ambiguus (Figure 13–1), this nucleus is not part of the special visceral motor column. This is because the sternocleidomastoid and trapezius muscles do not develop from the branchial arches. Unlike the nucleus ambiguus, which is under bilateral cortical control, the spinal accessory nucleus receives a predominantly unilateral cortical projection.

The spinal root of the spinal accessory nerve comprises many branches that leave the lateral margin of the spinal cord, between the dorsal and ventral roots (Figure 13–1). The branches ascend in the spinal canal

and join the fibers from the cranial root. After exiting the jugular foramen, the spinal root fibers separate from the cranial root fibers.

The General Visceral Motor Cell Column Contains Parasympathetic Preganglionic Neurons

The general visceral motor cell column contains neurons that regulate the function of various smooth muscle and exocrine glands. These neurons are part of the **parasympathetic nervous system**, a division of the **autonomic nervous system** (see Chapters 1 and 14). In contrast to the innervation of skeletal muscle, which is mediated by a single motor neuron (Figure 13–5A), the innervation of smooth muscle and glands is accomplished by two separate neurons: preganglionic and postganglionic neurons (Figure 13–5B; see also Figure 14–6). Parasympathetic preganglionic neurons are located in the various nuclei that comprise the general visceral motor cell column; these neurons also are found in the sacral spinal cord (see Chapter 14). Parasympathetic postganglionic neurons are located in **peripheral autonomic ganglia**.

The general visceral motor cell column, which is found lateral to the general somatic motor column, contains four nuclei, from rostral to caudal: **Edinger–Westphal**, **superior salivatory**, **inferior salivatory**, and **dorsal motor nucleus of the vagus**. (While most of the cranial parasympathetic preganglionic neurons are located in these nuclei, additional preganglionic neurons are located in and around the nucleus ambiguus.

Figure 13–5. Comparison of the motor projections of the somatic and autonomic nervous systems to the periphery. *A.* In the somatic nervous system, motor neurons in the central nervous system directly innervate skeletal muscle. *B.* In the autonomic nervous system, a preganglionic neuron in the central nervous system (i.e., central motor neuron) synapses on a postganglionic neuron, which, in turn, innervates the target organ.

A. Somatic nervous system

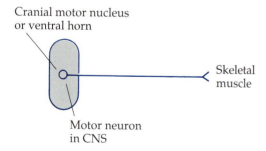

B. Autonomic nervous system

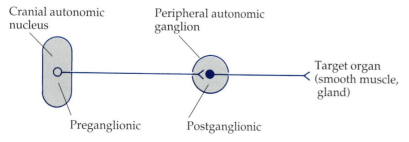

The axons of these neurons course in the vagus nerve.) The general visceral motor column is analogous to the **intermediolateral nucleus**, a column of sympathetic preganglionic neurons, in the spinal cord. The autonomic nervous system is discussed in Chapter 14 together with the hypothalamus, which regulates many autonomic functions.

The **Edinger–Westphal nucleus** is located in the midbrain and in the pretectal region, dorsal to the oculomotor nucleus (Figure 13–6). The proximity of the Edinger–Westphal and oculomotor nuclei makes it easy to remember that the parasympathetic preganglionic neurons in the Edinger–Westphal nucleus send their axons into the **oculomotor (III) nerve**. The preganglionic neurons in the Edinger–Westphal nucleus synapse on postganglionic neurons in the **ciliary ganglion**. These neurons, in turn, innervate the **ciliary muscle** and the **constrictor muscles of the iris**. Most of the neurons in the Edinger–Westphal nucleus synapse in the ciliary ganglion, whereas other neurons project axons to the spinal cord. These descending projection neurons may coordinate the functions of the parasympathetic and sympathetic divisions of the autonomic nervous system.

Figure 13–6. *A.* The projection of the Edinger–Westphal nucleus to the periphery and the efferent projections to the ciliary ganglion. *B.* The circuit for the pupillary light reflex is shown in relation to sections through the pretectal nuclei (*top*) and the oculomotor nucleus (*bottom*).

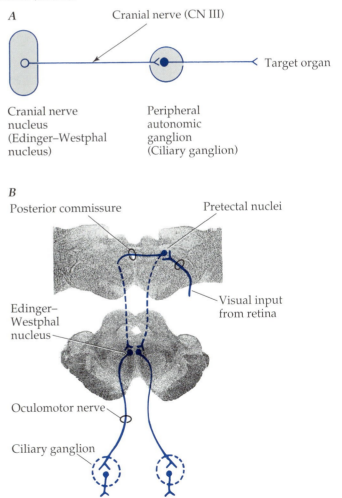

Parasympathetic preganglionic neurons in the midbrain are the efferent components of two important visual reflexes: the pupillary light reflex and the accommodation reflex. The **pupillary light reflex** is the constriction of the pupil that occurs when light hits the retina (Figure 13–6B). Visual input from the retina passes directly to the **pretectal nuclei** via the **brachium of the superior colliculus** (see Chapter 6). The pretectal nuclei, in turn, project bilaterally to the parasympathetic preganglionic neurons. The axons cross to the contralateral side in the **posterior commissure**.

Parasympathetic preganglionic neurons project to the ciliary ganglion through the **oculomotor nerve** and, from there, postganglionic neurons innervate the constrictor muscles of the iris. The bilateral projection of pretectal neurons to the parasympathetic preganglionic neurons in the Edinger–Westphal nucleus ensures that illumination of one eye causes constriction of the pupil on the ipsilateral side (direct response) as well as on the contralateral side (consensual response). **Pupillary dilation** is mediated either by inhibition of the neural circuit for pupillary constriction or by the separate control of the iris by the sympathetic component of the autonomic nervous system.

Parasympathetic preganglionic neurons of the midbrain participate in a second visual reflex, the **accommodation reflex**, which is the **increase in lens curvature that occurs during near vision**. This reflex is normally part of the **accommodation–convergence reaction**, a complex response that prepares the eyes for near vision by: (1) increasing lens curvature, (2) constricting the pupils, and (3) coordinating convergence of the eyes. These responses involve the integrated actions of the visual areas of the occipital lobe, along with motor neurons in the oculomotor nucleus that innervate the extraocular muscles and parasympathetic preganglionic neurons. Central nervous system pathology can distinguish different components of the various visual reflexes. For example, in neurosyphilis the accommodation reaction is preserved but the light reflex is impaired. Patients with this condition have a classic neurologic sign, the **Argyll–Robertson pupils**: their pupils are small and unreactive to light but get smaller to accommodation.

Parasympathetic preganglionic neurons are also located in three sets of nuclei of the caudal pons and medulla (Figure 13–1B). Neurons of the **superior salivatory nucleus** (1), which is located in the pons, and the **inferior salivatory nucleus** (2), which is located in the medulla, do not form a discrete cell column. The **dorsal motor nucleus of the vagus** (3) forms a column of neurons beneath the floor of the **fourth ventricle** in the medulla.

The axons of neurons of the **superior salivatory nucleus** course in the **intermediate nerve** (Figure 13–7). They synapse in two peripheral ganglia: (1) the **pterygopalatine** ganglion, where postganglionic neurons innervate the lacrimal glands and glands of the nasal mucosa; and (2) the **submandibular** ganglion, from which postganglionic parasympathetic neurons innervate the submandibular and sublingual salivary glands. The intermediate nerve is sometimes considered to be the "sensory" branch of the **facial nerve** because it contains afferent fibers, which are the axons of pseudounipolar neurons of the geniculate ganglion (see Chapters 8 and 12).

The inferior salivatory nucleus contains parasympathetic preganglionic neurons whose axons course in the **glossopharyngeal nerve** and synapse on postganglionic neurons in the **otic ganglion** (Figure 13–7). Parasympathetic postganglionic neurons in the otic ganglion, in turn, innervate the parotid gland, which secretes saliva.

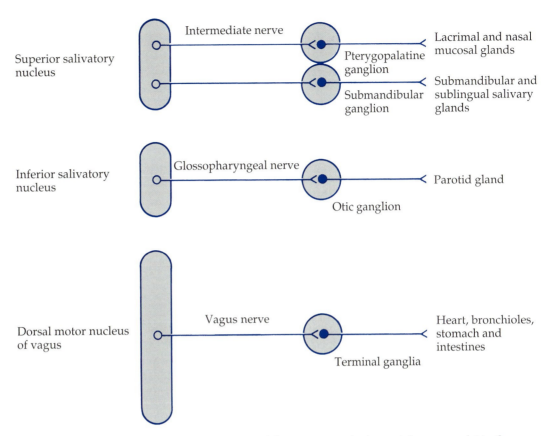

Figure 13–7. Organization of the parasympathetic cranial nerve nuclei in the pons and medulla, the peripheral ganglia to which they project, and the target organs.

The parasympathetic preganglionic neurons in the dorsal motor nucleus of the vagus nerve synapse in extracranial parasympathetic ganglia, called **terminal ganglia** (Figure 13–7). These ganglia are located in the viscera of the thoracic and abdominal cavities, including the gastrointestinal tract proximal to the splenic flexure of the colon. The functions of the vagal parasympathetic neurons include regulating heart rate, gastric motility, bronchial muscle control, and bronchial secretions. (The colon distal to the flexure is innervated by parasympathetic preganglionic neurons of the sacral spinal cord [see Figure 14–7].)

■ REGIONAL ANATOMY

The rest of this chapter focuses on the spatial relations between the cranial nerve nuclei and other important brain stem structures. In addition to learning the locations and connections of the cranial nerve motor nuclei, our goal is to obtain a three-dimensional view of brain stem structure. The levels of the transverse and sagittal sections that we will examine are shown in Figure 13–8 in relation to dorsal and ventral brain stem views.

The Spinal Accessory Nucleus Is Located at the Junction of the Spinal Cord and Medulla

The dominant structure in the section through the junction of the spinal cord and medulla (Figure 13–9) is the **pyramidal decussation,**

which can also be seen on the ventral brain stem view (Figure 13–8A). The **spinal accessory nerve** contains axons of motor neurons whose cell bodies are located in the **spinal accessory nucleus** (Figure 13–9). Recall that these motor neurons innervate the sternocleido-mastoid muscle and the upper part of the trapezius muscle. Comparison of this section with the one through the cervical enlargement (for example, see Figure AII–5) reveals the similarity in location of the spinal accessory nucleus, on the one hand, and ventral horn motor nuclei, on the other.

A Level Through the Midmedulla Reveals the Locations of Six Cranial Nerve Nuclei

Six cranial nerve nuclei are present in the midmedulla (Figure 13–10). All three motor nuclei—hypoglossal, dorsal motor nucleus of vagus, and nucleus ambiguus—are located medial to the **sulcus limitans**. In contrast, the three sensory nuclei—solitary, vestibular, and spinal trigeminal—are located medial to the sulcus (Figure 13–10).

The **hypoglossal** and **vagal** nuclei are found immediately beneath the floor of the fourth ventricle and are large enough to produce distinct bulges on the ventricular floor (Figure 13–8B). The hypoglossal nerve exits the brain stem immediately lateral to the pyramid (Figure 13–8A) and in cross section, a segment of hypoglossal nerve axons can be identified (Figure 13–10). Axons from the dorsal motor nucleus of the vagus also can be seen in Figure 13–10.

The **nucleus ambiguus** is located deeper within the medulla. Whereas the hypoglossal and vagal nuclei are relatively distinct, the precise location of nucleus ambiguus cannot be determined in myelin-stained sections; its approximate location is indicated in Figure 13–10.

The **vestibular nuclei** (Figure 13–10; see also Figure 13–12) participate in the reflex stabilization of eye movements, the **vestibulo-ocular reflex** (VOR). In this reflex, movements of the eyes compensate for head movements. The afferent limb of the reflex consists of the semicircular canals (see Chapter 7) and processing in the vestibular nuclei. The efferent limb involves parts of the reticular formation and the motor neurons innervating extraocular muscles. Neurons in the vestibular nuclei have direct projections to the reticular formation and to the three extraocular motor nuclei.

Infarction in the Territory of Different Arterial Branches Interrupts the Function of Specific Cranial Nerve Nuclei and Brain Stem Paths

In the medulla, different cranial nerve nuclei receive their arterial supply from specific branches of the vertebrobasilar system (Figure 13–11; see Figure 12–10). The medial portion of the medulla is supplied by branches of the main portion of the **vertebral artery**. This region contains the hypoglossal nucleus, the medial lemniscus, and the pyramid. Infarction of this region of the medulla produces three deficits. First, tongue muscles are paralyzed on the side of the lesion because the **hypoglossal motor neurons and axons** are destroyed. Second, tactile sensation, vibration sense, and limb proprioception sense on the side opposite the lesion are impaired because the **medial lemniscus** is affected. Third, muscles of the limb on the side opposite the lesion are weak because corticospinal axons in the **pyramid** are affected.

The dorsolateral portion of the medulla is supplied by the **posterior**

A

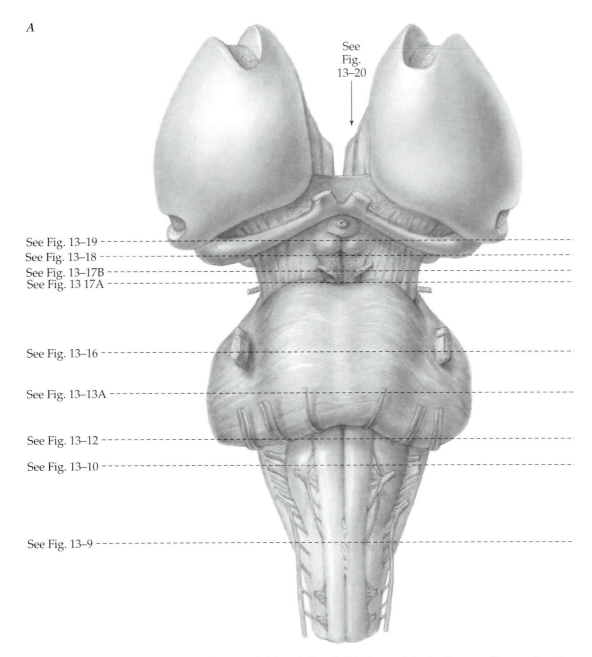

See
Fig.
13–20

See Fig. 13–19
See Fig. 13–18
See Fig. 13–17B
See Fig. 13 17A

See Fig. 13–16

See Fig. 13–13A

See Fig. 13–12

See Fig. 13–10

See Fig. 13–9

Figure 13–8. Ventral *(A)* and dorsal *(B)* views of the brain stem. Planes of section for various myelin-stained sections in latter parts of this chapter are shown.

inferior cerebellar artery (PICA) (Figure 13–11). Six key sensory and motor signs, which comprise the lateral medullary, or Wallenberg's, syndrome, can be produced when the territory of this artery becomes infarcted. Among these signs, three are associated with damage to different cranial nerve nuclei:

• Difficulty in swallowing and hoarseness result from lesions of the **nucleus ambiguus**. An associated change, the loss of the gag reflex,

B

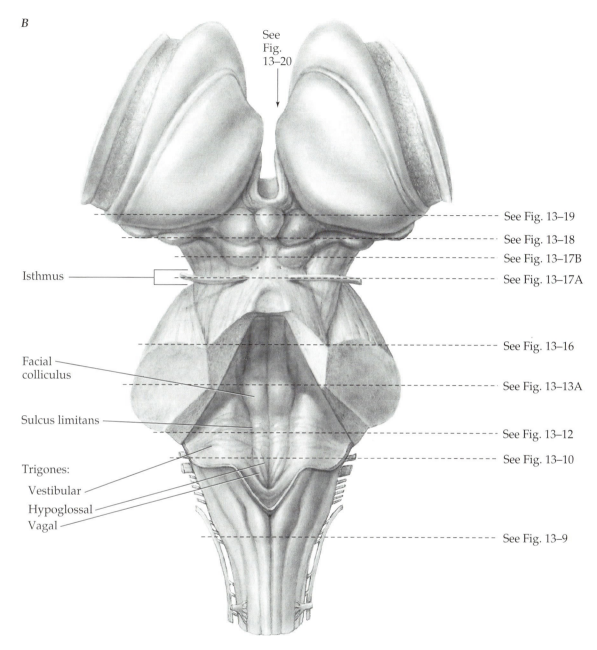

See
Fig.
13–20

- - - - - - - - - See Fig. 13–19

- - - - - - - - - See Fig. 13–18

- - - - - - - - - See Fig. 13–17B

Isthmus - - - - - - - - - - - - - - - - See Fig. 13–17A

- - - - - - - - - See Fig. 13–16

Facial
colliculus - - - - - - - - - - - - - - - See Fig. 13–13A

Sulcus limitans - - - - - - - - - - - - See Fig. 13–12

- - - - - - - - - See Fig. 13–10

Trigones:

Vestibular

Hypoglossal

Vagal - - - - - - - - - - - - - - - - - - See Fig. 13–9

Figure 13–8.   (continued)

is due either to lesions of the nucleus ambiguus—the efferent limb of
the reflex—or loss of pharyngeal sensation (IX)—the afferent limb.

• Dizziness or vertigo (described as the sense of the room whirling
around the patient) and nystagmus, or involuntary rhythmical oscillation of the eyes, are produced by **vestibular nuclear** lesions.

• Loss of pain and temperature senses on the ipsilateral face is due to
lesions of the **spinal trigeminal nucleus** and **tract**.

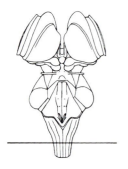

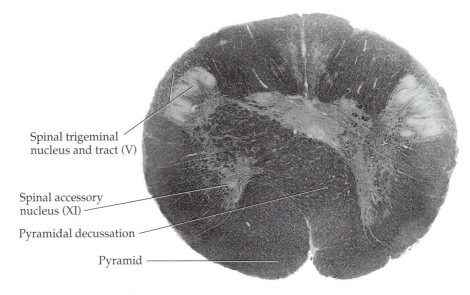

Spinal trigeminal
nucleus and tract (V)

Spinal accessory
nucleus (XI)

Pyramidal decussation

Pyramid

Figure 13–9. Myelin-stained transverse section at the level of the spinal
cord–medulla junction through the spinal accessory nucleus.

The remaining signs result from damage to ascending or descending
pathways that course through the dorsolateral medulla:

- Reduced pain and temperature senses on the contralateral limbs and
  trunk reflect lesions of the **anterolateral system**.
- Ipsilateral limb **ataxia** is due to lesions of the **inferior cerebellar
  peduncle**.
- Horner's syndrome results from damage to descending hypothalamic axons that regulate the sympathetic nervous system. (The precise
  location of these axons in the dorsolateral medulla is not known.)
  Horner's syndrome consists of pupillary constriction (due to unopposed actions of parasympathetic pupillary constrictors), pseudoptosis due to weakness of the tarsal muscle, a smooth muscle that

Figure 13–10. Myelin-stained transverse section through the hypoglossal nucleus
in the medulla.

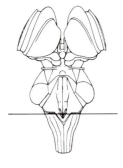

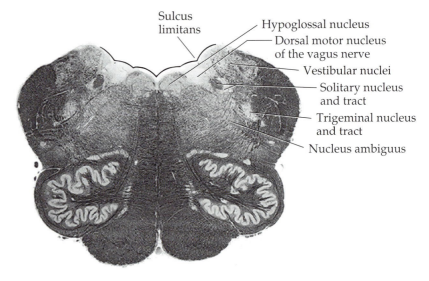

Sulcus
limitans

Hypoglossal nucleus

Dorsal motor nucleus
of the vagus nerve

Vestibular nuclei

Solitary nucleus
and tract

Trigeminal nucleus
and tract

Nucleus ambiguus

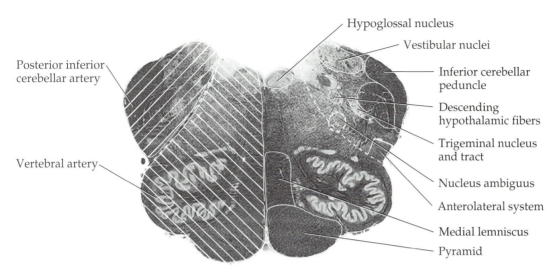

Figure 13–11. Arterial supply of the medulla. Occlusion of the posterior inferior cerebellar artery produces a complex set of neurological deficits, termed the lateral medullary syndrome (or Wallenberg's syndrome; see Figure 12–10). Occlusion of the vertebral artery can produce a discrete set of limb sensory and motor signs.

assists the action of the levator palpebrae muscle (ptosis is drooping of upper eyelid, due to levator palpebrae muscle weakness), reddening of facial skin (due to loss of sympathetic vasoconstrictor activity), and impaired sweating (due to loss of sympathetic control of the sweat glands).

The Glossopharyngeal Nerve Enters and Exits From the Rostral Medulla

The myelin-stained section through the rostral medulla (Figure 13–12) is through the glossopharyngeal nerve root. This cranial nerve can be seen at the lateral brain stem surface, interposed between the inferior cerebellar peduncle and the spinal trigeminal tract (Figure 13–12). The motor axons of the glossopharyngeal nerve originate from neurons in two nuclei: Motor neurons innervating striated muscle are located in the rostral portion of the **nucleus ambiguus** (motor neurons that innervate the stylopharyngeus muscle); autonomic motor neurons are located in the **inferior salivatory nucleus** (parasympathetic preganglionic neurons that innervate the otic ganglion).

The glossopharyngeal nerve also contains gustatory and viscerosensory afferent fibers that terminate in the solitary nucleus (see Figure 8–1) and general somatic afferents that terminate in the trigeminal spinal nucleus. From a clinical perspective, the glossopharyngeal nerve can be considered a sensory nerve because a unilateral lesion does not produce frank motor dysfunction (either somatic or visceral motor) on clinical examination. The approximate location of the solitary nucleus is shown in Figure 13–12. The other sensory nuclei seen in this rostral medullary slice are the spinal trigeminal nucleus, cochlear, and vestibular nuclei.

At this level, a large nucleus is located close to the midline beneath the ventricular floor, the **prepositus nucleus** (Figure 13–12). Because of its location, this nucleus can be mistaken for the hypoglossal nucleus. The prepositus nucleus, together with the vestibular nuclei, play a key role in regulating eye position and slow eye movements (see Box 13–1).

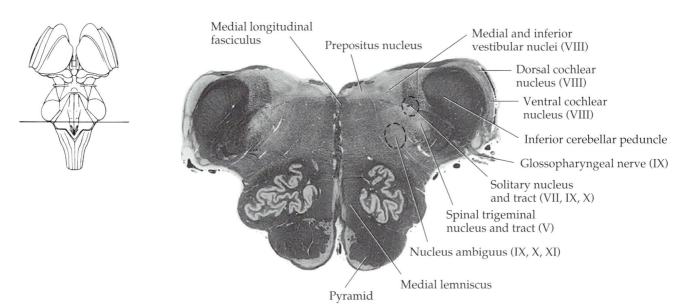

Figure 13–12. Myelin-stained transverse section at the level of exiting fibers of the glossopharyngeal (IX) nerve. Note that the cochlear nucleus contains two divisions (anteroventral and posteroventral).

The Fibers of the Facial Nerve Have a Complex Trajectory Through the Pons

The pontine section shown in Figure 13–13A cuts through portions of the facial nerve. The axons leave the facial nucleus and follow a path toward the floor of the fourth ventricle (Figure 13–13B). These fibers of the facial nerve are not seen in Figure 13–13A because they do not course in discrete and straight fascicles.

As the facial nerve fibers approach the ventricular floor, they first ascend close to the midline. Next, the fibers sweep around the medial, dorsal, and rostral aspects of the abducens nucleus. This component is termed the **genu** of the facial nerve and, with the abducens nucleus, forms the **facial colliculus**, a surface landmark on the pontine floor of the fourth ventricle (Figure 13–8B). The facial nerve fibers then run ventrally and caudally to exit the pons at the **pontomedullary junction**.

Eye Movement Deficits After an Abducens Nerve Lesion Differ From Those After a Lesion of the Abducens Nucleus

As fibers of the abducens nerve exit from the abducens nucleus (Figure 13–13), they course toward the ventral brain stem surface, medial to the central tegmental tract and lateral to the medial lemniscus. These fibers exit the pons medial to the facial nerve (Figures 13–8A and 13–13B) and innervate the **lateral rectus muscle** (Figure 13–14A).

Horizontal eye movements are controlled by the coordinated actions of the lateral and medial rectus muscles, extraocular muscles that are innervated by the abducens and oculomotor nuclei. For example, to look to the right, one must contract the right lateral rectus muscle together with the left medial rectus muscle. Special **internuclear neurons** in the abducens nucleus coordinate contraction of these two muscles (Figure 13–14B). These neurons intermingle among the lateral rectus motor neu-

A Medial longitudinal fasciculus

Facial colliculus and abducens nucleus (VI)

Superior and lateral vestibular nuclei

Fibers of CN VII

Spinal trigeminal nucleus and tract (V)

Facial nucleus (VII)

Fibers of abducens nerve(VI)

Central tegmental tract

Medial lemniscus

Paramedian pontine reticular formation

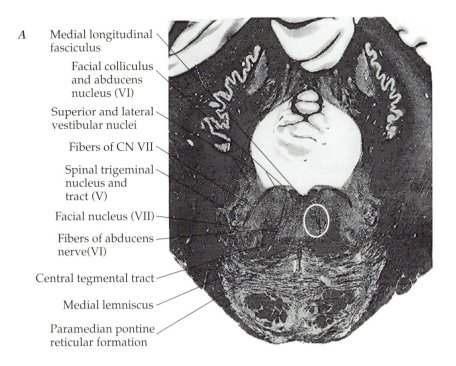

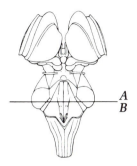

B

Medial longitudinal fasciculus

Facial colliculus: Genu of facial nerve Abducens nucleus

Facial nucleus

Facial nerve

Abducens nerve

Descending cortical fibers: Corticopontine Corticobulbar Corticospinal

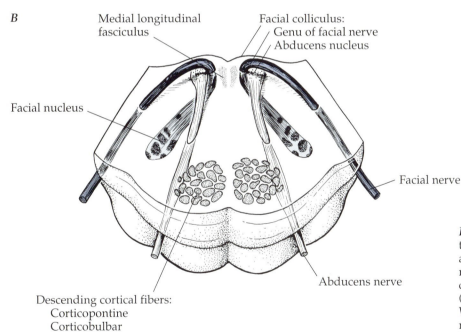

Figure 13–13. ***A.*** Myelin-stained transverse section through the pons, at the level of the genu of cranial nerve VII. ***B.*** The three-dimensional course of the facial nerve in the pons. (***B***, Adapted from Williams, P. L., and Warwick, R. 1975. Functional Neuroanatomy of Man. Philadelphia: W. B. Saunders.)

rons. Internuclear neurons transmit control signals from premotor structures, such as the **paramedian pontine reticular formation** (Figure 13–13A), to the contralateral oculomotor nucleus. The voluntary control of eye movements, which involve the coordinated actions of regions of the parietal and frontal lobe with the brain stem, is considered in Box 13–1. Internuclear axons decussate in the pons and ascend to the contralateral oculomotor nucleus in the **medial longitudinal fasciculus**. Lesions at different sites in the circuit for controlling horizontal eye movements produce distinct defects (Figure 13–14B and C):

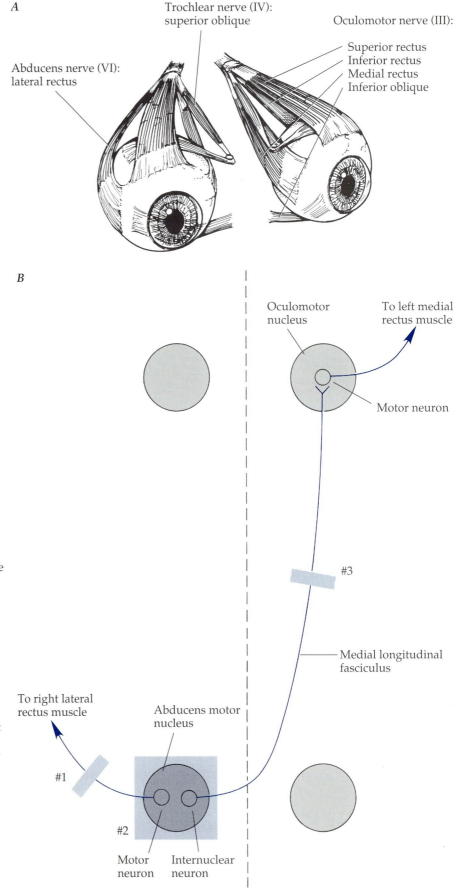

Figure 13–14. Brain stem mechanisms for controlling horizontal eye movements. *A.* The two eyes with the various extraocular muscles and their innervation patterns. Not shown is the levator palpebrae, which is an eyelid elevator innervated by cranial nerve III. The extraocular muscles of both eyes operate as three functional pairs. The lateral and medial rectus muscles move the eye horizontally. The superior and inferior rectus muscles elevate and depress the eye, respectively (most importantly when the eye is abducted). Finally, the superior and inferior oblique muscles depress and elevate the eye, but to a greater extent when the eye is adducted. *B.* Circuit for coordinating horizontal eye movements. *C.* The four pairs of eyes illustrate eye position when an individual is asked to look to the right: (*from top to bottom row*) normal control of eyes; with a lesion of the abducens nerve (lesion 1); with a lesion of the abducens nucleus (lesion 2); with a medial longitudinal fasciculus (MLF) lesion (lesion 3).

C   Attempt to gaze right

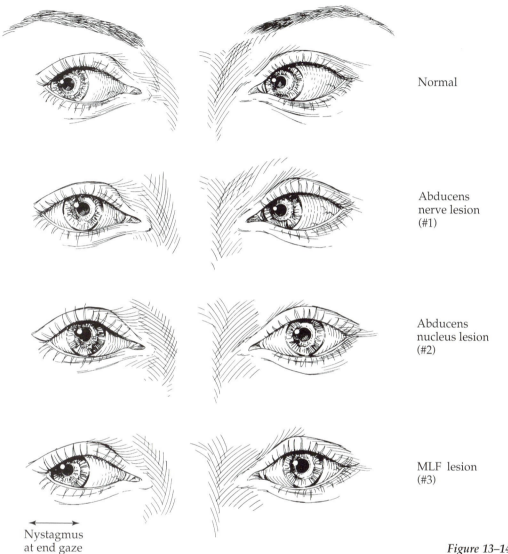

Normal

Abducens
nerve lesion
(#1)

Abducens
nucleus lesion
(#2)

MLF lesion
(#3)

Nystagmus
at end gaze

Figure 13–14.   *(continued)*

- A lesion of the abducens nerve only produces **paralysis of the ipsilateral lateral rectus muscle**, thereby preventing ocular abduction on the same side (Figure 13–14B, lesion 1). The unopposed action of the medial rectus muscle can cause the affected eye to be adducted at rest (not shown in figure).
- A lesion of the abducens nucleus produces two defects (Figure 13–14B, lesion 2). First, as with the nerve lesion, there is an inability to abduct the ipsilateral eye because of destruction of the lateral rectus motor neurons. Here, too, the resting position of the eye may be adducted because of the unopposed action of the medial rectus muscle. Second, the patient cannot contract the contralateral medial rectus muscle on horizontal gaze, and hence cannot gaze in the same direction as the side of the lesion. This is called a lateral gaze palsy and occurs because the lesion also destroys the **internuclear neurons**.

(Text continues on page 409).

Box 13–1 *The Voluntary and Reflexive Control of Eye Movements*

Eye movements are divided into two major categories: **rapid** and **slow**. Rapid eye movements are normally conjugate: The eyes move in tandem at the same speed and in the same direction. Rapid eye movements that bring the fovea to the image are termed **saccades**. Slow move-ments can be either conjugate, such as **smooth pursuit move-ments** for tracking a moving object, or disconjugate, such as **convergence**, when viewing an object at close distance. Eye movements are not controlled by descending pathways from the primary motor cortex, as are limb movements.

Saccades are triggered princi-pally by two cortical regions (Figure 13–15A). The (1) **frontal eye field**, a portion of cytoar-chitectonic area 8, is thought to be important in triggering intentional or voluntary sac-cades, the kind of saccades we make to look at objects of inter-est. The (2) **posterior parietal**

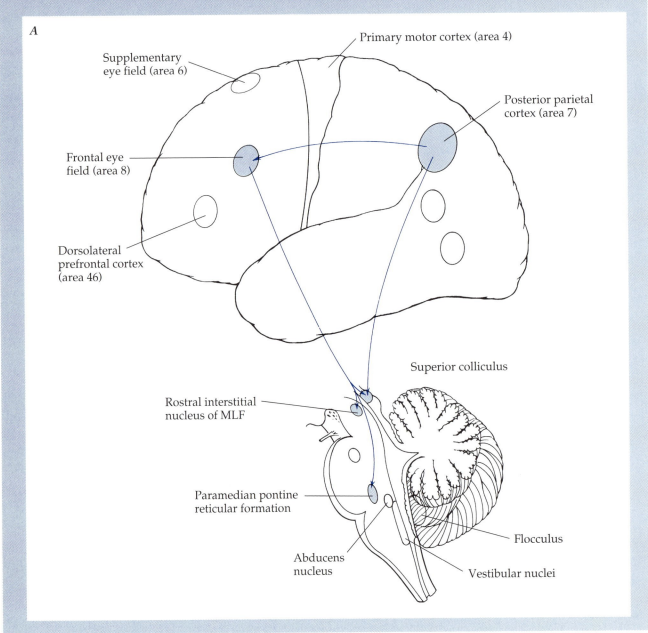

A

Supplementary eye field (area 6)

Primary motor cortex (area 4)

Posterior parietal cortex (area 7)

Frontal eye field (area 8)

Dorsolateral prefrontal cortex (area 46)

Superior colliculus

Rostral interstitial nucleus of MLF

Paramedian pontine reticular formation

Flocculus

Abducens nucleus

Vestibular nuclei

Box 13–1 (continued)

cortex, corresponding roughly to part of area 7, may trigger reflexive saccades, for example, when our gaze is automatically directed to a moving object or the origin of a loud sound.

Axons from the frontal eye field descend through the **anterior limb and genu of the internal capsule** to the brain stem.

For horizontal eye movements, the frontal eye fields project directly to a particular part of the contralateral reticular formation, the **paramedian pontine**

Figure 13–15. *A.* A lateral view of the cerebral cortex and midsagittal view of the brain stem shows the approximate location of structures involved in controlling rapid eye movements. *B.* Same as in *A*, but for slow eye movement control. Note that the flocculus is located more laterally than indicated in the figure. *C.* The dominant connections of brain stem premotor regions for rapid and slow eye movements to the three extraocular nuclei.

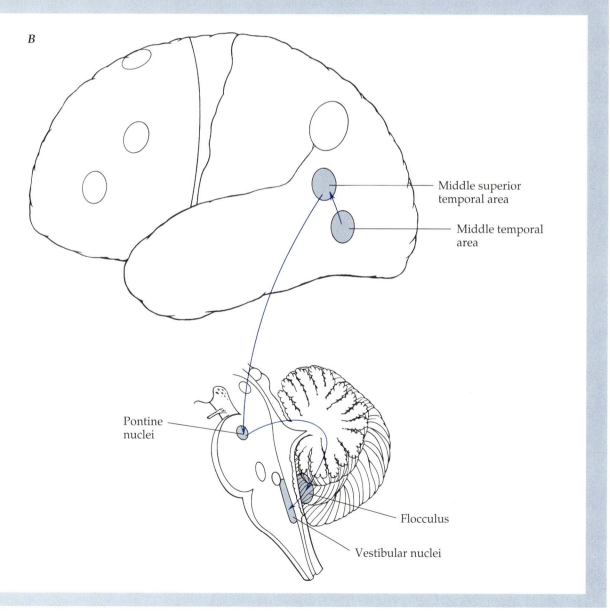

B

Middle superior temporal area

Middle temporal area

Pontine nuclei

Flocculus

Vestibular nuclei

Box 13–1   (continued)

reticular formation (PPRF). Neurons in the PPRF synapse on lateral rectus motor neurons, for ipsilateral ocular abduction. PPRF neurons also synapse on internuclear cells, which, in turn, synapse on contralateral medial rectus motor neurons for contralateral ocular adduction (Figure 13–14B and C). In contrast, for vertical eye movements, the rostral midbrain is essential. The key structure is the **rostral interstitial nucleus of the MLF** (Figure 13–15B; see also Figure 13–20), which projects to motor neurons in the oculomotor and trochlear nuclei (Figure 13–15C).

For the posterior parietal cortex, axons descend in the **posterior limb of the internal capsule**. Rather than contact neurons in the PPRF and rostral interstitial nucleus of the medial longitudinal fasciculus directly, as the frontal eye field, posterior parietal axons do so indirectly, through a synapse in the intermediate layers of the

ipsilateral **superior colliculus** (see Chapter 6). (The superficial layers of the superior colliculus receive visual input directly from retinal ganglion cells.) The superior colliculus, in turn, projects to the PPRF and the rostral interstitial nucleus of the medial longitudinal fasciculus.

Two other frontal lobe areas, the **supplementary eye field** and the **dorsolateral prefrontal cortex**, also participate in controlling rapid eye movements. The dorsolateral prefrontal cortex is thought to be involved in controlling the spatial aspects of saccades, especially to remembered targets. The supplementary eye field, on the other hand, may participate in the appropriate timing of saccades in relation to limb movements, such as looking toward an object to be grasped.

Slow eye movements have a remarkably different control circuit, one that involves higher-order **cortical visual areas** implicated in visual motion per-

ception and the **cerebellum**. The cortical control of **smooth pursuit** eye movements, which maintain the position of a moving visual image on the fovea, begins in the middle temporal (also termed V5) and middle superior temporal visual areas. From the cortex, axons descend in the **posterior limb of the internal capsule** to contact neurons of the **pontine nuclei**, which, in turn, project to the **flocculus** (see Chapter 10). This is part of the corticopontine projection (see Figure 9–10B). The output of the flocculus is directed to premotor neurons in the **vestibular nuclei**. All three extraocular nuclei receive input from the vestibular nuclei (Figure 13–15C); the vestibular axons course in the medial longitudinal fasciculus. Axons in the medial longitudinal fasciculus originating from the vestibular nuclei are also especially important in stabilizing eye position when the head is moved (vestibulo-ocular reflex).

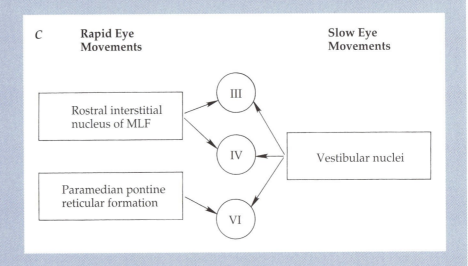

Figure 13–15.   (continued)

- A unilateral lesion of the medial longitudinal fasciculus (MLF) rostral to the abducens nucleus (Figure 13–14B, lesion 3; at level of pons in Figures 13–16 or 13–17A) produces **internuclear ophthalmoplegia**. This is characterized, on lateral gaze away from the side of the MLF lesion, by the lack of (or reduced) ability to contract the ipsilateral medial rectus muscle and thereby adduct that eye. In addition, there is nystagmus (more pronounced in the abducting eye) as a result of involvement of the axons of vestibular neurons, which also course in the MLF. A common neurological sign in patients with multiple sclerosis, a demyelinating disease, is internuclear ophthalmoplegia due to medial longitudinal fascicular lesion.

For lesions at sites 2 and 3, a clever way to verify that the affected medial rectus muscle is not paralyzed is to demonstrate that the patient can converge both eyes to view an object at close distance. This eye movement requires activation of both medial rectus muscles. The neural mechanisms that coordinate convergence involve the visual cortex and midbrain integrative centers, not the internuclear cells of the abducens nucleus.

The Motor Nucleus of the Trigeminal Nerve Is Located Medial to the Main Sensory Nucleus

The most rostral component of the special visceral motor cell column is the **trigeminal motor nucleus** (Figure 13–16). At this brain stem level, the sulcus limitans is indistinct. The mediolateral organization of motor and sensory nuclei is preserved, however, with the trigeminal motor nucleus located medial to the main trigeminal sensory nucleus. Identifying the **trigeminal root fibers** in Figure 13–16 helps us distinguish the trigeminal sensory from motor nuclei. The trigeminal mesencephalic

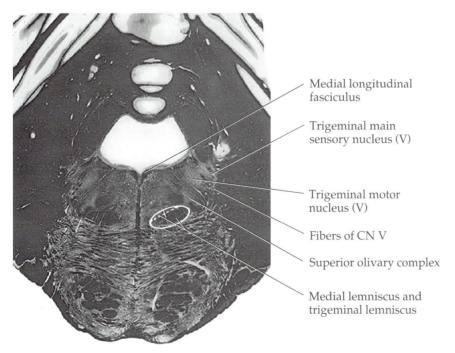

Medial longitudinal
fasciculus

Trigeminal main
sensory nucleus (V)

Trigeminal motor
nucleus (V)

Fibers of CN V

Superior olivary complex

Medial lemniscus and
trigeminal lemniscus

Figure 13–16. Myelin-stained transverse section through the pons, at the level of the main sensory and trigeminal motor nuclei.

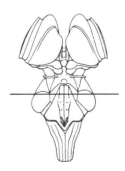

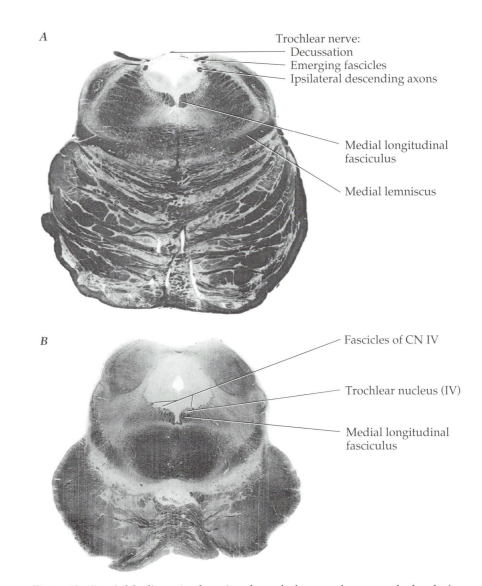

Figure 13–17. *A.* Myelin-stained section through the rostral pons, at the level of exiting trochlear nerve fibers. *B.* Myelin-stained section through the caudal midbrain at the level of the trochlear nucleus.

nucleus and tract, which are also located at this level, extend farther rostrally, where they can be readily identified (see below). The superior olivary complex, which receives input from the ventral cochlear nucleus (see Chapter 7), can also be seen in Figure 13–16.

The Trochlear Nerve Exits the Dorsal Surface of the Pons at the Level of the Isthmus

The junction of the pons and the midbrain is named the **isthmus** (Figures 13–8B and 13–17A) for the constriction in the diameter of the brain stem—especially noticeable during development (see Figure 2–13). The trochlear nerve exits the brain stem at this level. Two unusual features of trochlear nerve anatomy are apparent in Figure 13–17: **its emergence from the dorsal pontine surface** (see Figure 13–2B) and its **decussation**. Trochlear motor neurons are found in the **trochlear nucleus**, which is located in the caudal midbrain at the level of the inferior colliculus (Figure 13–17B). The trochlear nucleus is nested within the MLF. The axons of the trochlear motor neurons course caudally along the lateral margin of the cerebral aqueduct and fourth ventricle, in the **periaqueductal gray matter**. The axons decussate in the isthmus of the pons, dorsal to the cerebral aqueduct, and emerge from the dorsal brain stem surface. Some of the descending, decussating, and emerging fibers of the trochlear nerve can be seen in Figure 13–17A.

The Cranial Nerve Cell Columns Have a Dorsoventral Spatial Organization in the Midbrain

The **oculomotor nucleus**, which innervates extraocular muscles, and the **Edinger–Westphal nucleus**, which contains parasympathetic preganglionic neurons, are located at the level of the superior colliculus (Figure 13–18). Axons from these nuclei course through the red nucleus in their path to the periphery. The oculomotor nerve exits from the medial surface of the cerebral peduncle into the **interpeduncular fossa**.

The oculomotor nucleus innervates the medial, inferior, and superior rectus muscles, the inferior oblique muscle, and the levator palpebrae superioris muscle. The action of this latter muscle, an eyelid elevator, is assisted by the **tarsal muscle**, a smooth muscle under sympathetic nervous system control. Conditions that impair the functions of the sympathetic nervous system can produce **pseudoptosis**, resulting from weakness of the tarsal muscle. True ptosis is produced by weakness of the levator palpebrae muscle, such as from a neuromuscular disease like myasthenia gravis.

The **Edinger–Westphal nucleus** (Figures 13–18 and 13–19) mediates lens accommodation and pupillary constriction in response to light. It does this through a projection to parasympathetic postganglionic neurons in the ciliary ganglion. Earlier we saw that neurons in the **pretectal nuclei** (Figure 13–19) receive visual information from axons coursing in the brachium of the superior colliculus and transmit this information bilater-

Figure 13–18. Myelin-stained transverse sections through the rostral midbrain at the level of the superior colliculus.

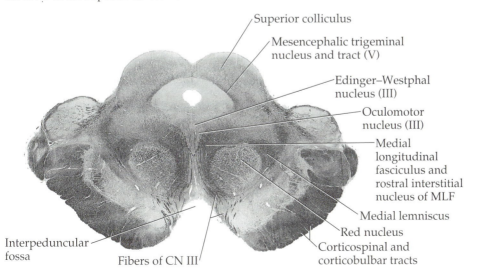
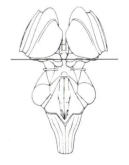

Superior colliculus

Mesencephalic trigeminal nucleus and tract (V)

Edinger–Westphal nucleus (III)

Oculomotor nucleus (III)

Medial longitudinal fasciculus and rostral interstitial nucleus of MLF

Medial lemniscus

Red nucleus

Corticospinal and corticobulbar tracts

Interpeduncular fossa

Fibers of CN III

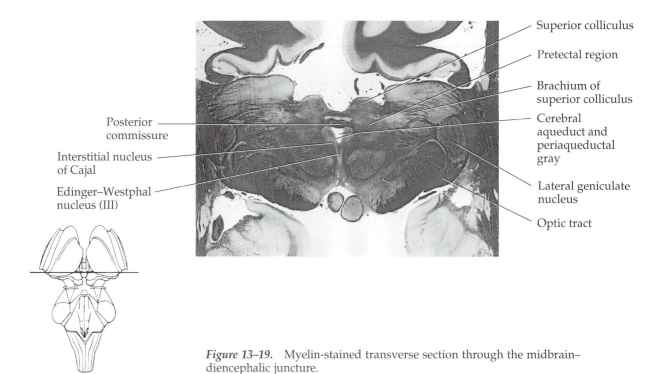

Posterior commissure

Interstitial nucleus of Cajal

Edinger–Westphal nucleus (III)

Superior colliculus

Pretectal region

Brachium of superior colliculus

Cerebral aqueduct and periaqueductal gray

Lateral geniculate nucleus

Optic tract

Figure 13–19. Myelin-stained transverse section through the midbrain–diencephalic juncture.

ally to neurons in the Edinger–Westphal nucleus (Figure 13–6). The decussating axons of pretectal neurons course in the **posterior commissure**. The interstitial nucleus of Cajal, which is thought to help coordinate eye and head movements, is located at this level along with the rostral portion of the superior colliculus.

Knowledge of regional midbrain anatomy is clinically important, because occlusion of the vascular supply to the midbrain produces a complex set of neurological deficits that disrupts eye movement control, facial muscle function, and limb movements. A lesion of the ventromedial midbrain, which is normally supplied by branches of the posterior cerebral artery, can cause an infarction in three key structures:

- **Extraocular motor neuron axons,** which course in the oculomotor (III) nerve. Damage produces a "down and out" resting eye position ipsilaterally, resulting from the unopposed actions of the lateral rectus muscle (producing the outward position) and the superior oblique muscle (producing the downward position). These muscles are innervated by the abducens (VI) and trochlear (IV) nerves, respectively.
- **Axons of the Edinger–Westphal nucleus,** which also course in the oculomotor nerve. Damage results in pupillary dilation because of the unopposed action of the sympathetic pupillary dilator fibers.
- **The basis pedunculi,** which contains the corticobulbar and corticospinal tracts. Damage results in limb and lower facial muscle weakness on the contralateral side. Limb tremor can also occur due to damage of the parvocellular division of the red nucleus and the cerebellothalamic fibers.

It is important to note that the mediolateral organization of the cranial nerve nuclei, which is characteristic of the medulla and pons, does not describe the organization in the midbrain. The spatial organization of the

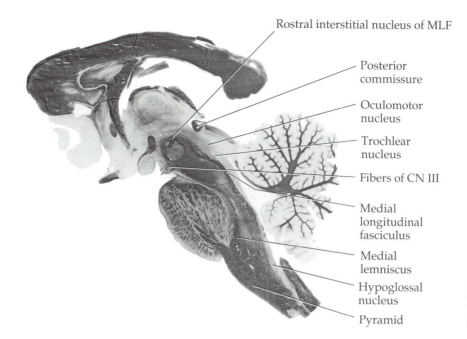

Rostral interstitial nucleus of MLF

Posterior commissure

Oculomotor nucleus

Trochlear nucleus

Fibers of CN III

Medial longitudinal fasciculus

Medial lemniscus

Hypoglossal nucleus

Pyramid

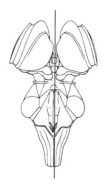

Figure 13–20. Myelin-stained sagittal section through the brain stem, close to the midline through nuclei of the general somatic motor column.

three cranial nerve nuclear columns in the midbrain is more like that of the spinal cord. As in the spinal cord, midbrain columns are oriented dorsal to ventral: general somatic afferent (mesencephalic trigeminal) nucleus, general visceral motor (Edinger–Westphal) nucleus, and general somatic motor (oculomotor) nucleus.

The Medial Longitudinal Fasciculus and Components of the General Somatic Motor Column Are Seen on a Midsagittal Section

Three of the four general somatic motor nuclei are seen on the sagittal section (Figure 13–20), from caudal to rostral: hypoglossal nucleus, trochlear nucleus, and oculomotor nucleus. The fourth, the abducens nucleus, is located lateral to the plane of section. The rostrocaudal course of the MLF can be identified in this section. In the caudal pons, the MLF is located immediately beneath the floor of the fourth ventricle. At progressively more rostral levels, it is displaced ventrally from the ventricular floor as the periaqueductal gray matter becomes larger. (Compare, for example, the location of the MLF in Figures 13–13 and 13–17.) In the midbrain, the MLF is further displaced by the trochlear and oculomotor nuclei. The path of the exiting oculomotor nerve fibers in the midbrain also can be identified. Fascicles of the oculomotor nerve can be seen exiting the ventral midbrain surface.

There are three separate columns of cranial nerve motor nuclei (Figure 13–1), from medial to lateral: **general somatic motor**, **special visceral motor**, and **general visceral motor**.

Summary

General Somatic Motor Nuclei

This is the most medial motor column and it comprises four nuclei, each of which contains motor neurons that innervate striated muscle derived from the **occipital somites**. The **oculomotor nucleus** (1) (Figures

13–2, 13–18, and 13–20) contains motor neurons whose axons course in the **oculomotor (III) nerve** and innervate the following extraocular muscles: **medial rectus**, **superior rectus**, **inferior rectus**, and **inferior oblique** (Figure 13–14A). The oculomotor nucleus also innervates the **levator palpebrae superioris** muscle (Figure 13–14A). The **trochlear nucleus** (2) (Figures 13–2, 13–17B, and 13–20), via the **trochlear (IV) nerve**, innervates the **contralateral superior oblique** muscle; the **abducens nucleus** (3) (Figures 13–2 and 13–13), via the **abducens (VI) nerve**, innervates the **lateral rectus** muscle. The extraocular motor nuclei receive an indirect projection from areas of the cerebral cortex rostral and medial to the primary motor cortex, the **frontal eye fields** and a portion of the **parietal lobe** (Figure 13–15). The **hypoglossal nucleus** (4) gives rise to axons that course in the **hypoglossal (XII) nerve** and innervate tongue muscles (Figures 13–3 and 13–10). The hypoglossal nucleus is the only nucleus of this column that receives a projection from the primary motor cortex. The extraocular nuclei receive input from brain stem premotor centers, the **paramedial pontine reticular formation**, the **rostral interstitial nucleus of the medial longitudinal fasciculus**, and the **vestibular nuclei**. The former two premotor regions receive a projection from the **frontal eye fields**.

Special Visceral Motor Nuclei

This column is displaced ventrally from the floor of the fourth ventricle (Figures 13–1 and 13–4). It contains three nuclei, each of which innervates striated muscles derived from the branchial arches. The **trigeminal motor nucleus** (1) (Figures 13–4 and 13–16) innervates the muscles of **mastication** via the **trigeminal (V) nerve**. This nucleus receives a **bilateral projection from the motor cortex**. The **facial nucleus** (2) (Figures 13–4 and 13–13) innervates the muscles of **facial expression**. The axons of facial motor neurons course in the **facial (VII) nerve**. Facial motor neurons that innervate upper face muscles receive a **bilateral projection** from the motor cortex, whereas motor neurons innervating lower face muscles receive a **contralateral projection** (Figure 13–4B). The **nucleus ambiguus** (3) (Figures 13–4 and 13–10) innervates the muscles of the **palate**, **pharynx**, and **larynx** predominantly via the **vagus (X) nerve** and to a lesser extent the **glossopharyngeal (IX) nerve** and the cranial root of the **spinal accessory (XI) nerve**. The **spinal accessory nucleus** (spinal root) is in line with the nucleus ambiguus but is not part of the special visceral motor column. It innervates the sternocleidomastoid and trapezius muscles via the **spinal accessory (XI) nerve** (Figure 13–9).

General Visceral Motor Nuclei

This column contains four nuclei (Figure 13–1). Each nucleus contains **parasympathetic preganglionic neurons** (Figure 13–5). The **Edinger–Westphal nucleus** (1) is located in the midbrain (Figures 13–6, 13–18, and 13–19). Its axons project via the **oculomotor nerve** to the **ciliary ganglion**, where postganglionic neurons innervate the constrictor muscles of the iris and the ciliary muscle. Axons from the **superior salivatory nucleus** (2) (Figures 13–1 and 13–7) course in the **intermediate nerve** (a branch of the **facial nerve**). Via synapses in the pterygopalatine and submandibular ganglia, the nucleus influences the **lacrimal gland** and **glands of the nasal mucosa**. The **inferior salivatory nucleus** (3) (Figures 13–1 and 13–7), via the **glossopharyngeal nerve**, synapses on postganglionic neurons in the otic ganglion. From there, postganglionic neurons innervate the **parotid gland**. Axons from the **dorsal motor nucleus of the vagus** (4) (Figures 13–1, 13–7, and 13–10) course in the periphery in the **vagus nerve** and innervate **terminal ganglia** in most of the thoracic and abdominal viscera (to the splenic flexure of the colon). ■

KEY STRUCTURES AND TERMS

sulcus limitans
facial colliculus
corticobulbar tract
occipital somites
general somatic motor
    oculomotor nucleus
    trochlear nucleus
    abducens nucleus
    hypoglossal nucleus
special visceral motor
    trigeminal motor nucleus
    facial motor nucleus
    nucleus ambiguus
spinal accessory nucleus
general visceral motor
    Edinger–Westphal
    superior salivatory
    inferior salivatory
    dorsal motor nucleus of the vagus
intermediolateral nucleus
otic ganglion

pterygopalatine ganglion
submandibular ganglion
terminal ganglia
pretectal nuclei
superior colliculus
brachium of the superior colliculus
posterior commissure
nucleus prepositus
internuclear neurons
paramedian pontine reticular
    formation
medial longitudinal fasciculus
frontal eye field
posterior parietal cortex
supplementary eye field
dorsolateral prefrontal cortex
rostral interstitial nucleus of the
    medial longitudinal
    fasciculus
cortical visual areas
pontine nuclei

flocculus
vestibular nuclei
periaqueductal gray matter
saccades
smooth pursuit movements
convergence
vertebral artery
posterior inferior cerebellar artery
pupillary light reflex
accommodation–convergence
    reaction
gag reflex
vestibulo-ocular reflex
lateral gaze palsy
internuclear ophthalmoplegia
lateral medullary syndrome
Horner's syndrome
Argyll–Robertson pupils
pseudoptosis

Selected Readings

Brodal, A. 1965. The Cranial Nerves: Anatomical and Anatomicoclinical Correlations. Oxford: Blackwell Scientific Publications.

Brodal, A. 1981. Neurological Anatomy. New York: Oxford University Press.

Büttner, U., and Büttner-Ennever, J. A. 1988. Present concepts of oculomotor organization. In Büttner-Ennever, J. A. (ed.), Neuroanatomy of the Oculomotor System. Amsterdam: Elsevier Science Publishers, pp. 3–164.

Patten, J. 1977. Neurological Differential Diagnosis. New York: Springer–Verlag, p. 292.

Pierrot-Deseilligny, C., and Gaymard, B. 1992. Eye movements. In Kennard, C. (ed.), Clinical Neurology. Edinburgh: Churchill Livingstone, pp. 27–56.

Reiner, A., Karten, H. J., Gamlin, P. D. R., et al. 1983. Parasympathetic ocular control: Functional subdivisions and circuitry of the avian nucleus of Edinger–Westphal. Trends Neurosci. 6:140–145.

Role, L., and Kelly, J. P. 1991. The brain stem: Cranial nerve nuclei and the monoaminergic systems. In Kandel, E. R., Schwartz, J. H., and Jessell, T. M. (eds.), Principles of Neural Science, 3rd ed. New York: Elsevier, pp. 684–699.

References

Akert, K., Glickman, M. A., Lang, W., et al. 1980. The Edinger–Westphal nucleus in the monkey. A retrograde tracer study. Brain Res. 184:491–498.

Büttner-Ennever, J. A., and Henn, V. 1976. An autoradiographic study of the pathways from the pontine reticular formation involved in horizontal eye movements. Brain Res. 108:155–164.

Carpenter, M. B., and Sutin, J. 1983. Human Neuroanatomy. Baltimore: Williams & Wilkins.

Ferner, H., and Staubestand, J. (eds.) 1983. Sobota Atlas of Human Anatomy, Vol. 1: Head, Neck, Upper Extremities. Baltimore: Urban & Schwartzenberg.

Lowey, A. D., Saper, C. B., and Yamondis, N. D. 1978. Re-evaluation of the efferent projections of the Edinger–Westphal nucleus in the cat. Brain Res. 141:153–159.

Simpson, J. I. 1984. The accessory optic system. Annu. Rev. Neurosci. 7:13–41.

Törk, I., McRitchie, D. A., Rikkard-Bell, G. C., and Paxinos, G. 1990. Autonomic regulatory centers in the medulla oblongata. In Paxinos, G. (ed.), The Human Nervous System. San Diego: Academic Press, pp. 221–259.

Williams, P. L., and Warwick, R. 1975. Functional Neuroanatomy of Man. Philadelphia: W. B. Saunders.

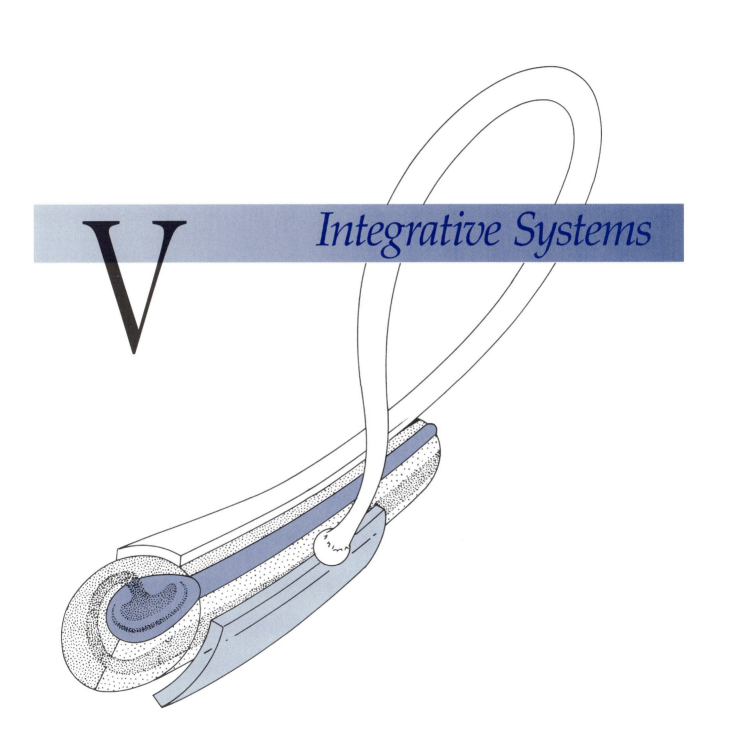

V   Integrative Systems

14

The Hypothalamus and the Regulation of Endocrine and Visceral Functions

T*HE HYPOTHALAMUS IS CRUCIAL* in maintaining normal organ function and it does so by integrating viscerosensory information, together with information about the individual's emotional state (see Chapter 15). Through its role in pituitary function and modulating the actions of the autonomic nervous system, the hypothalamus regulates virtually all body organs. The anatomical substrates of central neural control of endocrine and autonomic function are beginning to be unraveled, with the aid of techniques for assessing both the projections of hypothalamic neurons and their biochemistry. In additon to regulating bodily functions, another major function of the hypothalamus is to effect the behaviors necessary to meet such basic needs as feeding, drinking, and mating. The hypothalamus thus ensures survival both of the individual and its species.

In this chapter, we examine the anatomy and connections of the hypothalamus that are important for regulating endocrine and autonomic functions. The pituitary gland and neuroendocrine function are considered first. Next, the organization of the autonomic nervous system is surveyed, and then the control of autonomic function by the hypothalamus is examined. The role of the hypothalamus in motivational and appetitive behavior will be considered in Chapter 15 along with other brain structures that constitute the limbic system.

FUNCTIONAL ANATOMY OF THE NEUROENDOCRINE SYSTEMS

The Hypothalamus Is Divided Into Three Functionally Distinct Mediolateral Zones

The hypothalamus, a key component of the diencephalon, is located ventral to the thalamus (Figure 14–1). The third ventricle separates the two halves of the hypothalamus. On its medial, or ventricular surface, the hypothalamus is distinguished from the thalamus by a shallow groove, the **hypothalamic sulcus**. Anteriorly, the hypothalamus extends a bit

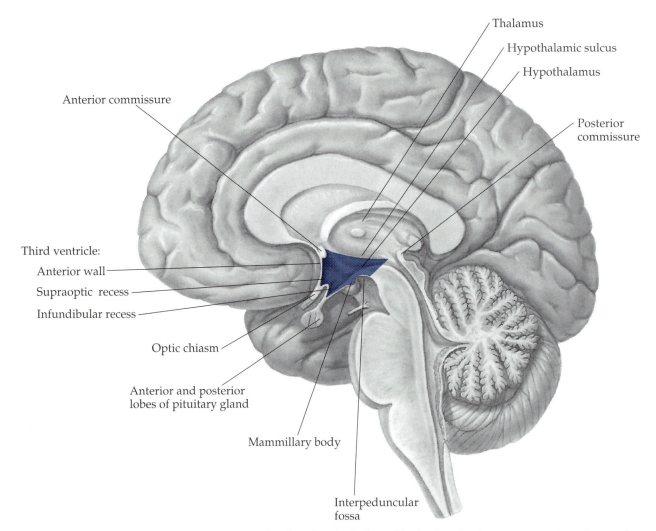

Figure 14–1. A midsagittal view of brain showing key structures in and around the hypothalamus.

beyond the anterior wall of the third ventricle (the lamina terminalis, see Chapter 2). The hypothalamus reaches as far caudally as the **mammillary bodies**, paired structures on the ventral hypothalamic surface (Figure 14–2).

The nuclei of the hypothalamus are organized into three mediolateral zones, as shown in the schematic three-dimensional view (Figure 14–3):

- The **periventricular zone** is the most medial and is comprised of thin nuclei that border the third ventricle. This zone is important in regulating the release of **endocrine hormones** from the anterior pituitary gland.
- The **middle zone** serves diverse functions. It contains nuclei that regulate the release of **vasopressin** and **oxytocin** from the posterior pituitary gland. It is also a major site for neurons that regulate the **autonomic nervous system**.
- The **lateral zone** contains neurons that integrate information from telencephalic limbic system structures and transmit this information to other parts of the hypothalamus, as well as to the midbrain. This

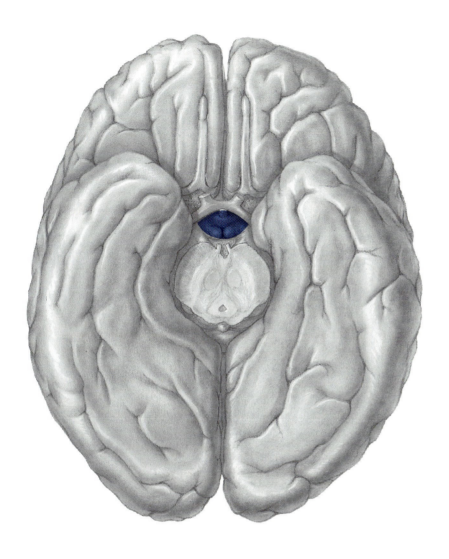

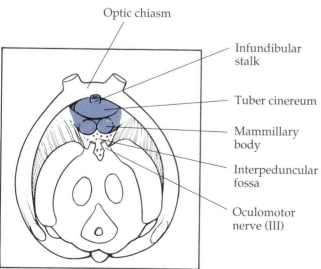

Optic chiasm

Infundibular
stalk

Tuber cinereum

Mammillary
body

Interpeduncular
fossa

Oculomotor
nerve (III)

Figure 14–2. The basal surface of the brain. The inset shows the key features of
the basal surface of the hypothalamus. The tuber cinereum is a swelling surrounding the base of the infundibular stalk and contains many hypothalamic
nuclei that regulate the release of anterior pituitary hormones.

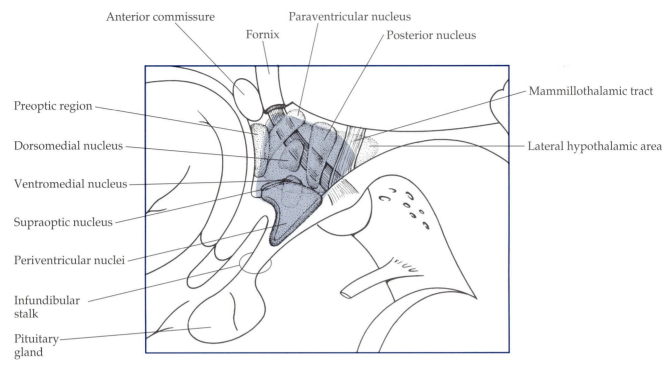

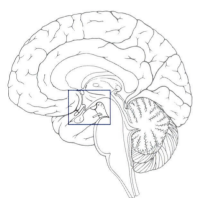

Figure 14–3. The major nuclei are illustrated in a cutaway view of the hypothalamus. The inset shows the region illustrated in the internal view. Note that the nuclei of the periventricular zone (tinted blue) are located immediately beneath the walls and floor of the third ventricle. Only a small portion of the nuclei in this zone is illustrated. The middle and lateral zones are the two other hypothalamic zones. (Adapted from Nauta, W. J. H., and Haymaker, W. 1969. Hypothalamic nuclei and fiber connections. In Haymaker, W., Anderson, E., and Nauta, W. J. H. (eds.), The Hypothalamus. Springfield, Ill.: Charles C. Thomas, pp. 136–209.)

zone is important in emotions and their behavioral expression. The lateral zone is separated from the medial zone by the **fornix,** a tract that interconnects limbic system structures. The lateral zone will be considered in Chapter 15 when we consider the limbic system.

Separate Parvocellular and Magnocellular Neurosecretory Systems Regulate Hormone Release From the Anterior and Posterior Lobes of the Pituitary

The pituitary gland (Figure 14–3) is connected to the ventral surface of the hypothalamus by the **infundibular stalk**. In humans, two major anatomical divisions of the pituitary gland mediate the release of distinct sets of hormones: the **anterior lobe** (or adenohypophysis; Table 14–1), and the **posterior lobe** (or neurohypophysis). A third lobe, the intermediate lobe, although prominent in many simpler mammals, is vestigial in humans.

Table 14–1. Anterior pituitary hormones and substances that control their release.

Hormone	Releasing hormone (RH)	Release-inhibiting hormone
Growth hormone	Growth hormone RH/ dopamine	Somatostatin
Luteinizing hormone	Gonadotropin RH	
Follicle-stimulating hormone	Gonadotropin RH	
Thyrotropin	Thyrotropin RH	
Prolactin	Prolactin RH	Dopamine
Adrenocorticotropic hormone	Corticotropin RH	
Melanocyte-stimulating hormone[1]	Corticotropin RH	

[1]In humans, the intermediate lobe of the pituitary gland is vestigial. Secretory cells containing melanocyte-stimulating hormone are located in the anterior lobe.

The lobes of the pituitary gland have different developmental histories. The posterior lobe develops from the **neuroectoderm**. In contrast, the anterior and intermediate lobes are of nonneural **ectodermal** origin, developing from a diverticulum in the roof of the developing oral cavity, called **Rathke's pouch**. Early in development, the ectodermal and neuroectodermal portions fuse to form a single structure.

The anterior and posterior lobes are parts of two distinct neurosecretory systems, and hormone release from these lobes is regulated by different populations of hypothalamic neurons. The anterior lobe is part of the **parvocellular neurosecretory system** (Figure 14–4A). **Small-diameter** hypothalamic neurons in numerous nuclei regulate anterior lobe hormone release by **neurovascular** rather than synaptic mechanisms. Specific chemicals (Table 14–1) are secreted into the **portal circulation** (Figure 14–5) of the pituitary gland. Parvocellular neurosecretory neurons are located in nuclei of the **periventricular zone**. By contrast, the posterior lobe is part of the **magnocellular neurosecretory system** (Figure 14–4B). Here, **large-diameter** hypothalamic neurons in two nuclei project their axons into the posterior lobe, where peptide hormones are released from their terminals directly onto capillaries of the systemic circulation. Magnocellular neurosecretory neurons are located in the **middle zone**.

Regulatory Peptides Released by Hypothalamic Neurons Into the Portal Circulation Control Secretion of Anterior Lobe Hormones

Anterior pituitary hormones are released from **epithelial secretory cells** into the systemic circulation. The process by which the hypothalamus stimulates anterior lobe secretory cells to release their hormones (or to inhibit release) is quite unlike mechanisms of neural action that we have considered so far. Rather than synapse on anterior lobe secretory cells, the hypothalamic parvocellular neurosecretory neurons terminate on capillaries of the **pituitary portal circulation** in the floor of the third ventricle (Figure 14–5).

A portal circulatory system is distinguished by the presence of separate **portal veins** interposed between two sets of capillaries. The first set is located in a region termed the **median eminence**, which is part of the proximal infundibular stalk. The portal veins are located in the distal part of the infundibular stalk. The second set of capillaries is found in the ante-

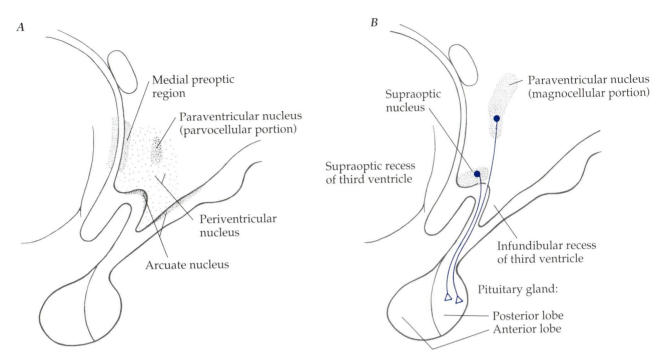

Figure 14–4. Midsagittal view of the region around the anterior wall of the third ventricle showing the location of neurons of the parvocellular system *(A)*. In part *B*, neurons constituting the magnocellular system are shown along with the path that their axons take to reach the posterior lobe of the pituitary gland.

rior pituitary. (In the systemic circulation, such as the vascular supply of the rest of the brain, capillary beds are interposed between arterial and venous systems.)

Parvocellular neurons release chemicals, most of which are peptides, that either promote (**releasing hormones**) or inhibit (**release-inhibiting hormones**) the release of hormones from anterior lobe secretory cells. These chemicals are listed in Table 14–1. Release or release-inhibiting hormones are carried to the **anterior lobe** in the portal veins (Figure 14–5), where they act directly on secretory cells.

An analogy can be drawn between the capillaries in the median eminence and the integrative function of spinal motor neurons (see Chapter 9). Separate descending pathways and interneuronal systems synapse on the spinal motor neuron. Thus the motor neuron is the "final common path" for the integration of neuronal information controlling skeletal muscle. The "final common path" for control of anterior lobe hormone release are the capillaries of the median eminence. This is because separate hypothalamic neurons secrete releasing or release-inhibiting hormones into the capillaries of the median eminence (Figure 14–5), and it is at this **vascular site** that summation of neurohormones occurs.

The distribution of neurons that project to the median eminence has been examined extensively in rodents. Although these neurons are widespread, the major sources are located in nuclei within the **periventricular zone** (Figure 14–4A). Among the major sources, and the hormones they release, are:

- The **arcuate nucleus**, which contains neurons that release gonadotropin-releasing hormone, luteinizing hormone-releasing hor-

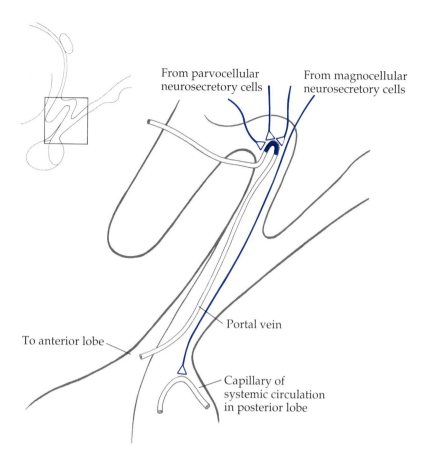

From parvocellular
neurosecretory cells

From magnocellular
neurosecretory cells

Portal vein

To anterior lobe

Capillary of
systemic circulation
in posterior lobe

Figure 14–5. The hypothalamus,
pituitary gland, and rostral and ventral portions of the third ventricle are
shown in this schematic drawing of
the midsagittal brain surface. The
region indicated by the box is
enlarged below to show the organization of the parvocellular and magnocellular neurosecretory systems in
relation to the portal circulation. The
region of the primary capillaries of the
hypophyseal portal system are indicated in dark blue. These vessels
derive from the superior hypophyseal
arteries, which are branches of the
internal carotid and posterior communicating arteries.

mone, corticotropin-releasing hormone, somatostatin, and adreno-
corticotropic hormone.

- Neurons in the portion of the **paraventricular nucleus that lies along
the third ventricle** contain corticotropin-releasing hormone.
- The **periventricular nucleus** provides gonadotropin-releasing hormone, luteinizing hormone–releasing hormone, and dopamine
(which inhibits prolactin release).
- The **medial preoptic area** contains parvocellular neurons that secrete
luteinizing hormone–releasing hormone.

In addition, there are extrahypothalamic sources of releasing and
release-inhibiting neurohormones. For example, the septal nuclei (see
Chapter 15) are a source of gonadotropin-releasing hormone. Interestingly,
most of these neurohormones (Table 14–1) are also found in hypothalamic
neurons that do not project to the median eminence. These neurohormones are found in neurons in other regions of the central nervous system
as well. This widespread distribution of neurohormones indicates that
they are **neuroactive compounds** at these other sites and not only chemicals that regulate anterior pituitary hormone release.

Individual neurons of the parvocellular system, as in the magnocellular system (see below), may synthesize and release more than one peptide. In certain groups of parvocellular neurons, for example, it is thought
that the synthesis of one or another peptide is regulated by circulating hormones in the blood. This is one way in which environmental factors, such
as prolonged exposure to stressful situations, may alter the neurohormone

composition in the portal circulation and thereby influence anterior pituitary hormone release.

Hypothalamic Neurons Project to the Posterior Lobe and Release Vasopressin and Oxytocin

Posterior pituitary hormones are the neurosecretory products of hypothalamic neurons, unlike anterior lobe hormones, which are the products of epithelial secretory cells. **Vasopressin**, a peptide consisting of nine amino acids, has numerous functions. It elevates blood pressure, for example, through its action on vascular smooth muscle. Vasopressin also promotes water reabsorption from the distal tubules of the kidney to reduce urine volume. Another name for vasopressin is antidiuretic hormone (ADH).

Oxytocin, which has a chemical structure nearly identical to that of vasopressin—differing by amino acids at only two sites—functions primarily to stimulate uterine contractions and to promote ejection of milk from the mammary glands. Despite the fact that oxytocin is best known for its actions on female organs, there do not seem to be major differences in the numbers and locations of oxytocin-containing neurons in the nervous systems of males and females (see below). Hence, it is likely that other important actions of this peptide will be discovered.

In the hypothalamus, both vasopressin and oxytocin are synthesized primarily in two nuclei, the **paraventricular nucleus** and the **supraoptic nucleus**. Experiments in animals have shown that the paraventricular nucleus comprises at least three distinct cell groups. As we saw above, there are parvocellular neurosecretory neurons in the portion of the nucleus that apposes the third ventricle. Located lateral to these are the **magnocellular neurons**, which synthesize and release the two posterior lobe neurohormones. A third neuron group gives rise to a descending brain stem and spinal projection, important for regulating autonomic nervous system functions (see next section). The supraoptic nucleus consists only of magnocellular neurons. The paraventricular and supraoptic nuclei are illustrated in Figure 14–4B, which is a midsagittal view of the hypothalamus.

Both vasopressin and oxytocin are synthesized from larger prohormone molecules. It was once thought that vasopressin was synthesized in one nucleus and oxytocin in the other. With the use of immunocytochemical techniques, however, it has been established that **different cells in each nucleus** produce one or the other hormone. The prohormone molecules from which vasopressin and oxytocin derive also contain proteins, called **neurophysins**. A physiological role for neurophysins, which are co-released with vasopressin and oxytocin, has not been identified.

The axons of the paraventricular and the supraoptic nuclei course in the **infundibular stalk** (Figures 14–3B and 14–4B) and do not make synaptic contacts with other neurons. Rather, they terminate on **fenestrated capillaries** in the **posterior lobe** of the pituitary (Figure 14–5). (Fenestrations, or pores, make capillaries leaky. Recall that in Chapter 4 we saw that the posterior lobe of the pituitary [see Figure 4–17] is one of the brain regions that lacks a blood–brain barrier. Thus, neurohormones can pass freely into the capillaries through the fenestrations.) The process by which these hypothalamic neurons release vasopressin or oxytocin from their terminals into the systemic circulation is similar to the release of neurotransmitters at synapses.

Immunocytochemical studies also have shown that magnocellular neurons, like their parvocellular counterparts, have a complex biochemistry and contain other peptides that have both central and peripheral actions. These other peptides also may be released into the circulation along with oxytocin or vasopressin and have coordinated actions on diverse structures. Vasopressin itself is an example of a brain peptide that has a diversity of coordinated functions at different sites. For example, it is a blood-borne hormone that influences the function of specific peripheral target organs, such as the kidney, and it is a neuroactive peptide involved in control of the autonomic nervous system (see below).

An understanding of the projections from other brain regions to magnocellular hypothalamic neurons provides insight into how the brain controls neurohormone release. For example, magnocellular neurons that contain vasopressin are important for regulating blood volume. These neurons receive inputs from three sources that each serve a related function.

First, magnocellular neurons receive an indirect projection from the **solitary nucleus.** This pathway conveys **baroreceptor** input from the glossopharyngeal and vagus nerves (see Chapter 8) to the hypothalamus, providing important afferent signals for controlling blood pressure and blood volume.

The second major input source is from the **circumventricular organs.** These structures do not have a blood–brain barrier. Two that project to the magnocellular nuclei are: the **subfornical organ** and the **organum vasculosum of the lamina terminalis** (see Chapter 4; Figure 4–17). As we saw in Chapter 4, the blood–brain barrier is a specific permeability barrier between capillaries in the central nervous system and the extracellular space. This barrier protects the brain from the influence of many neuroactive chemicals circulating in the blood. With no blood–brain barrier, these structures sense plasma osmolality and circulating chemicals and thereby can regulate blood pressure and blood volume through their hypothalamic projections.

The **preoptic region** provides the third input to the magnocellular neurons. This region is implicated in the central neural mechanisms for regulating the composition and volume of body fluids, and thus indirectly affects the control of blood pressure.

Peptidergic neurons have a remarkable capacity for plasticity. For example, damage to the infundibular stalk may interrupt the axons of magnocellular neurosecretory cells containing vasopressin as they pass to the posterior pituitary. This results in **diabetes insipidus**, in which excessive amounts of urine are produced. Fortunately the condition is temporary because the cells form a new, functional "posterior lobe."

FUNCTIONAL ANATOMY OF AUTONOMIC NERVOUS SYSTEM CONTROL

The other major role of the hypothalamus is regulating the **autonomic nervous system**. The autonomic nervous system controls the various organ systems of the body: cardiovascular and respiratory, gastrointestinal, exocrine, and urogenital. Two divisions of the autonomic nervous system—the **parasympathetic** and the **sympathetic nervous systems**—originate from different parts of the central nervous system. Similar to the control of skeletal muscle, visceral control by the sympathetic and parasympathetic systems relies both on relatively simple reflexes, involving the spinal cord and brain stem, and more complex control by higher levels of the central nervous system, including the hypothalamus.

A third division of the autonomic nervous system, the **enteric nervous system**, is located entirely in the periphery. This third system provides the intrinsic innervation of the gastrointestinal tract and mediates the complex coordinated reflexes for peristalsis. The enteric nervous system functions independent of the hypothalamus and the rest of the central nervous system.

We next review briefly the anatomical organization of the sympathetic and parasympathetic divisions. It is important to understand how these autonomic divisions connect to their target organs before we consider the higher-order regulation by the hypothalamus.

The Parasympathetic and Sympathetic Divisions of the Autonomic Nervous System Originate From Different Central Nervous System Locations

As we saw in Chapter 13, the innervation of body organs by the sympathetic and parasympathetic systems is fundamentally different from the innervation of skeletal muscle by the somatic nervous system (Figure 14–6). The innervation of skeletal muscle is mediated directly by motor neurons (Figure 14–6A) located in spinal and cranial nerve motor nuclei. For the autonomic innervation, two neurons link the central nervous system with organs in the periphery: the **preganglionic neuron**, and the **postganglionic neuron** (Figure 14–6B; see Figure 13–5).

The cell body of the preganglionic neuron is located in the central nervous system and its axon follows a tortuous course to the periphery.

Figure 14–6.   A. The circuit for peripheral innervation of skeletal muscle. *B.* The innervation of peripheral autonomic ganglia. Preganglionic autonomic neurons are located in the intermediate zone of the spinal cord. Their axons exit the spinal cord through the ventral roots and project to ganglia in the sympathetic trunk (paravertebral ganglia) through the spinal nerves and white rami. The axons of postganglionic neurons in the sympathetic ganglia course to the periphery through the gray rami and spinal nerves. The white and gray rami contain, respectively, the myelinated and unmyelinated axons of preganglionic and postganglionic autonomic neurons. A postganglionic neuron in a prevertebral ganglion is also shown with input from a preganglionic neuron. (*B*, Adapted from Appenzeller, O. 1986. Clinical Autonomic Failure: Practical Concepts. Amsterdam: Elsevier.)

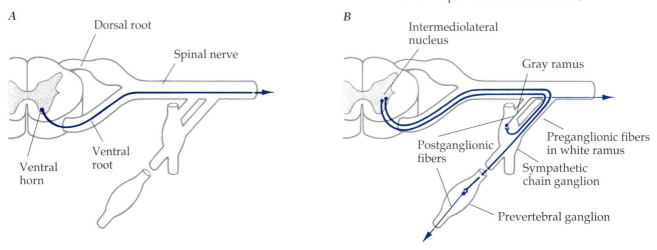

From the ventral root and through various peripheral neural conduits, the axon of the preganglionic neuron finally synapses on postganglionic neurons in **peripheral ganglia** (Figure 14–6B). A notable exception is the adrenal medulla, which receives direct innervation by preganglionic sympathetic neurons. This is related to the fact that adrenal medullary cells, like postganglionic neurons, develop from the neural crest (see Chapter 2).

There are two major differences in the neuroanatomical organization of the sympathetic and parasympathetic divisions (Figure 14–7). First is the location of the preganglionic neurons in the central nervous system;

Figure 14–7. Organization of the autonomic nervous system. The sympathetic nervous system is shown at left and the parasympathetic nervous system, at right. Note that the postganglionic neurons for the sympathetic nervous system are located in sympathetic trunk ganglia and prevertebral ganglia (e.g., celiac ganglion). The postganglionic neurons for the parasympathetic nervous system are located in terminal ganglia which are located close to the target organ. (Adapted from Schmidt, R. F., and Thews, G. (eds.) 1983. Human Physiology. Berlin: Springer.)

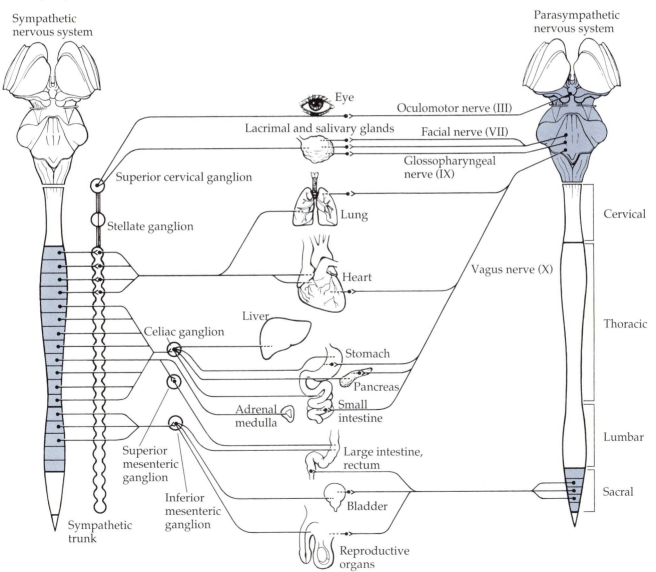

second is the location of the peripheral ganglia. **Sympathetic preganglionic neurons** are found in the intermediate zone of the spinal cord, between the **first thoracic and third lumbar** segments. Most of the neurons are located in the **intermediolateral nucleus** (also called **intermediolateral cell column** because, like Clarke's column, this nucleus has an extensive rostrocaudal organization).

In contrast, parasympathetic preganglionic neurons are found in the **brain stem** and the **second through fourth sacral** spinal cord segments. The parasympathetic brain stem nuclei were described in Chapter 13 when the cranial nerve nuclei were discussed. Most preganglionic neurons are located in the Edinger–Westphal nucleus, the superior salivatory nucleus, the inferior salivatory nucleus, and the dorsal motor nucleus of the vagus. Others are scattered in the reticular formation. The parasympathetic preganglionic neurons in the sacral spinal cord are found in the intermediate zone, at sites analogous to those of sympathetic preganglionic neurons.

The second major difference in the neuroanatomy of the sympathetic and parasympathetic divisions is the location of the peripheral ganglia in which the postganglionic neurons are located. Parasympathetic ganglia, often called **terminal ganglia**, are located on or near the target organ. In contrast, sympathetic ganglia are found at some distance from the target organs. Postganglionic sympathetic neurons are located in the **paravertebral ganglia**, part of the sympathetic trunk, and in **prevertebral ganglia** (Figure 14–7).

Descending Projections From the Hypothalamus Regulate Autonomic Function

How does the hypothalamus regulate the functions of the autonomic nervous system? The answer, perhaps surprising, is related to how the brain controls voluntary movement. As we saw in Chapter 9, distinct areas of the cerebral cortex and brain stem nuclei give rise to the descending motor pathways that regulate the excitability of motor neurons and interneurons (Figure 14–8A). These spinal projections transmit control signals to steer voluntary movements and regulate spinal reflexes. Visceral motor functions—mediated by the autonomic nervous system—are subjected to a similar control by the brain (Figure 14–8B). The descending autonomic pathways originate from the hypothalamus and various brain stem nuclei.

The major hypothalamic nucleus for controlling sympathetic and parasympathetic functions is the **paraventricular nucleus** (Figure 14–9). The neurotransmitters used by this pathway include **vasopressin** and **oxytocin**, the same peptides released by the magnocellular neurosecretory system. The neurons giving rise to the descending path, however, are distinct from those projecting to the posterior pituitary. This pathway descends laterally through the hypothalamus and brain stem. In the hypothalamus, axons course in the **medial forebrain bundle** (MFB), which is located in the lateral zone. The descending axons leave the bundle and then run in the **dorsolateral tegmentum** in the midbrain, pons, and medulla (Figure 14–9). As we will see below, lesions of the lateral brain stem tegmentum can produce characteristic autonomic changes because of damage to these descending hypothalamic axons.

The descending autonomic pathway synapses on brain stem parasympathetic nuclei, such as the dorsal motor nucleus of the vagus, spinal sympathetic neurons in the intermediolateral nucleus of the tho-

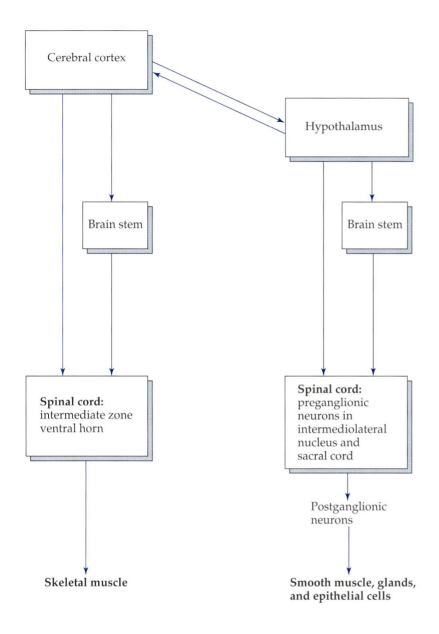

Figure 14–8. Organization of descending pathways controlling voluntary movement *(left)* and visceromotor function *(right)*.

racic and lumbar segments, and spinal parasympathetic neurons in the sacral cord (Figure 14–9).

Other hypothalamic sites contribute axons to the descending visceromotor pathways. These areas include neurons in the lateral hypothalamic zone, the dorsomedial hypothalamic nucleus, and the posterior hypothalamus. In addition, these areas have strong projections to brain stem nuclei. Whereas some of these areas project laterally through the hypothalamus and brain stem, en route to the autonomic nuclei, others project more medially. One such medial hypothalamic path is the dorsal longitudinal fasciculus. Throughout its course, the dorsal longitudinal fasciculus travels in close proximity to the ventricular system.

In addition to the hypothalamus, numerous brain stem nuclei help regulate the autonomic nervous system. They do so by projecting to other brain stem nuclei implicated in viscerosensory functions and visceromotor control, as well as by projecting directly to brain stem and spinal cord autonomic nuclei:

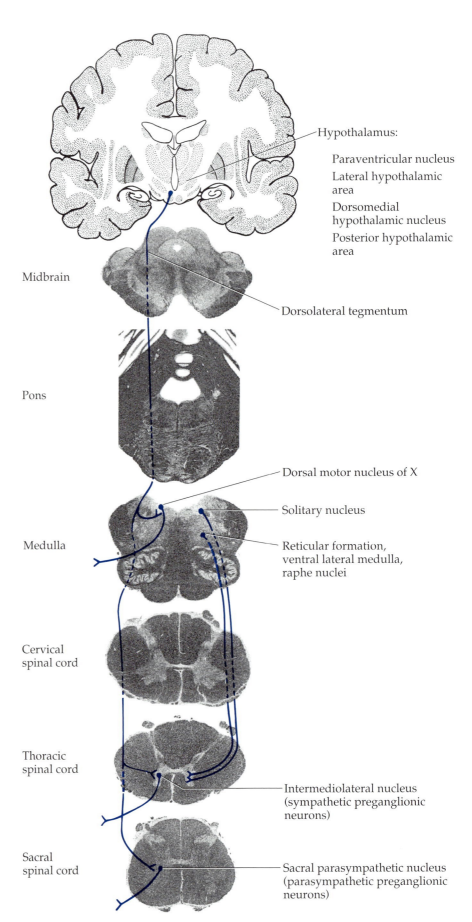

Hypothalamus:

Paraventricular nucleus

Lateral hypothalamic
area

Dorsomedial
hypothalamic nucleus

Posterior hypothalamic
area

Midbrain

Dorsolateral tegmentum

Pons

Dorsal motor nucleus of X

Solitary nucleus

Medulla

Reticular formation,
ventral lateral medulla,
raphe nuclei

Cervical
spinal cord

Thoracic
spinal cord

Intermediolateral nucleus
(sympathetic preganglionic
neurons)

Sacral
spinal cord

Sacral parasympathetic nucleus
(parasympathetic preganglionic
neurons)

Figure 14–9. Regions of origin,
course, and termination sites of
descending hypothalamic pathways.

- The **solitary nucleus** (see Figure 14–18C), in addition to its role in chemosensory mechanisms, has a component that projects to the intermediolateral nucleus. Recall that the solitary nucleus relays viscerosensory information from the glossopharyngeal and vagus nerves to the hypothalamus, as well as to the **parabrachial nucleus** (see Figure 14–18B), the thalamus, and other forebrain structures (see Chapter 8).

- Neurons in the **ventrolateral medulla** (see Figure 14–18C) give rise to an **adrenergic** projection to brain stem and spinal autonomic nuclei. These neurons are thought to play an important role in regulating blood pressure.

- Neurons of the **pontomedullary reticular formation** have strong projections to autonomic preganglionic neurons in the brain stem and spinal cord. Because many of these neurons also project to spinal motor and premotor neurons, they may coordinate complex behavioral responses such as defense reactions that involve both visceral and somatic changes. For example, when we are startled by an unexpected, loud noise, our blood pressure rises.

- The **raphe nuclei**, which use serotonin as their neurotransmitter, receive strong inputs from the hypothalamus and, in turn, project to spinal autonomic nuclei. The projections of the raphespinal system are also thought to be important in suppressing dorsal horn pain transmission (see Chapter 5) in relation to the emotional state of the individual.

■ REGIONAL ANATOMY

The mediolateral functional organization of the hypothalamus was briefly considered earlier in the chapter. The three zones—periventricular, middle, and lateral—are located at all anterior–posterior levels of the hypothalamus (see Figures 14–12, 14–15, and 14–17). To better formulate an understanding of regional anatomy, we will now also consider three anterior-to-posterior portions of the hypothalamus. It should be noted that although the boundaries between these three regions are based on landmarks on the ventral brain surface, the nuclei included within each region depends on the plane of section.

- The **anterior** part of the hypothalamus, located dorsal and rostral to the optic chiasm (see inset to Figure 14–12), includes the **preoptic region**. The preoptic region extends rostral to the lamina terminalis.

- The **middle** hypothalamus (see Figure 14–15) is between the optic chiasm and the mammillary bodies. This portion contains the tuber cinereum (Latin for "gray swelling"), from which the pituitary stalk arises.

- The **posterior** portion (see Figure 14–17) includes the mammillary bodies and the structures dorsal to them.

The Preoptic Region Influences Release of Reproductive Hormones From the Anterior Pituitary

Once considered separate from the hypothalamus, the preoptic region is now generally thought to be the most anterior part of the hypothalamus. This modern view derives from an understanding of the connections and functions of the preoptic region, which are similar to the rest of the hypothalamus. Figure 14–10 is a section through the **preoptic region**, which contains neurons that synthesize gonadotropin-releasing hormone. These neurons are believed to regulate pituitary release of reproductive hormones since they project to the **median eminence.** (The section shown in Figure 14–10 also cuts through the **supraoptic recess** of the third ventricle.)

Nuclei in the preoptic region and anterior hypothalamus of animals show sexual dimorphism (i.e., morphologic differences in males and females). In the rat, gender affects the size of a sexually dimorphic nucleus as well as the architecture of neurons within the nucleus. Moreover, the size of this nucleus is dependent on perinatal exposure to gonadal steroids. This is an interesting example of how sexual differentiation alters brain morphology. In humans, identification of sexual dimorphism in the hypothalamus and other forebrain regions is controversial. At present, evidence for and against sex differences in the preoptic region and anterior hypothalamus has been published. Part of the problem in identifying sex differences is that the human preoptic region has a complex organization, with numerous small and sometimes poorly differentiated nuclei (Figure 14–11). One of the nuclei reported to show sexual dimorphism in the human is part of the interstitial nuclei of the anterior hypothalamus (Figure 14–11). An important challenge for neuroscience is to resolve the question of sexual dimorphism in the human hypothalamus.

The Supraoptic and Paraventricular Nuclei Comprise the Magnocellular Neurosecretory System

The paraventricular and supraoptic nuclei are located in the anterior region (Figures 14–10 and 14–12). These are the two **magnocellular** nuclei; they release vasopressin and oxytocin in the posterior lobe of the pituitary (Figure 14–4A). The axons from the magnocellular nuclei course through the median eminence, en route to the posterior lobe. However, the axons are segregated in an internal zone of the median eminence from the axons and terminals of the parvocellular neurons, which are located in an external zone.

Figure 14–10. Myelin-stained coronal section through the anterior hypothalamus showing the preoptic region.

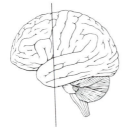

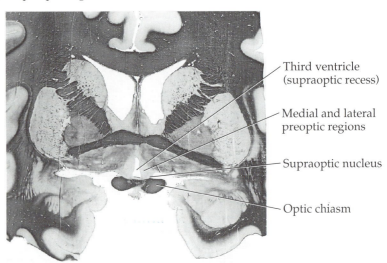

Third ventricle
(supraoptic recess)

Medial and lateral
preoptic regions

Supraoptic nucleus

Optic chiasm

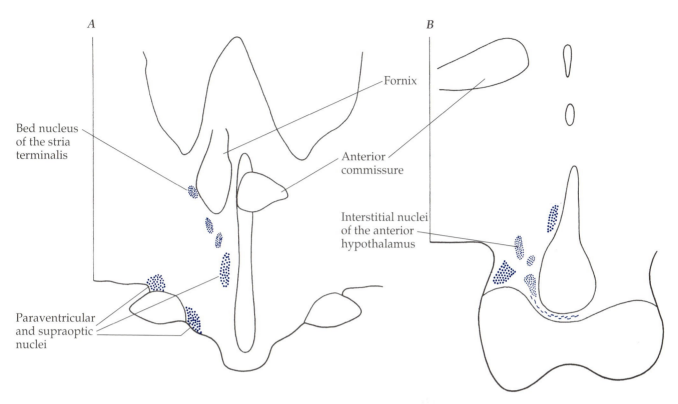

Figure 14–11. Nuclei of the human forebrain reported to be sexually dimorphic. *A.* Drawing of section through anterior commissure (similar to level shown in Figure 14–13). *B.* Drawing of section through optic chiasm (similar to level shown in Figure 14–10). The interstitial nuclei of the anterior hypothalamus consist of a set of four small nuclei scattered throughout the anterior hypothalamus and preoptic area. (From Swaab, D. F., and Hoffman, M. A. 1995)

Recall that the paraventricular nucleus has a complex organization. It contains three major functional subdivisions (Figure 14–12):

- The **parvocellular division**, apposed to the third ventricle, projects to the median eminence (Figure 14–4A).
- The **magnocellular division** projects to the posterior lobe (Figure 14–4B).
- A separate **autonomic division** projects to brain stem and spinal cord nuclei containing autonomic preganglionic neurons (Figure 14–9).

A common feature of paraventricular nucleus biochemistry is that many neurons in each subdivision contain vasopressin or oxytocin. Release of vasopressin or oxytocin at the various target sites of neurons in the paraventricular nucleus may subserve similar sets of functions, for example, in regulating blood pressure and blood volume.

The paraventricular and supraoptic nuclei derive from the same group of embryonic neurons. Their locations in the mature brain reflect the complex migration that neuroblasts often undergo. Accessory magnocellular neurosecretory neurons bridge the gap between the paraventricular and supraoptic nuclei (Figure 14–12).

The **suprachiasmatic nucleus**, which is also located at this level (Figure 14–12), functions as the "master clock" for circadian rhythms. It receives a direct projection from the **retina**, thereby allowing visual stimuli to synchronize the internal clock (or circadian rhythm) of the body. The

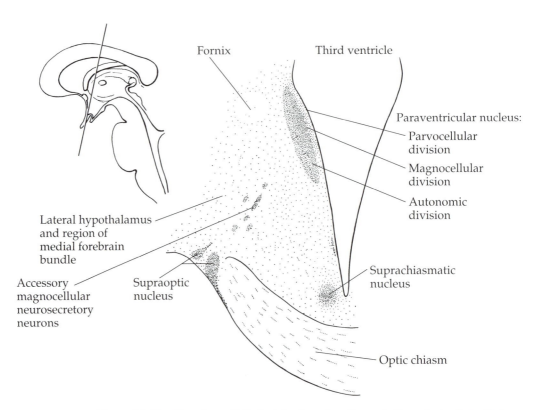

Figure 14–12. Drawing of Nissl-stained section through the anterior hypothalamus (optic chiasm). The inset shows the plane of section. (Adapted from Clarke, W. E. LeGros. 1938. Morphological aspects of the hypothalamus. In Clarke, W. E. LeGros, Beattie, J., Riddoch, G., et al. (eds.), The Hypothalamus: Morphological, Functional, Clinical and Surgical Aspects. Edinburgh: Oliver & Boyd, pp. 2–68).

suprachiasmatic nucleus controls circadian rhythms both through local connections with other hypothalamic nuclei more directly involved in behavior, for example, the paraventricular nucleus, as well as through projections to the **pineal gland** and other extrahypothalamic structures. The clinical significance of normal circadian rhythms and the function of the suprachiasmatic nucleus are just beginning to be appreciated. For example, defects in circadian rhythms are believed to underlie certain forms of depression and sleeping disorders.

The Parvocellular Neurosecretory Neurons Project to the Median Eminence

The **median eminence**, which contains the primary capillaries of the hypophyseal portal system, is located in the proximal portion of the infundibular stalk (or infundibulum, Figure 14–3). The myelin-stained section in Figure 14–13 transects this region, although the median eminence is not differentiated. A midsagittal MRI through the pituitary gland is shown in Figure 14–14. The infundibular stalk connects the basal hypothalamic surface with the pituitary gland. Release and release-inhibiting hormones secreted by the parvocellular neurosecretory neurons pass directly into the portal circulation through fenestrations, or pores, in the capillaries of the median eminence. The median eminence is one central nervous system site where the blood–brain barrier is absent (see Figure 4–17).

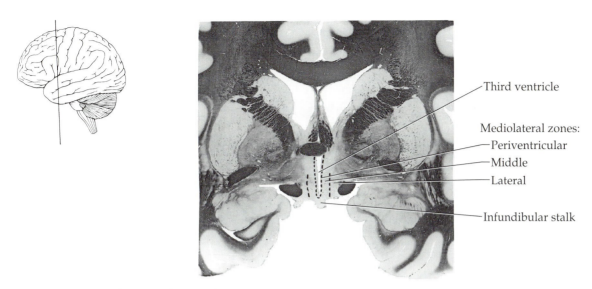

Third ventricle

Mediolateral zones:
Periventricular
Middle
Lateral

Infundibular stalk

Figure 14–13. Myelin-stained coronal section through the infundibular stalk (infundibulum).

The three mediolateral zones are shown in Figure 14–13. The **arcuate nucleus** is located in the middle hypothalamic region (Figure 14–15). Parvocellular neurons in the arcuate nucleus contain various releasing and release-inhibiting hormones. In addition, many neurons in the arcuate nucleus contain β-**endorphin**, an endogenous opiate that is cleaved from the large peptide **pro-opiomelanocortin** (POMC). Some of these neurons may play a role in opiate analgesia because they project to the periaqueductal gray matter, where electrical stimulation produces analgesia (see Chapter 5).

The **ventromedial hypothalamic nucleus** is located in the middle region of the hypothalamus. This nucleus receives input from a major limbic system structure, the **amygdala** (see Chapter 15), and is important in

Figure 14–14. A midsagittal MRI through the human pituitary gland. The posterior lobe *(arrow)* produces a bright signal. The thin infundibular stalk connects the basal surface of the hypothalamus with the pituitary. (From Sartor, K. 1992.)

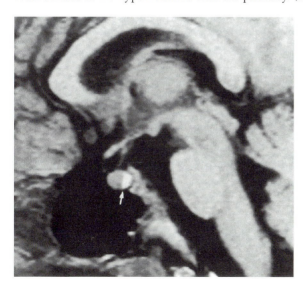

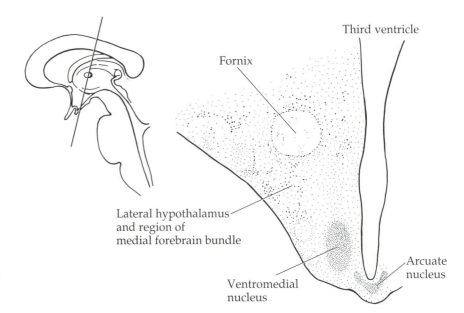

Figure 14–15. Drawings of Nissl-stained section through the middle hypothalamus. The inset shows the plane of section. (Adapted from Clark, W. E. LeGros. 1938. Morphological aspects of the hypothalamus. In Clarke, W. E. LeGros, Beattie, J., Riddoch, G., et al. (eds.), The Hypothalamus: Morphological, Functional, Clinical and Surgical Aspects. Edinburgh: Oliver & Boyd, pp. 2–68.)

regulating appetite and other consummatory behaviors. Many hypothalamic neurons in the lateral zone (Figure 14–15) also have widespread **projections to the cerebral cortex**. These neurons, which use **acetylcholine** as well as other neurochemicals as their transmitters, are thought to play a role in regulating cortical excitability. In this regard, they are similar to cholinergic neurons in the basal nucleus (see Figure 3–17A). In Alzheimer's disease, cholinergic neurons in the hypothalamus, basal nucleus, and other forebrain sites undergo degeneration.

The Posterior Hypothalamus Contains the Mammillary Bodies

A section through the posterior hypothalamus (Figures 14–14, 14–16, and 14–17) reveals the mammillary nuclei (or bodies). Each mammillary body contains two nuclei: the prominent **medial mammillary nucleus** and the smaller lateral mammillary nucleus. Remarkably, the mammillary bodies, the principal component of the posterior hypothalamus, establish virtually no intrahypothalamic connections. They receive their major input from the **fornix** (Figure 14–3), a tract that originates from the hippocampal formation.

The efferent projections of the mammillary bodies are carried primarily in the **mammillothalamic tract**, which projects to the anterior nuclei of the thalamus (see Figure AII–19). The mammillary bodies also have a descending projection to the midbrain and pons, the mammillotegmental tract. Whereas the mammillothalamic tract originates both from the medial and lateral mammillary nuclei, the mammillotegmental tract originates only from the lateral nucleus. The outputs of the mammillary bodies are considered part of the limbic system and will be discussed further in Chapter 15.

Other nuclei in the posterior hypothalamus, for example, nuclei located in the lateral hypothalamus, do not contribute in a major way to neuroendocrine function. Rather, this region plays a role in regulating autonomic functions and mediating integrated behavioral responses to

A

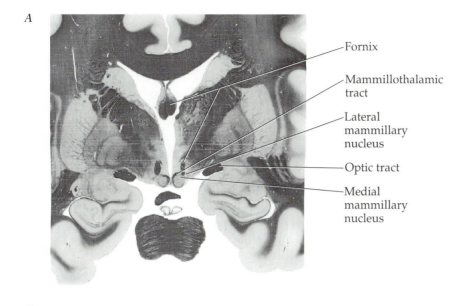

Fornix

Mammillothalamic tract

Lateral mammillary nucleus

Optic tract

Medial mammillary nucleus

B

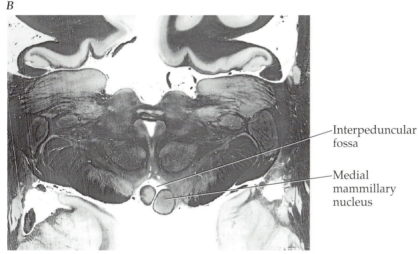

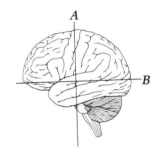

Interpeduncular fossa

Medial mammillary nucleus

Figure 14–16. Myelin-stained coronal section through the mammillary bodies *(A)* and transverse section through the junction of the midbrain and diencephalon *(B)*. In *B,* the mammillary bodies are located in the interpeduncular fossa, separated from the rest of the diencephalon. This is because the mammillary bodies extend from the basal surface of the diencephalon.

environmental stimuli. For example, the posterior hypothalamus is important in conserving body heat, which includes mediation of vasoconstriction and shivering in response to low temperatures.

Descending Autonomic Fibers Course in the Periaqueductal Gray Matter and in the Dorsolateral Tegmentum

Hypothalamic regulation of the autonomic nervous system is mediated, at least in part, by direct projections to brain stem parasympathetic nuclei, sympathetic neurons in the intermediolateral nucleus in thoracic and lumbar spinal segments, and parasympathetic neurons in the intermediate zone of the sacral spinal cord. The major path out of the hypothalamus taken by the autonomic pathway is through the **medial forebrain bundle** (MFB), which is in the lateral zone. This pathway contains axons from diverse sources including ascending and descending connections between the brain stem, the hypothalamus, and the cerebral hemisphere. Neurons in the lateral zone are not organized into distinct nuclei, but are interspersed along the MFB. The MFB becomes even more scat-

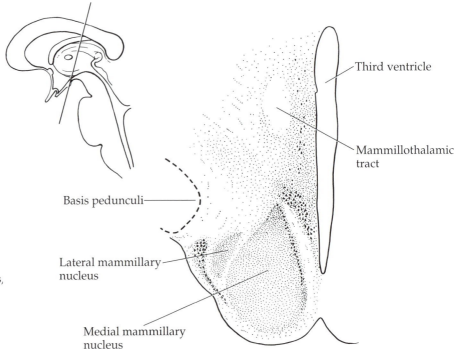

Figure 14–17. Drawings of Nissl-stained section through the posterior hypothalamus (mammillary bodies). The inset shows the plane of section. (Adapted from Clark, W. E. LeGros. 1938. Morphological aspects of the hypothalamus. In Clark, W. E. LeGros, Beattie, J., Riddoch, G., et al. (eds.), The Hypothalamus: Morphological, Functional, Clinical and Surgical Aspects. Edinburgh: Oliver & Boyd, pp. 2–68.)

Labels in figure: Third ventricle; Mammillothalamic tract; Basis pedunculi; Lateral mammillary nucleus; Medial mammillary nucleus

tered caudal to the hypothalamus, in the brain stem. (The term medial forebrain bundle is not applied to the brain stem segment.) In the brain stem, the descending autonomic pathway courses in the dorsolateral tegmentum (Figure 14–18).

Another hypothalamic pathway, the **dorsal longitudinal fasciculus**, contains ascending viscerosensory and descending fibers. This path courses within the gray matter along the wall of the third ventricle, in the midbrain periaqueductal gray matter and the gray matter in the floor of the fourth ventricle. Although diffuse in the diencephalon and midbrain, fibers constituting this path can be identified in the pons and in the medulla (in the dorsal portion of the hypoglossal nucleus; Figure 14–18C).

*Dorsolateral Brain Stem Lesions Interrupt
Descending Sympathetic Fibers*

Damage to the dorsolateral pons or medulla can produce **Horner's syndrome**, a disturbance in which the functions of the sympathetic nervous system become impaired. Surprisingly, parasympathetic functions are spared (see below). Such damage typically occurs as a consequence of occlusion of the **posterior inferior cerebellar artery** (see Figure 4–3). The most common signs of Horner's syndrome and their causes are:

- **Ipsilateral pupillary constriction (miosis)**, resulting from the unopposed action of the pupillary constrictor innervation by Edinger–Westphal nucleus (see Chapter 13).
- **Partial dropping of the eyelid** (pseudoptosis), produced by removal of the sympathetic control of the smooth muscle assisting the action of the levator palpebrae muscle (tarsal muscle).
- **Decreased sweating** and **increased warmth and redness of the ipsilateral face**, related to reduced sympathetic control of facial blood flow.

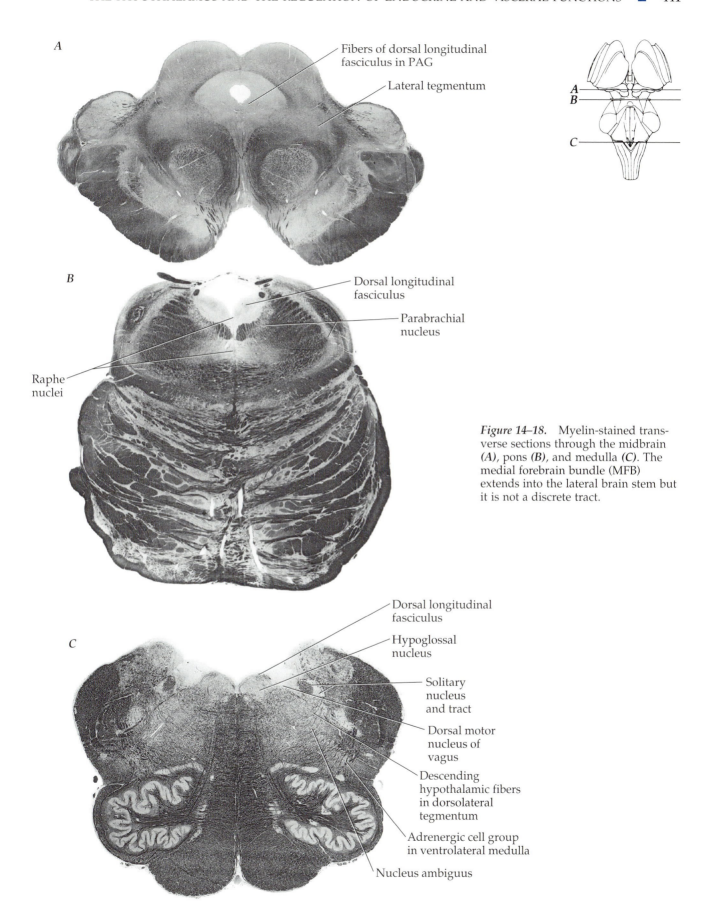

A

Fibers of dorsal longitudinal
fasciculus in PAG

Lateral tegmentum

B

Dorsal longitudinal
fasciculus

Parabrachial
nucleus

Raphe
nuclei

Figure 14–18. Myelin-stained transverse sections through the midbrain *(A)*, pons *(B)*, and medulla *(C)*. The medial forebrain bundle (MFB) extends into the lateral brain stem but it is not a discrete tract.

C

Dorsal longitudinal
fasciculus

Hypoglossal
nucleus

Solitary
nucleus
and tract

Dorsal motor
nucleus of
vagus

Descending
hypothalamic fibers
in dorsolateral
tegmentum

Adrenergic cell group
in ventrolateral medulla

Nucleus ambiguus

Unfortunately, Horner's syndrome alone provides little information to the clinician for localizing the site of a lesion. This is because the syndrome can be produced by a lesion anywhere along the descending autonomic fibers from the hypothalamus, through the dorsolateral brain stem, to the spinal cord (see next section). In fact, Horner's syndrome can even be produced by a lesion in the periphery, where axons of the sympathetic postganglionic neurons course to reach the head. How can the clinician distinguish between damage to one or another level? The answer lies in identifying other neurological signs that may accompany Horner's syndrome. For example, a medullary lesion that produces Horner's syndrome also will produce other signs associated with the **lateral medullary syndrome** (see Chapter 13; Figure 13–11). By contrast, a spinal cord lesion producing Horner's syndrome will also cause paralysis because the descending autonomic pathway is near the axons of the lateral corticospinal tract (Figure 14–19A) (see Chapter 9).

A question regarding the descending autonomic projection is why sympathetic, but not parasympathetic, functions are affected by a dorsolateral tegmental lesion. The most likely answer is that the hypothalamic

Figure 14–19. Myelin-stained transverse sections through the thoracic *(A)* and sacral *(B)* spinal cord. Inset shows configuration of intermediolateral cell column.

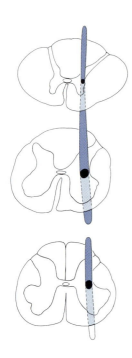

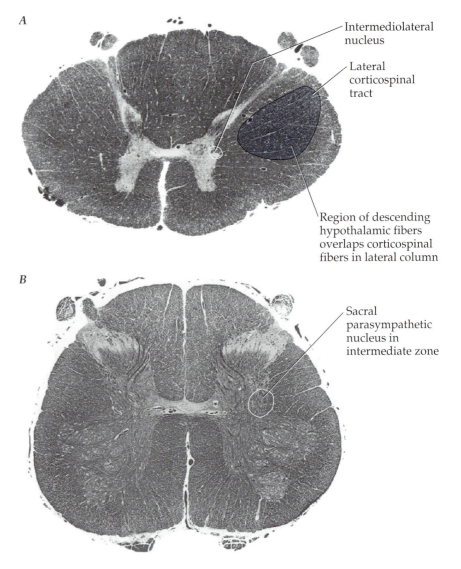

Intermediolateral nucleus

Lateral corticospinal tract

Region of descending hypothalamic fibers overlaps corticospinal fibers in lateral column

Sacral parasympathetic nucleus in intermediate zone

projections to parasympathetic nuclei, such as the dorsal vagal motor nucleus, are more bilateral than the sympathetic projections. Following a unilateral lesion, there remains an intact pathway on the contralateral side that may assume the functions of the damaged pathway. Moreover, many sympathetic nervous system functions, such as regulating skin arterial perfusion, are mediated by the innervation from the ipsilateral nervous system, whereas many of the functions of the parasympathetic system, such as gastrointestinal and bladder functions, are bilateral.

Preganglionic Neurons Are Located in the Lateral Intermediate Zone of the Spinal Cord

The descending autonomic fibers from the hypothalamus course in the lateral column of the spinal cord (Figure 14–19) and terminate in the intermediolateral nucleus (or cell column) of the thoracic and lumbar cord (Figure 14–19A) and the intermediate zone of the second through fourth sacral segments (Figure 14–19B). These sites in the spinal gray matter are where most of the autonomic preganglionic neurons are located. Additional preganglionic neurons are scattered medially in the intermediate zone. At certain thoracic levels, the intermediolateral nucleus extends into the lateral column (Figure 14–19A), which explains why this region is sometimes called the **intermediate horn** of the spinal cord gray matter. The inset shows the columnar shape of the intermediolateral nucleus. This organization is similar to that of Clarke's nucleus (see Figure 10–7) and the cranial nerve nuclei (see Figure 12–4).

General Hypothalamic Anatomy

The hypothalamus regulates the neuroendocrine and autonomic nervous systems. It is a part of the diencephalon, and it is bounded by the **lamina terminalis** rostrally, the **hypothalamic sulcus** dorsally, and the **internal capsule** laterally (Figure 14–1). The hypothalamus has a mediolateral anatomical and functional organization, with separate **periventricular, medial, and lateral zones** (Figure 14–3).

Neuroendocrine Control

Neuroendocrine control by the hypothalamus is mediated by separate **parvocellular** and **magnocellular neurosecretory systems**, which control hormone release from the anterior and posterior pituitary, respectively (Figure 14–4).

Parvocellular neurosecretory neurons (Figure 14–4A) regulate anterior lobe hormone release by secreting **releasing** or **release-inhibiting hormones** (Table 14–1) into the **portal circulation** in the **median eminence** (Figure 14–5). The major parvocellular nuclei, which are largely located in the periventricular zone, are: **periventricular nuclei**, **arcuate nucleus**, **paraventricular (medial part, only) nucleus**, and **medial preoptic region**. Additional hypothalamic and extrahypothalamic sites project to the median eminence and release gonadotropin-releasing hormones.

Two nuclei form the magnocellular system: the magnocellular division of the **paraventricular nucleus** and the **supraoptic nucleus** (Figures 14–3, 14–4B, and 14–10). Magnocellular neurons in these nuclei project their axons into the **infundibular stalk**, which connects the pituitary with

Summary

the brain (Figure 14–3). Their termination site is the posterior lobe, where they release **vasopressin** and **oxytocin** directly into the systemic circulation. Separate neurons in the paraventricular and supraoptic nuclei synthesize either vasopressin or oxytocin. Both parvocellular and magnocellular neurons co-localize neuroactive peptides.

Autonomic Nervous System and Visceromotor Functions

There are three anatomical components of the autonomic nervous system: **sympathetic division**, **parasympathetic division**, and **enteric nervous system**, which is the intrinsic innervation of the gut. For both the sympathetic and the parasympathetic divisions, two neurons link the central nervous system with their target organs (Figure 14–6B): a **preganglionic neuron**, located in the central nervous system, and a **postganglionic neuron**, located in peripheral ganglia (Figure 14–7). The sympathetic division originates from the spinal cord, between the **first thoracic and third lumbar** segments (Figure 14–7). Preganglionic neurons of this division are located in the **intermediolateral nucleus** (Figure 14–19A). The parasympathetic division originates from the **brain stem** and the **sacral spinal cord**. There are four parasympathetic nuclei in the brain stem containing preganglionic neurons (see Chapter 13): Edinger–Westphal nucleus, superior salivatory nucleus, inferior salivatory nucleus, and dorsal motor nucleus of the vagus. The lateral intermediate zone of the **second through fourth sacral** segments contains parasympathetic preganglionic neurons (Figure 14–19B).

Hypothalamic control of the autonomic nervous system is through descending pathways whose axons synapse on preganglionic neurons (Figures 14–8 and 14–9). The major source of this projection is the autonomic division of the **paraventricular nucleus**. This hypothalamic path courses in the **medial forebrain bundle** (Figures 14–12 and 14–15), located laterally in the hypothalamus, and its caudal extension in the lateral tegmentum of the brain stem (Figure 14–18) and the lateral column of the spinal cord (Figure 14–19A). Disruption of axons of this pathway at any level can produce **Horner's syndrome**. The hypothalamus also projects to other sites important in visceral sensory and motor function: **parabrachial nucleus**, **solitary nucleus**, raphe nuclei, and reticular formation (Figure 14–18). ■

KEY STRUCTURES AND TERMS

periventricular zone
middle zone
lateral zone
pituitary gland
    anterior lobe (or
         adenohypophysis)
    posterior lobe (or
         neurohypophysis)
Rathke's pouch
parvocellular neurosecretory system
    portal circulation
magnocellular neurosecretory system
median eminence
releasing hormones
release-inhibiting hormones
vasopressin (ADH)
oxytocin
β-endorphin
pro-opiomelanocortin (POMC)
arcuate nucleus

paraventricular nucleus
    parvocellular part
    magnocellular part
    autonomic part
supraoptic nucleus
medial mammillary nucleus
suprachiasmatic nucleus
medial preoptic area
periventricular nucleus
ventromedial hypothalamic nucleus
subfornical organ
organum vasculosum of the lamina
    terminalis
ventrolateral medulla
solitary nucleus
pontomedullary reticular formation
raphe nuclei
pineal gland
medial forebrain bundle
dorsolateral tegmentum

fornix
mammillothalamic tract
autonomic nervous system
    parasympathetic division (brain
        stem; S2–S4)
    sympathetic division (T1–L2)
    enteric nervous system
intermediolateral nucleus
preganglionic neuron
postganglionic neuron
peripheral ganglia
lateral medullary syndrome
Horner's syndrome
    ipsilateral miosis
    pseudoptosis
    decreased sweating and
        vasodilation of ipsilateral
        face

Selected Readings

Appenzeller, O. 1986. Clinical Autonomic Failure: Practical Concepts. Amsterdam: Elsevier.

Dodd, J., and Role, L. W. 1991. The autonomic nervous system. In Kandel, E. R., Schwartz, J. H., and Jessell, T. M. (eds.), Principles of Neural Science, 3rd ed. New York: Elsevier, pp. 761–775.

Gershon, M. 1981. The enteric nervous system. Annu. Rev. Neurosci. 4:227–272.

Kupferman, I. 1991. Hypothalamus and limbic system: Peptidergic neurons, homeostasis, and emotional behavior. In Kandel, E. R., Schwartz, J. H., and Jessell, T. M. (eds.), Principles of Neural Science, 3rd ed. New York: Elsevier, pp. 735–749.

Kupferman, I. 1991. Hypothalamus and limbic system: Motivation. In Kandel, E. R., Schwartz, J. H., and Jessell, T. M. (eds.), Principles of Neural Science, 3rd ed. New York: Elsevier, pp. 750–760.

Nauta, W. J. H., and Haymaker, W. 1969. Hypothalamic nuclei and fiber connections. In Haymaker, W., Anderson, E., and Nauta, W. J. H. (eds.), The Hypothalamus. Springfield, Ill.: Charles C. Thomas, pp. 136–209.

Silverman, A. J., and Zimmerman, E. A. 1983. Magnocellular neurosecretory system. Annu. Rev. Neurosci. 6:357–380.

Swaab, D. F., and Hofman, M. A. 1995. Sexual differentiation of the human hypothalamus in relation to gender and sexual orientation. Trends Neurosci. 18:264–270.

Swanson, L. W. 1986. Organization of mammalian neuroendocrine system. In Bloom, F. E. (ed.), Intrinsic Regulatory Systems of the Brain. Bethesda, Md.: American Physiological Society, pp. 317–363.

Swanson, L. W., and Mogenson, G. J. 1981. Neural mechanisms for the functional coupling of autonomic, endocrine and somatomotor responses in adaptive behavior. Brain Res. Rev. 3:1–34.

Swanson, L. W., and Sawchencko, P. E. 1983. Hypothalamic integration: Organization of the paraventricular and supraoptic nuclei. Annu. Rev. Neurosci. 6:269:324.

References

Cechetto, D. F., and Saper, C. B. 1988. Neurochemical organization of the hypothalamic projection to the spinal cord in the rat. J. Comp. Neurol. 272:579–604.

Clarke, W. E. LeGros. 1938. Morphological aspects of the hypothalamus. In Clark, W. E. LeGros, Beattie, J., Riddoch, G., et al. (eds.), The Hypothalamus: Morphological, Functional, Clinical and Surgical Aspects. Edinburgh: Oliver & Boyd, pp. 2–68.

Holstege, G. 1987. Some anatomical observations on the projections from the hypothalamus to brainstem and spinal cord: An HRP and autoradiographic tracing study in the cat. J. Comp. Neurol. 260:98–126.

Lechan, R. M., Nestler, J. L., and Jacobson, S. 1982. The tuberoinfundibular system of the rat as demonstrated by immunohistochemical localization of retrogradely transported wheat germ agglutinin (WGA) from the median eminence. Brain Res. 245:1–15.

Loewy, A. D., Saper, C. B., and Yamondis, N. D. 1978. Re-evaluation of the efferent projections of the Edinger–Westphal nucleus in the cat. Brain Res. 141:153–159.

Nathan, P. W., and Smith, R. C. 1986. The location of descending fibres to sympathetic neurons supplying the eye and sudomotor neurons supplying the head and neck. J. Neurol. Neurosurg. Psych. 49:187–194.

Saper, C. B. 1985. Organization of cerebral cortical afferent systems in the rat. II. Hypothalamocortical projections. J. Comp. Neurol. 237:21–46.

Saper, C. B. 1990. Hypothalamus. In Paxinos, G. (ed.), The Human Nervous System. San Diego: Academic Press, pp. 389–413.

Saper, C. B., Loewy, A. D., Swanson, L. W., and Cowan, W. M. 1976. Direct hypothalamo-autonomic connections. Brain Res. 117:305–312.

Sartor, K. 1992. MR Imaging of the Skull and Brain. Berlin: Springer.

Schmidt, R. F., and Thews, G. (eds.) 1983. Human Physiology. Berlin: Springer.

Swanson, L. W., and Kuypers, H. G. J. M. 1980. The paraventricular nucleus of the hypothalamus: Cytoarchitectonic subdivisions and organization of projections to the pituitary, dorsal vagal complex, and spinal cord as demonstrated by retrograde fluorescence double-labeling methods. J. Comp. Neurol. 1984:555–570.

Veazey, R. B., Amaral, D. G., and Cowan, M. W. 1982. The morphology and connections of the posterior hypothalamus in the cynomolgus monkey (Macaca fascicularis). II. Efferent connections. J. Comp. Neurol. 207:135–156.

Watson, R. E. Jr., Hoffmann, G. E., and Wiegand, S. J. 1986. Sexually dimorphic opioid distribution in the preoptic area: Manipulation by gonadal steroids. Brain Res. 398:157–163.

15

The Limbic System

FROM A HISTORICAL PERSPECTIVE, KNOWLEDGE of the regional anatomy of the cerebral hemisphere has helped us understand the anatomical substrates of emotion, learning, and memory. In the 19th century, the French neurologist Pierre Paul Broca first noted that C-shaped structures on the medial brain surface played an important role in emotions. As we saw in the early chapters, these structures include the hippocampal formation and amygdala, as well as the cingulate and parahippocampal gyri. Broca named this region **le grande lobe limbique** (*limbus* is Latin for "border") because these structures encircled the diencephalon and thus bordered the cerebral cortex.

Also during the 19th century, the German neuroanatomist, Alois Alzheimer had recognized characteristic pathologic changes in the brain that were associated with dementia. These changes were most notable in the hippocampal formation. Thus, during this period the groundwork was laid implicating structures of the limbic lobe in diverse brain functions, such as thoughts, memories, and aspects of our personality.

It was not until 1937, however, that James Papez, a neuroanatomist at Cornell University, suggested that a complex set of specific connections between structures of the limbic lobe formed an anatomical circuit for emotion, much like neural circuits for sensory or motor function. In post mortem examination of the brains of victims of psychiatric disease, Papez noted degenerative changes in such structures as the hippocampus and the mammillary bodies as well as the thalamus and cingulate cortex. He proposed that these diverse telencephalic and diencephalic structures were linked by a set of unidirectional connections. As the cortical structures were thought to be important in subjective emotional experience, subcortical limbic system structures, such as the hypothalamus (see Chapter 14) and amygdala, were thought to mediate their behavioral expression. While modern research suggests a role in learning, memory, and cognition for many of the structures Papez identified—in particular the hippocampal formation—his idea marshaled in a new era of research on the emotional systems of the brain.

In this chapter we will examine the structure and connections of the brain regions collectively termed the limbic system. These regions include diverse portions of the cerebral hemispheres, diencephalon, and midbrain (Table 15–1). The function of these structures are key to normal human behavior. Who we are—our memories, our unique personality, our thoughts—in large measure are determined by the functions of the diverse brain regions that comprise the limbic system. Indeed, dysfunction of many of these structures is implicated in virtually all psychiatric disease.

We first consider the components of the limbic system in relation to their generalized functions and interconnections. We focus on the neural systems thought to be important for emotions, learning, and memory. Later in this chapter we examine limbic system components in relation to their spatial interrelations.

■ FUNCTIONAL ANATOMY OF THE LIMBIC SYSTEM

The limbic system has tremendous anatomical and functional diversity (Table 15–1, page 454), so much so that modern research is shaping a view of multiple distinct circuits involved in separate, but overlapping, functions. There are two key subcortical structures, the **hippocampal formation** and the **amygdala**, and each forms distinct circuits with the rest of the brain. Hippocampal circuits are made with diverse telencephalic and diencephalic structures; these circuits are essential for consolidating short-term memory into long-term memory and for spatial memory. Amygdalar circuits appear to be preferentially involved in emotions and their overt behavioral expressions, such as rage. These circuits ultimately influence the effector systems of the brain: the neuroendocrine, autonomic regulatory, and somatic motor systems. The functions of amygdalar circuits are therefore **similar to the functions originally proposed for the entire limbic system.**

There is, however, considerable overlap in the functions of the amygdala and hippocampal formation and the other structures they engage. Many of the limbic system components, including many of the other structures listed in Table 15–1 (page 454), work together in a more general and integrative way in **cognition.**

An even greater diversity of limbic system function is appreciated when we consider that there is a striking, and largely inexplicable, association between limbic system structures and processing of chemical signals for olfaction. As we saw in Chapter 8, the olfactory bulb projects directly to a component of the **amygdala** and to the **piriform cortex**, part of the limbic association cortex. In fact, various components of the limbic system are often referred to as the **rhinencephalon**, or "nose brain." Projections from the olfactory bulb are a major input to the limbic system of many mammals, for example, rodents and carnivores. In these creatures, much of what is termed emotional behavior, for example, fear or sexual behavior, is strongly affected by olfactory cues, or pheromones, released by members of the species. In nonhuman primates, the input to limbic system structures appears to be dominated not by olfactory signals but rather by connections from association areas of the cerebral cortex. It is also perplexing that whales and other cetaceans do not have a sense of smell; they are anosmic, yet their brains have a well-developed limbic system.

Components of the Limbic System Are C-shaped

The major telencephalic components of the limbic system form a C-shaped configuration, similar to that of the caudate nucleus, a part of the basal ganglia (see Chapter 11). A C shape results from the extensive development of the forebrain (see Chapter 2). The **C-shaped telencephalic**

components of the limbic system are: (1) the limbic association cortex (Figures 15–1 and 15–2); (2) the hippocampal formation together with its efferent pathway, the fornix (Figure 15–3); and (3) part of the amygdala and one of its output pathways, the stria terminalis (see Figure 15–6). These three sets of structures have connections with other telencephalic parts of the limbic system—including the septal nuclei and ventral striatum—as well as the diencephalon and midbrain (see Table 15–1, page 454).

The Limbic Association Cortex Is Located on the Medial Surface of the Frontal, Parietal, and Temporal Lobes

There are three major association areas of the cortex: (1) parietal temporal occipital area, (2) prefrontal association cortex, and (3) limbic association cortex. The limbic association cortex receives information primarily from higher-order sensory areas and from the two other association cortical areas. Then the limbic association cortex conveys this information to the hippocampal formation and the amygdala. The information that the amygdala and hippocampal formation receive from the cortex is not the same, however. The modality of sensory information projecting to the amygdala is preserved. This allows the amygdala to link particular stimuli, like seeing an object, with particular emotions. On the other hand, the hippocampal formation receives integrated sensory information from mul-

Figure 15–1. Midsagittal view of the right cerebral hemisphere, with brain stem removed. The limbic association cortex is indicated by the dotted regions.

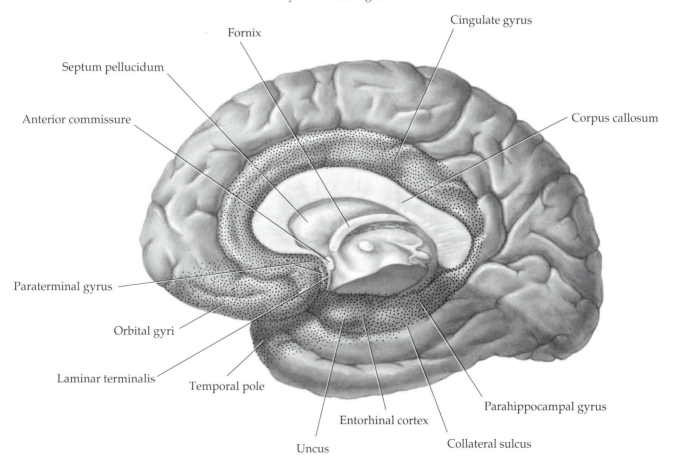

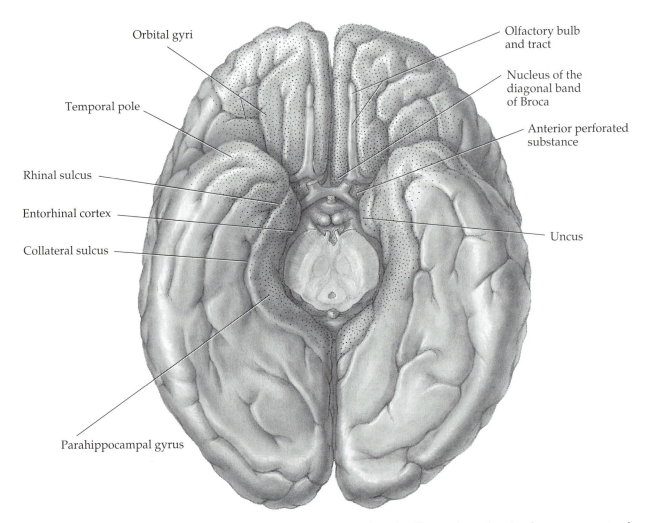

Figure 15–2. Ventral surface of cerebral hemisphere showing key components of the limbic association cortex (dotted area) as well as other basal forebrain structures.

tiple sensory modalities. This integrated information is thought to reflect more complex features of the environment, such as spatial relationships. For example, when we see a snake we may become threatened and fearful. Visual pathways through the ventral portion of the temporal lobe, or the **ventral stream for object vision** (see Figure 6–19B), convey information about the snake to the amygdala. The amygdala uses this information to organize our response, both the emotions we feel and our overt behavior, to this potential danger. The hippocampal formation is thought to be important in learning the complex environmental setting, or context, in which the snake was seen.

The limbic association cortex consists of morphologically and functionally diverse regions on four sets of gyri on the medial and orbital surfaces of the cerebral hemisphere (Figures 15–1 and 15–2): the cingulate gyrus, the parahippocampal gyrus, the medial orbital gyri, and the gyri of the temporal pole. Together, the **cingulate and parahippocampal gyri** form a ring of cortex that partially encircles the corpus callosum, diencephalon, and midbrain (Figure 15–1). The **cingulum** (or cingulum bundle) is a collection of axons that courses in the white matter deep within

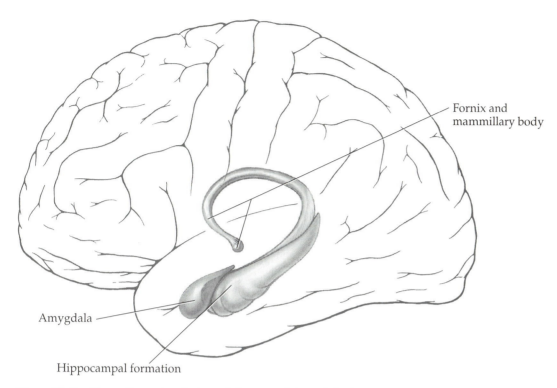

Fornix and
mammillary body

Amygdala

Hippocampal formation

Figure 15–3. Three-dimensional view of the amygdala and the hippocampal formation. The fornix, which is the output pathway of the hippocampal formation, is also illustrated as well as a target to which it projects, the mammillary body.

the cingulate and parahippocampal gyri. Cortical association fibers course in the cingulum and terminate in the parahippocampal gyrus.

Rostral to this cortical ring are the **medial orbital gyri of the frontal lobe** and the cortex of the **temporal pole**. On the ventral brain surface (Figure 15–2), the lateral boundary of the limbic association cortex corresponds approximately to the **collateral sulcus**. Most of the limbic association cortex is either allocortex or neocortex that is morphologically distinct from that located on the lateral surface of the cerebral hemisphere (see Figure 3–15).   .

The Hippocampal Formation Plays a Role in Memory Consolidation

The second C-shaped component of the limbic system is the **hippocampal formation** and its efferent pathway, the **fornix** (Figure 15–3). The first important insights into the function of the hippocampal formation were obtained by studying the behavior of patients whose medial temporal lobe had been ablated to ameliorate the symptoms of temporal lobe epilepsy. In one of the most extensively examined cases, a patient, "H.M.," had this region removed bilaterally. After surgery, H.M. lost the capacity for consolidating **short-term memory** into long-term memory, but retained the memory of events that occurred before the lesion. This loss is attributable to a lesion of the hippocampal formation, a common site of damage in other patients who had undergone similar operations.

On the medial brain surface, the hippocampal formation and fornix form a concentric ring that is within the limbic association cortex and sur-

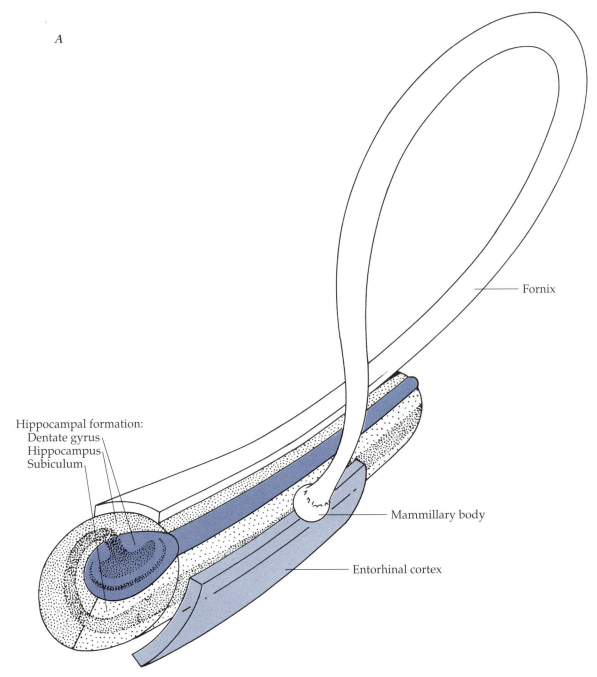

A

Hippocampal formation:
Dentate gyrus
Hippocampus
Subiculum

Fornix

Mammillary body

Entorhinal cortex

Figure 15–4. Schematic views of the hippocampal formation and fornix. *A.* The general spatial relations of components of the hippocampal formation, its efferent pathway (fornix), and the entorhinal cortex. *B.* Simplified serial circuit from entorhinal cortex to the hippocampal formation. Two outputs are shown: the fornix, which has a major projection to the septal nucleus and mamillary body, and the projection back to entorhinal cortex.

rounds the diencephalon and midbrain (Figures 15–1 and 15–3). Although the hippocampal formation typically is considered a subcortical structure because it is located beneath the medial surface of the temporal lobe, it is comprised of primitive **archicortex** (see below).

The **hippocampal formation** consists of three components, each with distinctive morphologies and connections (Figure 15–4; Table 15–1 on page 454): the **subiculum**, the **hippocampus** proper, and the **dentate gyrus**. (The

B

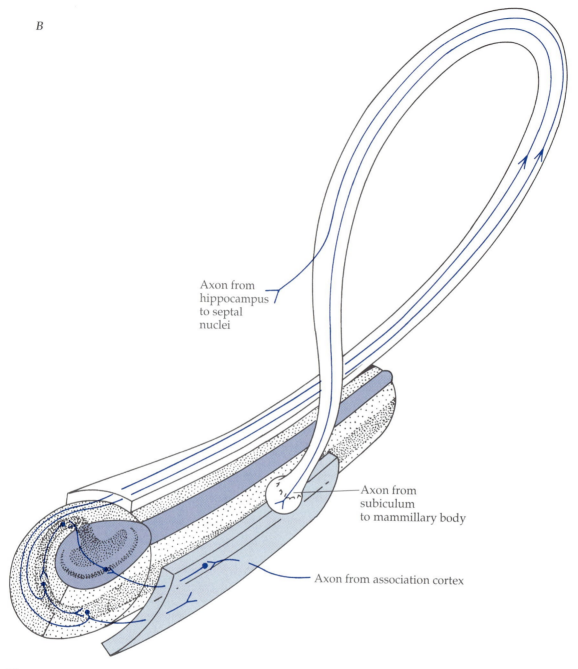

Axon from hippocampus to septal nuclei

Axon from subiculum to mammillary body

Axon from association cortex

Figure 15–4.   (continued)

nomenclature of the hippocampal formation is variable and exactly which components are included in this term may differ depending on the source.) The three hippocampal formation components are roughly organized as strips running rostrocaudally within the temporal lobe that together form a cylinder (Figure 15–4A). We will see below that during development (see Figure 15–14) these strips fold upon one another in a complex manner to assume their mature configuration, which resembles a "jelly-roll" pastry.

Table 15–1. Components of the limbic system.

Major brain division	Structure	Component part
Cerebral hemisphere (telencephalon)	Limbic association cortex	Orbito-frontal Cingulate Entorhinal Temporal pole
	Hippocampal formation	Hippocampus (Ammon's horn) Subiculum Dentate gyrus
	Amygdaloid complex	Corticomedial Basolateral Central nucleus[1]
	Ventral striatum	Nucleus accumbens Olfactory tubercle Ventromedial caudate and putamen
Diencephalon	Thalamus	Anterior nucleus Medial dorsal nucleus Midtine nuclei
	Hypothalamus	Mammillary nuclei Ventromedial nucleus Lateral hypothalamic area
	Epithalamus[2]	Habenula
Midbrain	Portions of the periaqueductal gray matter and reticular formation	

[1]the bed nucleus of stria terminalis is largely included within the division of the central nucleus.

[2]In addition to the two major divisions of the diencephalon, there is a third division that includes the pineal gland, located along the midline, and the bilaterally paired habenula nuclei.

The hippocampal formation receives its major input from a portion of the **limbic association cortex** termed the **entorhinal cortex** (Figures 15–1 and 15–4B). This region, located on the parahippocampal gyrus adjacent to the hippocampal formation, collects information from other parts of the limbic association cortex as well as other association areas (Figure 15–5A).

The output neurons of the hippocampal formation are pyramidal neurons, and they are located in the hippocampus and subiculum. (The projection of the dentate gyrus is entirely within the hippocampal formation.) Pyramidal neurons have axon collaterals that collect on the surface of the hippocampal formation. Eventually these axons form a compact fiber bundle, the **fornix** (Figure 15–4), that projects to other subcortical telencephalic and diencephalic structures. Two output systems can be distinguished, one from the hippocampus and the other from the subiculum. Although these systems are involved in the cognitive aspects of learning and memory, it is not yet understood how their functions differ.

From the subiculum, axons synapse in the **mammillary bodies** of the hypothalamus (Figure 15–5B). This projection completes an anatomical loop: Via the **mammillothalamic tract**, the mammillary body projects to the **anterior nuclei of the thalamus**, which, in turn, project to the **cingulate**

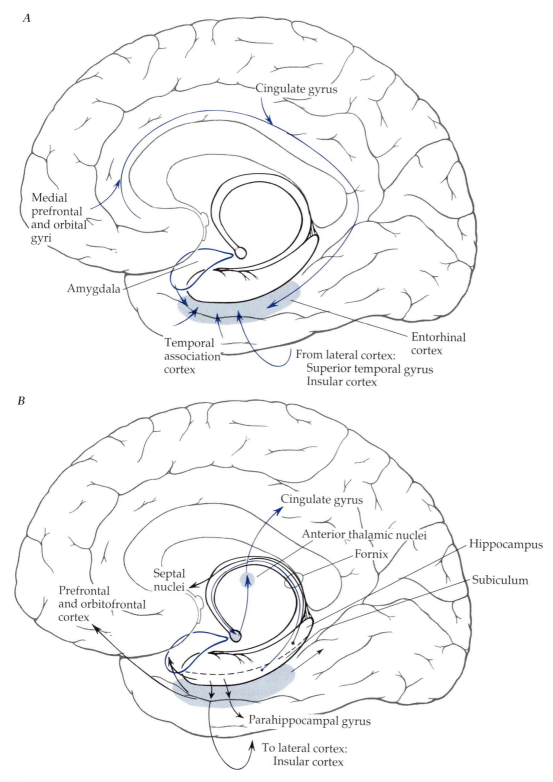

A

Cingulate gyrus

Medial prefrontal and orbital gyri

Amygdala

Temporal association cortex

From lateral cortex: Superior temporal gyrus Insular cortex

Entorhinal cortex

B

Cingulate gyrus

Anterior thalamic nuclei

Fornix

Hippocampus

Septal nuclei

Subiculum

Prefrontal and orbitofrontal cortex

Parahippocampal gyrus

To lateral cortex: Insular cortex

Figure 15–5. Principal afferent connections *(A)* and efferent projections *(B)* of the hippocampal formation. Inputs from cingulate gyrus and other association areas of the cerebral cortex are transmitted to the hippocampal formation from the entorhinal cortex. Efferent projections from the subiculum and hippocampus to the rostral diencephalon and telencephalon are located in the fornix.

gyrus (Figure 15–5B). The cingulate gyrus is a part of the limbic association cortex, which provides information to the entorhinal cortex; this information is the major input to the hippocampal formation. The pathway from the subiculum to the mammillary body and back to the cingulate gyrus is the circuit postulated by Papez to play an important role in emotion. It is now known that the circuit named in his honor is part of a complex network of **bidirectional connections** and that many components of this network play a more important role in **memory** than emotions. For example, profound memory loss is a key sign of **Korsakoff's syndrome**. In this condition, believed to result from thiamin deficiency accompanying alcoholism, the mammillary bodies as well as portions of the medial thalamus are destroyed.

From the hippocampus, axons synapse in the **septal nuclei**, located more rostrally in the forebrain (Figure 15–5B). Little is known of the function of septal nuclei in humans. In a fascinating series of experiments in the early 1950s, it was discovered that laboratory rats, when given the choice of receiving either electrical stimulation of the septal nuclei or food and water, preferred the electrical stimulation! Investigators reasoned that this region is a "pleasure center" that likely plays an important role in consummatory behaviors, such as reproductive behaviors or feeding. The septal nuclei give rise to a cholinergic (see Figure 3–17) and a GABAergic projection, via the fornix, back to the hippocampal formation. This septal projection is important in regulating hippocampal activity during certain active behavorial states.

The fornix is an extremely large tract, with over one million heavily myelinated axons on each side. This number is comparable to the number of myelinated axons in one medullary pyramid or an optic nerve. Despite its size, a major target of axons of the fornix is the ipsilateral mammillary body, whose output is also highly focused, on the **anterior thalamic nuclei**. This raises the question: How can the hippocampal formation, with such a focused subcortical projection, have a generalized role in memory? One answer is that the fornix is not the only major output of the hippocampal formation. The subiculum also projects back to the entorhinal cortex, which, in turn, has diverse efferent corticocortical connections to the prefrontal cortex, orbitofrontal cortex, parahippocampal gyrus, cingulate gyrus, and insular cortex (Figure 15–5B). Collectively, these cortical areas also have widespread projections. Because the entorhinal cortex has widespread projections to cortical association areas, the hippocampal formation can influence diverse regions of the temporal, parietal, and frontal lobes. The divergence in the cortical output of the hippocampal formation parallels the widespread convergence of its inputs, also via the entorhinal cortex, from association areas.

Despite our knowledge of such connections and circuitry, we have little insight into the specific functions of the hippocampal formation. The intrinsic circuitry of the hippocampal formation is considered in Box 15–1. Although we know that the strength of synaptic connections in parts of this circuit can be modified by neuronal activity, it is not yet understood what information is modified and how this synaptic plasticity helps the hippocampus consolidate short-term into long-term memory.

The Amygdaloid Nuclear Complex Contains Three Major Functional Divisions

The amygdaloid complex (or simply termed **amygdala**) is a collection of morphologically, histochemically, and functionally diverse nuclei.

Located largely within the rostral temporal lobe (Figure 15–3), the main portion of the amygdala is almond-shaped (*amygdala* is Greek for "almond"). One of its output pathways, however, the **stria terminalis**, and one of its component nuclei, the **bed nucleus of the stria terminalis**, are C-shaped (Figure 15–6). Axons of the other output path of the amygdala, the **ventral amygdalofugal pathway**, take a somewhat more direct route to their targets.

The amygdala is key to our emotional experiences. What stimuli we respond to, how our overt responses to these stimuli are organized, as well as the internal responses of our body's organs, are all dependent on this subcortical structure. Following damage to the amygdala in nonhuman primates, threatening objects no longer elicit fear, or food is no longer distinguished from nonfood items. Conversely, electrical stimulation of the intact amygdala, depending on the particular site, evokes diverse visceral and defense reactions in carnivores.

The numerous nuclei of the amygdala can be divided into three principal groups (Figure 15–6): basolateral, central, and corticomedial. Each group has different connections and functions.

The Basolateral Nuclei Are Reciprocally Connected With the Cerebral Cortex

The **basolateral nuclei** (Figure 15–6A) comprise the largest division of the amygdala in the primate brain. These nuclei are thought to play a key role in attaching emotional significance to a stimulus. The basolateral nuclei receive information about the modality and particular characteristics of a stimulus from higher-order sensory cortical areas in the temporal and insular cortex and from association cortex. There are four major outputs of the basolateral nuclei: the cortex, basal nucleus (of Meynert), thalamus, and the central amygdala nucleus. The major efferent connections are directed back to the cerebral cortex, either directly or indirectly. The cortical areas receiving a direct projection from the basolateral amygdala include: limbic association cortex (cingulate gyrus, temporal pole, medial orbitofrontal cortex) and the prefrontal cortex. The amygdala also projects directly to allocortex of the **hippocampal formation,** which is thought to be important in learning the emotional significance of complex stimuli, or the context in which emotionally charged stimuli are experienced. In addition, the basolateral division has extensive subcortical projections that give rise to indirect connections to the cortex. Via the **ventral amygdalofugal pathway,** the basolateral amygdala projects to the thalamic relay nucleus for association areas in the frontal lobe, the **medial dorsal nucleus**. It also has a major projection to cholinergic forebrain neurons located in the **basal nucleus** (of Meynert), which itself has widespread cortical projections (see next section below and Figure 3–17A). Neurons of the basolateral nuclei also project to the central amygdala nucleus (see below), which is important in mediating behavioral responses to emotional stimuli.

The Central Nucleus Projects to Brain Stem and Spinal Autonomic Nuclei

The **central nucleus** (Figure 15–6B) is key to mediating our emotional responses. In regulating the autonomic nervous system, the central nucleus receives viscerosensory input from brain stem nuclei, in particular the **solitary nucleus** and the **parabrachial nucleus** (see Chapter 8). In turn, the central nucleus projects via the **ventral amygdalofugal pathway** to the **dorsal**

A Basolateral nuclei

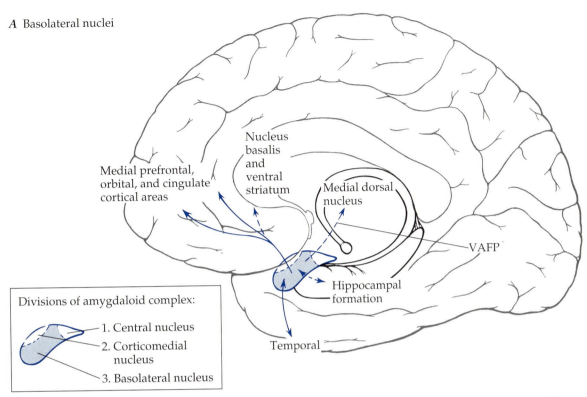

Divisions of amygdaloid complex:

1. Central nucleus
2. Corticomedial nucleus
3. Basolateral nucleus

Figure 15–6. Principal connections of the amygdaloid complex. The inset shows schematically the three divisions of the amygdaloid complex. *A.* The basolateral nuclei are reciprocally connected with the cortex of the temporal lobe, including higher-order sensory areas and association cortex. The basolateral amygdala also projects to the medial dorsal nucleus of the thalamus, basal nucleus, and the ventral striatum. *B.* The central nucleus receives input from the brain stem, especially visceral afferent relay nuclei (solitary nucleus and parabrachial nucleus). The targets of its efferent projections include the hypothalamus and autonomic nuclei in the brain stem. *C.* The corticomedial nuclei have reciprocal connections with the olfactory bulb and efferent projections via the stria terminalis to the ventromedial nucleus of the hypothalamus.

motor nucleus of the vagus as well as other brain stem parasympathetic nuclei and nearby portions of the reticular formation. The central nucleus also regulates the autonomic nervous system through hypothalamic projections (see Chapter 14). As we saw above, the central nucleus receives an input from the basolateral nucleus. This path brings sensory information to the central nucleus to help shape our responses to emotional stimuli.

The Corticomedial Nuclei Are Reciprocally Connected With Olfactory Structures

As we saw in Chapter 8, the corticomedial nuclei receive olfactory information from the olfactory bulb (Figure 15–6C). Although the piriform cortex is thought to be important in olfactory perception, in animals, the corticomedial nuclei are thought to play a role in behaviors that are triggered by olfactory stimuli, such as sexual responses. The corticomedial division also projects to the **ventromedial nucleus** of the hypothalamus, predominantly via the **stria terminalis**. The ventromedial nucleus mediates diverse functions associated with appetitive behaviors, such as eating. The corticomedial division may transmit important information about

B Central Nuclei

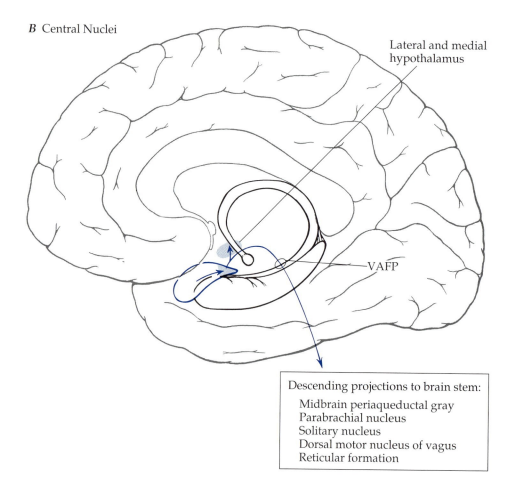

Lateral and medial
hypothalamus

VAFP

Descending projections to brain stem:
Midbrain periaqueductal gray
Parabrachial nucleus
Solitary nucleus
Dorsal motor nucleus of vagus
Reticular formation

C Corticomedial nuclei

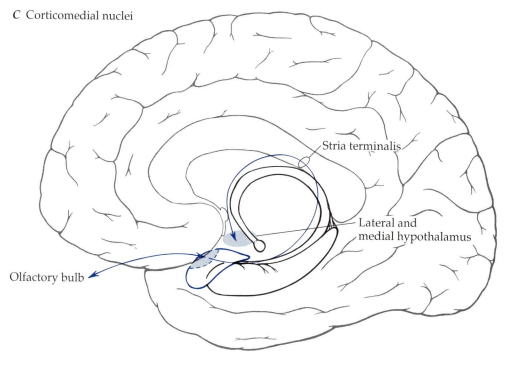

Stria terminalis

Lateral and
medial hypothalamus

Olfactory bulb

Figure 15–6. (continued)

how foods smell to portions of the hypothalamus directly involved in regulating food intake. Hence, a pleasant food aroma stimulates the appetite, whereas an unpleasant odor quells it.

There Are Connections Between Components of the Limbic System and the Effector Systems

The limbic system is difficult to study, in part because of the bewilderingly large number of interconnections between its many structures. When we studied the motor systems, we also noted rich interconnections. These interconnections reflected the many capabilities of motor control that humans and animals possess. For example, the projection of primary motor cortex to the cervical spinal cord steers reaching movements, whereas the projections to the reticular formation are thought to regulate balance and postural changes during limb movement.

What might be the function of the myriad interconnections within the limbic system? Many of the connections of the limbic system relate to the behavioral expression of emotions. Complex polysynaptic pathways ultimately link limbic system structures with the **three effector systems for the behavioral expression of emotion**: the endocrine, autonomic, and somatic motor systems (Figure 15–7).

Paths by which the limbic system may influence pituitary hormone secretion involve indirect connections between the amygdala and the periventricular hypothalamus. One such path, for example, involves the projection from the corticomedial amygdala to the ventromedial nucleus (Figure 15–7A). This nucleus, in turn, projects to a key component of the parvocellular neurosecretory system, the **arcuate nucleus** (see Chapter 14).

The visceral consequences of emotions are mediated by direct and indirect connections to nuclei of the autonomic nervous system. As we saw above, the central amygdaloid nucleus projects directly to brain stem and spinal autonomic centers (Figure 15–7B). The amygdala also affects autonomic function indirectly, through projections to the hypothalamus. Connections with the **lateral hypothalamus** influence autonomic function through various mechanisms, including neural circuits of the reticular formation and other parts of the hypothalamus. Recall that the hypothalamus, including part of the paraventricular nucleus and the lateral hypothalamus, gives rise to descending pathways that regulate autonomic function (see Figure 14–9).

Most of the overt behavioral signs of emotion, such as *flight or fight* reactions, are mediated by the actions of the limbic system on the **somatic motor systems**, especially the reticulospinal tracts. For example, there are direct (and indirect) projections from the hippocampus, septal nuclei, and amygdala to the lateral hypothalamus, which, in turn, can influence the reticulospinal system (Figure 15–7C). These connections may be important in triggering stereotypic defensive reactions. Experimental studies in animals have also shown that the periaqueductal gray matter mediates motor behaviors that are typical of particular species, such as growling and hissing in carnivores. The periaqueductal gray matter receives inputs from the central amygdala nucleus as well as the hypothalamus. The limbic system can also influence somatic motor functions in more complex and behaviorally flexible ways through the **limbic loop of the basal ganglia,** which includes the ventral striatum, ventral pallidum, and the thalamic medial dorsal nucleus. Cortical inputs to this loop derive from the limbic association areas and the hippocampal formation. As noted in Chapter 11, the

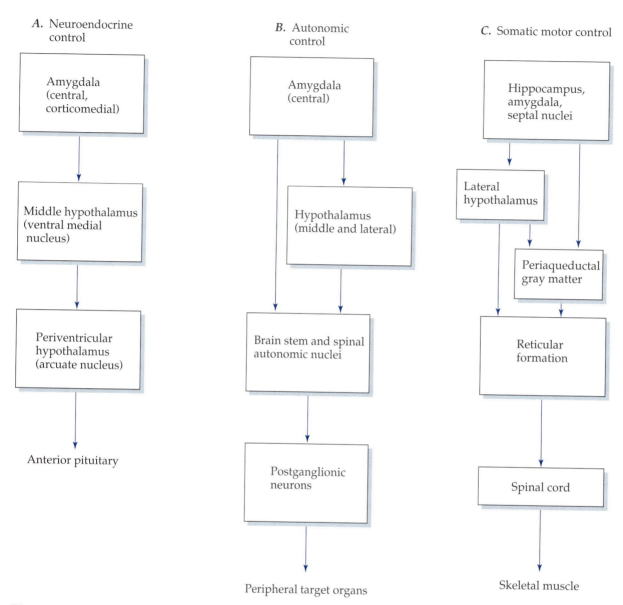

Figure 15–7. Relations between the limbic system and effector systems. *A.* Neuroendocrine control is mediated by the amygdala via the periventricular hypothalamus. *B.* Autonomic control is mediated by both the amygdala and the lateral hypothalamus, via descending pathways that originate from the central nucleus of the amygdala and the middle and lateral hypothalamus. *C.* Somatic motor control is mediated by relatively direct projections to the reticular formation, for stereotypic behaviors, and through more complex telencephalic and diencephalic circuitry (not shown), for more flexible control.

output of the limbic loop is to the limbic association areas of the frontal lobe (see Figure 11–3).

All Major Neurotransmitter Regulatory Systems Have Projections to the Limbic System

Whereas most brain regions receive an innervation by one or more of the major neurotransmitter regulatory systems (see Chapter 3; Figure

3–17), the innervation of the limbic system appears to be particularly important for normal thoughts, moods, and behaviors. We draw this conclusion because many of the drugs used to treat psychiatric illness, the disorders of thought and mood, affect selectively one of the neurotransmitter systems. These neurotransmitter systems have direct and widespread connections with the limbic system.

- The **midbrain dopaminergic** projections originate from the **ventral tegmental area** and the **substantia nigra pars compacta** (see Figure 15–17). Coursing through the **medial forebrain bundle** and **nigrostriatal tract**, the dopaminergic fibers synapse on neurons in the: prefrontal association area, limbic association cortex in the medial frontal lobe, cingulate gyrus, striatum, amygdala, and hippocampal formation. Many antipsychotic drugs are dopamine receptor blockers, and excessive dopamine transmission in limbic structures may contribute to schizophrenia.
- **Serotonergic** projections to limbic system structures of the telencephalon and diencephalon originate from the **dorsal and median raphe nucleus** (see Figure 15–17). Coursing within three tracts—medial forebrain bundle, dorsal longitudinal fasciculus, and medial longitudinal fasciculus—the ascending serotonergic projection synapses on neurons in the amygdala, hippocampal formation, striatum, and cerebral cortex. Drugs that block serotonin reuptake mechanisms are effective in treating mood disorders, including anxiety and obsessive–compulsive disorders.
- The **noradrenergic** projection, which originates from the **locus ceruleus** (see Figure 15–17), influences the entire cerebral cortex, including the limbic association areas, as well as limbic and other subcortical structures. This system, together with the serotonergic system, may play a role in depression.
- The **cholinergic** projection originates from large neurons located near the ventral telencephalic surface. The neurons are found in the **basal nucleus**, the **medial septal nucleus**, and the **nucleus of the diagonal band** (of Broca) (see Figure 15–9). There are additional cholinergic cell groups with widespread cortical projections in the brain stem near the **pedunculopontine tegmental nucleus** (see Figure 15–17) and lateral hypothalamus. Targets of this projection include the entire neocortex (including the limbic association cortex), the amygdala, and the hippocampal formation. Alzheimer's disease, characterized by progressive dementia, begins with a loss of these basal forebrain cholinergic neurons. As the disease progresses, other neurotransmitter systems are also affected.

■ **REGIONAL ANATOMY**

Knowing the three-dimensional configuration of individual limbic system structures is essential for understanding their location in two-dimensional slices. As noted earlier in this chapter, three components of the limbic system have a C shape: (1) the limbic association cortex, especially the cingulate and parahippocampal gyri (Figures 15–1 and 15–2); (2) the hippocampal formation and its output pathway, the fornix (Figure 15–3); and (3) part of the amygdala and one of its pathways, the stria terminalis (Figures 15–3 and 15–6). As a consequence of their C shape, a

coronal section through the cerebral hemisphere may transect these structures twice: first **dorsally** and then **ventrally**. In horizontal sections, C-shaped structures are located rostrally and caudally (see Figure 15–13).

The Nucleus Accumbens and Olfactory Tubercle Comprise Part of the Basal Forebrain

Sections through the rostral forebrain cut through components of the limbic loop of the basal ganglia. The input side of the loop (see Figure 11–3) is the **ventral striatum,** consisting of the **nucleus accumbens**, the olfactory tubercles, and the ventromedial parts of the caudate nucleus and putamen (Figure 15–8). The ventral striatum receives information from all of the nuclear groups of the amygdala as well as from the hippocampal formation and limbic association cortex. The output nucleus of the limbic loop is the **ventral pallidum**, which, in turn, projects to parts of the **medial dorsal nucleus** of the thalamus (see Figure 15–11B) and from there to the **limbic association cortex** (medial orbitofrontal and anterior cingulate cortex). The ventral striatum also has direct projections to the amygdala. Recall that the dorsal parts of the striatum are important in skeletal motor and oculomotor functions and cognition. Their outputs are focused on the internal and external segments of the globus pallidus and the substantia nigra pars reticulata.

Other than receiving olfactory input from the olfactory tract, little is known of the functions of the **olfactory tubercle**. The olfactory tubercle corresponds to the region of the **anterior perforated substance** (see Atlas, Figure AI–3). This is where penetrating branches of the middle and anterior cerebral arteries (the lenticulostriate arteries) enter the basal brain surface to supply parts of the basal ganglia and internal capsule. This slice in Figure 15–8 also cuts through the most anterior portions of the cingulate and parahippocampal gyri.

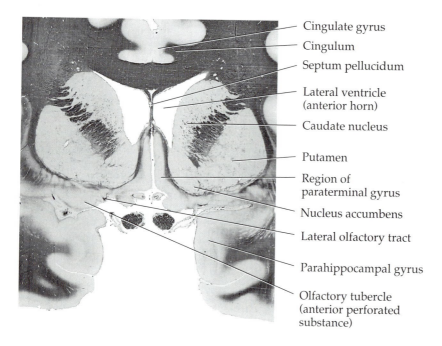

Cingulate gyrus

Cingulum

Septum pellucidum

Lateral ventricle (anterior horn)

Caudate nucleus

Putamen

Region of paraterminal gyrus

Nucleus accumbens

Lateral olfactory tract

Parahippocampal gyrus

Olfactory tubercle (anterior perforated substance)

Figure 15–8. Myelin-stained coronal section through the rostral forebrain.

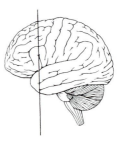

Basal Forebrain Cholinergic Systems Have Diffuse Limbic and Neocortical Projections

The septal nuclei are found adjacent to the **septum pellucidum** (Figures 15–9 and 15–10), a nonneural structure that separates the anterior horns of the lateral ventricles of the two cerebral hemispheres. Animal studies have revealed that the **septal nuclei** (Figure 15–9) consist of separate medial and lateral components. In the human the lateral septal nucleus may correspond to neurons located near the ventricular surface whereas the medial septal nucleus corresponds to those near the septum pellucidum. Moreover, these medial cells are continuous with the gray matter on the medial surface of the cerebral hemisphere, just rostral to the lamina terminalis (see Chapter 2). This region, termed the **paraterminal gyrus**, merges with the nucleus of the diagonal band of Broca, which is located on the basal forebrain surface (Figure 15–1; also see Atlas, Figure AII–23).

The lateral septal nucleus is a target of the projection from the hippocampus and subiculum, via the fornix. The medial septal nucleus receives its major input from the lateral septal nucleus, and, in turn, projects:

- via the **fornix**, to the **hippocampal formation**
- via the **medial forebrain bundle**, to the **midbrain**
- via the **stria medullaris**, a tract located in the wall of the third ventricle (see Figure 15–16A), to a portion of the diencephalon termed the **habenula**. (The habenula, located lateral and ventral to the pineal gland [see Atlas, Figure AI–7], is part of a limbic circuit with the midbrain medial dopaminergic and the serotonergic systems [see Figure 15–17].)

As we saw earlier, one of the transmitters used by the medial septal nucleus is **acetylcholine**. In fact, neurons of the medial septal nucleus form a continuous band of large cholinergic neurons with those of the **diagonal band** and, more laterally and caudally, the **basal nucleus** (Figure

Figure 15–9. Myelin-stained coronal section through the septal nuclei, basal nucleus, and amygdaloid complex.

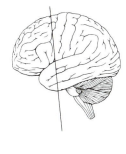

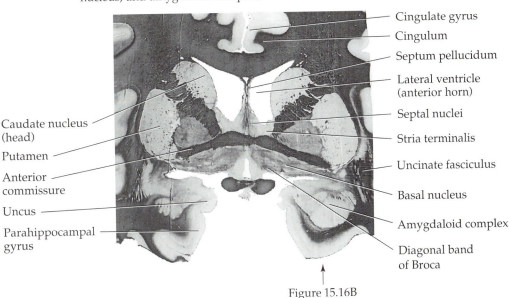

Caudate nucleus (head)

Putamen

Anterior commissure

Uncus

Parahippocampal gyrus

Cingulate gyrus

Cingulum

Septum pellucidum

Lateral ventricle (anterior horn)

Septal nuclei

Stria terminalis

Uncinate fasciculus

Basal nucleus

Amygdaloid complex

Diagonal band of Broca

Figure 15.16B

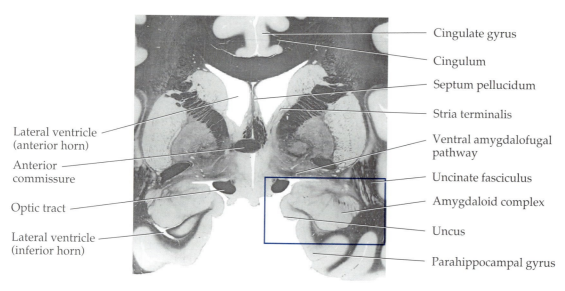

Cingulate gyrus

Cingulum

Septum pellucidum

Stria terminalis

Ventral amygdalofugal pathway

Uncinate fasciculus

Amygdaloid complex

Uncus

Parahippocampal gyrus

Lateral ventricle (anterior horn)

Anterior commissure

Optic tract

Lateral ventricle (inferior horn)

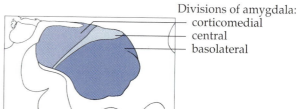

Divisions of amygdala:
corticomedial
central
basolateral

Figure 15–10. Myelin-stained coronal section through the column of fornix and amygdala. The inset shows the approximate location of the nuclear groups in the amygdalar complex.

15–9). The basal nucleus is located within the **substantia innominata**, the region ventral to the anterior commissure and lying on the basal forebrain surface. Still more large cholinergic neurons are dispersed between the lamina of the globus pallidus and putamen and adjacent to the internal capsule.

There is a **mediolateral organization** of the cortical projections from the medial septal nucleus, the nucleus of the diagonal band, and the basal nucleus. The medial portion of this basal forebrain cholinergic cell group (medial septal nucleus, the nucleus of the diagonal band, and the medial part of the basal nucleus) projects to the hippocampal formation through the fornix and to the medial surface of the hemisphere through the **cingulum bundle**. The lateral portion of the cell group (lateral part of the basal nucleus) projects to lateral cortex via the **external capsule**. The basal forebrain cholinergic neurons excite their neocortical and allocortical targets through **muscarinic receptors**; such responses to acetylcholine may facilitate cortical responses to other inputs. These cholinergic neurons, through widespread projections to allocortical and neocortical structures, may also modulate overall cortical excitability.

The Cingulum Courses Beneath the Cingulate and Parahippocampal Gyri

Two cortical limbic areas, the cingulate gyrus and the parahippocampal gyrus, are seen in the series of coronal sections (Figures 15–8 through 15–12): The cingulate gyrus is located dorsally and the parahippocampal gyrus, ventrally. The pathway that connects regions of the

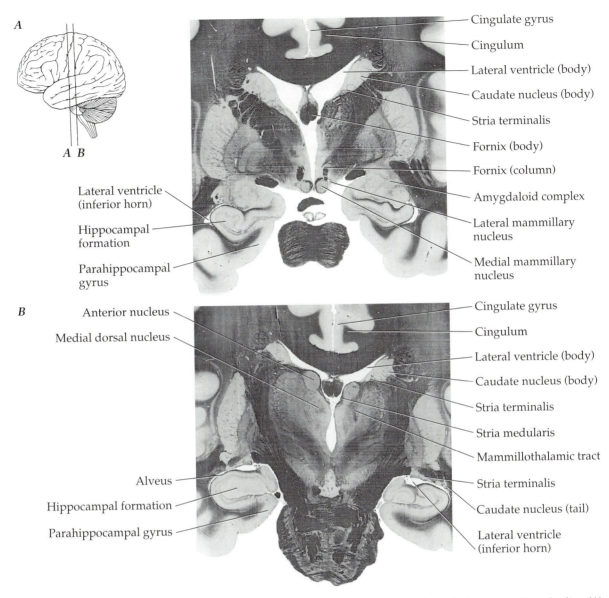

Figure 15–11. Myelin-stained coronal section through the mammillary bodies **(A)** and through the mammillothalamic tract **(B)**. In **B**, the mammillothalamic tract is seen on the right side only, because the section is asymmetric.

orbitofrontal gyri and the cingulate gyrus with the parahippocampal gyrus, including the **entorhinal cortex**, is termed the **cingulum**. This path is located beneath the cingulate gyrus (Figure 15–11). Unlike the cingulum, another limbic system cortical association pathway, the **uncinate fasciculus** (Figures 15–9 and 15–10), has a more direct (i.e., not C-shaped) trajectory for interconnecting anterior portions of the temporal lobe with medial orbital gyri of the frontal lobe.

The Three Nuclear Divisions of the Amygdala Are Revealed in Coronal Section

The amygdala is located in the rostral temporal lobe deep to the parahippocampal gyrus (Figures 15–9, 15–10, and 15–11A). The amygdala

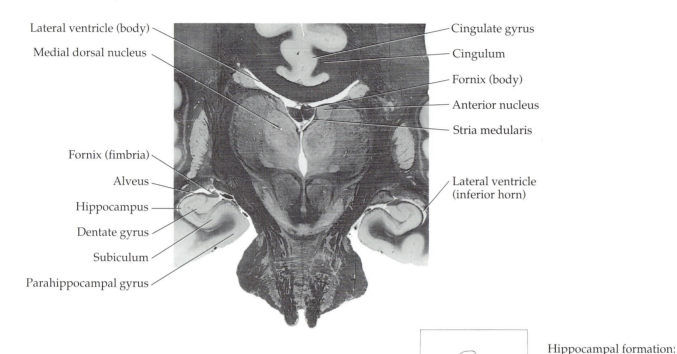

Lateral ventricle (body)
Medial dorsal nucleus
Fornix (fimbria)
Alveus
Hippocampus
Dentate gyrus
Subiculum
Parahippocampal gyrus

Cingulate gyrus
Cingulum
Fornix (body)
Anterior nucleus
Stria medularis
Lateral ventricle (inferior horn)

Hippocampal formation:
Dentate gyrus
Hippocampus
Subiculum

Figure 15–12. Myelin-stained coronal section through the medial dorsal nucleus of the thalamus. The divisions of the hippocampal formation are shown.

is rostral and slightly dorsal to the hippocampal formation. (Compare the parasagittal section in Figure 15–16B with the drawing in Figure 15–3.) The laterally placed arrow in Figure 15–9 shows the approximate plane of section in Figure 15–16B. The amygdala, together with the rostral hippocampal formation, form the uncus (Figures 15–1, 15–2, and 15–10). Expanding space-occupying lesions above the cerebellar tentorium (see Figure 4–14), especially those of the temporal lobe, may cause the uncus to become displaced medially. This **uncal herniation** compresses midbrain structures, ultimately resulting in coma and even death. Initially uncal herniation can compress the oculomotor nerves, which exit from the ventral midbrain surface. This results in third nerve dysfunction (palsy).

The three divisions of the amygdala are schematically depicted in the inset to Figure 15–10. The **corticomedial** division of the amygdala merges with the overlying cortex of the medial temporal lobe. This division receives a major input directly from the **olfactory bulb**. The two other nuclear divisions, **basolateral** and **central**, are also shown. The **bed nucleus of the stria terminalis** is the C-shaped nuclear component of the amygdala. It has connections with brain stem autonomic and visceroafferent nuclei and thus is similar to the central nuclear group. A portion of the bed nucleus of the stria terminalis is thought to be sexually dimorphic.

The Stria Terminalis and the Ventral Amygdalofugal Pathway Are the Two Output Pathways of the Amygdala

The **stria terminalis** carries output from the amygdala, predominantly from the corticomedial nuclei. In coronal section (Figures 15–9 through 15–11), the stria terminalis is found medial to the caudate nucleus

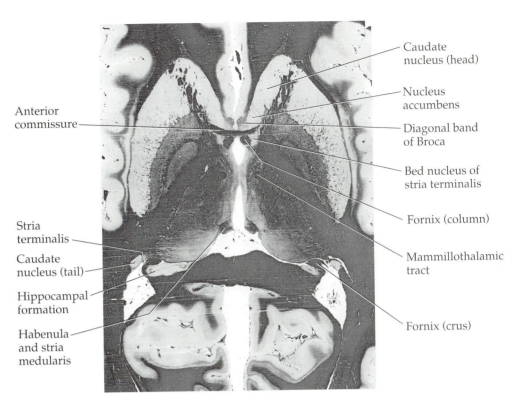

Anterior commissure

Caudate nucleus (head)

Nucleus accumbens

Diagonal band of Broca

Bed nucleus of stria terminalis

Fornix (column)

Mammillothalamic tract

Stria terminalis

Caudate nucleus (tail)

Hippocampal formation

Habenula and stria medularis

Fornix (crus)

Figure 15–13. Myelin-stained horizontal section through the anterior commissure.

in the roof of the inferior horn of the lateral ventricle and the floor of the body and anterior horn of the lateral ventricle. In the horizontal section (Figure 15–13), it is located rostrally (where the bed nucleus is more prominent) and caudally (where the stria is more prominent) rather than dorsally and ventrally.

The stria terminalis and its bed nucleus have a C shape, following that of the lateral ventricle and the caudate nucleus. These limbic system structures lie in a shallow groove formed at the junction of the thalamus and the caudate nucleus, termed the terminal sulcus. Running along with the stria terminalis and bed nucleus is the **thalamostriate vein** (or terminal vein), which drains portions of the thalamus and caudate nucleus. The stria terminalis does not stain darkly because its axons are not heavily myelinated. A major target of the axons running in the stria terminalis is the **ventral medial nucleus of the hypothalamus**, important in feeding.

The other efferent path of the amygdala, the **ventral amygdalofugal pathway** (Figure 15–10), runs ventral to the anterior commissure and globus pallidus (see Chapter 11). The projections of the central and basolateral nuclei course primarily in this efferent pathway. There are three major targets of the ventral pathway:

- The **medial dorsal nucleus** of the thalamus (Figures 15–11B and 15–12) links the basolateral amygdala indirectly with the prefrontal and orbitofrontal cortex.
- The **basal forebrain**, including the ventral striatum and the cholinergic neurons of the basal nucleus and nucleus of the diagonal band of Broca, link the amygdala with the cortex indirectly.
- The **brain stem**, which contains parasympathetic preganglionic nuclei, receives a projection from the central nucleus.

The Hippocampal Formation Is Located in the Floor of the Inferior Horn of the Lateral Ventricle

Coronal sections through the temporal lobe, from rostral to caudal, slice first through the amygdala, then through both the amygdala and hippocampal formation and finally through the hippocampal formation alone (see Figures 15–10, 15–11A, and 15–11B for these rostrocaudal relationships). The hippocampal formation forms part of the **floor of the inferior horn of the lateral ventricle**. In coronal section (e.g., Figure 15–12), the hippocampal formation is located ventrally and the fornix, dorsally. In horizontal section (Figure 15–13) the hippocampal formation (which here is quite small) is caudal and the fornix, rostral. In Chapter 2, we saw that early in brain development, the hippocampal formation is located dorsal to the corpus callosum; later, it is as if it were "dragged" into the temporal lobe. The minuscule portion of the hippocampal formation located dorsal to the corpus callosum in the mature brain is termed the indusium gresium (see Atlas, Figure II–16).

During development, the hippocampal formation also undergoes an **infolding into the temporal lobe** (Figure 15–14). The simple sequence of the component parts of the temporal lobe, from the parahippocampal gyrus on the lateral surface to the dentate nucleus on the medial surface, becomes more complex later in development. As the **hippocampal sulcus** forms, the dentate gyrus and the subiculum become apposed; there is actually fusion of the pial surfaces of these two structures through which a hippocampal afferent path (the perforant path) courses (see below).

The Hippocampal Formation Is Archicortex and Has a Laminar Organization

The hippocampal formation is **archicortex**, with three principal cell layers (see Figure 3–15). It should be recalled that archicortex is a type of allocortex and the other type of cortex is neocortex (e.g., primary somatic sensory cortex). Neocortex has at least six cell layers, whereas allocortex is more variable. Parts of the hippocampal formation have a layering pattern that rivals the cerebellum in geometric regularity. As with the cerebellum, know-

Figure 15–14. Schematic of hippocampal formation at two stages of development (*A, B*) and in maturity (*C*). (Adapted from Williams, P. L., and Warwick, R. 1975. Functional Neuroanatomy of Man. Philadelphia: W. B. Saunders.)

A   *B*   *C*

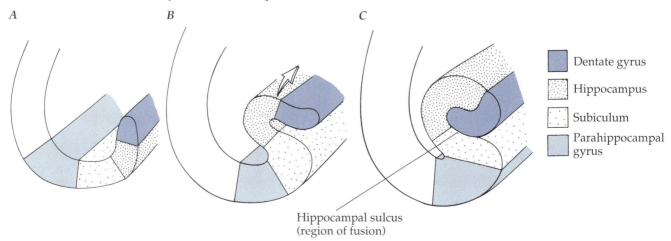

Dentate gyrus

Hippocampus

Subiculum

Parahippocampal gyrus

Hippocampal sulcus (region of fusion)

Box 15–1. *Information Flow Through the Hippocampal Formation*

The dentate gyrus, hippocampus, and subiculum are separate processing stages in a sequence of intrinsic connections within the hippocampal formation. The flow of information through the hippocampal formation is largely **unidirectional** (Figure 15–15). The simplest circuit consists of a serial processing chain of four sets of neurons. Input from the entorhinal cortex is first projected to the dentate gyrus (1), which, in turn, projects to neurons in two portions of the hippocampus (2 and 3), and from there to the subiculum (4). This is shown in relation to the three-dimensional organization of these structures in Figure 15–15A.

Knowledge of the cytoarchitecture of the hippocampus is important for understanding its intrinsic connections. The hippocampus has three cytoarchitectonic divisions (Figure 15–15).

These divisions are abbreviated CA for cornus ammonis, or Ammon's horn. (To early anatomists, the hippocampal formation together with the fornix looked like the horns of a ram.) The basic circuitry is superimposed on the cytoarchitecture of the hippocampal formation and entorhinal cortex in the schematic diagram in Figure 15–15B.

Pyramidal cells of the entorhinal cortex send their axons to the dentate gyrus to synapse on granule cells. Granule cell axons, termed **mossy fibers**, synapse on pyramidal cells of the CA3 region of the hippocampal formation, which in turn send their axons (called the **Schaefer collaterals**) to pyramidal cells of the CA1 region. (These axon collaterals spare the CA2 region.) The subiculum receives the next projection in the sequence, from the CA1 region, and it projects back to the entorhinal cortex. This

forms a closed anatomical loop.

A more complex, parallel set of projections from entorhinal cortex has now been identified. In addition to projecting to the dentate gyrus, the entorhinal cortex also has direct projections to the CA1 and CA3 regions of the hippocampus as well as to the subiculum. These parallel paths through the hippocampal formation may carry different kinds of information and thus comprise distinct processing circuits. These serially-ordered and parallel sets of connections within the hippocampal formation are entirely located within discrete rostrocaudal slices (Figure 15–15A). What is the significance of this arrangement? Tracer experiments conducted in animals reveal that inputs to different slices derive from populations of neurons located in different rostrocaudal locations in the entorhinal cortex (Figure 15–15A). These entorhinal neu-

Figure 15–15. Intrinsic hippocampal circuitry. *A.* Schematic three-dimensional view of the hippocampal formation, fornix, and entorhinal cortex. The hippocampal formation and entorhinal cortex are divided into discrete slices to illustrate that intrinsic circuitry is largely within discrete rostrocaudal regions. *B.* Nissl-stained transverse section of human hippocampal formation, parahippocampal gyrus, and ventral temporal lobe. *C.* Schematic diagram of the layers of the hippocampus and subiculum and the circuitry of the hippocampal formation. (*B,* Courtesy of Dr. David Amaral, State University of New York at Stony Brook; *C,* Adapted from Zola-Morgan, S., Squire, L. R., and Amaral, D. G. 1986. Human amnesia and medial temporal lobe region: Enduring memory impairment following a bilateral lesion limited to field CA1 of the hippocampus. J. Neurosci. 6:2950–2967.)

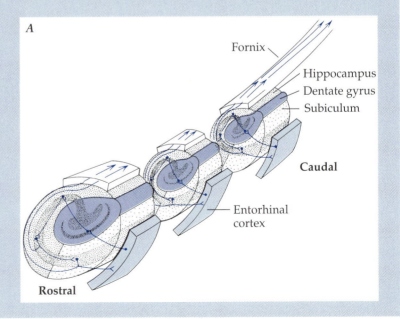

A

Fornix

Hippocampus

Dentate gyrus

Subiculum

Caudal

Entorhinal cortex

Rostral

Box 15–1 (continued)

rons, in turn, receive input from different parts of association cortex. In this way, it is believed that different rostrocaudal circuits in the hippocampal formation operate on different kinds of incoming information.

The functions of a circuit in one slice are linked with those of circuits located in other rostrocaudal slices by **association connections** within the hippocampal formation. Moreover, both sides of the hippocampal formation are interconnected through commissural neurons whose axons course in the ventral portion of the fornix. It is not yet understood how the myriad connections of the entorhinal cortex and hippocampal formation are organized to play a role in memory consolidation, spatial memory, and other aspects of cognition. There is, however, an important clue. It has been shown that the efficacy of many synapses in the hippocampal formation can be modified under various experimental conditions. An important challenge is to identify under which behavioral conditions such plasticity is normally expressed.

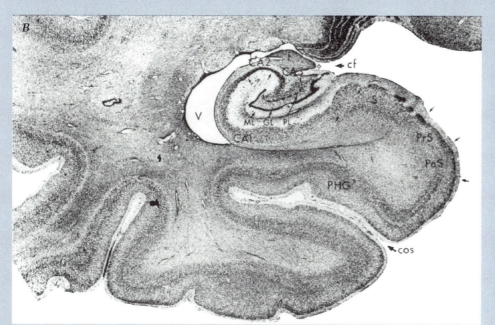

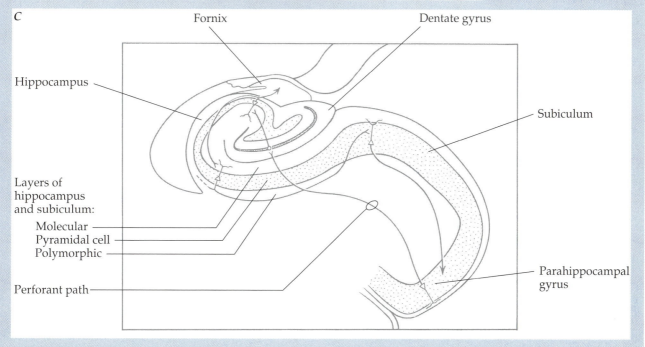

ing hippocampal cytoarchitecture provides insight into its synaptic organization as well as the intrinsic and extrinsic connectivity (see Figure 15–15).

The three divisions of the hippocampal formation—the **dentate gyrus**, **hippocampus**, and **subiculum**—are shown in the inset in Figure 15–12. Each division has three principal cell layers. The dentate gyrus contains the molecular, granule cell, and polymorphic layers. In the molecular layer are the apical dendrites of granule cells and other processes, but few cell bodies. Granule cells, which are the projection neurons of the dentate gyrus, are in the second layer. Their axons synapse on other neurons of the hippocampal formation. The polymorphic layer contains interneurons. The three layers of the hippocampus and subiculum are analogous to those of the dentate gyrus. The important difference is that the granule cell layer is replaced by the pyramidal layer, which contains **pyramidal cells**, the projection neurons of the hippocampus and subiculum. Box 15–1 considers the intrinsic hippocampal circuitry in detail.

Pyramidal cells of the hippocampus and subiculum have extrinsic connections, sending their axons to distant subcortical targets. For example, the mammillary bodies receive a projection from pyramidal cells of the subiculum. These axons course in the fornix; other axons in the fornix terminate in the lateral septal nucleus, anterior thalamic nuclei, amygdala, and nucleus accumbens. The extrinsic projections of the hippocampus also course through the fornix; the major target is the lateral septal nucleus. The subiculum also has extensive projection to the entorhinal cortex (see Box 15–1).

A Sagittal Cut Through the Mammillary Bodies Reveals the Fornix and Mammillothalamic Tract

Structures that have a C shape are oriented approximately in the sagittal plane. The sagittal section in Figure 15–16A is located close to the midline and transects the fornix, although not through its entire length. The sagittal section in Figure 15–16B is located farther laterally and cuts through the long axis of the hippocampal formation.

Pyramidal cell axons of the hippocampus and subiculum form the **alveus** (Figure 15–15B), the myelinated envelope surrounding the hippocampal formation. Alvear axons collect on the medial side of the hippocampal formation to form the first of the four anatomical parts of the fornix, termed the **fimbria**. The other three parts—the **crus** (where the axons are separate from the hippocampal formation), the **body** (where the axons from both sides join at the midline), and the **column** (where axons descend toward their targets)—bring the axons of the fornix to neurons in the diencephalon and rostral telencephalon.

The body and column of the fornix can be seen in Figure 15–16A. Note how the column of the fornix descends **caudal to the anterior commissure** to terminate in the **mammillary body**; this is the **postcommissural fornix** (see also Figure 15–13). As we saw in Chapter 14, the mammillary body is comprised of the medial and lateral mammillary nuclei (Figure 15–11A). Although the fornix terminates in both components, the **mammillothalamic tract** originates only from the medial mammillary nucleus. Axons of the mammillothalamic tract also can be seen leaving the mammillary body in Figure 15–16A. These axons are coursing toward the **anterior thalamic nuclei** (Figure 15–11B). In addition to axons of the mammillothalamic tract, there are also axons that descend from the mammillary bodies to the midbrain and rostral pontine reticular formation. This contingent is termed the **mammillotegmental tract** and originates from the lateral mammillary nucleus (Figure 15–11A).

A

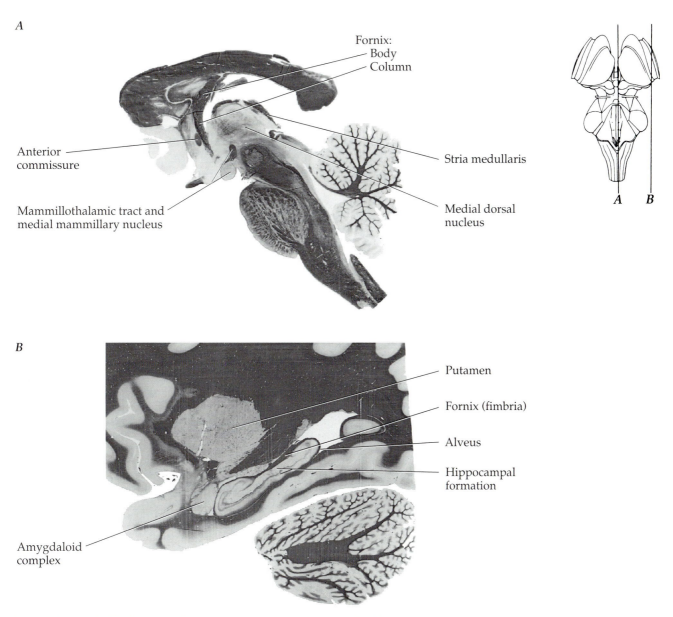

Fornix:
Body
Column

Anterior
commissure

Stria medullaris

Mammillothalamic tract and
medial mammillary nucleus

Medial dorsal
nucleus

A *B*

B

Putamen

Fornix (fimbria)

Alveus

Hippocampal
formation

Amygdaloid
complex

Figure 15–16. *A.* Myelin-stained sagittal section through the cerebral hemisphere, diencephalon, and brain stem close to midline. *B.* A parasagittal section through the amygdaloid complex and hippocampal formation.

Fibers of the fornix also terminate in locations other than the mammillary bodies. For example, some of these fibers terminate directly in the anterior thalamic nuclei. Moreover, rostral to the anterior commissure, the **precommissural fornix**, which is smaller than the postcommissural portion, courses away from the midline. (It cannot be seen in this section.) The precommissural fornix, which contains the axons from both the subiculum and hippocampus, terminates in the lateral septal nucleus. A portion of the **stria medullaris**, which has a predominantly rostrocaudal course, is also revealed in this section (Figure 15–16A). Earlier we saw that the medial septal nucleus sends axons into the stria medullaris. These axons synapse in the habenula (see Figures AI–7 and AII–18).

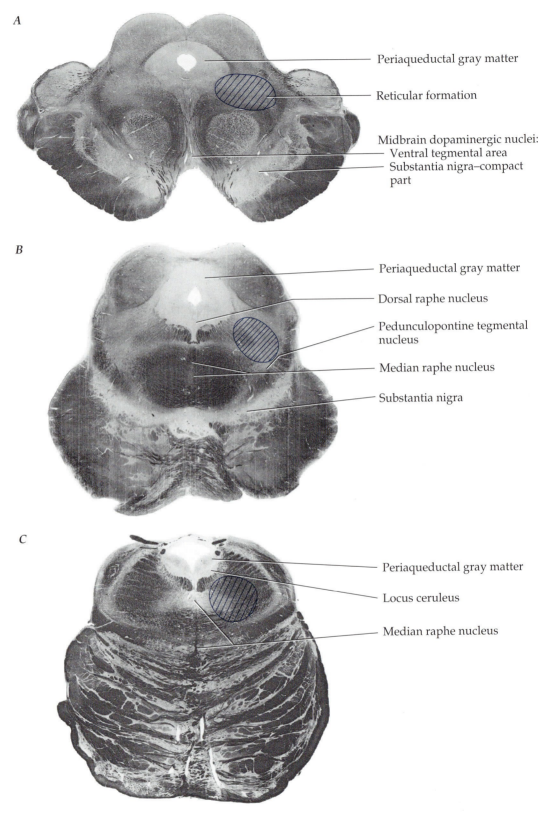

A

Periaqueductal gray matter

Reticular formation

Midbrain dopaminergic nuclei:
Ventral tegmental area
Substantia nigra–compact part

B

Periaqueductal gray matter

Dorsal raphe nucleus

Pedunculopontine tegmental nucleus

Median raphe nucleus

Substantia nigra

C

Periaqueductal gray matter

Locus ceruleus

Median raphe nucleus

Figure 15–17. Components of the brain stem related to the limbic system. Myelin-stained sections through the rostral midbrain *(A)*, caudal midbrain *(B)*, and rostral pons *(C)*. The reticular formation is indicated by hatched regions.

Nuclei in the Brain Stem Link Telencephalic and Diencephalic Limbic Structures With the Autonomic Nervous System and the Spinal Cord

The **limbic midbrain area** is the caudal part of a complex system of connections believed to be important in the behavioral expression of emotions, such as the response of the body to stress, and its reaction to pain, pleasure, and satiety. This area includes the **periaqueductal gray matter** and various nuclei of the **reticular formation** (Figure 15–17). Septal neurons project to the midbrain reticular formation via neurons of the **lateral hypothalamus**. Neurons of the lateral hypothalamus are interspersed throughout the **medial forebrain bundle** (see Chapter 14). From these midbrain regions, the actions of neurons in wide areas of the reticular formation can be modified by the limbic system. The hypothalamus also projects to the periaqueductal gray matter. In Chapter 5, we considered the projection of the periaqueductal gray matter to the raphe nuclei (Figure 15–17), which in turn gives rise to a spinal cord projection for regulating pain transmission.

General Anatomy of the Limbic System

The limbic system comprises a set of structures located predominantly on the **medial surface** of the cerebral hemisphere (Figures 15–1 and 15–2). The diverse functions of the limbic system include important roles in **memory**, **emotion**, **control of visceral functions**, and **olfaction**. Many of the structures have a **C-shaped configuration**. There are three C-shaped components to the limbic system (Figures 15–1 through 15–5): (1) **limbic association cortex**, (2) **hippocampal formation** and **fornix**, and (3) part of the **amygdala** (bed of the stria terminalis) and the **stria terminalis**.

Limbic Association Cortex

The limbic cortical areas include (Figures 15–1 and 15–2): the **medial orbital gyri** of the frontal lobe, the **cingulate gyrus** in the frontal and parietal lobes, the **parahippocampal gyrus** in the temporal lobe, and the cortex of the **temporal pole**. The limbic cortical areas receive input from higher-order sensory areas in the temporal lobe as well as from the **prefrontal association cortex** and the **parietal temporal occipital association area**. The two principal pathways carrying cortical association axons to and from other limbic system structures are the **cingulum** (Figure 15–8) (located beneath the cingulate gyrus, Figure 15–9) and the **uncinate fasciculus** (Figure 15–9). Limbic association cortex has a different cytoarchitecture compared with other cortical regions. The cortex on the external surface of the parahippocampal gyrus lateral to the **collateral sulcus** (Figure 15–2) has at least six layers (**neocortex**), whereas the cortex medial to the sulcus is more variable and typically has fewer than six cell layers (**allocortex**) (Figure 15–12).

Hippocampal Formation

The **hippocampal formation** (Figure 15–3) includes three cytoarchitectonically distinct subdivisions (Figures 15–4 and 15–15): the **dentate gyrus**, the **hippocampus**, and the **subiculum**. Collectively these regions

Summary

constitute the **archicortex**, a type of primitive allocortex. **Memory disorders** are a characteristic feature of hippocampal formation lesions. The limbic association cortex provides the major input to the hippocampal formation. The **entorhinal cortex**, a specific portion of the rostral parahippocampal gyrus, projects directly to the hippocampal formation (Figure 15–5A). Other portions of the limbic association cortex influence the hippocampal formation **indirectly**, via the entorhinal cortex. The dentate gyrus, hippocampus, and subiculum are separate processing stages in a sequence of intrinsic connections in the hippocampal formation (Figures 15–4B and 15–15). The flow of information through the hippocampal formation is largely unidirectional.

Hippocampal efferents originate from the subiculum and the hippocampus proper; the dentate gyrus projects only to the hippocampus. Cortical projections from the subiculum terminate in the entorhinal cortex, and from there information is widely distributed throughout the cerebral cortex. Subcortical projections are via the **fornix**, which has four component parts, from caudal and inferior to rostral (Figures 15–4 and 15–13): **fimbria**, **crus**, **body**, and **column**. Most of the axons in the fornix are those of **pyramidal cells** of the subiculum and hippocampus. Axons from the **subiculum** synapse in the **mammillary body** (Figures 15–5B, 15–11, and 15–16A). These axons course in the postcommissural fornix (Figure 15–13 and 15–16A). The projection to the mammillary body is part of an anatomical loop (**Papez's circuit**): the mammillary bodies project, via the **mammillothalamic tract** (Figures 15–11A and 15–16A), to the **anterior thalamic nuclei** (Figure 15–11B), which in turn project to the **cingulate gyrus** (Figures 15–1, and 15–8 through 15–11). The subiculum also projects to the anterior thalamic nuclei directly. The hippocampus projects, via the precommissural fornix, to the **lateral septal nucleus** (Figures 15–5B and 15–10). The **medial septal nucleus**, which contains cholinergic GABAergic neurons, receives its input from the lateral septal nucleus and projects back to the **hippocampal formation**, via the **fornix**.

Amygdala

There are three major nuclear divisions of the amygdaloid complex (Figures 15–6 and 15–10) which collectively are involved in **emotions and their behavioral expression**, regulating **appetitive** behaviors, control of **visceral function**, and **olfaction** (Figure 15–6). The **basolateral division** (1) receives a major input from the **cerebral cortex** and projects to the **medial dorsal nucleus** of the thalamus, **basal nucleus**, **ventral striatum**, as well as back to the **cortex** (temporal and orbital frontal association areas). The **central nucleus** (2) is reciprocally connected with **visceral sensory** and **visceral motor nuclei** of the brain stem. The **corticomedial division** (3) receives direct olfactory input. This division may play a role in appetitive behaviors through its projection to the **ventromedial nucleus** of the hypothalamus.

The amygdala has two output pathways: (1) the **stria terminalis** (Figures 15–6 and 15–10), which is C-shaped, carries the efferent projection primarily from the **corticomedial division**, and (2) the **ventral amygdalofugal pathway** (Figure 15–10) carries the efferents from the **central nucleus**, which descend to the **brain stem**, and those from the **basolateral nucleus**, which ascends to the **thalamus**, the **ventral striatum**, and the **basal nucleus** (Figure 15–10). The bed nucleus of the stria terminalis runs along with the stria. ■

KEY STRUCTURES AND TERMS

limbic association cortex
  cingulate gyrus
  parahippocampal gyrus
    entorhinal cortex
    medial orbital gyri of the frontal
      lobe
  temporal pole
cingulum
uncinate fasciculus
piriform cortex
paraterminal gyrus
collateral sulcus
limbic loop of the basal ganglia
  ventral striatum
  olfactory tubercle
  ventral pallidum
hippocampal formation
  subiculum
  hippocampus
  dentate gyrus
archicortex
hippocampal sulcus
alveus
fornix
  fimbria
  crus

body
column
postcommissural fornix
precommissural fornix
amygdala
  basolateral nuclei
  central nucleus
  corticomedial nuclei
bed nucleus of the stria terminalis
stria terminalis
anterior commissure
ventral amygdalofugal pathway
septal nuclei
  lateral septal nucleus
  medial septal nucleus
limbic midbrain area
periaqueductal gray matter
reticular formation
habenula
stria medullaris
lateral hypothalamus
medial forebrain bundle
mammillary bodies
mammillothalamic tract
anterior thalamic nuclei
medial dorsal nucleus

septum pellucidum
prefrontal cortex
medial dorsal nucleus
olfactory bulb
ventromedial hypothalamic nucleus
arcuate nucleus
substantia innominata
solitary nucleus
parabrachial nucleus
dorsal motor nucleus of the vagus
intermediolateral nucleus
dopamine
  ventral tegmental area
  substantia nigra pars compacta
serotonin
  dorsal raphe nucleus
norepinephrine
  locus ceruleus
acetylcholine
  basal nucleus
  medial septal nucleus
  nucleus of the diagonal band (of
    Broca)
Korsakoff's syndrome
uncal herniation

Selected Readings

Amaral, D. G. 1987. Memory: Anatomical organization of candidate brain regions. In Plum, R. (ed.), Handbook of Physiology. Section 1: The Nervous System. Vol. V. Higher Functions of the Brain. Bethesda, Md.: American Physiological Society, pp. 211–294.

Amaral, D. G. 1993. Emerging principles of intrinsic hippocampal organization. Curr. Opin. Neurobiol. 3:225–229.

Andersen, N. C. 1988. Brain imaging: Applications in psychiatry. Science 239:1381–1388.

Andreasen, N. C. 1994. The mechanisms of schizophrenia. Curr. Opin. Neurobiol. 4:245–251.

Cleghorn, J. M., Zipursky, R. B., and List, S. J. 1991. Structural and functional brain imaging in schizophrenia. J. Psychiatr. Neurosci. 16:53–74.

Kandel, E. R. 1991. Cellular mechanisms of learning and the biological basis of individuality. In Kandel, E. R., Schwartz, J. H., and Jessell, T. M. (eds.), Principles of Neural Science, 3rd ed. New York: Elsevier, pp. 1009–1031.

Kandel, E. R. 1991. Disorders of thought: Schizophrenia. In Kandel, E. R., Schwartz, J. H., and Jessell, T. M. (eds.), Principles of Neural Science, 3rd ed. New York: Elsevier, pp. 853–868.

Kandel, E. R. 1991. Disorders of mood: Depression, mania, and anxiety disorders. In Kandel, E. R., Schwartz, J. H., and Jessell, T. M. (eds.), Principles of Neural Science, 3rd ed. New York: Elsevier, pp. 869–883.

Kupferman, I. 1991. Hypothalamus and limbic system: Motivation. In Kandel, E. R., Schwartz, J. H., and Jessell, T. M. (eds.), Principles of Neural Science, 3rd ed. New York: Elsevier, pp. 751–760.

Kupferman, I. 1991. Hypothalamus and limbic system: Peptidergic neurons, homeostasis, and emotional behavior. In Kandel, E. R., Schwartz, J. H., and Jessell, T. M. (eds.), Principles of Neural Science, 3rd ed. New York: Elsevier, pp. 736–749.

LeDoux, J. E. 1991. Emotion and the limbic system concept. Concepts in Neuroscience 2:169–199.

LeDoux, J. E. 1994. Emotion, memory and the brain. Scientific American 270:50–57.

Price, J. L., Russchen, F. T., and Amaral D. G. 1987. The limbic region. II: The amygdaloid complex. In Björklund, A., Hökfelt, T., and Swanson, L. W. (eds.), Handbook of Chemical Neuroanatomy. Vol. 5. Integrated Systems of the CNS, Part I. New York: Elsevier, pp. 279–388.

Swanson, L. W., and Mogenson, G. J. 1981. Neural mechanisms for the functional coupling of autonomic, endocrine and somatomotor responses in adaptive behavior. Brain Res. Rev. 3:1–34.

References

Amaral, D. G. 1987. Memory: Anatomical organization of candidate brain regions. In Plum, F. (ed.), Handbook of Physiology, Section 1, Vol. 1, Part 2. Bethesda, Md.: American Physiological Society, pp. 211–294.

Amaral, D. G., and Insausti, R. 1990. Hippocampal formation. In Paxinos, G. (ed.), The Human Nervous System. San Diego: Academic Press, pp. 711–755.

Andy, O. J., and Stephan, H. 1968. The septum of the human brain. J. Comp. Neurol. 133:383–410.

Bietz, A. J. 1990. Central gray. In Paxinos, G. (ed.), The Human Nervous System. San Diego: Academic Press, pp. 307–320.

Carlsen, J., and Heimer, L. 1988. The basolateral amygdaloid complex as a cortical-like structure. Brain Res. 441:377–380.

DeOlmos, J. S. 1990. Amygdala. In Paxinos, G. (ed.), The Human Nervous System. San Diego: Academic Press, p. 583–710.

Duvernoy, H. M. 1988. The Human Hippocampus: An Atlas of Applied Anatomy. Munich: J. F. Bergmann Verlag, p. 166.

Hedren, J. C., Strumble, R. G., Whitehouse, P. J., et al. 1984. Topography of the magnocellular basal forebrain system in the human brain. J. Neuropath. Expt. Neurol. 43:1–21.

Holstege, G. 1990. Subcortical limbic system projections to caudal brainstem and spinal cord. In Paxinos, G. (ed.), The Human Nervous System. San Diego: Academic Press, pp. 261–286.

LeDoux, J. E. 1992. Emotion and the amygdala. In Appleton, J. P. (ed.), The Amygdala: Neurobiological Aspects of Emotion, Memory, and Mental Dysfunction. New York: Wiley-Liss, Inc., pp. 339–351.

Levitt, P. 1984. A monoclonal antibody to limbic system neurons. Science 223:299–301.

Millhouse, O. E., and DeOlmos, J. 1983. Neuronal configurations in lateral and basolateral amygdala. Neurosci. 10:1269–1300.

Naidich, T. P., Daniels, D. L., Haughton, V. M., et al. 1987. Hippocampal formation and related structures of the limbic lobe: Anatomical–MR correlations. Part I. Surface features and coronal sections. Neuroradiology 162:747–754.

Naidich, T. P., Daniels, D. L., Haughton, V. M., et al. 1987. Hippocampal formation and related structure of the limbic lobe: Anatomical–MR correlations. Part II. Sagittal sections. Neuroradiology 162:755–761.

Nauta, W. J. H., and Haymaker, W. 1969. Hypothalamic nuclei and fiber connections. In Haymaker, W., Anderson, E., and Nauta, W. J. H. (eds.), The Hypothalamus. Springfield, Ill.: Charles C Thomas, pp. 136–209.

Nieuwenhuys, R., Voogd, J., and van Huijzen, C. 1988. The Human Central Nervous System: A Synopsis and Atlas, 3rd ed. Berlin: Springer-Verlag.

Papez, J. W. 1937. A proposed mechanism of emotion. Arch. Neurol. Psych. 38:725–743.

Pfefferbaum, A., and Zipursky, R. B. 1991. Neuroimaging in schizophrenia. Schizophrenia Res. 4:193–208.

Price, J. L., and Amaral, D. G. 1981. An autoradiographic study of the projections of the central nucleus of the monkey amygdala. J. Neurosci. 1:1242–1259.

Williams, P. L., and Warwick, R. 1975. Functional Neuroanatomy of Man. Philadelphia: W. B. Saunders.

Zola-Morgan, S., Squire, L. R., and Amaral, D. G. 1986. Human amnesia and the medial temporal region: Enduring memory impairment following a bilateral lesion limited to field CA1 of the hippocampus. J. Neurosci. 6:2950–2967.

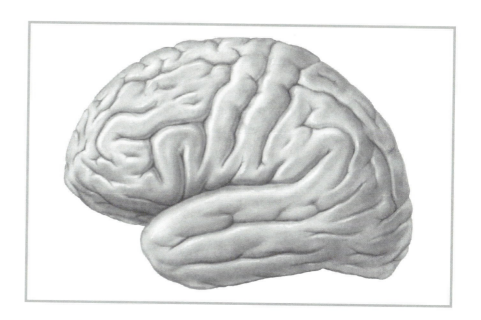

VI

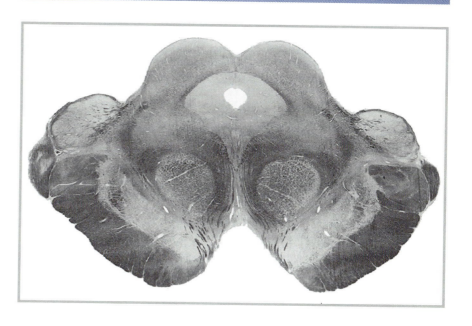

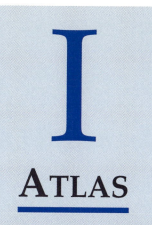

I

ATLAS

Surface Topography of the Central Nervous System

The surface topography atlas is a collection of drawings of the brain and rostral spinal cord. The various views are based on specimens and brain models. Key features are labeled on an accompanying line drawing of each view.

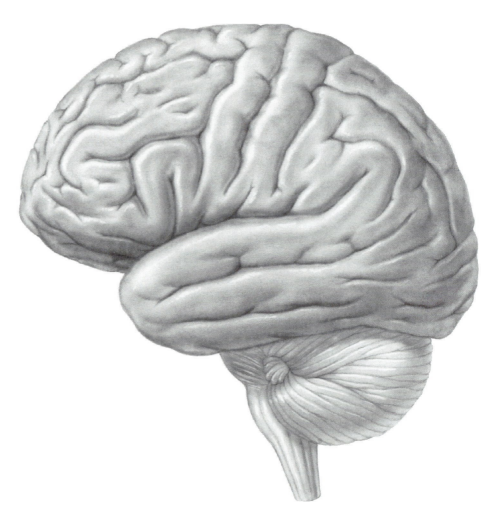

Figure AI–1. Lateral surface of the cerebral hemisphere, brain stem, cerebellum, and rostral spinal cord.

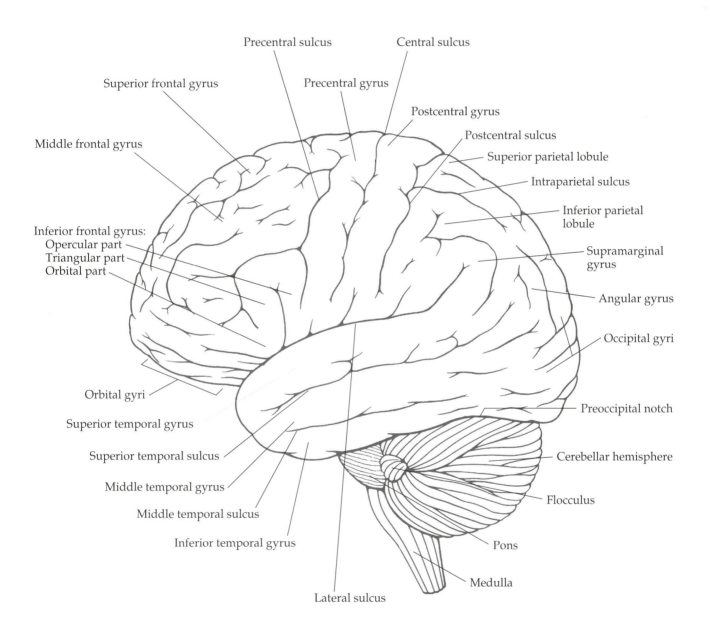

Precentral sulcus

Central sulcus

Superior frontal gyrus

Precentral gyrus

Postcentral gyrus

Middle frontal gyrus

Postcentral sulcus

Superior parietal lobule

Intraparietal sulcus

Inferior parietal lobule

Inferior frontal gyrus:
Opercular part
Triangular part
Orbital part

Supramarginal gyrus

Angular gyrus

Occipital gyri

Orbital gyri

Preoccipital notch

Superior temporal gyrus

Cerebellar hemisphere

Superior temporal sulcus

Flocculus

Middle temporal gyrus

Middle temporal sulcus

Pons

Inferior temporal gyrus

Medulla

Lateral sulcus

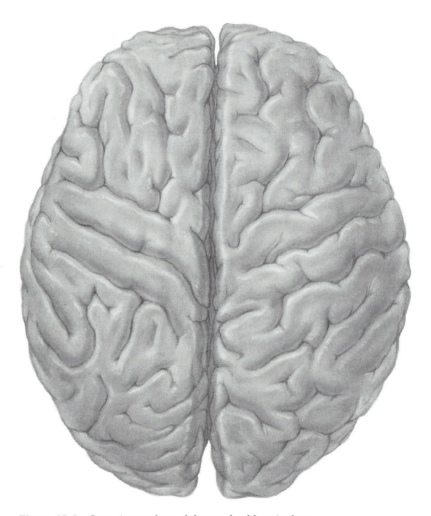

Figure AI–2. Superior surface of the cerebral hemisphere.

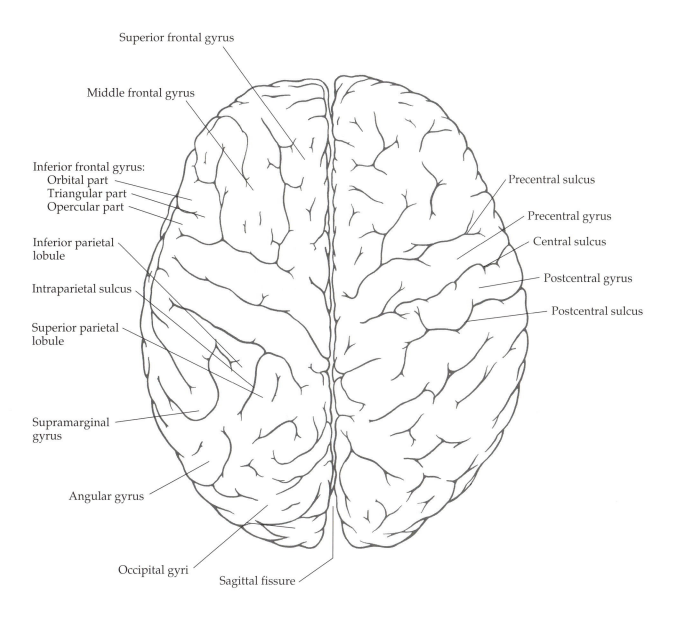

Superior frontal gyrus

Middle frontal gyrus

Inferior frontal gyrus:
Orbital part
Triangular part
Opercular part

Inferior parietal lobule

Intraparietal sulcus

Superior parietal lobule

Supramarginal gyrus

Angular gyrus

Occipital gyri

Sagittal fissure

Precentral sulcus

Precentral gyrus

Central sulcus

Postcentral gyrus

Postcentral sulcus

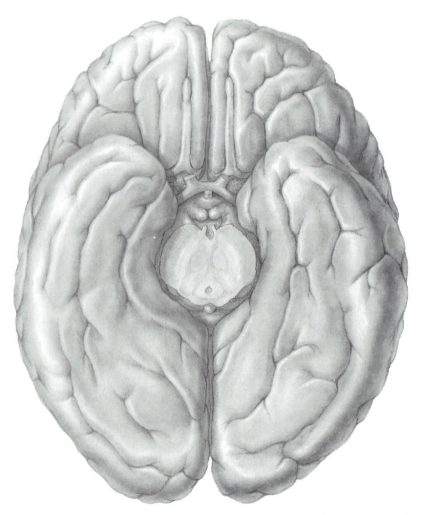

Figure AI–3. Inferior surface of the cerebral hemisphere and diencephalon. The brain stem is transected at the rostral midbrain.

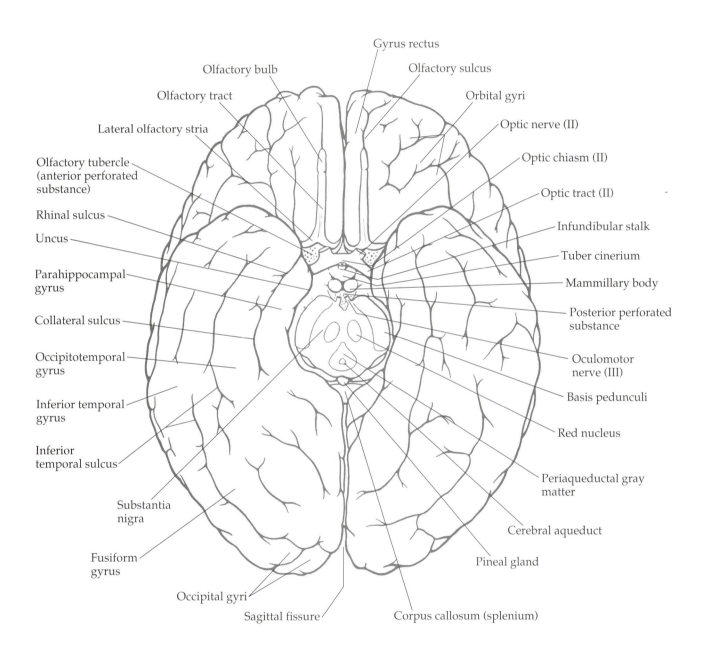

Gyrus rectus

Olfactory bulb

Olfactory tract

Olfactory sulcus

Orbital gyri

Lateral olfactory stria

Optic nerve (II)

Olfactory tubercle
(anterior perforated
substance)

Optic chiasm (II)

Optic tract (II)

Rhinal sulcus

Infundibular stalk

Uncus

Tuber cinerium

Parahippocampal
gyrus

Mammillary body

Collateral sulcus

Posterior perforated
substance

Occipitotemporal
gyrus

Oculomotor
nerve (III)

Inferior temporal
gyrus

Basis pedunculi

Inferior
temporal sulcus

Red nucleus

Substantia
nigra

Periaqueductal gray
matter

Fusiform
gyrus

Cerebral aqueduct

Occipital gyri

Pineal gland

Sagittal fissure

Corpus callosum (splenium)

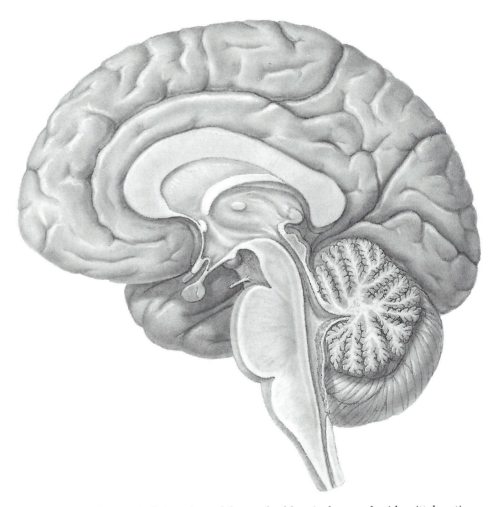

Figure AI–4. Medial surface of the cerebral hemisphere and midsagittal section through the diencephalon, brain stem, cerebellum, and rostral spinal cord.

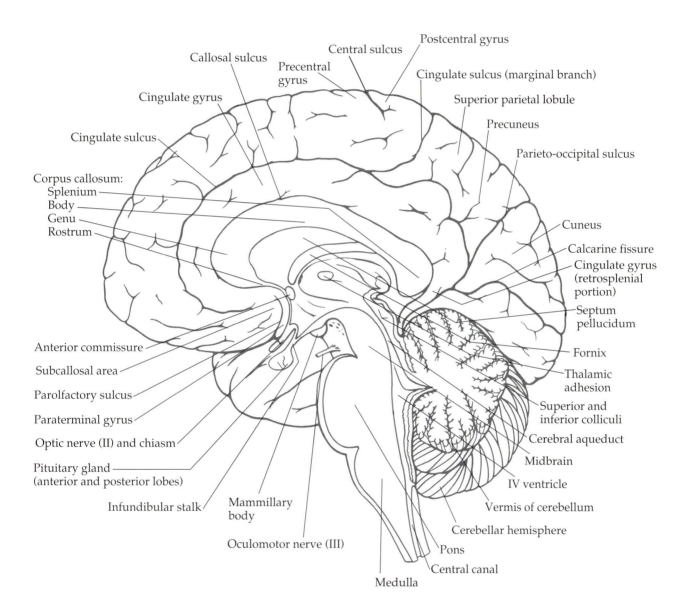

Callosal sulcus

Central sulcus

Postcentral gyrus

Precentral
gyrus

Cingulate sulcus (marginal branch)

Cingulate gyrus

Superior parietal lobule

Precuneus

Cingulate sulcus

Parieto-occipital sulcus

Corpus callosum:
Splenium
Body
Genu
Rostrum

Cuneus

Calcarine fissure

Cingulate gyrus
(retrosplenial
portion)

Septum
pellucidum

Anterior commissure

Fornix

Subcallosal area

Thalamic
adhesion

Parolfactory sulcus

Superior and
inferior colliculi

Paraterminal gyrus

Cerebral aqueduct

Optic nerve (II) and chiasm

Midbrain

Pituitary gland
(anterior and posterior lobes)

IV ventricle

Infundibular stalk

Vermis of cerebellum

Mammillary
body

Cerebellar hemisphere

Oculomotor nerve (III)

Pons

Central canal

Medulla

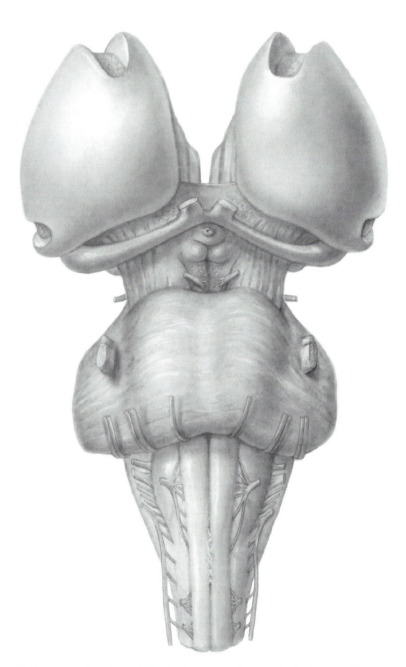

Figure AI–5. Ventral surface of the brain stem and rostral spinal cord. The striatum and diencephalon are also shown.

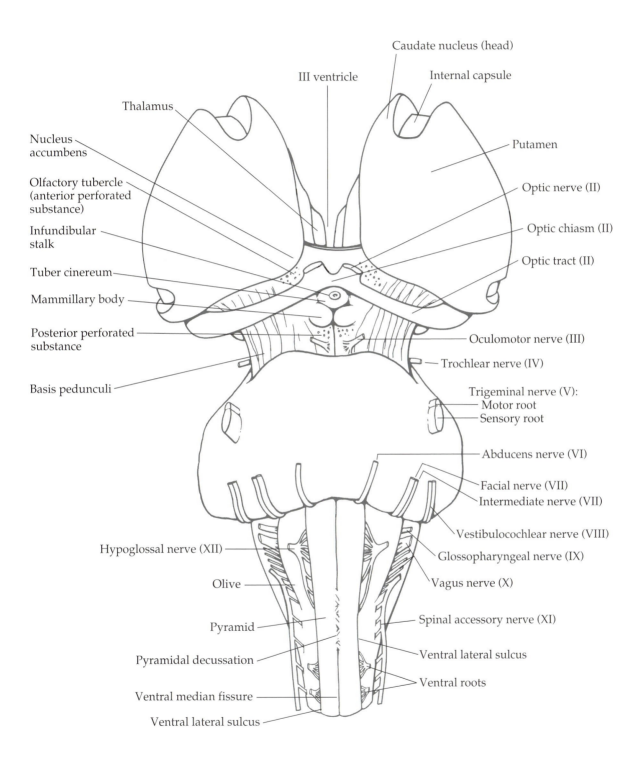

Caudate nucleus (head)

III ventricle

Internal capsule

Thalamus

Nucleus accumbens

Putamen

Olfactory tubercle (anterior perforated substance)

Optic nerve (II)

Infundibular stalk

Optic chiasm (II)

Optic tract (II)

Tuber cinereum

Mammillary body

Posterior perforated substance

Oculomotor nerve (III)

Trochlear nerve (IV)

Basis pedunculi

Trigeminal nerve (V):
Motor root
Sensory root

Abducens nerve (VI)

Facial nerve (VII)
Intermediate nerve (VII)

Vestibulocochlear nerve (VIII)

Hypoglossal nerve (XII)

Glossopharyngeal nerve (IX)

Vagus nerve (X)

Olive

Pyramid

Spinal accessory nerve (XI)

Ventral lateral sulcus

Pyramidal decussation

Ventral roots

Ventral median fissure

Ventral lateral sulcus

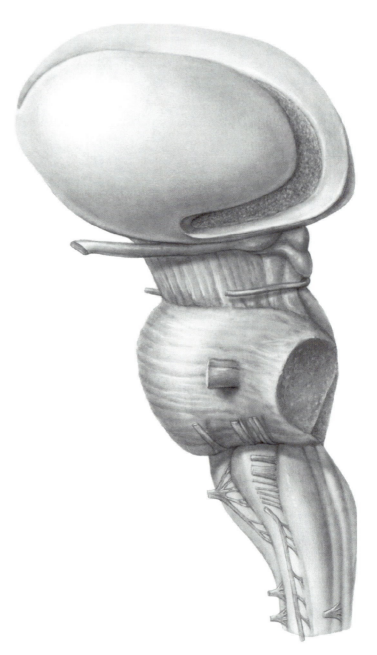

Figure AI–6. Lateral surface of the brain stem and rostral spinal cord. The striatum and diencephalon are also shown.

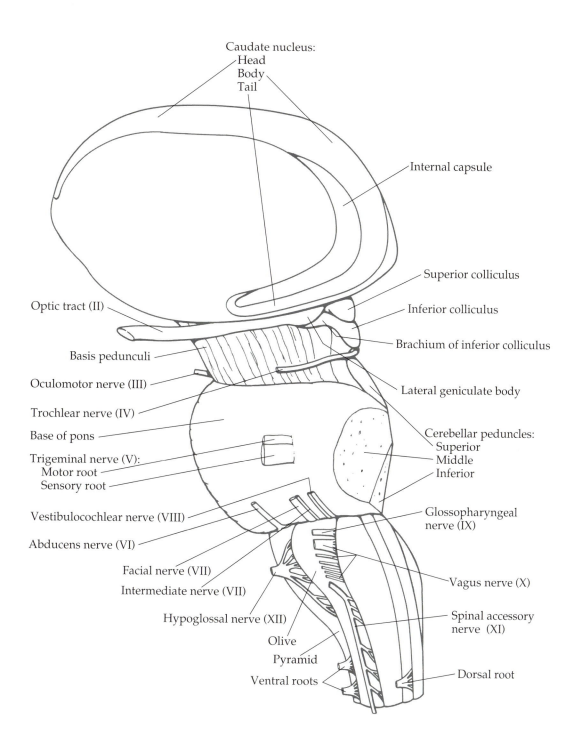

Caudate nucleus:
Head
Body
Tail

Internal capsule

Superior colliculus

Inferior colliculus

Optic tract (II)

Brachium of inferior colliculus

Basis pedunculi

Lateral geniculate body

Oculomotor nerve (III)

Trochlear nerve (IV)

Cerebellar peduncles:
Superior
Middle
Inferior

Base of pons

Trigeminal nerve (V):
Motor root
Sensory root

Vestibulocochlear nerve (VIII)

Glossopharyngeal
nerve (IX)

Abducens nerve (VI)

Facial nerve (VII)

Vagus nerve (X)

Intermediate nerve (VII)

Hypoglossal nerve (XII)

Spinal accessory
nerve (XI)

Olive

Pyramid

Ventral roots

Dorsal root

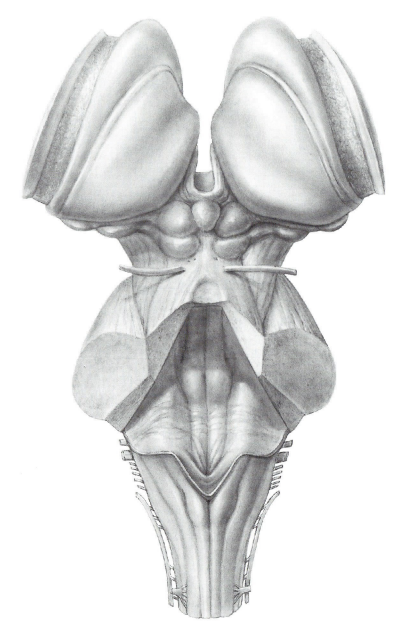

Figure AI–7. Dorsal surface of the brain stem and rostral spinal cord. The striatum and diencephalon are also shown. The cerebellum was removed to reveal the structure of the floor of the fourth ventricle.

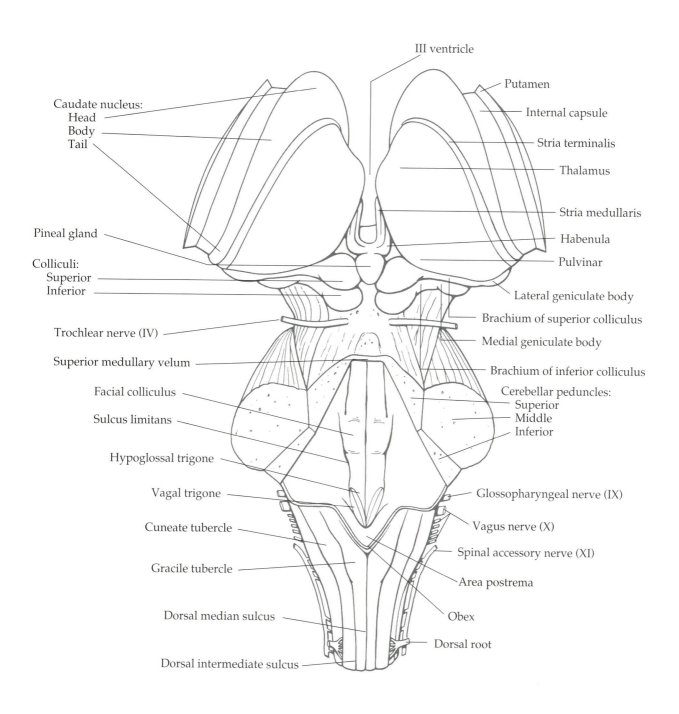

III ventricle

Caudate nucleus:
Head
Body
Tail

Putamen

Internal capsule

Stria terminalis

Thalamus

Pineal gland

Stria medullaris

Habenula

Pulvinar

Colliculi:
Superior
Inferior

Lateral geniculate body

Brachium of superior colliculus

Trochlear nerve (IV)

Medial geniculate body

Superior medullary velum

Brachium of inferior colliculus

Facial colliculus

Cerebellar peduncles:
Superior
Middle
Inferior

Sulcus limitans

Hypoglossal trigone

Vagal trigone

Glossopharyngeal nerve (IX)

Cuneate tubercle

Vagus nerve (X)

Spinal accessory nerve (XI)

Gracile tubercle

Area postrema

Dorsal median sulcus

Obex

Dorsal root

Dorsal intermediate sulcus

References

Braak, H., Braak, E. 1976. Architectonics of the Human Telencephalic Cortex. Berlin: Springer-Verlag.

Carpenter, M. B., and Sutin, J. 1983. Human Neuroanatomy. Baltimore: Williams & Wilkins.

Crosby, E. C., Humphrey, T., and Lauer, E. W. 1962. Correlative Anatomy of the Nervous System. New York: Macmillan.

Ferner, H., and Staubesand, J. 1983. Sobotta Atlas of Human Anatomy. Baltimore: Urban & Schwartzenberg.

Nieuwenhuys, R., Voogd, J., and van Huijzen, Chr. 1988. The Human Central Nervous System, 3rd ed. Berlin: Springer-Verlag.

Williams, P. L., and Warwick, R. 1975. Functional Neuroanatomy of Man. Philadelphia: Saunders.

Zilles, K. 1990. Cortex. In: Paxinos, G. (ed.), The Human Central Nervous System. San Diego: Academic Press.

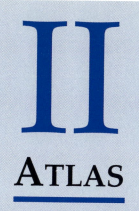

II

ATLAS

Myelin-Stained Sections Through the Central Nervous System

The atlas of myelin-stained sections through the central nervous system is in three planes: *transverse, horizontal*, and *sagittal*. (See Figure 1–13 for schematic views of these planes of sections.) Transverse sections through the cerebral hemispheres and diencephalon are termed *coronal* sections because they are approximately parallel to the coronal suture. These sections also cut the brain stem, but *parallel to its long axis*. In addition, there are three sections cut in planes oblique to the transverse and horizontal sections.

In this atlas, each level through the central nervous system is printed without labeled structures as well as with labels on an accompanying photograph (printed at reduced contrast to preseve the essence of the structure). Typically, the border of a structure is indicated either when the structure's location is extremely important for understanding the functional consequences of brain trauma, or the structure is clearly depicted on the section and it is didactically important to emphasize the border. Axons of cranial nerves and primary afferent fibers are indicated by bold lines to distinguish them from the other fibers.

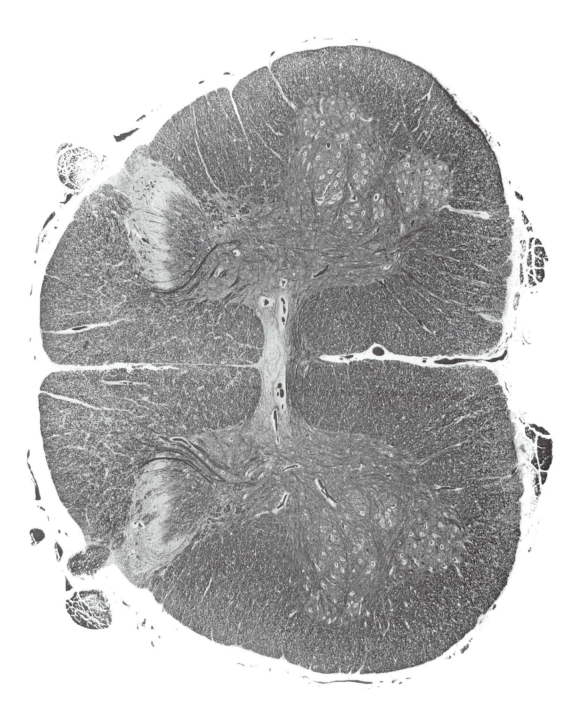

Figure AII–1. Transverse section of the first sacral segment (S1) of the spinal cord. (×20)

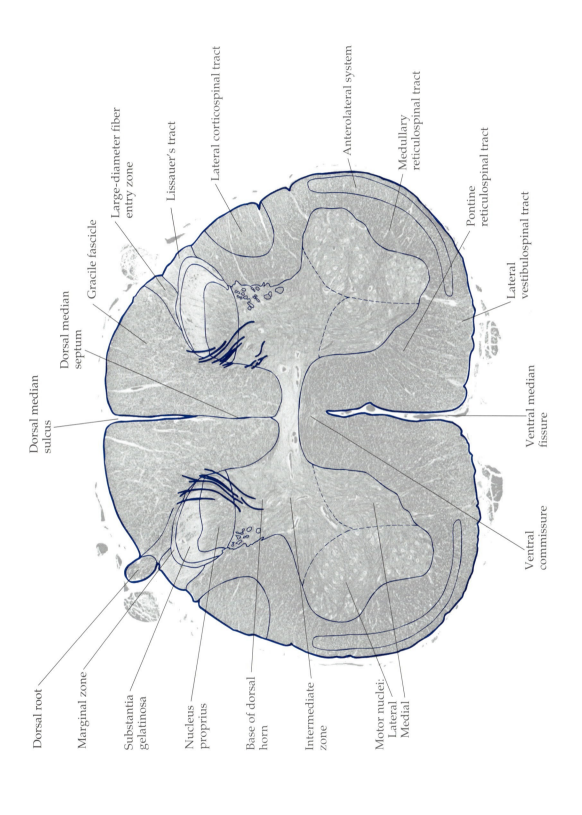

Dorsal median sulcus

Dorsal median septum

Gracile fascicle

Large-diameter fiber entry zone

Lissauer's tract

Lateral corticospinal tract

Anterolateral system

Medullary reticulospinal tract

Pontine reticulospinal tract

Lateral vestibulospinal tract

Ventral median fissure

Ventral commissure

Motor nuclei:
Lateral
Medial

Intermediate zone

Base of dorsal horn

Nucleus proprius

Substantia gelatinosa

Marginal zone

Dorsal root

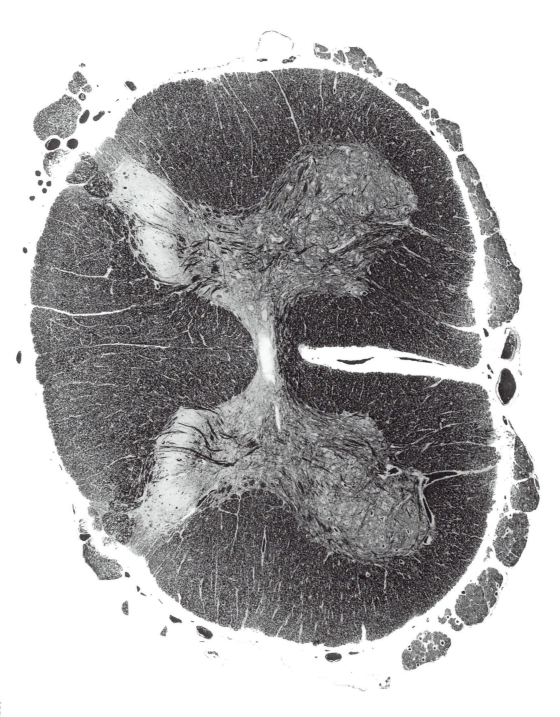

Figure AII–2. Transverse section of the second lumbar segment (L2) of the spinal cord. (×18)

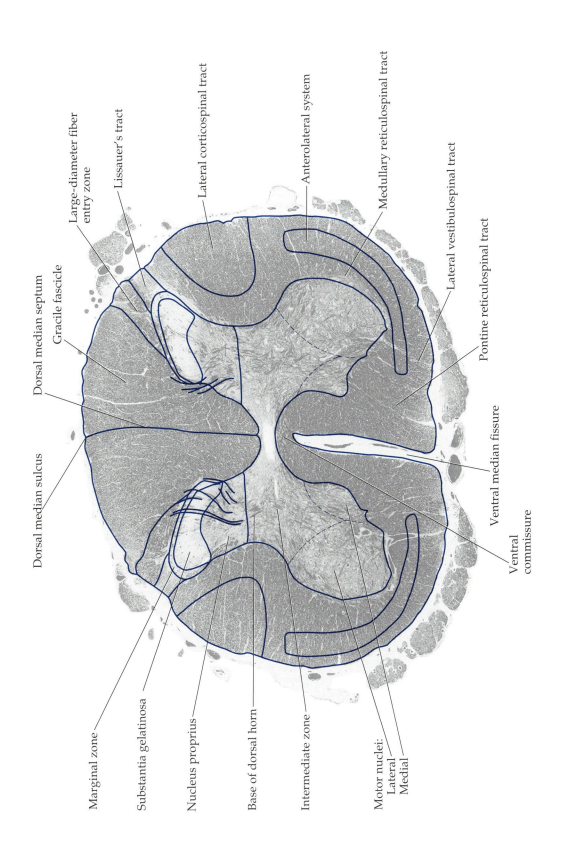

Dorsal median septum

Large-diameter fiber entry zone

Lissauer's tract

Lateral corticospinal tract

Anterolateral system

Medullary reticulospinal tract

Lateral vestibulospinal tract

Pontine reticulospinal tract

Gracile fascicle

Dorsal median sulcus

Marginal zone

Substantia gelatinosa

Nucleus proprius

Base of dorsal horn

Intermediate zone

Motor nuclei:
Lateral
Medial

Ventral commissure

Ventral median fissure

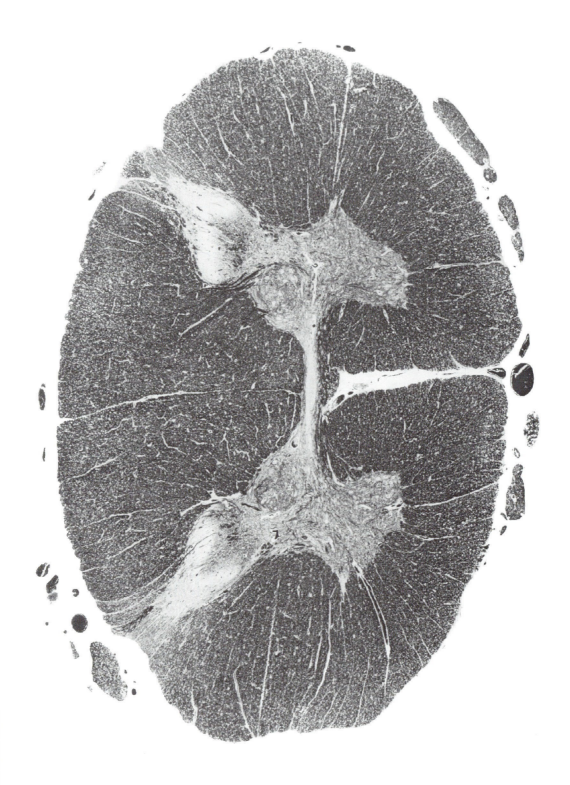

Figure AII–3. Transverse section of the first lumbar segment (L1) of the spinal cord. (×21)

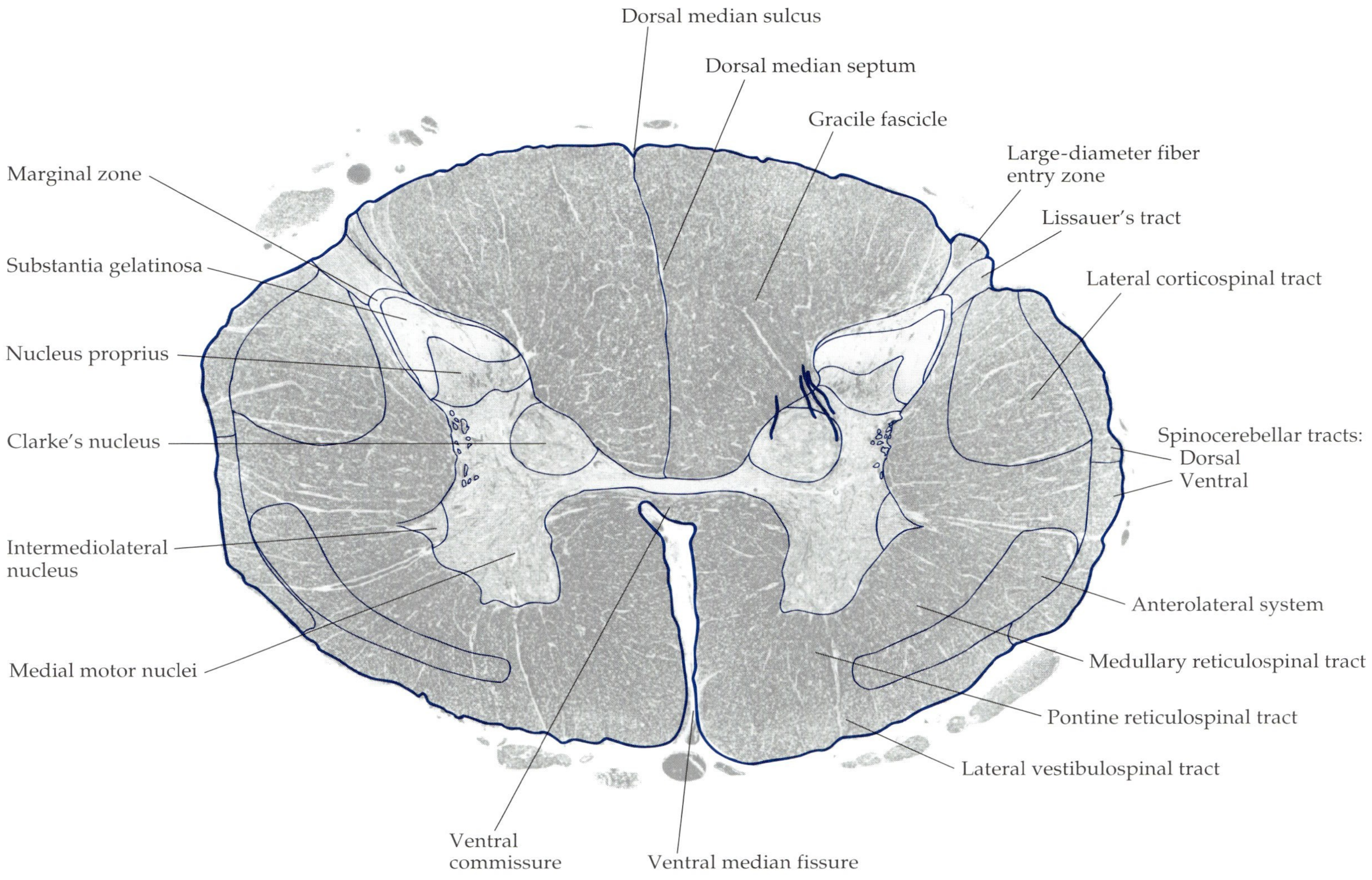

Dorsal median sulcus

Dorsal median septum

Gracile fascicle

Large-diameter fiber entry zone

Lissauer's tract

Lateral corticospinal tract

Spinocerebellar tracts:
Dorsal
Ventral

Anterolateral system

Medullary reticulospinal tract

Pontine reticulospinal tract

Lateral vestibulospinal tract

Ventral median fissure

Ventral commissure

Medial motor nuclei

Intermediolateral nucleus

Clarke's nucleus

Nucleus proprius

Substantia gelatinosa

Marginal zone

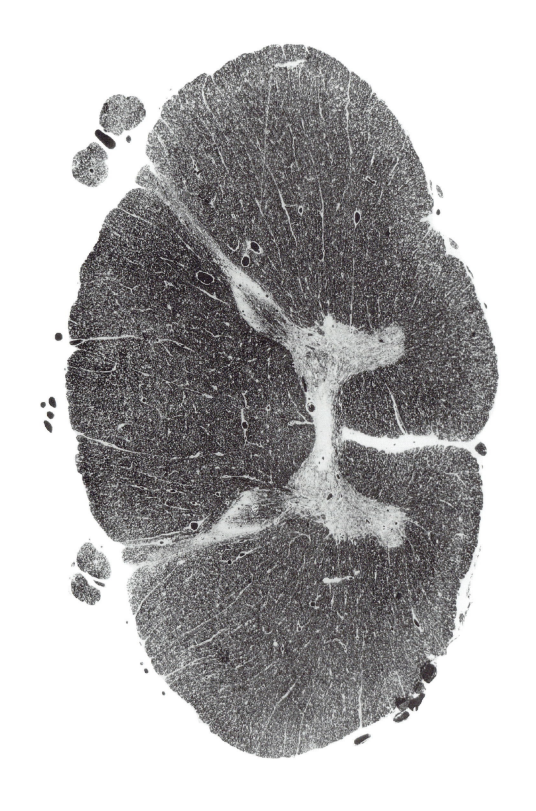

Figure AII-4. Transverse section of the third thoracic segment (T3) of the spinal cord. (×23)

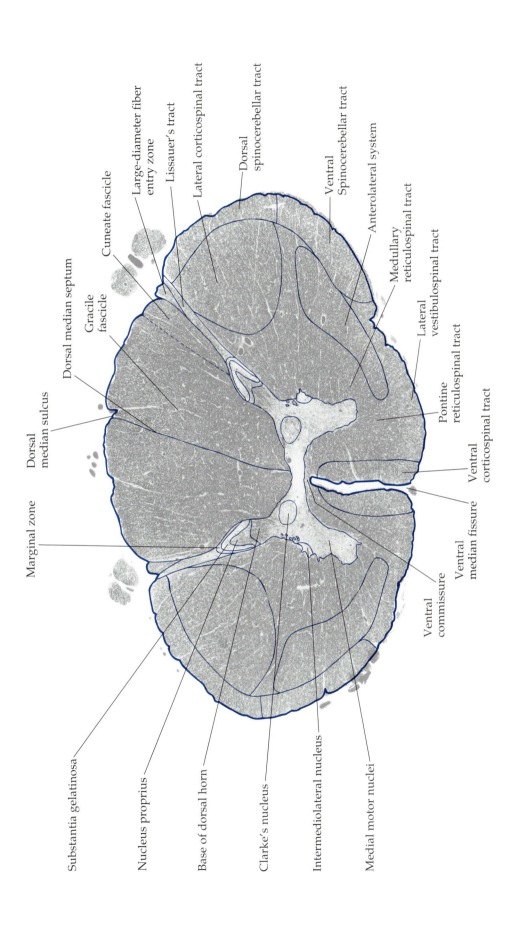

Substantia gelatinosa

Nucleus proprius

Base of dorsal horn

Clarke's nucleus

Intermediolateral nucleus

Medial motor nuclei

Marginal zone

Dorsal median sulcus

Dorsal median septum

Gracile fascicle

Cuneate fascicle

Large-diameter fiber entry zone

Lissauer's tract

Lateral corticospinal tract

Dorsal spinocerebellar tract

Ventral Spinocerebellar tract

Anterolateral system

Medullary reticulospinal tract

Lateral vestibulospinal tract

Pontine reticulospinal tract

Ventral corticospinal tract

Ventral median fissure

Ventral commissure

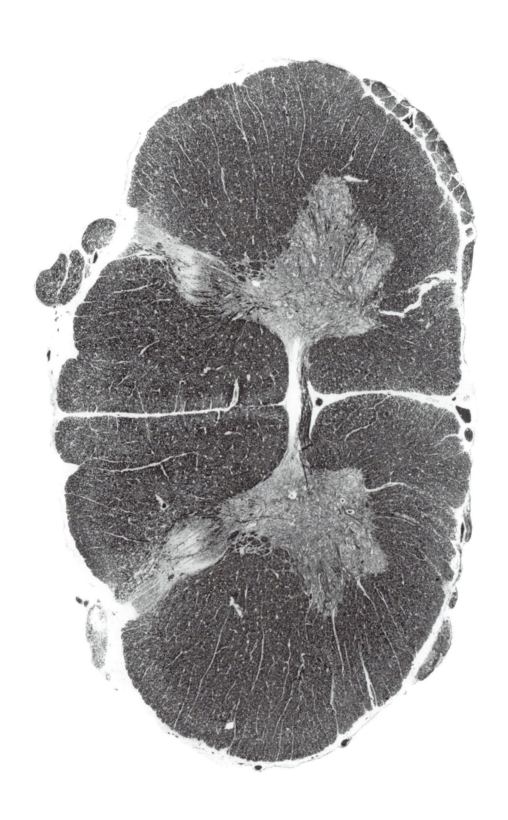

Figure AII–5. Transverse section of the seventh cervical segment (C7) of the spinal cord. (×16).

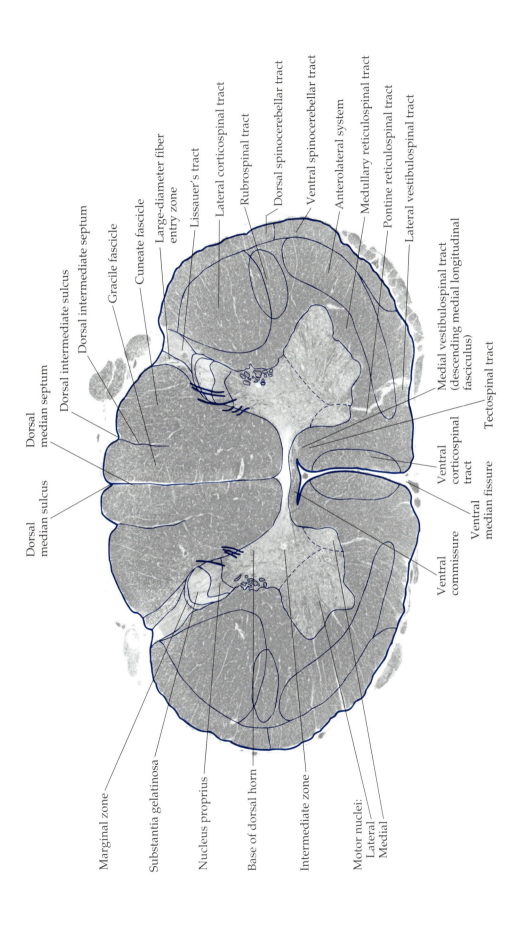

Dorsal
median sulcus

Dorsal
median septum

Dorsal intermediate sulcus

Dorsal intermediate septum

Gracile fascicle

Cuneate fascicle

Large-diameter fiber
entry zone

Lissauer's tract

Lateral corticospinal tract

Rubrospinal tract

Dorsal spinocerebellar tract

Ventral spinocerebellar tract

Anterolateral system

Medullary reticulospinal tract

Pontine reticulospinal tract

Lateral vestibulospinal tract

Medial vestibulospinal tract
(descending medial longitudinal
fasciculus)

Tectospinal tract

Ventral
corticospinal
tract

Ventral
median fissure

Ventral
commissure

Marginal zone

Substantia gelatinosa

Nucleus proprius

Base of dorsal horn

Intermediate zone

Motor nuclei:
    Lateral
    Medial

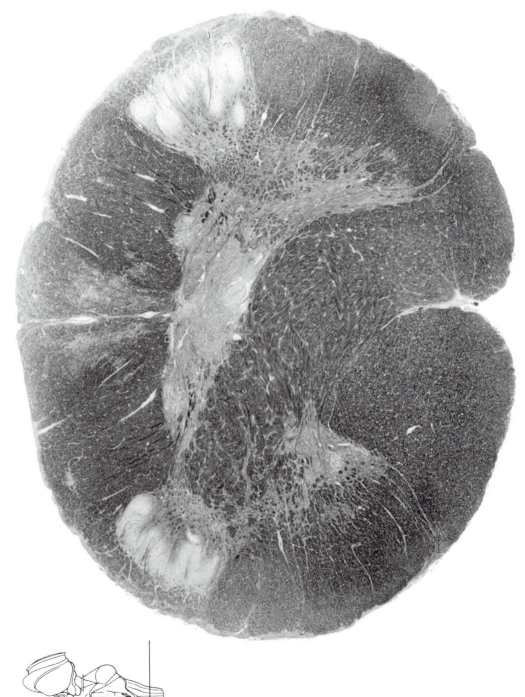

Figure AII–6. Transverse section of the caudal medulla at the level of the pyramidal (motor) decussation and the spinal (caudal) trigeminal nucleus. (×17)

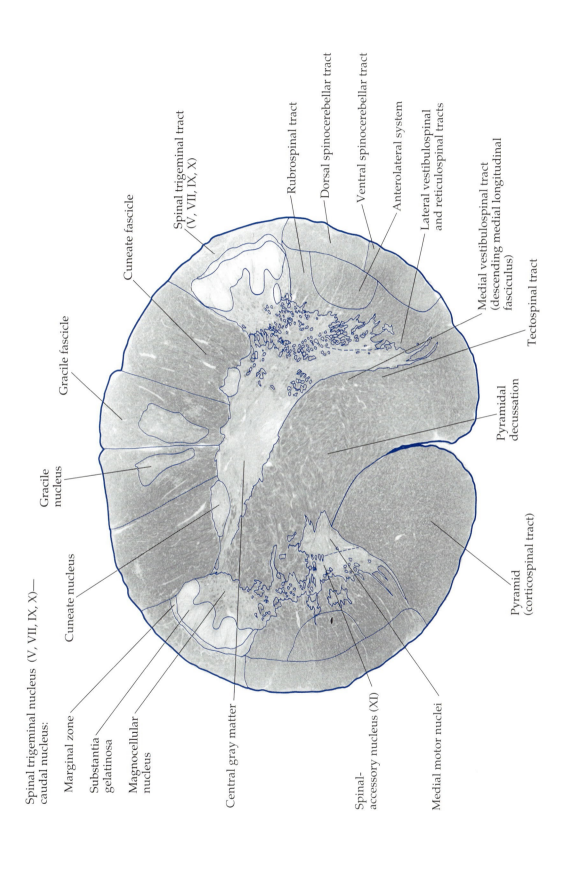

Spinal trigeminal nucleus (V, VII, IX, X)—caudal nucleus:

Marginal zone

Substantia gelatinosa

Magnocellular nucleus

Gracile nucleus

Cuneate nucleus

Cuneate fascicle

Spinal trigeminal tract (V, VII, IX, X)

Gracile fascicle

Rubrospinal tract

Dorsal spinocerebellar tract

Ventral spinocerebellar tract

Anterolateral system

Lateral vestibulospinal and reticulospinal tracts

Medial vestibulospinal tract (descending medial longitudinal fasciculus)

Tectospinal tract

Pyramidal decussation

Central gray matter

Spinal-accessory nucleus (XI)

Medial motor nuclei

Pyramid (corticospinal tract)

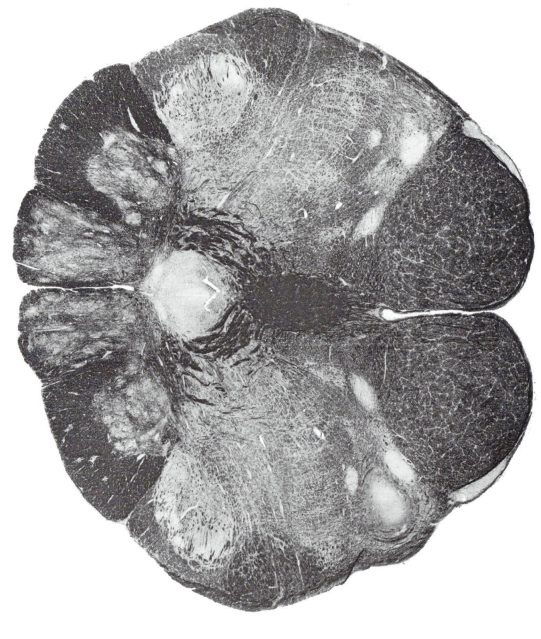

Figure AII–7. Transverse section of
the medulla at the level of the dorsal
column nuclei and the somatic sensory decussation. (×12)

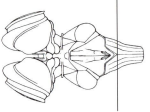

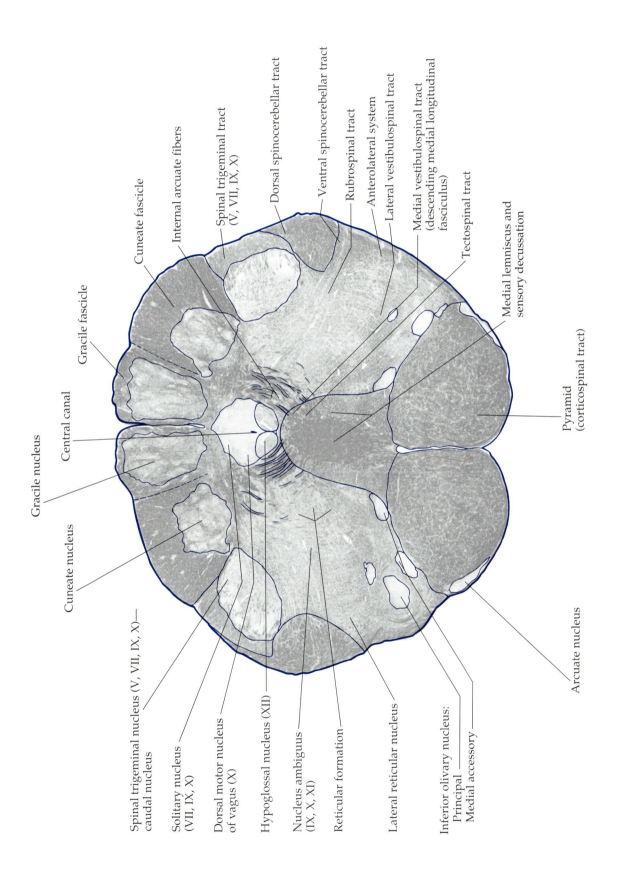

Gracile fascicle

Cuneate fascicle

Internal arcuate fibers

Spinal trigeminal tract (V, VII, IX, X)

Dorsal spinocerebellar tract

Ventral spinocerebellar tract

Rubrospinal tract

Anterolateral system

Lateral vestibulospinal tract

Medial vestibulospinal tract (descending medial longitudinal fasciculus)

Tectospinal tract

Medial lemniscus and sensory decussation

Central canal

Gracile nucleus

Cuneate nucleus

Spinal trigeminal nucleus (V, VII, IX, X)—caudal nucleus

Solitary nucleus (VII, IX, X)

Dorsal motor nucleus of vagus (X)

Hypoglossal nucleus (XII)

Nucleus ambiguus (IX, X, XI)

Reticular formation

Lateral reticular nucleus

Inferior olivary nucleus:
Principal
Medial accessory

Arcuate nucleus

Pyramid (corticospinal tract)

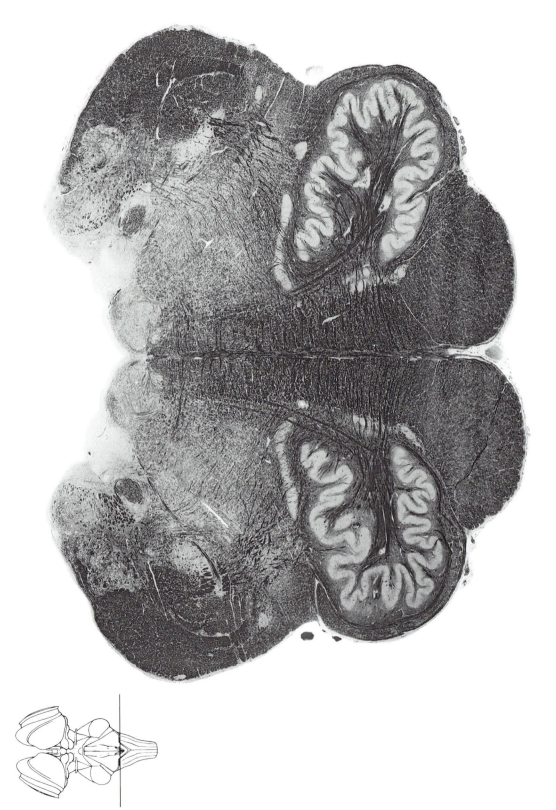

Figure AII–8. Transverse section of the medulla through the hypoglossal nucleus. (×9)

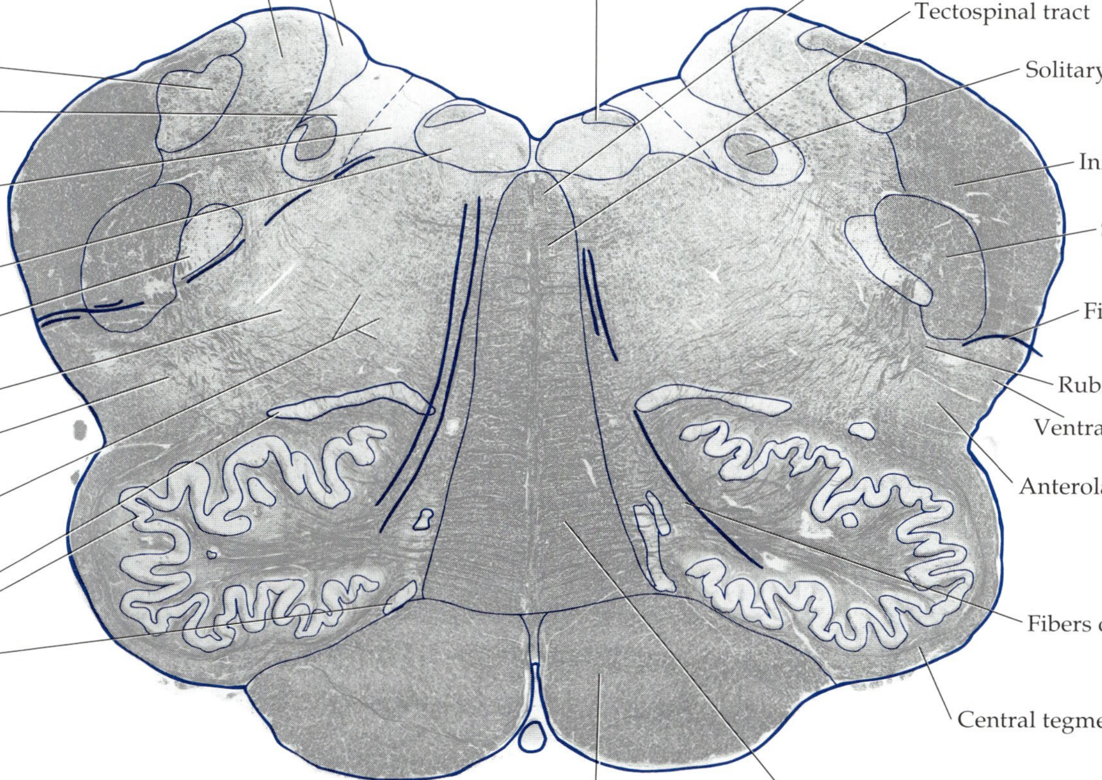

Dorsal longitudinal
fasciculus

Medial longitudinal fasciculus

Tectospinal tract

Solitary tract (VII, IX, X)

Inferior cerebellar peduncle

Spinal trigeminal tract
(V, VII, IX, X)

Fibers of vagus nerve (X)

Rubrospinal tract

Ventral spinocerebellar tract

Anterolateral system

Fibers of hypoglossal nerve (XII)

Central tegmental tract

Medial lemniscus

Pyramid

Vestibular nuclei (VIII):
Medial
Inferior

Accessory cuneate nucleus

Solitary nucleus
(VII, IX, X)

Dorsal motor nucleus
of vagus (X)

Hypoglossal nucleus (XII)

Spinal trigeminal nucleus
(V, VII, IX, X)—
interpolar nucleus

Nucleus ambiguus
(IX, X, XI)

Lateral reticular
nucleus

Reticular formation

Inferior olivary nucleus:
Dorsal accessory
Principal
Medial accessory

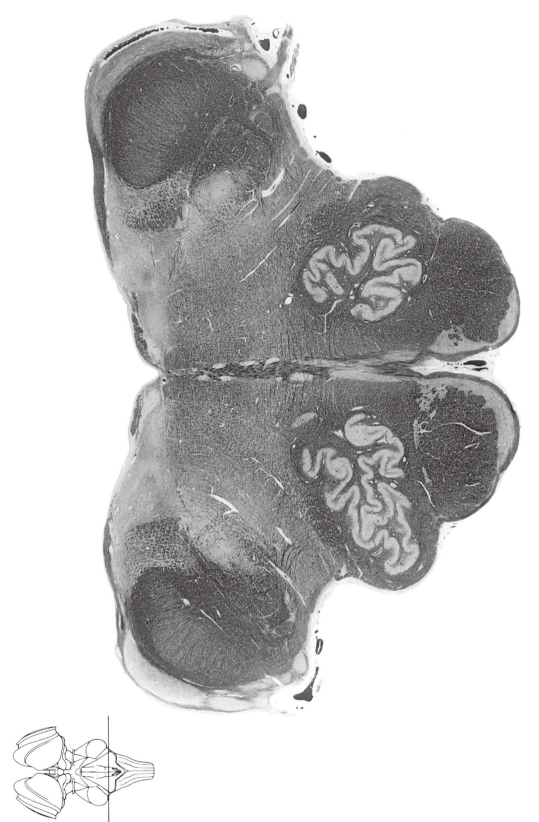

Figure AII–9. Transverse section of the rostral medulla through the cochlear nuclei. (×9).

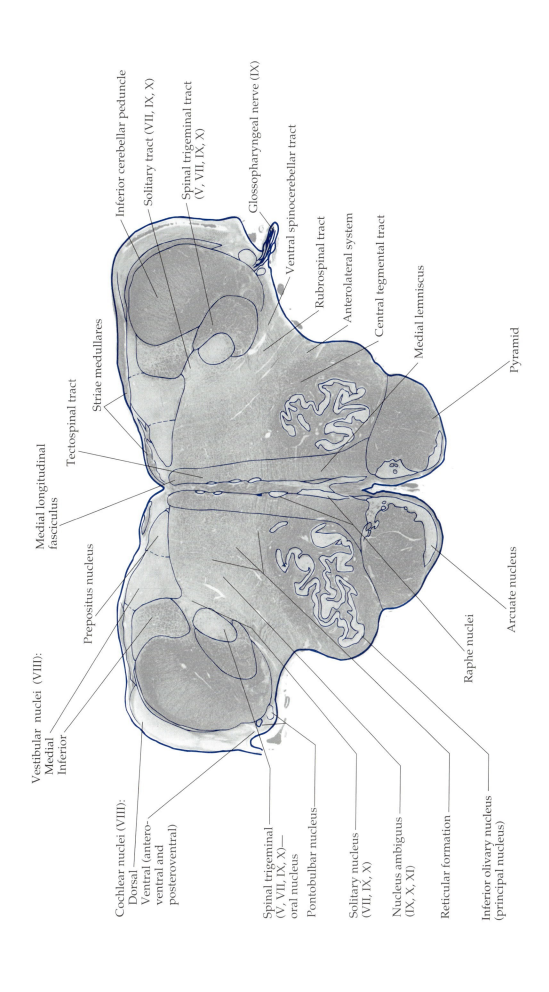

Vestibular nuclei (VIII):
Medial
Inferior

Medial longitudinal
fasciculus

Tectospinal tract

Striae medullares

Prepositus nucleus

Inferior cerebellar peduncle

Solitary tract (VII, IX, X)

Spinal trigeminal tract
(V, VII, IX, X)

Glossopharyngeal nerve (IX)

Ventral spinocerebellar tract

Rubrospinal tract

Anterolateral system

Central tegmental tract

Medial lemniscus

Pyramid

Arcuate nucleus

Raphe nuclei

Cochlear nuclei (VIII):
Dorsal
Ventral (antero-
ventral and
posteroventral)

Spinal trigeminal
(V, VII, IX, X)—
oral nucleus

Pontobulbar nucleus

Solitary nucleus
(VII, IX, X)

Nucleus ambiguus
(IX, X, XI)

Reticular formation

Inferior olivary nucleus
(principal nucleus)

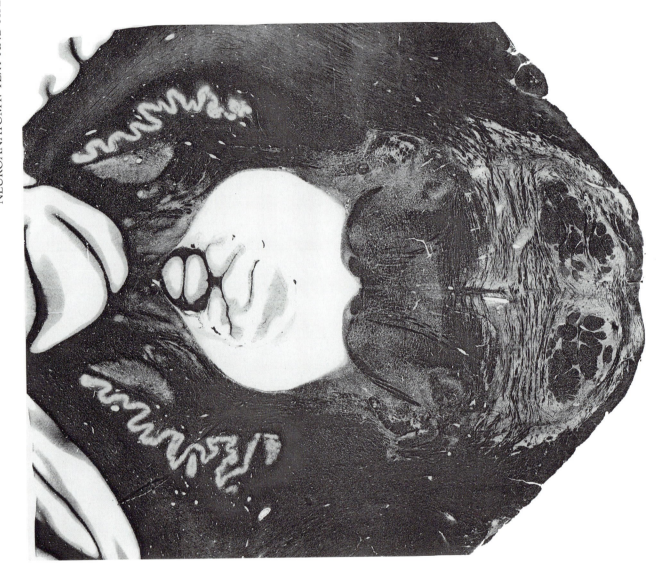

Figure AII–10. Transverse section of the pons at the level of the genu of the facial nerve and the deep cerebellar nuclei. (×4.3)

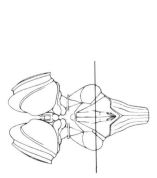

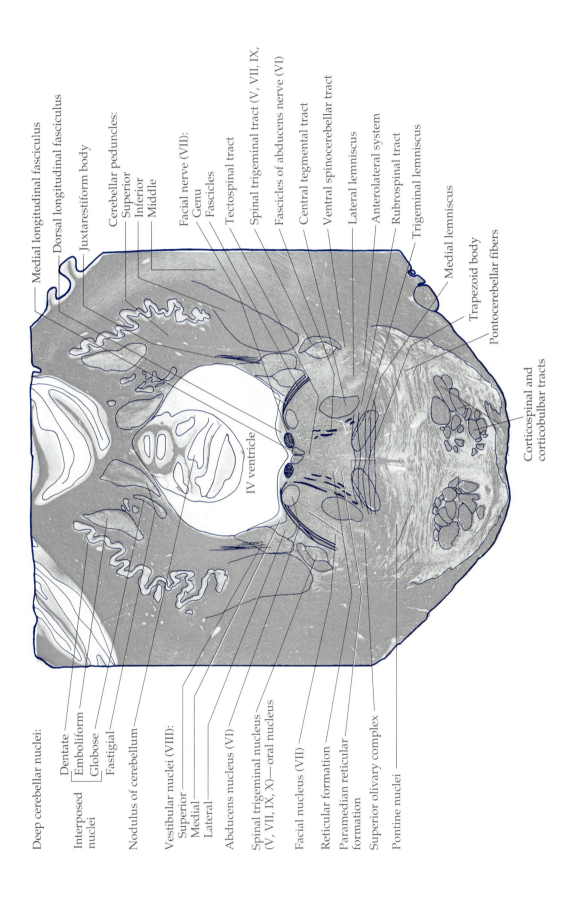

Medial longitudinal fasciculus

Dorsal longitudinal fasciculus

Juxtarestiform body

Cerebellar peduncles:
Superior
Inferior
Middle

Facial nerve (VII):
Genu
Fascicles

Tectospinal tract

Spinal trigeminal tract (V, VII, IX,

Fascicles of abducens nerve (VI)

Central tegmental tract

Ventral spinocerebellar tract

Lateral lemniscus

Anterolateral system

Rubrospinal tract

Trigeminal lemniscus

Medial lemniscus

Trapezoid body

Pontocerebellar fibers

Corticospinal and
corticobulbar tracts

IV ventricle

Deep cerebellar nuclei:
Dentate
Interposed ⌈ Emboliform
nuclei ⌊ Globose
Fastigial

Nodulus of cerebellum

Vestibular nuclei (VIII):
Superior
Medial
Lateral

Abducens nucleus (VI)

Spinal trigeminal nucleus
(V, VII, IX, X)—oral nucleus

Facial nucleus (VII)

Reticular formation

Paramedian reticular
formation

Superior olivary complex

Pontine nuclei

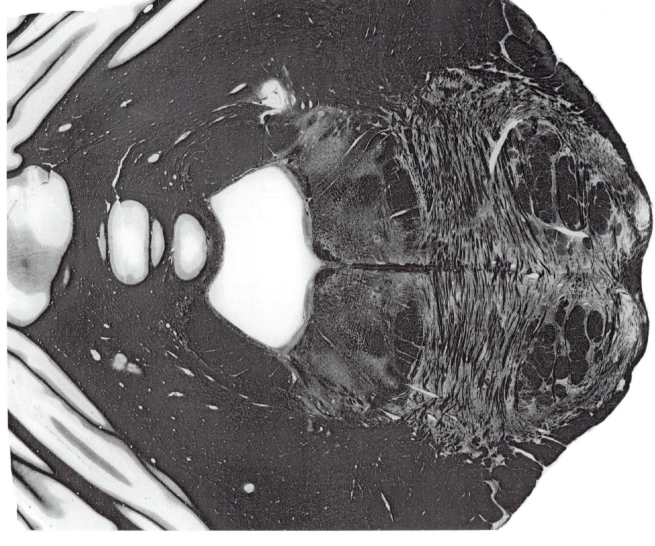

Figure AII–11. Transverse section of the pons through the main trigeminal sensory nuclei. (×10)

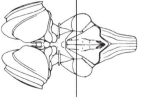

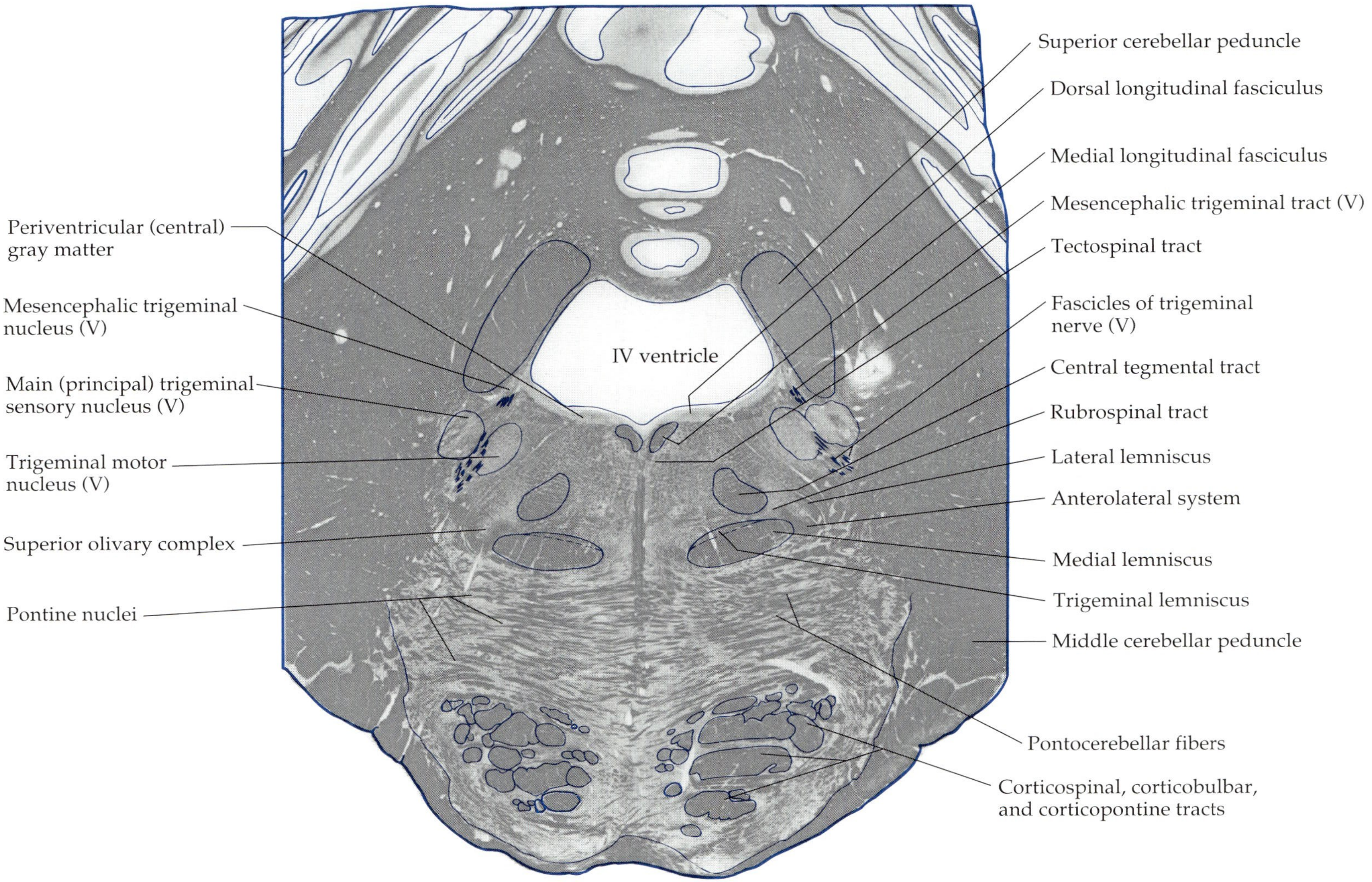

Superior cerebellar peduncle

Dorsal longitudinal fasciculus

Medial longitudinal fasciculus

Mesencephalic trigeminal tract (V)

Tectospinal tract

Fascicles of trigeminal nerve (V)

Central tegmental tract

Rubrospinal tract

Lateral lemniscus

Anterolateral system

Medial lemniscus

Trigeminal lemniscus

Middle cerebellar peduncle

Pontocerebellar fibers

Corticospinal, corticobulbar, and corticopontine tracts

IV ventricle

Periventricular (central) gray matter

Mesencephalic trigeminal nucleus (V)

Main (principal) trigeminal sensory nucleus (V)

Trigeminal motor nucleus (V)

Superior olivary complex

Pontine nuclei

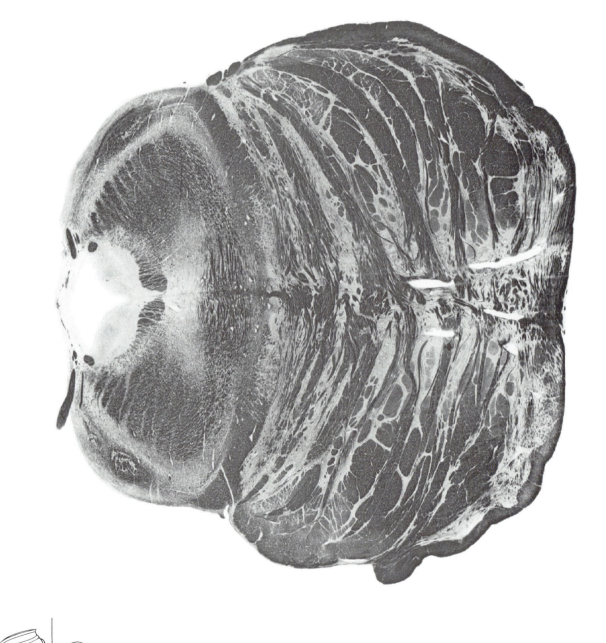

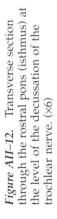

Figure AII–12. Transverse section through the rostral pons (isthmus) at the level of the decussation of the trochlear nerve. (×6)

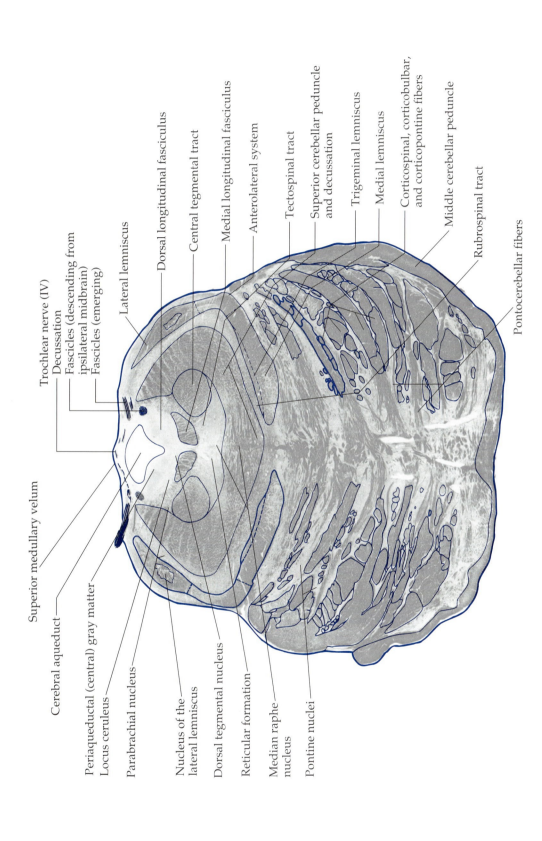

Superior medullary velum

Cerebral aqueduct

Periaqueductal (central) gray matter
Locus ceruleus

Parabrachial nucleus

Nucleus of the
lateral lemniscus

Dorsal tegmental nucleus

Reticular formation

Median raphe
nucleus

Pontine nuclei

Trochlear nerve (IV)
Decussation
Fascicles (descending from
ipsilateral midbrain)
Fascicles (emerging)

Lateral lemniscus

Dorsal longitudinal fasciculus

Central tegmental tract

Medial longitudinal fasciculus

Anterolateral system

Tectospinal tract

Superior cerebellar peduncle
and decussation

Trigeminal lemniscus

Medial lemniscus

Corticospinal, corticobulbar,
and corticopontine fibers

Middle cerebellar peduncle

Rubrospinal tract

Pontocerebellar fibers

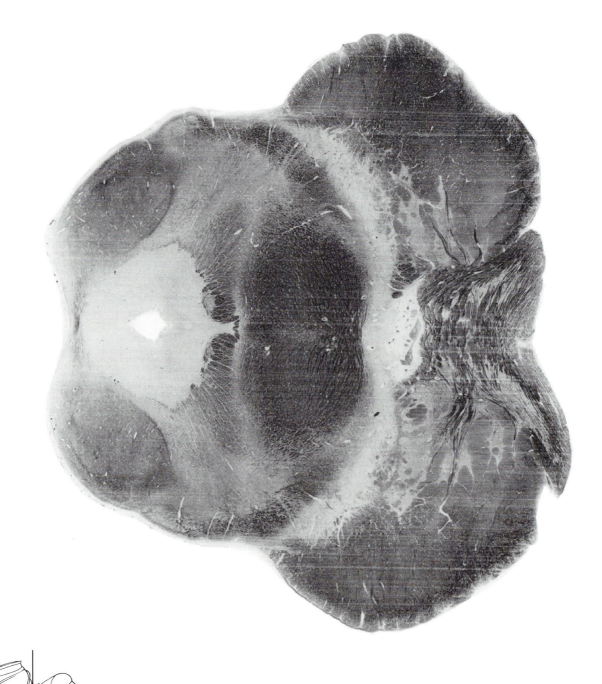

Figure AII–13. Transverse section of the caudal midbrain at the level of the inferior colliculus. (×5.6)

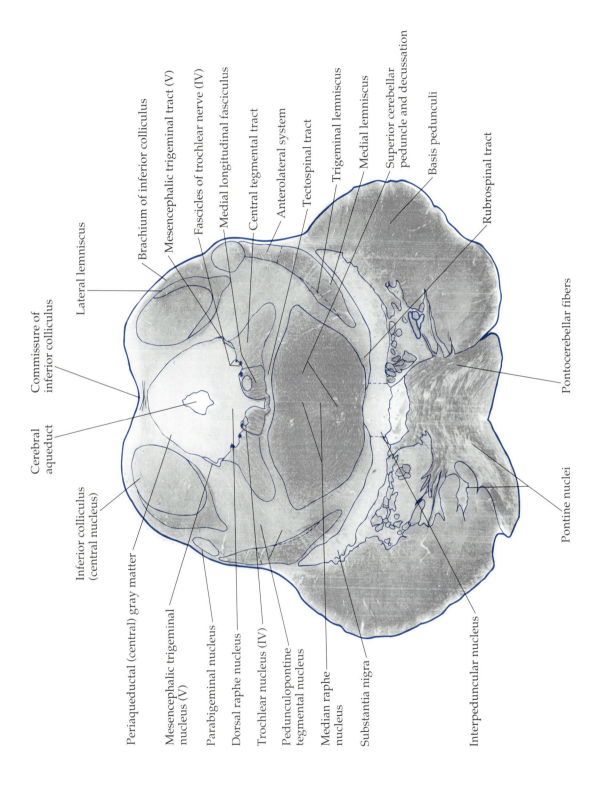

Periaqueductal (central) gray matter

Mesencephalic trigeminal nucleus (V)

Parabigeminal nucleus

Dorsal raphe nucleus

Trochlear nucleus (IV)

Pedunculopontine tegmental nucleus

Median raphe nucleus

Substantia nigra

Interpeduncular nucleus

Pontine nuclei

Pontocerebellar fibers

Rubrospinal tract

Basis pedunculi

Superior cerebellar peduncle and decussation

Medial lemniscus

Trigeminal lemniscus

Tectospinal tract

Anterolateral system

Central tegmental tract

Medial longitudinal fasciculus

Fascicles of trochlear nerve (IV)

Mesencephalic trigeminal tract (V)

Brachium of inferior colliculus

Lateral lemniscus

Commissure of inferior colliculus

Cerebral aqueduct

Inferior colliculus (central nucleus)

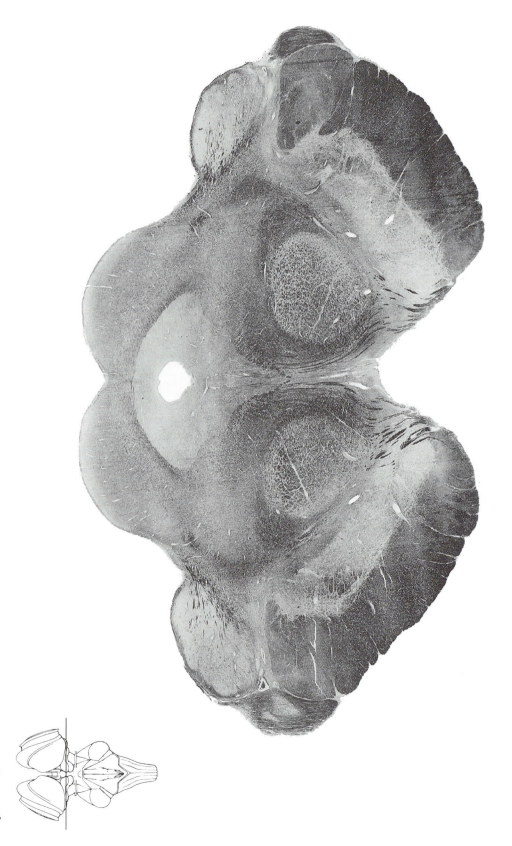

Figure AII-14. Transverse section of the rostral midbrain at the level of the superior colliculus. (×5.0)

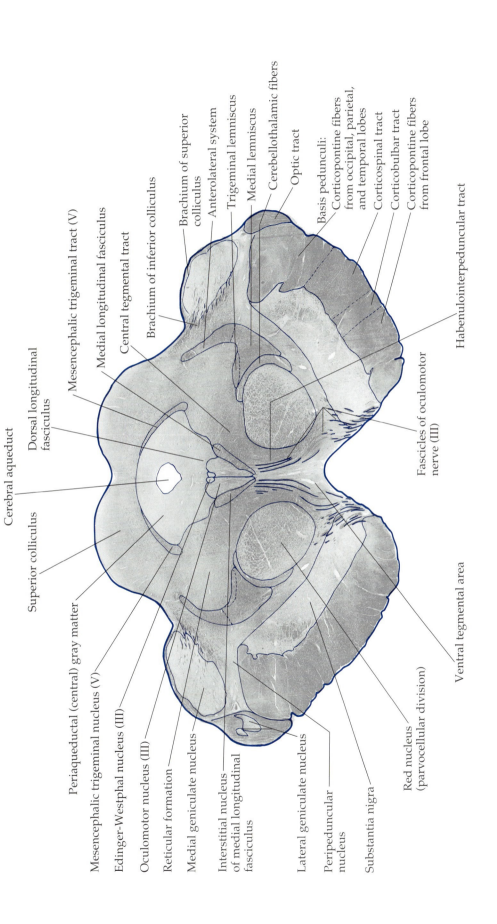

Cerebral aqueduct

Dorsal longitudinal
fasciculus

Mesencephalic trigeminal tract (V)

Medial longitudinal fasciculus

Central tegmental tract

Brachium of inferior colliculus

Brachium of superior
colliculus

Anterolateral system

Trigeminal lemniscus

Medial lemniscus

Cerebellothalamic fibers

Optic tract

Basis pedunculi:

Corticopontine fibers
from occipital, parietal,
and temporal lobes

Corticospinal tract

Corticobulbar tract

Corticopontine fibers
from frontal lobe

Habenulointerpeduncular tract

Superior colliculus

Periaqueductal (central) gray matter

Mesencephalic trigeminal nucleus (V)

Edinger-Westphal nucleus (III)

Oculomotor nucleus (III)

Reticular formation

Medial geniculate nucleus

Interstitial nucleus
of medial longitudinal
fasciculus

Lateral geniculate nucleus

Peripeduncular
nucleus

Substantia nigra

Red nucleus
(parvocellular division)

Ventral tegmental area

Fascicles of oculomotor
nerve (III)

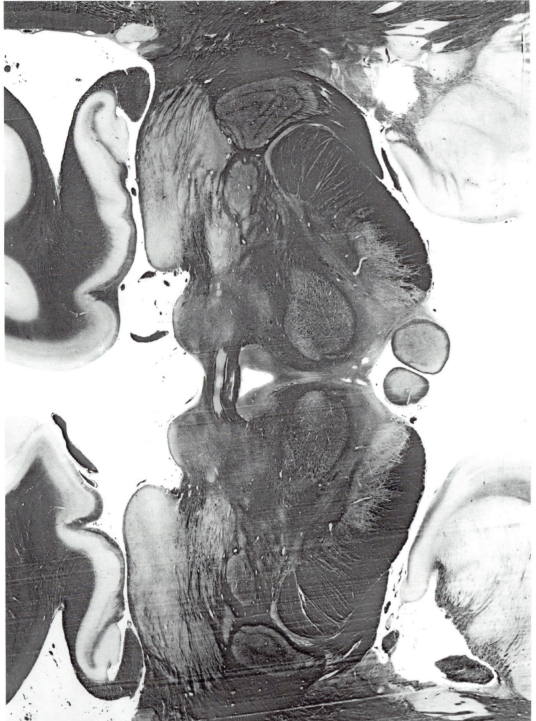

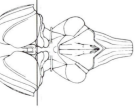

Figure AII–15. Transverse section of the juncture of the midbrain and diencephalon. (×3.3)

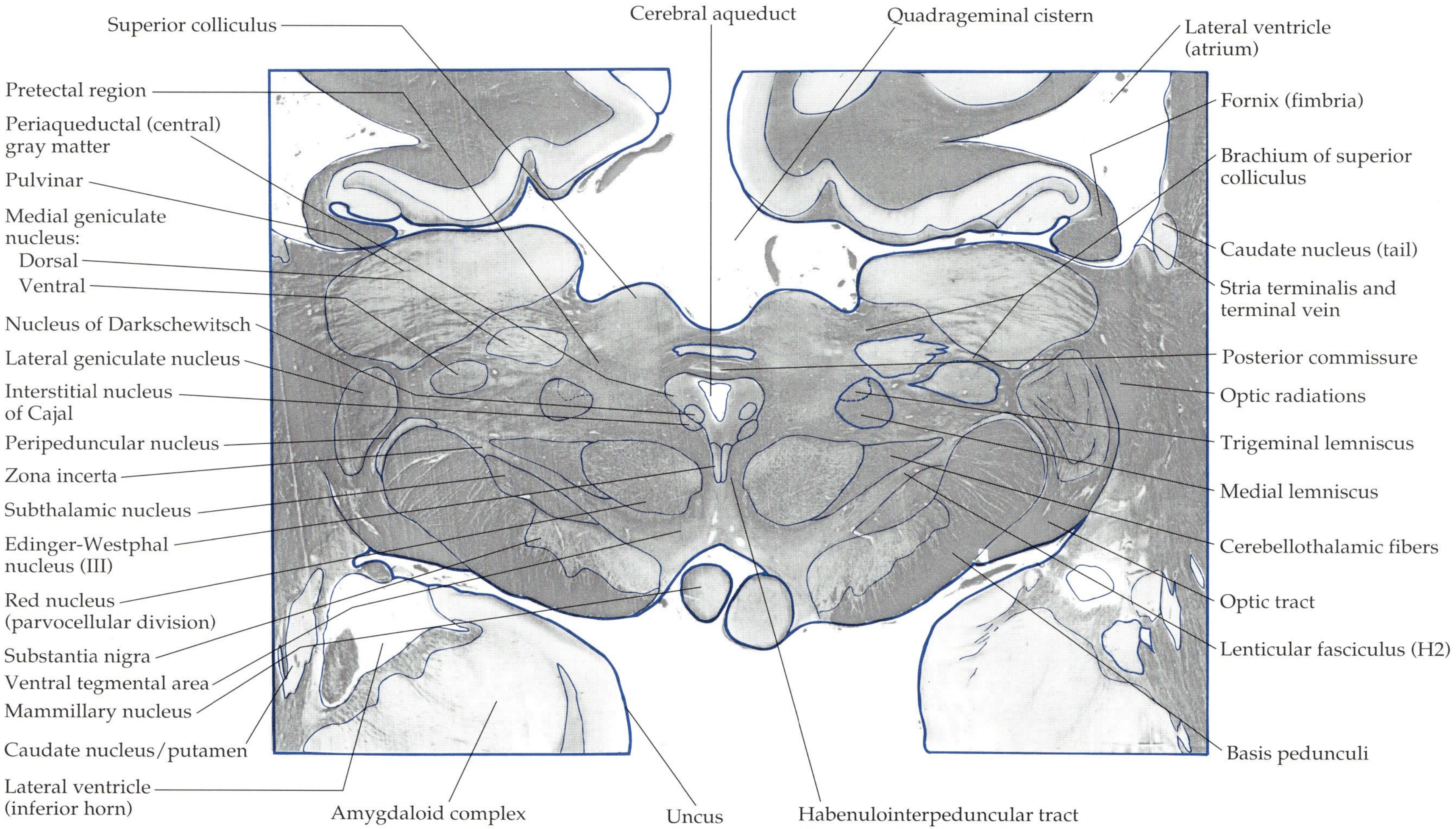

Lateral ventricle (atrium)

Fornix (fimbria)

Brachium of superior colliculus

Caudate nucleus (tail)

Stria terminalis and terminal vein

Posterior commissure

Optic radiations

Trigeminal lemniscus

Medial lemniscus

Cerebellothalamic fibers

Optic tract

Lenticular fasciculus (H2)

Basis pedunculi

Quadrageminal cistern

Cerebral aqueduct

Habenulointerpeduncular tract

Superior colliculus

Uncus

Amygdaloid complex

Pretectal region

Periaqueductal (central) gray matter

Pulvinar

Medial geniculate nucleus:
Dorsal
Ventral

Nucleus of Darkschewitsch

Lateral geniculate nucleus

Interstitial nucleus of Cajal

Peripeduncular nucleus

Zona incerta

Subthalamic nucleus

Edinger-Westphal nucleus (III)

Red nucleus (parvocellular division)

Substantia nigra

Ventral tegmental area

Mammillary nucleus

Caudate nucleus/putamen

Lateral ventricle (inferior horn)

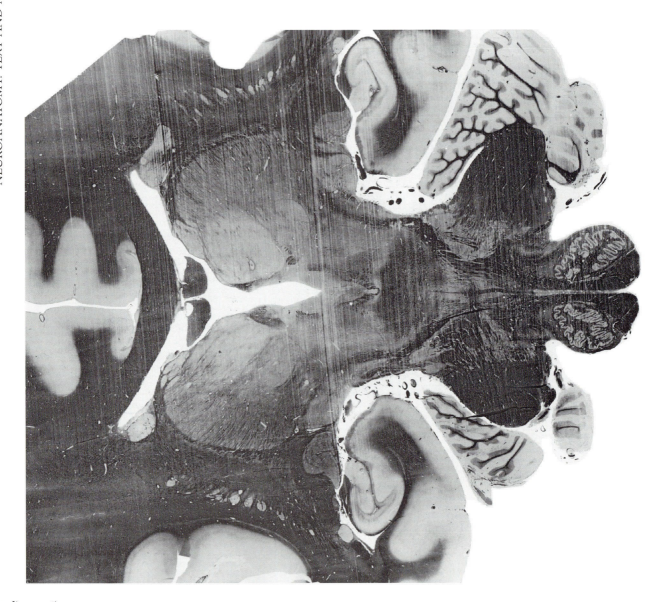

Figure AII–16. Coronal section of the diencephalon and cerebral hemisphere through the posterior limb of the internal capsule and the medial and lateral geniculate nuclei. The midbrain and pontine tegmentum, lateral cerebellum, and the ventral medulla are also shown. (×2.1)

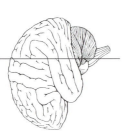

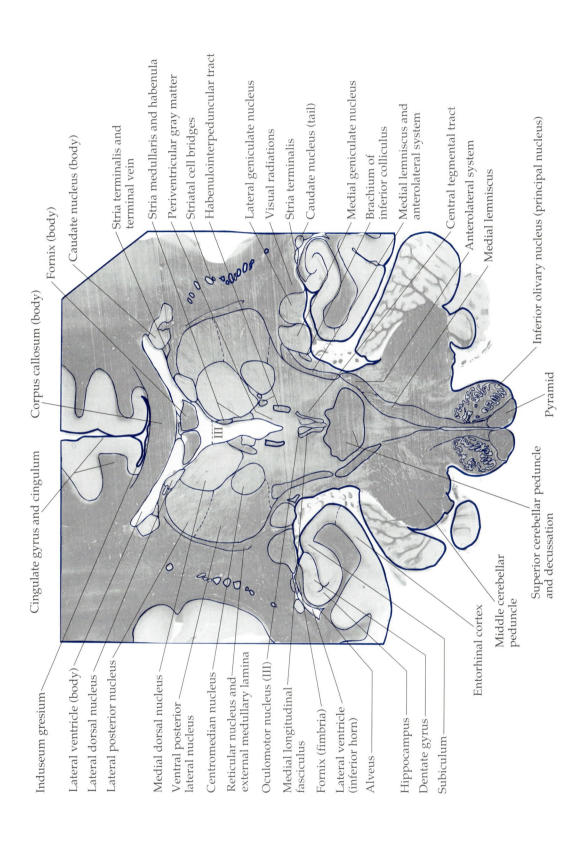

Induseum gresium

Cingulate gyrus and cingulum

Lateral ventricle (body)

Lateral dorsal nucleus

Lateral posterior nucleus

Corpus callosum (body)

Fornix (body)

Caudate nucleus (body)

Stria terminalis and
terminal vein

Stria medullaris and habenula

Periventricular gray matter

Striatal cell bridges

Habenulointerpeduncular tract

Lateral geniculate nucleus

Visual radiations

Stria terminalis

Caudate nucleus (tail)

Medial geniculate nucleus

Brachium of
inferior colliculus

Medial lemniscus and
anterolateral system

Central tegmental tract

Anterolateral system

Medial lemniscus

Inferior olivary nucleus (principal nucleus)

Pyramid

Superior cerebellar peduncle
and decussation

Middle cerebellar
peduncle

Entorhinal cortex

Subiculum

Dentate gyrus

Hippocampus

Alveus

Lateral ventricle
(inferior horn)

Fornix (fimbria)

Medial longitudinal
fasciculus

Oculomotor nucleus (III)

Reticular nucleus and
external medullary lamina

Centromedian nucleus

Ventral posterior
lateral nucleus

Medial dorsal nucleus

III

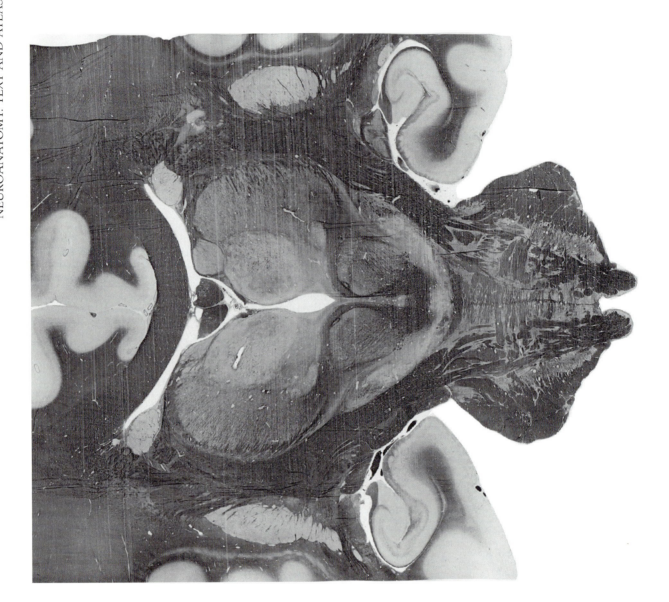

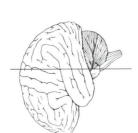

Figure AII–17. Coronal section of the diencephalon and cerebral hemisphere through the posterior limb of the internal capsule and and ventral posterior nucleus. The midbrain tegmentum and base of the pons are also shown. (×2.3)

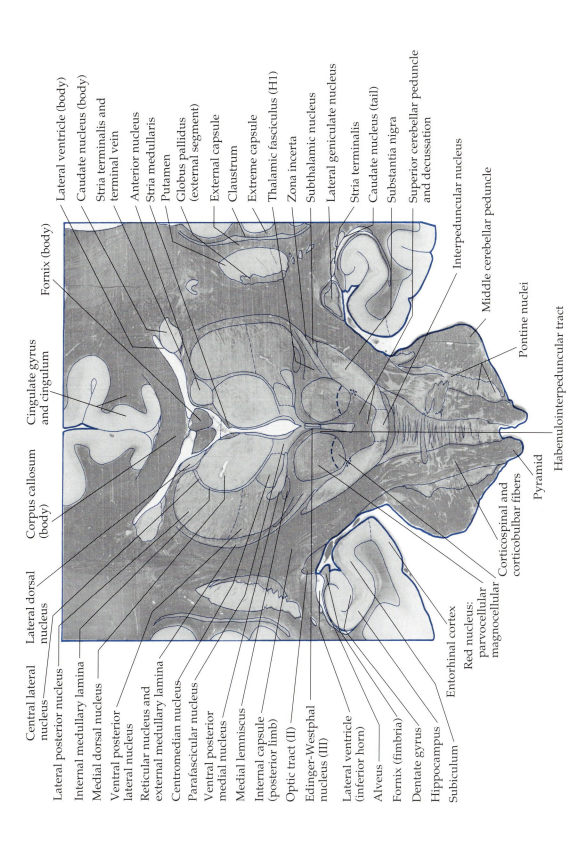

Central lateral
nucleus

Lateral dorsal
nucleus

Corpus callosum
(body)

Cingulate gyrus
and cingulum

Fornix (body)

Lateral ventricle (body)

Caudate nucleus (body)

Stria terminalis and
terminal vein

Anterior nucleus

Stria medullaris

Putamen

Globus pallidus
(external segment)

External capsule

Claustrum

Extreme capsule

Thalamic fasciculus (H1)

Zona incerta

Subthalamic nucleus

Lateral geniculate nucleus

Stria terminalis

Caudate nucleus (tail)

Substantia nigra

Superior cerebellar peduncle
and decussation

Interpeduncular nucleus

Middle cerebellar peduncle

Pontine nuclei

Habenulointerpeduncular tract

Pyramid

Corticospinal and
corticobulbar fibers

Red nucleus:
parvocellular
magnocellular

Entorhinal cortex

Subiculum

Hippocampus

Dentate gyrus

Fornix (fimbria)

Alveus

Lateral ventricle
(inferior horn)

Edinger-Westphal
nucleus (III)

Optic tract (II)

Internal capsule
(posterior limb)

Medial lemniscus

Ventral posterior
medial nucleus

Parafascicular nucleus

Centromedian nucleus

Reticular nucleus and
external medullary lamina

Ventral posterior
lateral nucleus

Medial dorsal nucleus

Internal medullary lamina

Lateral posterior nucleus

Figure AII–18. Oblique section of the cerebral hemisphere and diencephalon through the optic chiasm and tracts. (×2.3)

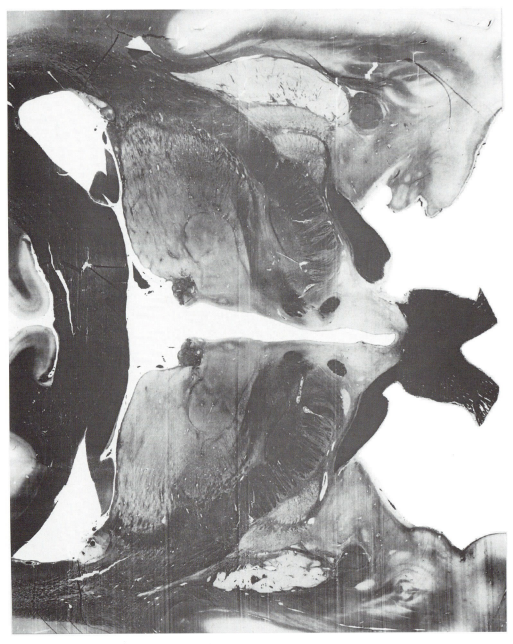

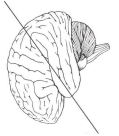

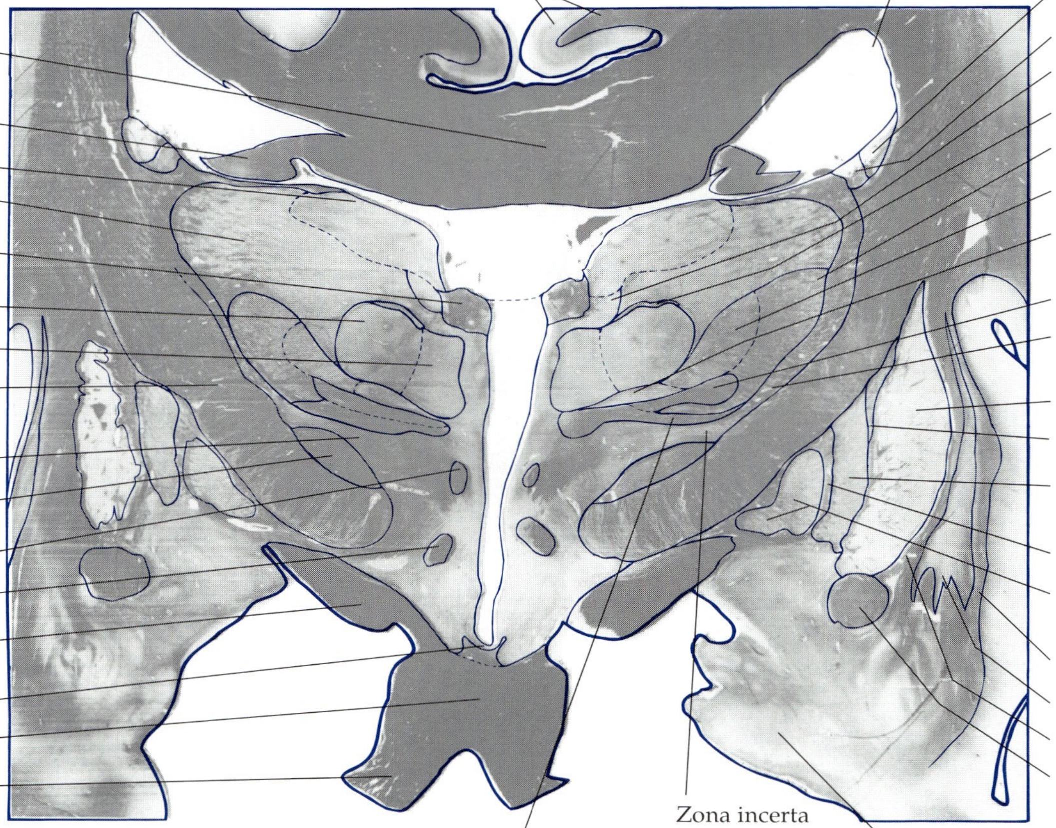

Corpus callosum
(splenium)

Fornix (crus)

Pulvinar

Lateral posterior nucleus

Habenula and stria
medullaris

Centromedian nucleus

Parafascicular nucleus

Internal capsule
(posterior limb)

Lenticular fasciculus (H2)

Subthalamic nucleus

Mammillothalamic tract

Fornix (column)

Optic tract (II)

Supraoptic decussation

Optic chiasm (II)

Optic nerve (II)

Cingulate gyrus and cingulum

Lateral ventricle (body)

Caudate nucleus (body)

Stria terminalis and terminal vein

Medial dorsal nucleus

Internal medullary lamina

Ventral posterior lateral nucleus

Ventral posterior medial nucleus

Ventral posterior medial nucleus
(parvocellular part)

Medial lemniscus

Reticular nucleus
and external medullary lamina

Putamen

Lateral medullary lamina

Globus pallidus (external
segment)

Medial medullary lamina

Globus pallidus (internal
segment)

Extreme capsule

Claustrum

External capsule

Anterior commissure

Amygdaloid complex

Zona incerta

Thalamic fasciculus (H1)

Figure AII–19. Coronal section of the diencephalon and cerebral hemisphere through the posterior limb of the internal capsule and anterior thalamic nuclei. The ventral midbrain and ventral pons are also shown. (×2.2)

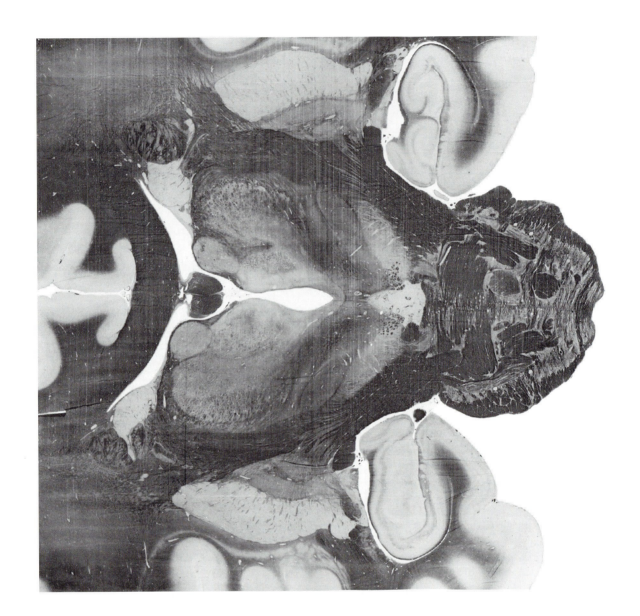

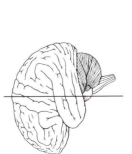

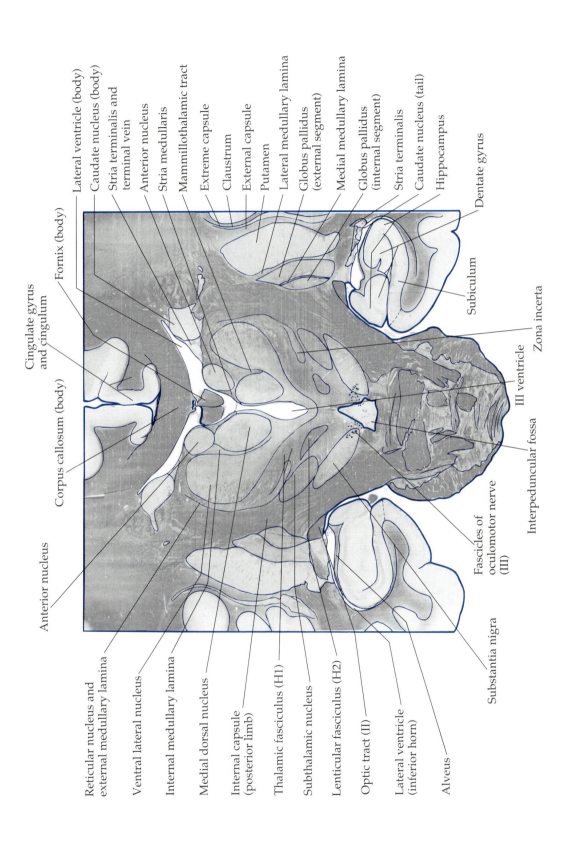

Cingulate gyrus
and cingulum

Fornix (body)

Lateral ventricle (body)
Caudate nucleus (body)
Stria terminalis and
terminal vein
Anterior nucleus
Stria medullaris
Mammillothalamic tract
Extreme capsule
Claustrum
External capsule
Putamen
Lateral medullary lamina
Globus pallidus
(external segment)
Medial medullary lamina
Globus pallidus
(internal segment)
Stria terminalis
Caudate nucleus (tail)
Hippocampus

Dentate gyrus

Subiculum

Zona incerta

III ventricle

Anterior nucleus

Corpus callosum (body)

Reticular nucleus and
external medullary lamina
Ventral lateral nucleus
Internal medullary lamina
Medial dorsal nucleus
Internal capsule
(posterior limb)
Thalamic fasciculus (H1)
Subthalamic nucleus
Lenticular fasciculus (H2)
Optic tract (II)
Lateral ventricle
(inferior horn)
Alveus

Substantia nigra

Fascicles of
oculomotor nerve
(III)

Interpeduncular fossa

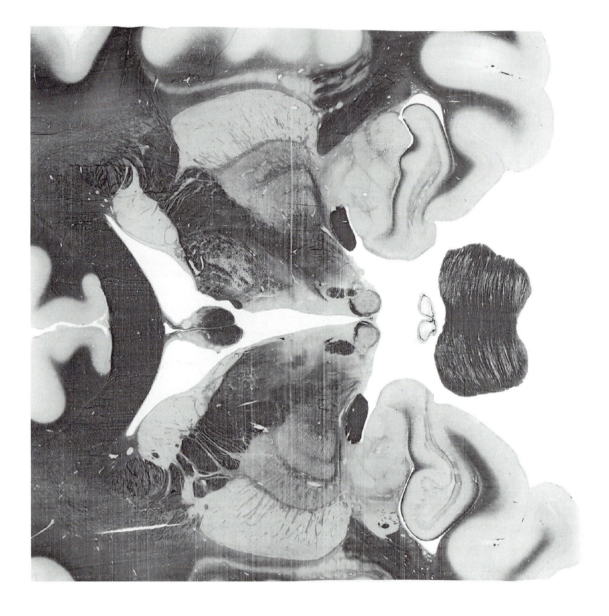

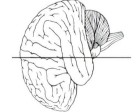

Figure AII–20.   Coronal section of the cerebral hemisphere and the diencephalon through the interventricular foramen. The base of the pons is also shown. (×2.1)

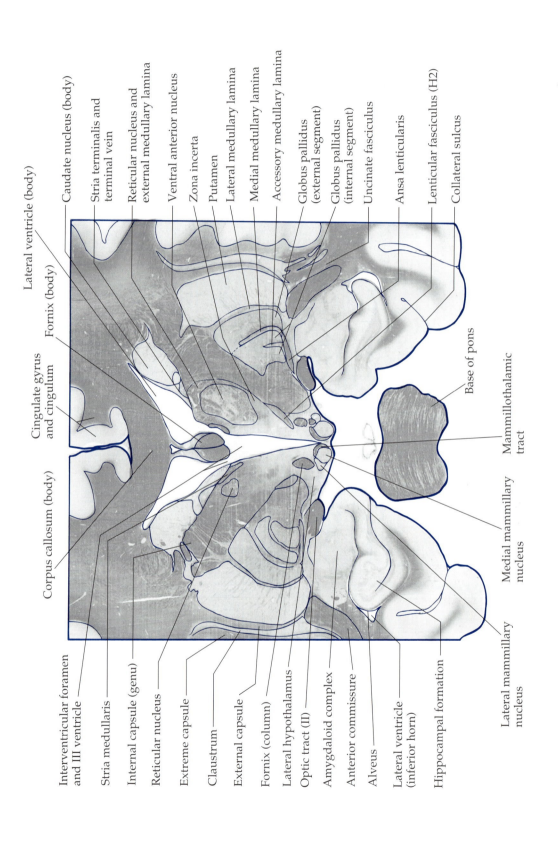

Lateral ventricle (body)

Caudate nucleus (body)

Stria terminalis and terminal vein

Reticular nucleus and external medullary lamina

Ventral anterior nucleus

Zona incerta

Putamen

Lateral medullary lamina

Medial medullary lamina

Accessory medullary lamina

Globus pallidus (external segment)

Globus pallidus (internal segment)

Uncinate fasciculus

Ansa lenticularis

Lenticular fasciculus (H2)

Collateral sulcus

Fornix (body)

Cingulate gyrus and cingulum

Corpus callosum (body)

Base of pons

Mammillothalamic tract

Medial mammillary nucleus

Lateral mammillary nucleus

Interventricular foramen and III ventricle

Stria medullaris

Internal capsule (genu)

Reticular nucleus

Extreme capsule

Claustrum

External capsule

Fornix (column)

Lateral hypothalamus

Optic tract (II)

Amygdaloid complex

Anterior commissure

Alveus

Lateral ventricle (inferior horn)

Hippocampal formation

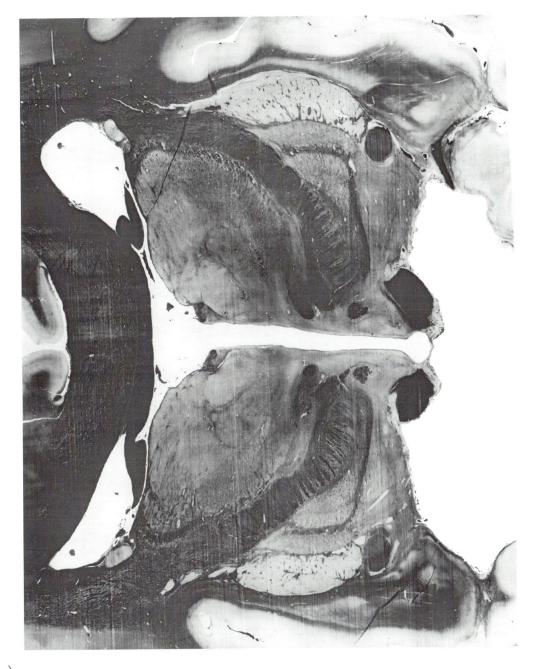

Figure AII–21. Oblique section of the cerebral hemisphere and diencephalon through the ansa lenticularis and optic tract. (×2.4)

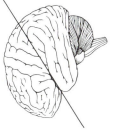

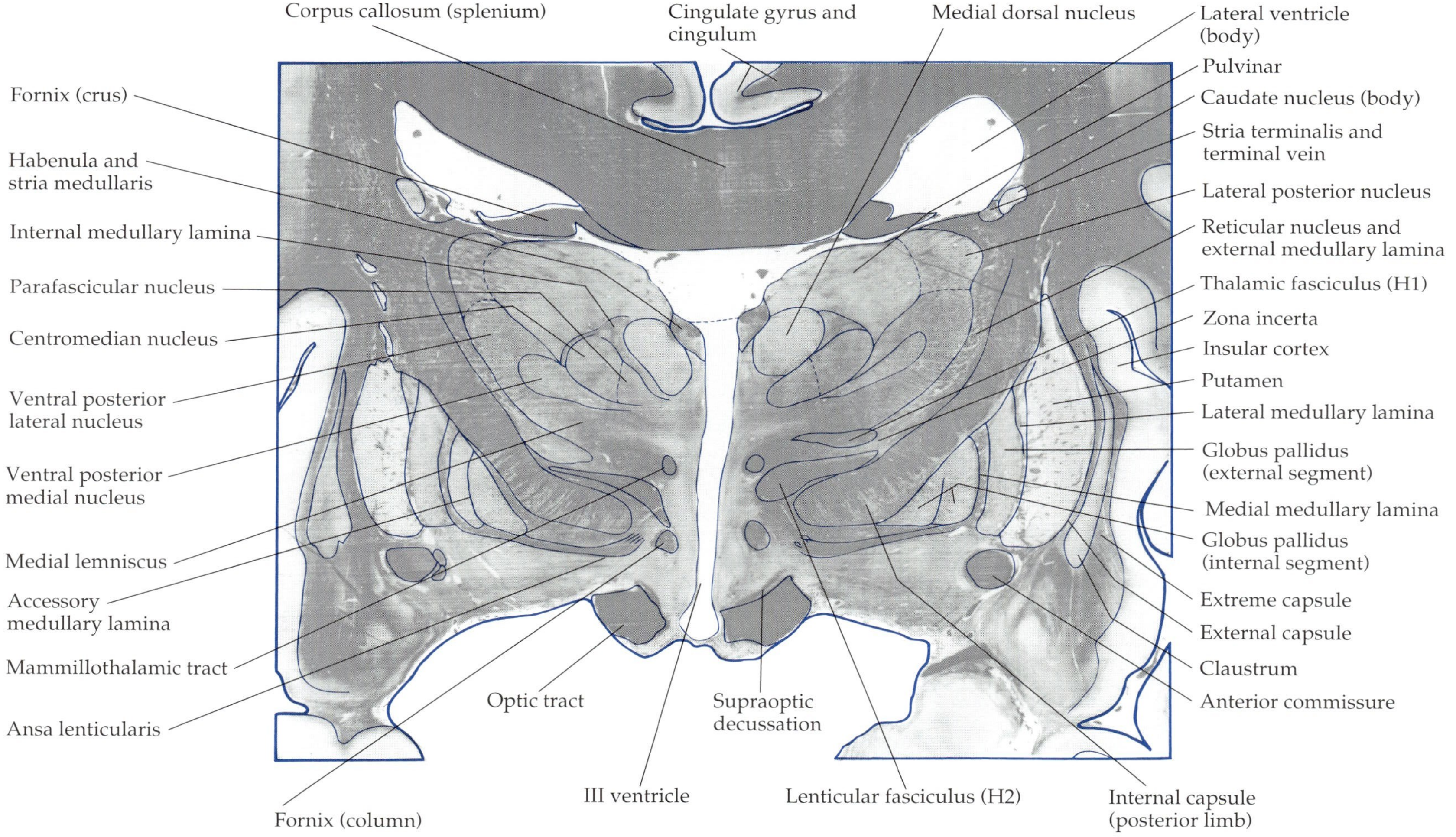

Corpus callosum (splenium)

Cingulate gyrus and cingulum

Medial dorsal nucleus

Lateral ventricle (body)

Pulvinar

Caudate nucleus (body)

Stria terminalis and terminal vein

Lateral posterior nucleus

Reticular nucleus and external medullary lamina

Thalamic fasciculus (H1)

Zona incerta

Insular cortex

Putamen

Lateral medullary lamina

Globus pallidus (external segment)

Medial medullary lamina

Globus pallidus (internal segment)

Extreme capsule

External capsule

Claustrum

Anterior commissure

Internal capsule (posterior limb)

Fornix (crus)

Habenula and stria medullaris

Internal medullary lamina

Parafascicular nucleus

Centromedian nucleus

Ventral posterior lateral nucleus

Ventral posterior medial nucleus

Medial lemniscus

Accessory medullary lamina

Mammillothalamic tract

Ansa lenticularis

Fornix (column)

Optic tract

III ventricle

Supraoptic decussation

Lenticular fasciculus (H2)

Figure AII–22. Coronal section of the cerebral hemisphere through the anterior limb of the internal capsule, columns of the fornix, and amygdaloid complex. (×2.2)

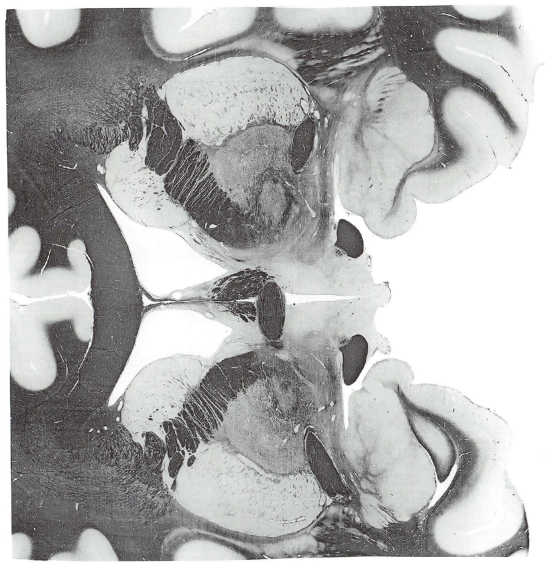

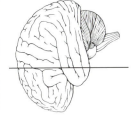

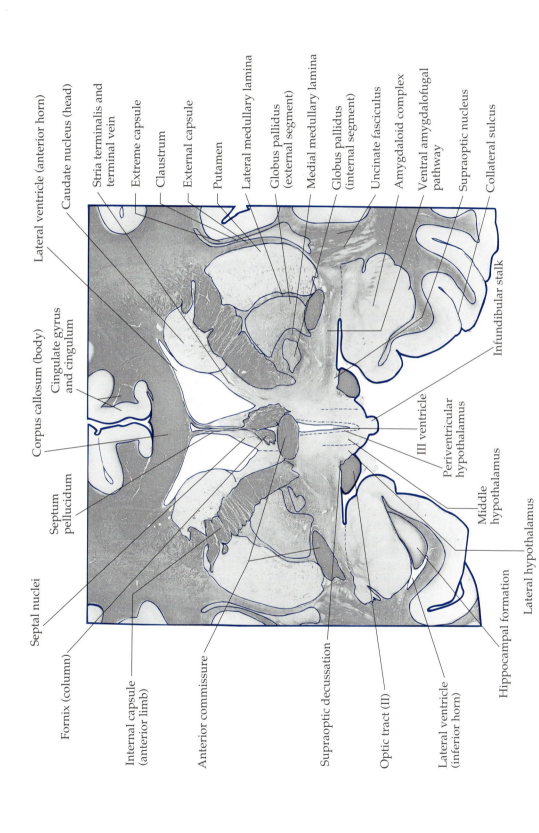

Septal nuclei

Corpus callosum (body)

Cingulate gyrus
and cingulum

Lateral ventricle (anterior horn)

Caudate nucleus (head)

Stria terminalis and
terminal vein

Extreme capsule

Claustrum

External capsule

Putamen

Lateral medullary lamina

Globus pallidus
(external segment)

Medial medullary lamina

Globus pallidus
(internal segment)

Uncinate fasciculus

Amygdaloid complex

Ventral amygdalofugal
pathway

Supraoptic nucleus

Collateral sulcus

Septum
pellucidum

Fornix (column)

Internal capsule
(anterior limb)

Anterior commissure

Supraoptic decussation

Optic tract (II)

Lateral ventricle
(inferior horn)

Hippocampal formation

Lateral hypothalamus

Middle
hypothalamus

Periventricular
hypothalamus

III ventricle

Infundibular stalk

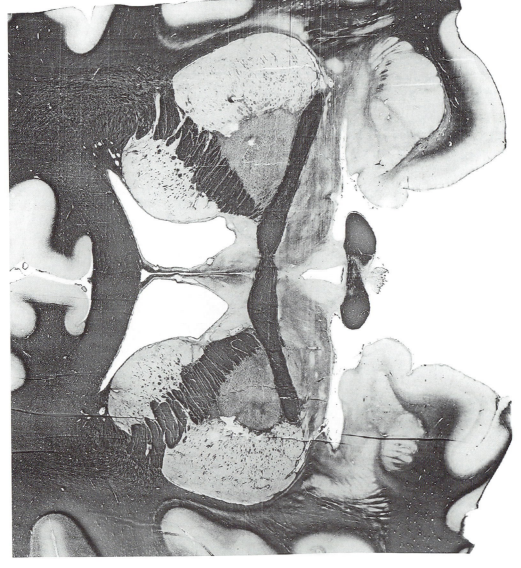

Figure AII–23. Coronal section of the cerebral hemisphere through the anterior limb of the internal capsule, anterior commissure, and optic chiasm. (×2.2)

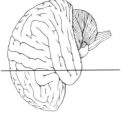

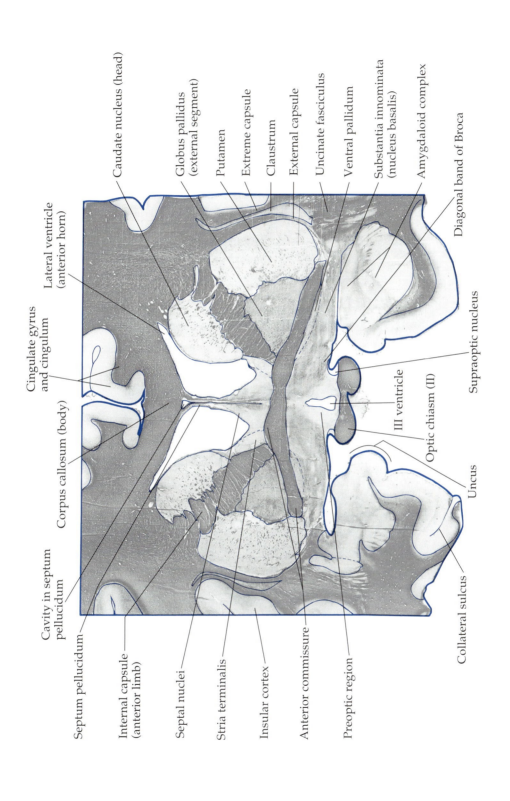

Cingulate gyrus
and cingulum

Lateral ventricle
(anterior horn)

Caudate nucleus (head)

Globus pallidus
(external segment)

Putamen

Extreme capsule

Claustrum

External capsule

Uncinate fasciculus

Ventral pallidum

Substantia innominata
(nucleus basalis)

Amygdaloid complex

Diagonal band of Broca

Corpus callosum (body)

Cavity in septum
pellucidum

Septum pellucidum

Internal capsule
(anterior limb)

Septal nuclei

Stria terminalis

Insular cortex

Anterior commissure

Preoptic region

Optic chiasm (II)

III ventricle

Supraoptic nucleus

Uncus

Collateral sulcus

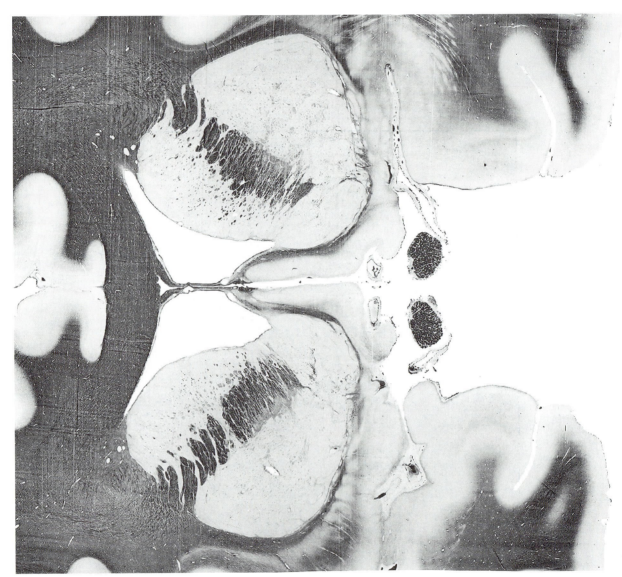

Figure AII–24.   Coronal section of the cerebral hemisphere through the anterior limb of the internal capsule and the head of caudate nucleus. (×2.4)

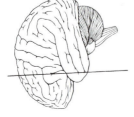

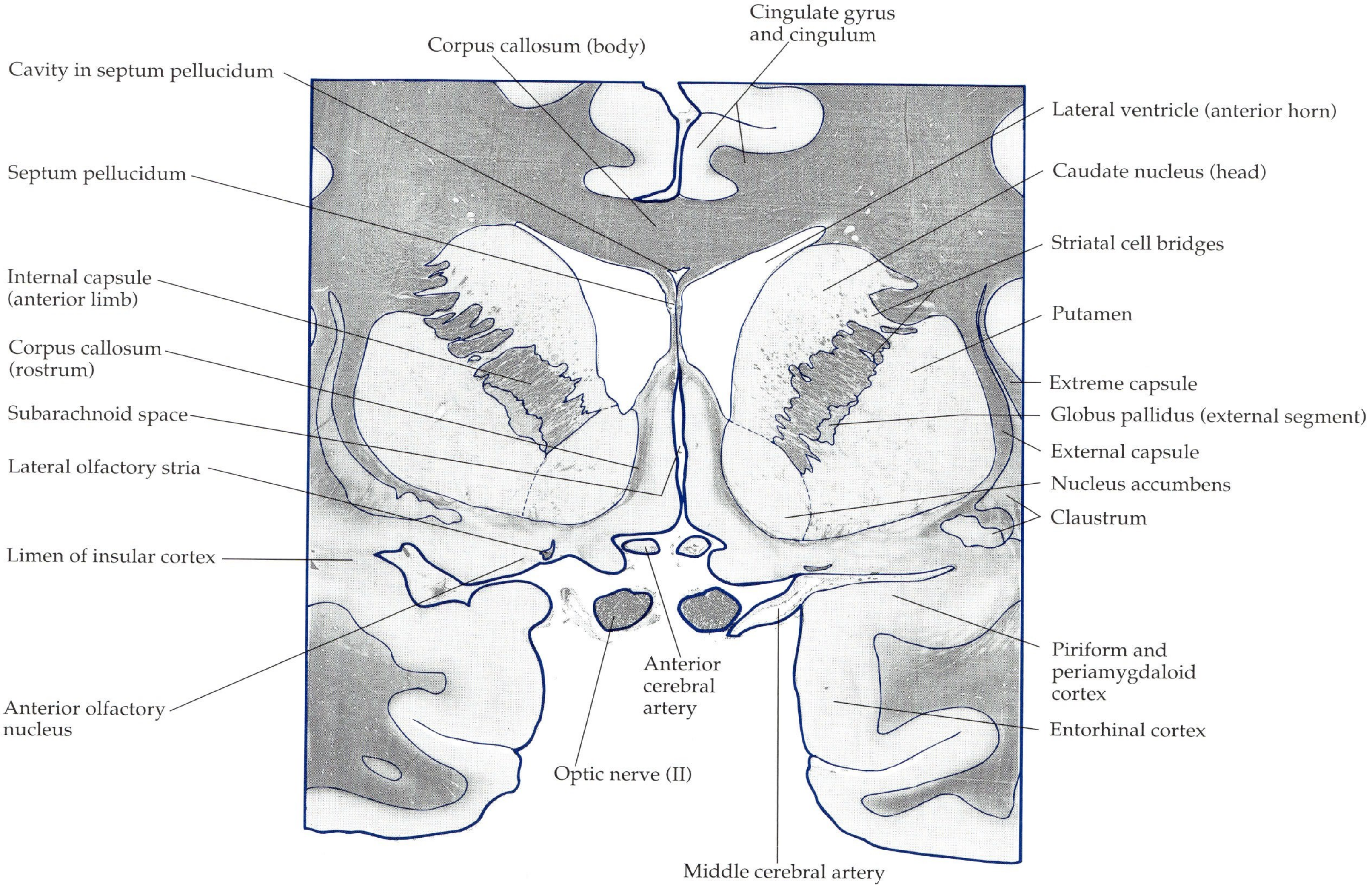

Cavity in septum pellucidum

Septum pellucidum

Internal capsule (anterior limb)

Corpus callosum (rostrum)

Subarachnoid space

Lateral olfactory stria

Limen of insular cortex

Anterior olfactory nucleus

Cingulate gyrus and cingulum

Corpus callosum (body)

Lateral ventricle (anterior horn)

Caudate nucleus (head)

Striatal cell bridges

Putamen

Extreme capsule

Globus pallidus (external segment)

External capsule

Nucleus accumbens

Claustrum

Piriform and periamygdaloid cortex

Entorhinal cortex

Anterior cerebral artery

Optic nerve (II)

Middle cerebral artery

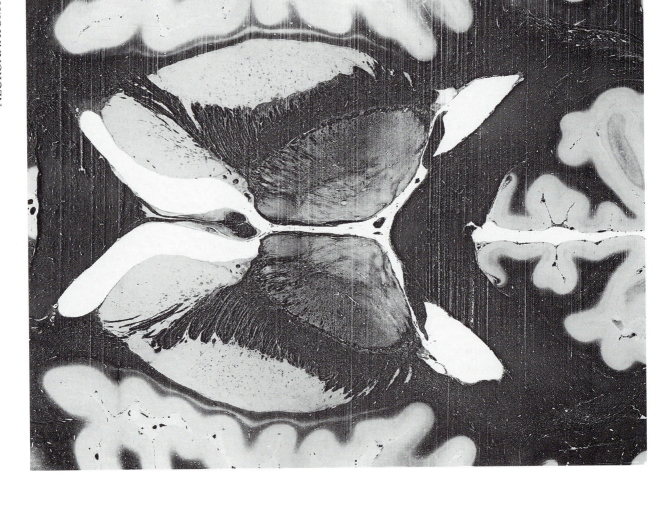

Figure AII–25. Horizontal section of the cerebral hemisphere and diencephalon through the anterior thalamic nuclei. (×1.9)

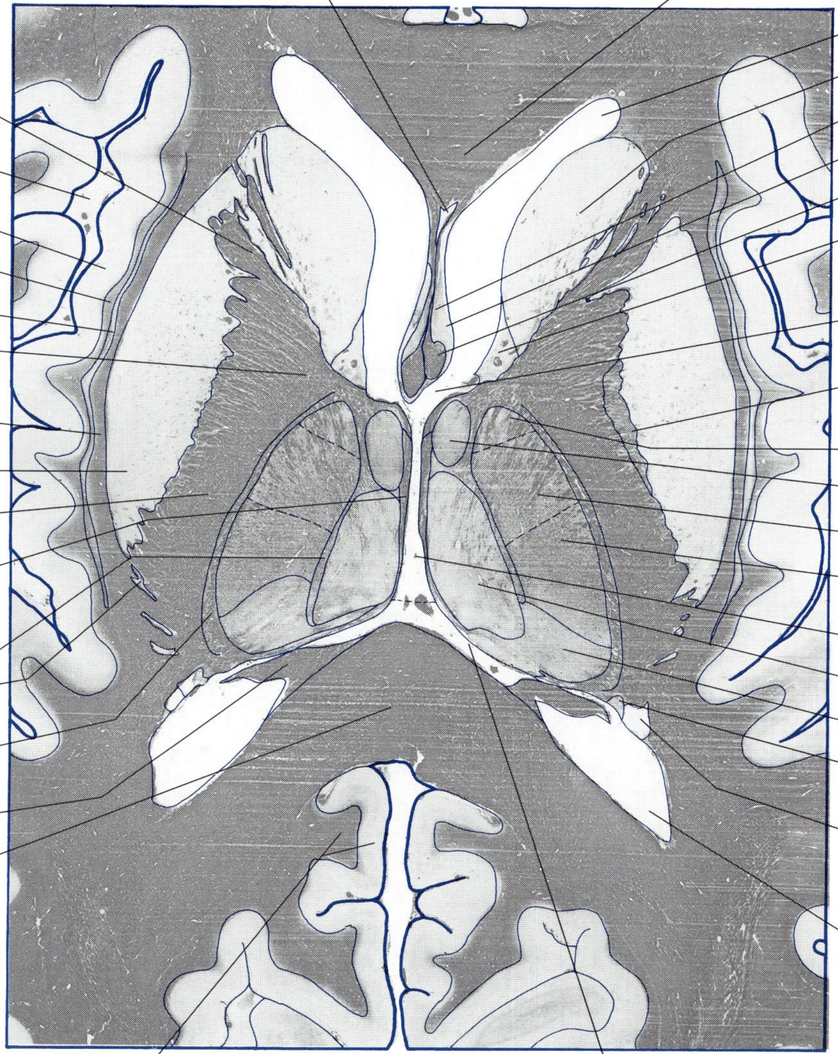

Corpus callosum (genu)

Lateral ventricle (anterior horn)

Caudate nucleus (head)

Septum pellucidum

Septal nuclei

Fornix (body)

Stria terminalis and terminal vein

Interventricular foramen (of Monro)

Globus pallidus (external segment)

Ventral anterior nucleus

Anterior nucleus

Ventral lateral nucleus

Lateral posterior nucleus

III ventricle

Medial dorsal nucleus

Pulvinar

Stria terminalis and terminal vein

Caudate nucleus (tail)

Lateral ventricle (atrium)

Cavity in septum pellucidum

Subarachnoid space

Cingulate gyrus and cingulum

Internal capsule (anterior limb)

Lateral sulcus

Insular cortex

Extreme capsule

Claustrum

Internal capsule (genu)

External capsule

Putamen

Internal capsule (posterior limb)

Stria medullaris

Internal medullary lamina

Striatal cell bridges

Reticular nucleus and external medullary lamina

Fornix (crus)

Corpus callosum (splenium)

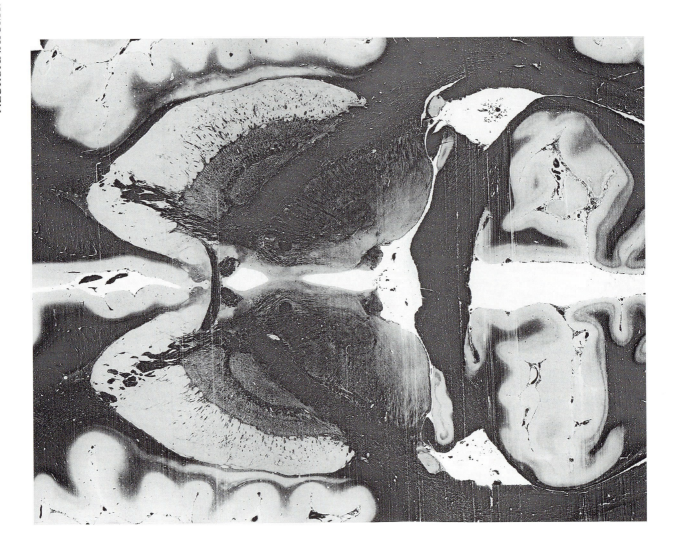

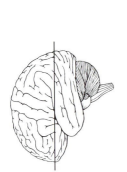

Figure AII–26. Horizontal section of the cerebral hemisphere and diencephalon at the level of the anterior commissure. (×1.9)

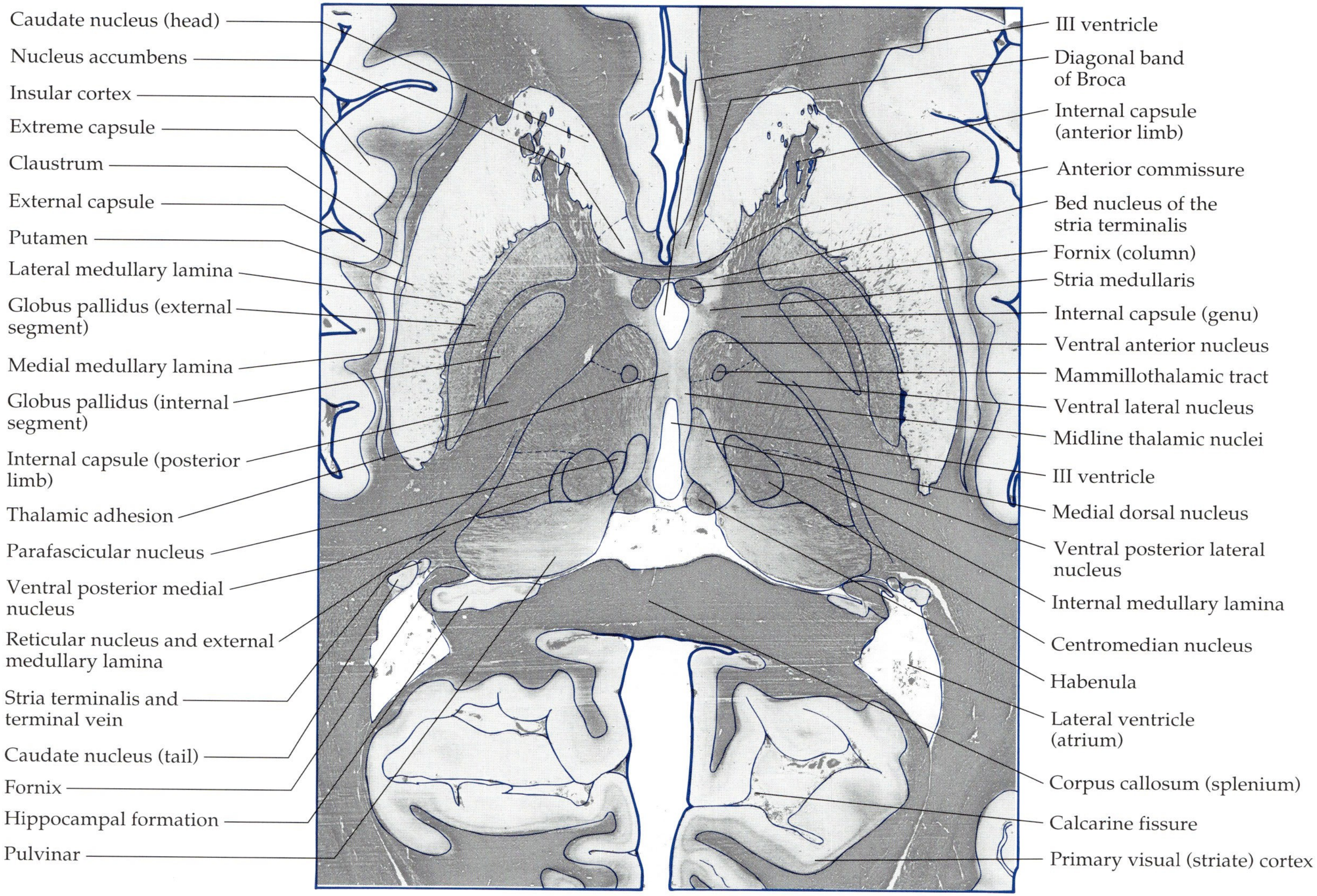

Caudate nucleus (head)

Nucleus accumbens

Insular cortex

Extreme capsule

Claustrum

External capsule

Putamen

Lateral medullary lamina

Globus pallidus (external segment)

Medial medullary lamina

Globus pallidus (internal segment)

Internal capsule (posterior limb)

Thalamic adhesion

Parafascicular nucleus

Ventral posterior medial nucleus

Reticular nucleus and external medullary lamina

Stria terminalis and terminal vein

Caudate nucleus (tail)

Fornix

Hippocampal formation

Pulvinar

III ventricle

Diagonal band of Broca

Internal capsule (anterior limb)

Anterior commissure

Bed nucleus of the stria terminalis

Fornix (column)

Stria medullaris

Internal capsule (genu)

Ventral anterior nucleus

Mammillothalamic tract

Ventral lateral nucleus

Midline thalamic nuclei

III ventricle

Medial dorsal nucleus

Ventral posterior lateral nucleus

Internal medullary lamina

Centromedian nucleus

Habenula

Lateral ventricle (atrium)

Corpus callosum (splenium)

Calcarine fissure

Primary visual (striate) cortex

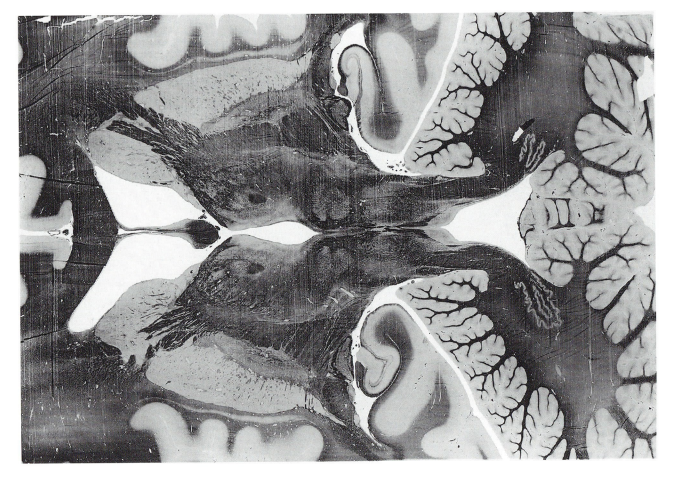

Figure AII–27. Oblique section of the cerebral hemisphere, diencephalon, brain stem, and cerebellum. (×1.6)

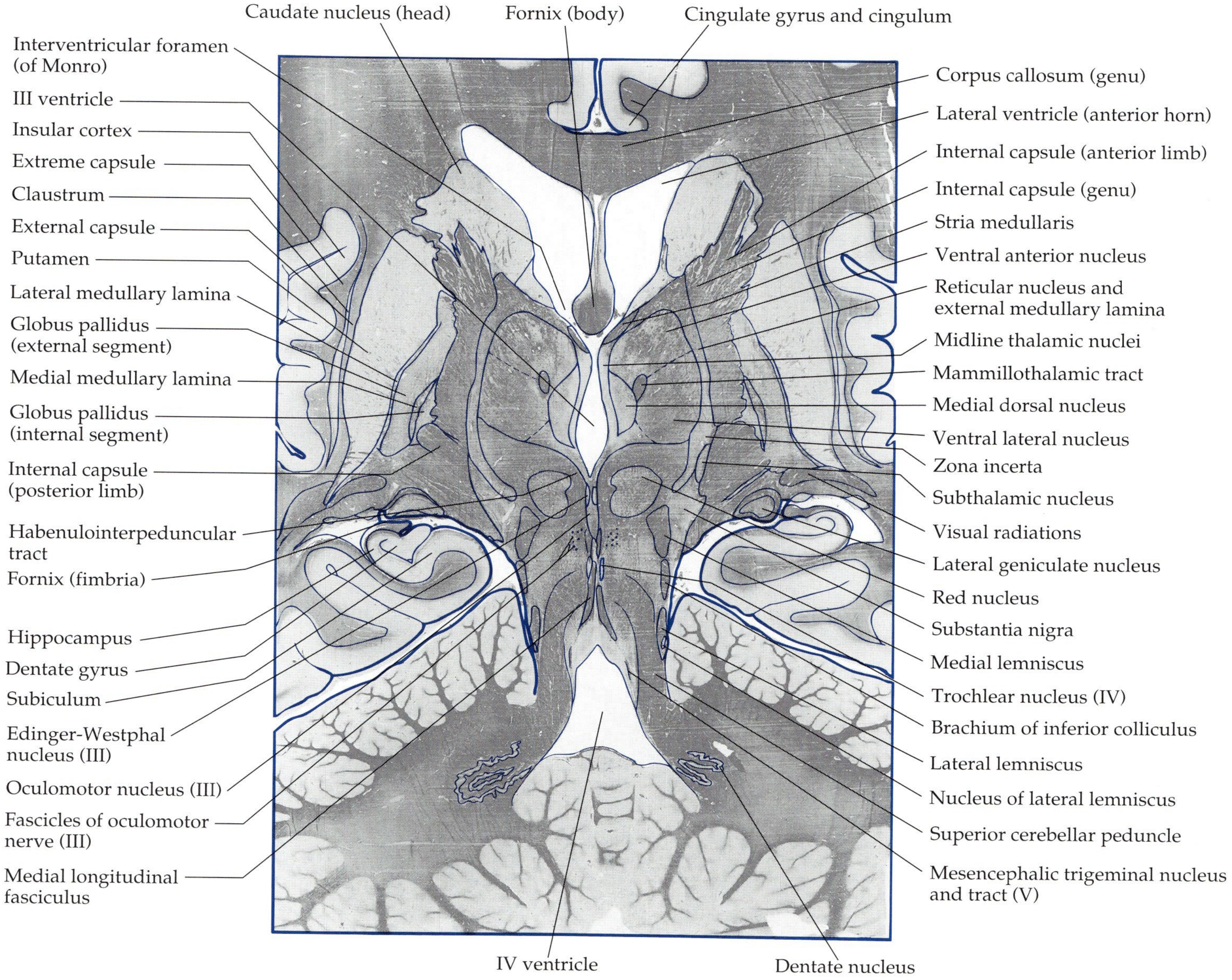

Caudate nucleus (head)   Fornix (body)   Cingulate gyrus and cingulum

Interventricular foramen (of Monro)
III ventricle
Insular cortex
Extreme capsule
Claustrum
External capsule
Putamen
Lateral medullary lamina
Globus pallidus (external segment)
Medial medullary lamina
Globus pallidus (internal segment)
Internal capsule (posterior limb)
Habenulointerpeduncular tract
Fornix (fimbria)
Hippocampus
Dentate gyrus
Subiculum
Edinger-Westphal nucleus (III)
Oculomotor nucleus (III)
Fascicles of oculomotor nerve (III)
Medial longitudinal fasciculus

Corpus callosum (genu)
Lateral ventricle (anterior horn)
Internal capsule (anterior limb)
Internal capsule (genu)
Stria medullaris
Ventral anterior nucleus
Reticular nucleus and external medullary lamina
Midline thalamic nuclei
Mammillothalamic tract
Medial dorsal nucleus
Ventral lateral nucleus
Zona incerta
Subthalamic nucleus
Visual radiations
Lateral geniculate nucleus
Red nucleus
Substantia nigra
Medial lemniscus
Trochlear nucleus (IV)
Brachium of inferior colliculus
Lateral lemniscus
Nucleus of lateral lemniscus
Superior cerebellar peduncle
Mesencephalic trigeminal nucleus and tract (V)

Dentate nucleus

IV ventricle

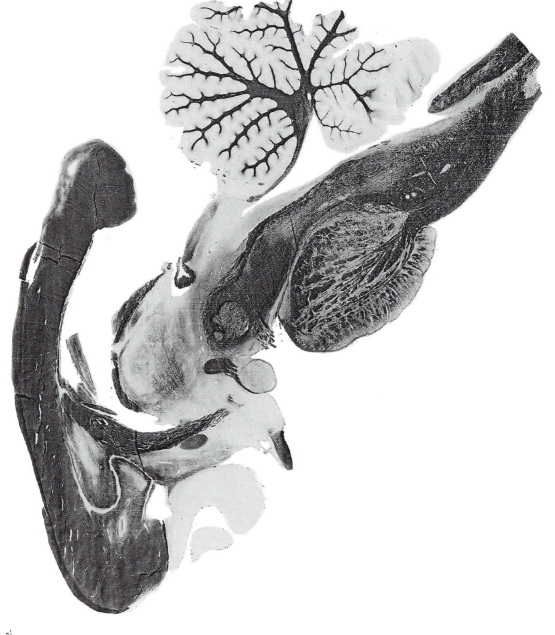

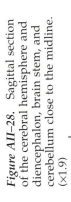

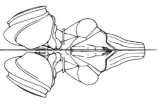

Figure AII–28. Sagittal section of the cerebral hemisphere and diencephalon, brain stem, and cerebellum close to the midline. (×1.9)

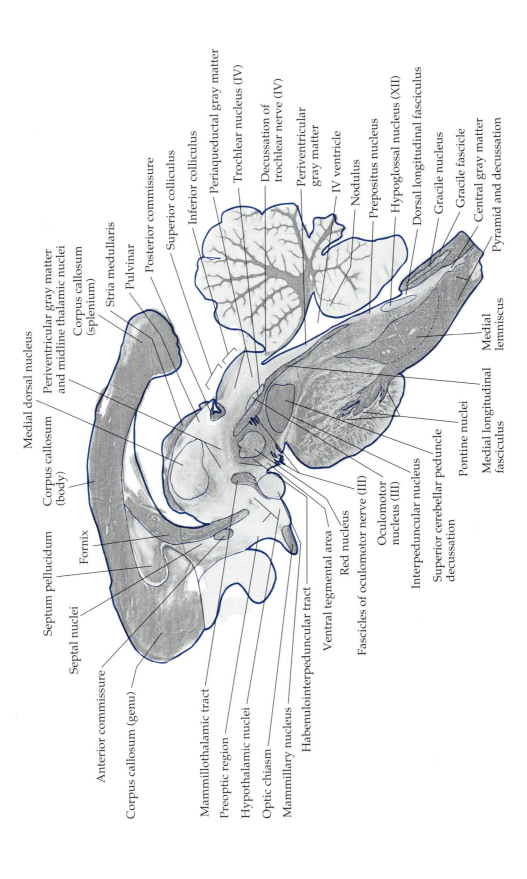

Medial dorsal nucleus

Periventricular gray matter
and midline thalamic nuclei

Corpus callosum
(splenium)

Stria medullaris

Pulvinar

Posterior commissure

Superior colliculus

Inferior colliculus

Periaqueductal gray matter

Trochlear nucleus (IV)

Decussation of
trochlear nerve (IV)

Periventricular
gray matter

IV ventricle

Nodulus

Prepositus nucleus

Hypoglossal nucleus (XII)

Dorsal longitudinal fasciculus

Gracile nucleus

Gracile fascicle

Central gray matter

Pyramid and decussation

Medial
lemniscus

Pontine nuclei

Medial longitudinal
fasciculus

Superior cerebellar peduncle
decussation

Interpeduncular nucleus

Oculomotor
nucleus (III)

Fascicles of oculomotor nerve (III)

Red nucleus

Ventral tegmental area

Habenulointerpeduncular tract

Mammillary nucleus

Optic chiasm

Hypothalamic nuclei

Preoptic region

Mammillothalamic tract

Corpus callosum (genu)

Anterior commissure

Fornix

Septal nuclei

Septum pellucidum

Corpus callosum
(body)

Medial dorsal nucleus

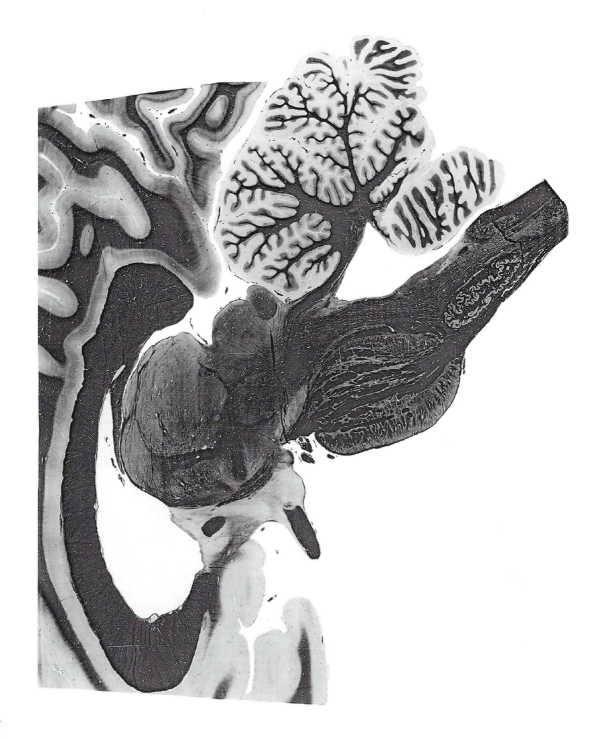

Figure AII–29. Sagittal section of the cerebral hemisphere, diencephalon, brain stem, and cerebellum through the mammillothalamic tract and anterior thalamic nucleus. (×1.8)

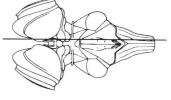

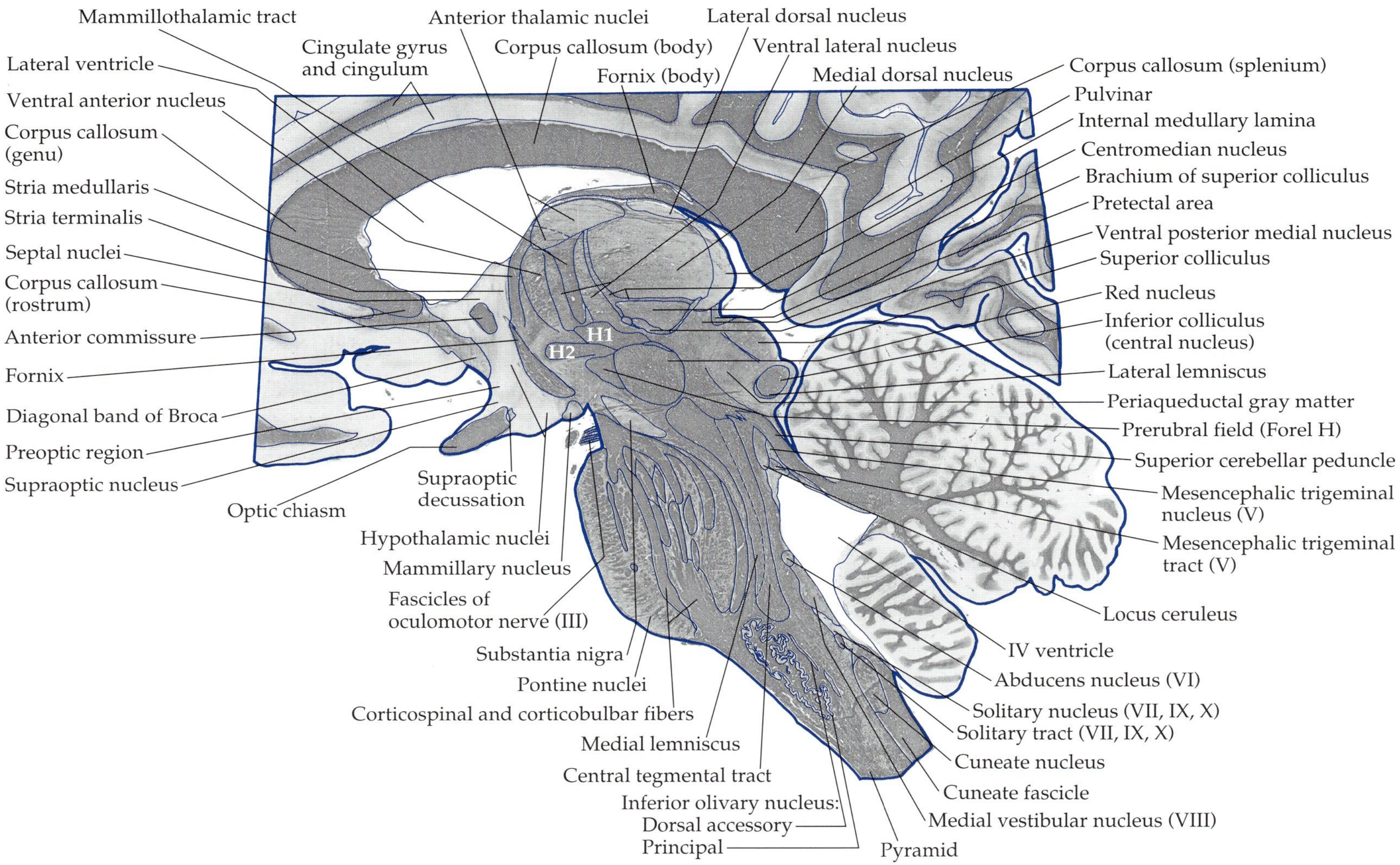

Corpus callosum (splenium)
Pulvinar
Internal medullary lamina
Centromedian nucleus
Brachium of superior colliculus
Pretectal area
Ventral posterior medial nucleus
Superior colliculus
Red nucleus
Inferior colliculus (central nucleus)
Lateral lemniscus
Periaqueductal gray matter
Prerubral field (Forel H)
Superior cerebellar peduncle
Mesencephalic trigeminal nucleus (V)
Mesencephalic trigeminal tract (V)
Locus ceruleus

Medial dorsal nucleus
Ventral lateral nucleus
Lateral dorsal nucleus
Anterior thalamic nuclei
Mammillothalamic tract

IV ventricle
Abducens nucleus (VI)
Solitary nucleus (VII, IX, X)
Solitary tract (VII, IX, X)
Cuneate nucleus
Cuneate fascicle
Medial vestibular nucleus (VIII)
Pyramid

Cingulate gyrus and cingulum
Corpus callosum (body)
Fornix (body)

H1
H2

Inferior olivary nucleus:
Dorsal accessory
Principal
Central tegmental tract
Medial lemniscus
Pontine nuclei
Corticospinal and corticobulbar fibers
Substantia nigra
Fascicles of oculomotor nerve (III)
Mammillary nucleus
Hypothalamic nuclei
Supraoptic decussation

Lateral ventricle
Ventral anterior nucleus
Corpus callosum (genu)
Stria medullaris
Stria terminalis
Septal nuclei
Corpus callosum (rostrum)
Anterior commissure
Fornix
Diagonal band of Broca
Preoptic region
Supraoptic nucleus

Optic chiasm

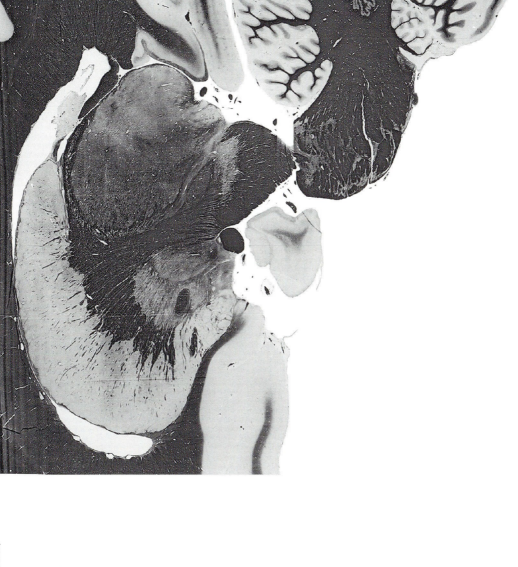

Figure AII–30. Sagittal section of the cerebral hemisphere, diencephalon, brain stem, and cerebellum through the ventral posterior lateral nucleus and the dentate nucleus. (×1.9)

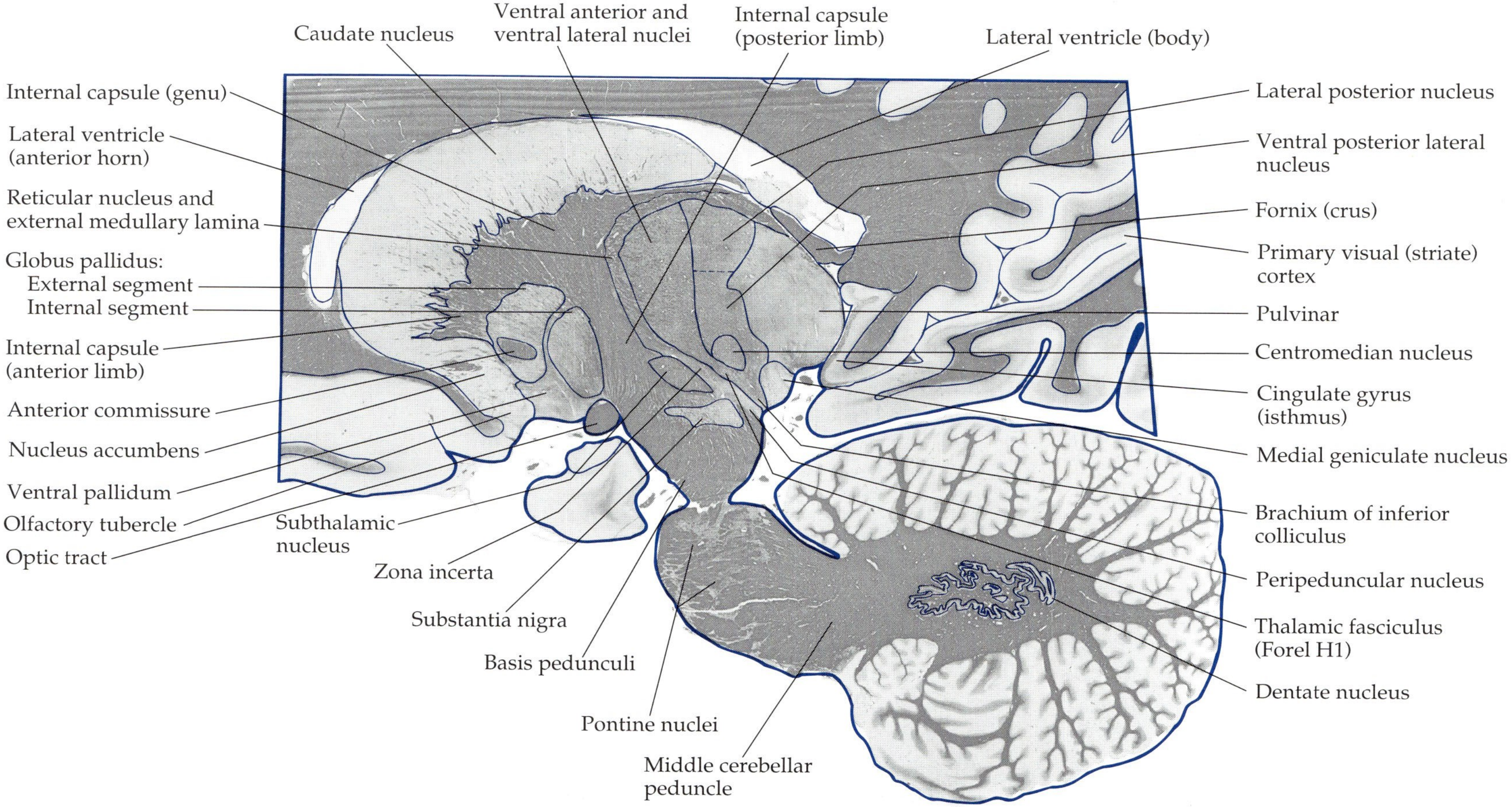

Lateral posterior nucleus

Ventral posterior lateral nucleus

Fornix (crus)

Primary visual (striate) cortex

Pulvinar

Centromedian nucleus

Cingulate gyrus (isthmus)

Medial geniculate nucleus

Brachium of inferior colliculus

Peripeduncular nucleus

Thalamic fasciculus (Forel H1)

Dentate nucleus

Lateral ventricle (body)

Internal capsule (posterior limb)

Ventral anterior and ventral lateral nuclei

Caudate nucleus

Internal capsule (genu)

Lateral ventricle (anterior horn)

Reticular nucleus and external medullary lamina

Globus pallidus:
External segment
Internal segment

Internal capsule (anterior limb)

Anterior commissure

Nucleus accumbens

Ventral pallidum

Olfactory tubercle

Optic tract

Subthalamic nucleus

Zona incerta

Substantia nigra

Basis pedunculi

Pontine nuclei

Middle cerebellar peduncle

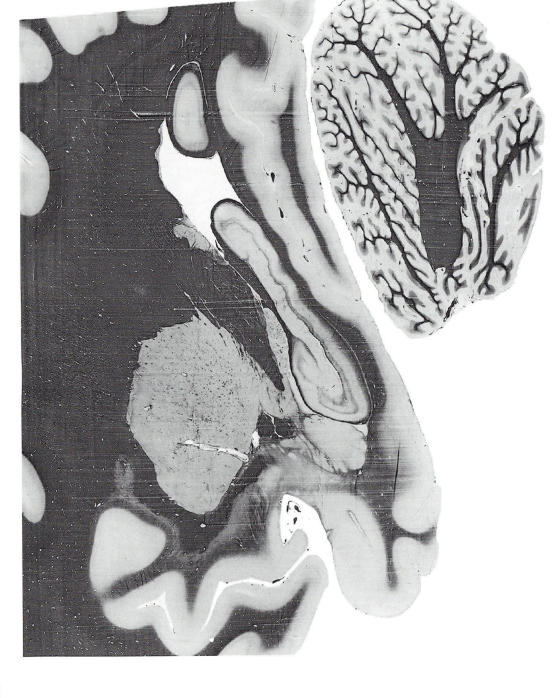

Figure AII–31. Sagittal section of the cerebral hemisphere and cerebellum through the amygdaloid complex and hippocampal formation. (×1.9)

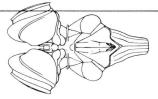

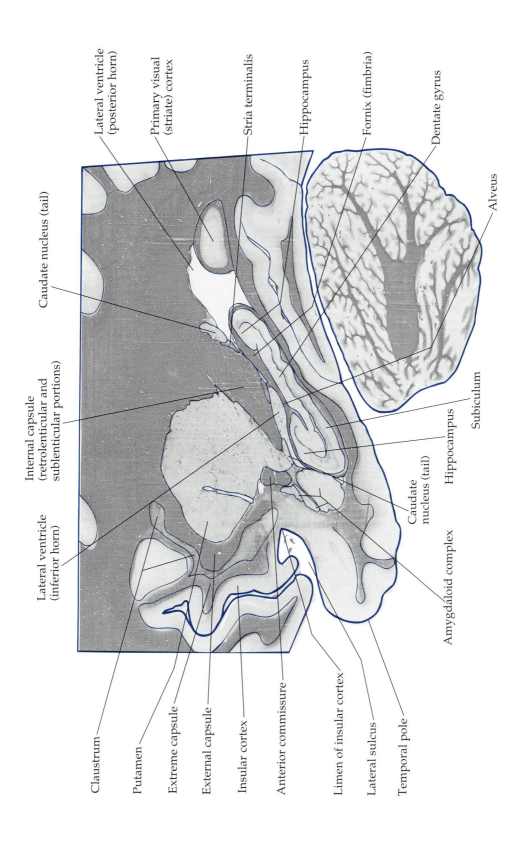

Caudate nucleus (tail)

Lateral ventricle (posterior horn)

Primary visual (striate) cortex

Stria terminalis

Hippocampus

Fornix (fimbria)

Dentate gyrus

Alveus

Internal capsule (retrolenticular and sublenticular portions)

Lateral ventricle (inferior horn)

Claustrum

Putamen

Extreme capsule

External capsule

Insular cortex

Anterior commissure

Limen of insular cortex

Lateral sulcus

Temporal pole

Amygdaloid complex

Caudate nucleus (tail)

Hippocampus

Subiculum

References

Alheld, G. F., Heimer, L., Switzer, R. C. III. 1990. Basal Ganglia. In Paxinos, G. (ed.), The Human Central Nervous System. San Diego: Academic Press, pp. 483–582.

Amaral, D. G., Insausti, R. 1990. Hippocampal Formation. In Paxinos, G. (ed.), The Human Central Nervous System. San Diego: Academic Press, pp. 711–755.

Andy, O. J., and Stephan, H. 1968. The septum of the human brain. J. Comp. Neurol. 133:383–410.

Bruce, A. 1901. A Topographical Altas of the Spinal Cord. London: Williams and Norgate.

Carpenter, M. B., and Sutin, J. 1983. Human Neuroanatomy. Baltimore: Williams & Wilkins.

Crosby, E. C., Humphrey, T., and Lauer, E. W. 1962. Correlative Anatomy of the Nervous System. New York: Macmillan.

DeArmond, S. J., Fusco, M. M., and Dewey, M. M. 1976. Structure of the Human Brain. New York: Oxford University Press.

De Olmos, J. S. 1990. Amygdala. In Paxinos, G. (ed.), The Human Central Nervous System. San Diego: Academic Press.

Haines, D. 1983. Neuroanatomy: An Atlas of Structures, Sections, and Systems. Baltimore: Urban & Schwarzenberg.

Hirai, T., Jones, E. G. 1989. A new parcellation of the human thalamus on the basis of histochemical staining. Brain Research Rev. 14:1–34.

Martin, G. F., Holstege, G., Mehler, W. R. 1990. Reticular formation of the pons and medulla. In Paxinos, G. (ed.), The Human Central Nervous System. San Diego: Academic Press.

Nathan, P. W., and Smith, M. C. 1955. Long descending tracts in man. I. Review of present knowledge. Brain 78:248–303.

Nathan, P. W., and Smith, M. C. 1982. The rubrospinal and central tegmental tracts in man. Brain 105:223–269.

Olszewski, J., and Baxter, D. (eds.). 1982. Cytoarchitecture of the Human Brain Stem. Vol. I: Head, Neck, Upper Extremities. Basel: S. Karger.

Paxinos, G., Török, I., Halliday, G., Mehler, W. R. 1990. Human homologs to brainstem nuclei identified in other animals as revealed by acetylcholinesterase activity. In Paxinos, G. (ed.), The Human Central Nervous System. San Diego: Academic Press, pp. 149–202.

Price, J. L. 1990. Olfactory System. In Paxinos G. (ed.), The Human Central Nervous System. San Diego: Academic Press, pp. 979–998.

Riley, H. A. 1943. An Atlas of the Basal Ganglia, Brain Stem and Spinal Cord. Baltimore: Williams & Wilkins.

Schaltenbrand, G., and Wahren, W. 1977. Atlas for Stereotaxy of the Human Brain. Chicago: Georg Thieme.

Williams, P. L., and Warwick, R. 1975. Functional Neuroanatomy of Man. Philadelphia: Sauders.

Index

Page numbers followed by *t* and *f* indicate tables and figures, respectively. Page numbers in italics indicate Atlas figures.